ENDOCRINOLOGY

ENDOCRINOLOGY

Basic and Clinical Principles

Edited by

P. MICHAEL CONN

*Oregon Regional Primate Research Center,
Beaverton, and Oregon Health Sciences University,
Portland, OR*

SHLOMO MELMED

*Cedars Sinai Medical Center and
UCLA School of Medicine, Los Angeles, CA*

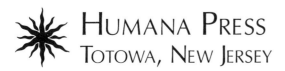

HUMANA PRESS
TOTOWA, NEW JERSEY

Library of Congress Cataloging-in-Publication Data

Endocrinology: basic and clinical principles/edited by P. Michael Conn, Shlomo Melmed.
    p. cm.
  Includes bibliographical references and index.
  ISBN 0-89603-349-X (alk. paper)
  1. Endocrinology.   2. Hormones.   I. Conn, P. Michael.
II. Melmed, Shlomo.
  [DNLM: 1. Hormones. 2. Endocrinology. WK 102 E576 1997]
QP187.E555 1997
612.4--dc20
DNLM/DLC   96-43898
for Library of Congress   CIP

PREFACE

Endocrinology: Basic and Clinical Principles aims to provide a comprehensive knowledge base for the clinical science of endocrinology. The challenge in its presentation was to produce a volume that was timely, provided integration of scientific and clinical principles, and yet was limited to 500 pages. This length makes the volume suitable as a text; and the timeliness we have striven for allows the book to serve as an off-the-shelf reference. Our goal was achieved largely through the selection of authors who are both expert writers and teachers. Tables and illustrative matter were used optimally to present information in a concise and comparative format.

Endocrinology: Basic and Clinical Principles will be useful to physicians and scientists as well as to students who wish to have a high-quality, current reference to the general field of endocrinology. The use of an outline system and a comprehensive index will allow readers to locate promptly topics of particular interest. Key references are provided throughout for individuals requiring more in-depth information. The volume comprehensively covers the entire spectrum of endocrinology, even including nonmammalian systems and plants, coverage rarely included in similar volumes.

The editors wish to express appreciation to our distinguished chapter authors for their efforts, as well as diligently meeting publication deadlines and to the staff at Humana Press for their cooperation and useful suggestions.

P. Michael Conn
Shlomo Melmed

CONTENTS

CONTRIBUTORS

DANIEL G. BICHET • *Clinical Research Unit, Hospital du Sacre-Coeur de Montreal, Canada*

GLENN D. BRAUNSTEIN • *Department of Medicine, Cedars-Sinai Medical Center, Los Angeles, CA*

GREGORY BRENT • *Division of Endocrinology, West Los Angeles VA Medical Center, Los Angeles, CA*

JOHN R. G. CHALLIS • *Department of Physiology, University of Toronto, Ontario, Canada*

JULIE CHAO • *Endocrine-Hypertension Division, Brigham and Women's Hospital, Harvard Medical School, Boston, MA*

LEE CHAO • *Endocrine-Hypertension Division, Brigham and Women's Hospital, Harvard Medical School, Boston, MA*

GEORGE P. CHROUSOS • *NICHD, National Institutes of Health, Bethesda, MD*

P. MICHAEL CONN • *Oregon Regional Primate Research Center, Beaverton, and Oregon Health Sciences University, Portland, OR*

ALAN C. DALKIN • *Department of Internal Medicine, University of Virginia Health Science Center, Charlottesville, VA*

ROBERT FRASER • *Division of Geriatric Medicine, St. Louis University School of Medicine, St. Louis, MO*

LARRY I. GILBERT • *Department of Biology, University of North Carolina, Chapel Hill, NC*

MICHAEL S. HARBUZ • *Department of Medicine, Bristol Royal Infirmary, Bristol, UK*

GEOFFREY N. HENDY • *Department of Medicine, Royal Victoria Hospital, Montreal, Canada*

PETER KRISTOFFERSEN • *Max Planck Institute, Koln, Germany*

KEN S. KORACH • *Laboratory of Reproductive and Developmental Toxicology, NIEHS, Research Triangle Park, NC*

JONATHAN LINDZEY • *Laboratory of Reproductive and Developmental Toxicology, NIEHS, Research Triangle Park, NC*

STAFFORD L. LIGHTMAN • *Department of Medicine, Bristol Royal Infirmary, Bristol, UK*

JOHN S. MARSHALL • *Department of Internal Medicine, University of Virginia Health Science Center, Charlottesville, VA*

KELLY E. MAYO • *Department of Biochemistry, Northwestern University, Evanston, IL*

DONALD A. MCCLAIN • *Division of Endocrinology, University of Mississippi, Jackson, MS*

JOHN MCCRACKEN • *Worcester Foundation for Experimental Biology, Shrewsbury, MA*

BRUCE S. MCEWEN • *Laboratory of Neuroendocrinology, Rockefeller University, New York, NY*

SHLOMO MELMED • *Division of Endocrinology, Cedars-Sinai Medical Center, UCLA School of Medicine, Los Angeles, CA*

JOHN E. MORLEY • *Division of Geriatric Medicine, St. Louis University School of Medicine, St. Louis, MO*

KLAUS PALME • *Max Planck Institute, Koln, Germany*

LIN PEI • *Division of Endocrinology, Cedars-Sinai Medical Center, UCLA School of Medicine, Los Angeles, CA*

WILLIAM J. RAUM • *Division of Endocrinology, Harbor-UCLA Medical Center, Torrance, CA*

CHRISTOPHER REDHEAD • *Max Planck Institute, Koln, Germany*

PETER ROTWEIN • *Department of Medicine, Washington University School of Medicine, St. Louis, MO*

WILLIS K. SAMSON • *Department of Physiology, University of North Dakota, School of Medicine, Grand Forks, ND*

ILAN SHIMON • *Division of Endocrinology, Cedars-Sinai Medical Center, UCLA School of Medicine, Los Angeles, CA*

BRYAN L. SPANGELO • *Department of Chemistry, University of Nevada/Las Vegas, Las Vegas, NV*

ELIOT SPINDEL • *Oregon Regional Primate Research Center, Beaverton, OR*

FREDRICK STORMSHAK • *Department of Animal Science, Oregon State University, Corvallis, OR*

CONSTANTINE A. STRATAKIS • *National Institutes of Health, Bethesda, MD*

GORDON H. WILLIAMS • *Endocrine-Hypertension Division, Brigham and Women's Hospital, Harvard Medical School, Boston, MA*

GARY A. WITTERT • *Division of Geriatric Medicine, St. Louis University School of Medicine, St. Louis, MO*

RICHARD J. WURTMAN • *Department of Food Sciences, Massachusetts Institute of Technology, Cambridge, MA*

IRINA V. ZHDANOVA • *MIT Clinical Research Center, Massachusetts Institute of Technology, Cambridge, MA*

PART I

INTRODUCTION

1 Introduction to Endocrinology

P. Michael Conn, PhD

CONTENTS

1. INTRODUCTION

The earliest bacterial fossil dates back about 3 billion years. This was a simpler time! Communications between cells were more modest than those required to maintain a multicellular organism and were probably focused on the ability to signal the presence of beneficial substances (food) or deleterious substances (toxins) in the local environment.

2. DEFINITIONS

Substances that provide the chemical basis for communication between cells are called "hormones." This word, coined by Bayliss and Starling, was originally used to describe the products of ductless glands released into the general circulation in order to respond to changes in homeostasis. "Hormone" has taken on a broader usage in recent years. Sometimes hormones are released into portal (closed) circulatory systems and have local actions. The word "paracrine" is used to describe the release of locally acting substances. This word also describes local hormone action as the diffusion of gastrin acts on neighboring cells. Hormonal substances released by an animal that influence responses in another animal are referred to as "pheromones."

Sometimes the word "hormone" is used as a reference to substances in plants (phytohormones) or in invertebrates that have open "circulatory" systems very different from those found in vertebrates. On other occasions, growth factors are (appropriately) called hormones, since they mediate signaling between cells. In recent years, the word has become a catch-all to describe substances released by one cell that provoke a response in another cell even when the messenger substance does not enter the general circulation. The science of endocrinology has broad coverage indeed!

3. HORMONES CONVEY INFORMATION THAT REGULATES CELL PROCESSES

Characteristically, hormones transmit information about the status of one organ to another, regulating corrective actions to maintain homeostasis. For example, elevated glucose in the blood signals the pancreas to release insulin. Insulin travels through the circulation signaling target cells in the liver and fat cells to increase their permeability to glucose; processed sugar is stored in cells as blood levels drop.

From: *Endocrinology: Basic and Clinical Principles* (P. M. Conn and S. Melmed, eds.), Humana Press Inc., Totowa, NJ.

In order to be effective, hormones must not be degraded too quickly (that is, before arrival at the target site). If degradation is too slow, on the other hand, the information conveyed will be outdated and may evoke an inappropriate response. Accordingly, it is not surprising that different hormones have varying half-lives in the circulation depending, in part, on the distance that the signal must travel and the nature of the information to be conveyed.

Concentrations of hormones are sensed by receptors, usually proteins, located on the surface (i.e., plasma membrane) or inside target cells. Receptors bind their respective hormone ligands with high affinity and specificity. Although estrogen and testosterone are chemically similar, for example, receptors must distinguish between them because they mediate very different cellular responses indeed. When hormone receptors are situated on the surface of target cells and the response involves intracellular changes (evoking secretion, for example), transduction of the hormonal message must occur. Such transduction molecules are called second messengers of hormone action.

It is a general truth that the chemical structures of hormones do not change markedly during evolution; instead, nature identifies and conserves molecules that already have informational value and develops systems that utilize that information. Steroids, thyroid hormones, and peptides are present in some species that do not utilize them for the same endocrine purposes as do mammals.

4. IDENTIFYING HORMONES

The effects of ablation of endocrine organs have been documented back to the time of Aristotle (384–322 BC), who described changes in secondary sex characteristics and loss of reproductive capacity associated with castration in men. Much insight into the role of endocrine substances has come from disease states, surgical errors, and animal experimentation in which damage to endocrine organs is correlated with particular phenotypic changes in the organism.

Ancient medical procedures prevalent in many cultures are based on the premise that administration of extracts from healthy organs aids in the recovery of diseased organs. This practice may be viewed as a predecessor to hormone replacement therapy. Restoration of function by supplements derived from healthy endocrine organs administered to animals with endocrine ablations has formed the basis of discovering active principles of the endocrine system.

In the mid-1800s, Berthold showed that the effects of castration in avians could be reversed by placement of a testis in the body cavity. Since the transplant was ectopic and not innervated, he concluded that the testes released a substance that controlled secondary sex characteristics.

A few years later, Claude Bernard, providing evidence to support a model of homeostasis, showed that the liver could release sugar to the blood. From the mid-1850s to the 20th century, endocrinology grew at a dramatic pace. Assays became more sensitive and specific; biosynthetic and genetic engineering techniques now allow synthesis of biologically active and highly purified hormones.

5. HORMONE-DERIVED DRUGS

The identification of new hormonal activities often follows a similar pattern. The observation is made that damage to a particular gland is associated with loss of a certain function. Efforts are then focused on isolating the active principle from the gland. The active principle is then administered to restore the function to the animal or patient who has ablated glandular function. The development of drugs is usually directed toward preparing purified fractions that can be used in replacement therapy. The hormone itself and, ultimately, chemical analogs can now readily be synthesized. Analogs can be designed to possess desirable properties, such as prolonged circulation half-lives, chemical stability, or specific receptor or tissue targeting. Availability of purified fractions or synthetic preparations often spawns studies designed to understand the cellular and molecular basis of hormone action. This information is then used to design even more useful drugs that recognize the target cell receptor with higher specificity and affinity; antagonists can also be prepared that block the receptor or its signaling. The science of endocrinology is poised to take advantage of our understanding of intricate second messenger systems, sensitive and precise assay systems (radioimmunoassays, bioassays, radioligand assays), and advances in structural and functional molecular biology. As the tools of endocrinology have become more precise, we have discovered that even the brain and the heart possess substantial endocrine functions.

6. ENDOCRINOLOGY AS A LEAD SCIENCE

Endocrinology continues to be a lead science. Many Nobel Prizes recognize the contributions of endocrinologists. The first cloned gene products to reach the clinical drug market were endocrine substances. Many advances in our understanding of cellular transduction systems, receptor binding, and physiological regulation are derivative of the studies conducted in endocrine laboratories. Why is this so?

A likely answer is found by understanding that endocrinologists study the actions of specific chemicals that cause cells to undergo specific and (usually) easily quantifiable and regulated responses. These are very simple, basic, and well-defined processes. Accordingly, clear and interpretable experiments can be designed at a complexity ranging from molecular to physiological. This is part of the general appeal and high level of achievement of this science—and much of the reason that those who call themselves endocrinologists have made a major contribution to our understanding of biological processes.

HORMONE SECRETION AND ACTION

2 Receptors

Molecular Mediators of Hormone Action

Kelly E. Mayo, PhD

CONTENTS

1. INTRODUCTION

The appropriate proliferation and differentiation of cells during development, and the maintenance of cellular homeostasis in the adult require a continuous flow of information to the cell. This is provided either by diffusible signaling molecules, or by direct cell–cell and cell–matrix interactions. All cells utilize a wide variety of signaling molecules and signal transduction systems to communicate with one another, but within the vertebrate endocrine system, it is the secreted hormones that are classically associated with cellular signaling. Hormones are chemical messengers produced from the endocrine glands that act either locally or at a distance to regulate the activity of a target cell. As discussed in detail elsewhere within this volume, prominent groups of hormonal agents include the peptide hormones, the steroid, retinoid and thyroid hormones, the growth factors, the cytokines, the pheromones, and the neurotransmitters or neuromodulators.

Endocrine signaling molecules exert their effects by interacting with specific receptor proteins that are generally coupled to one or more intracellular effector sys-

From: *Endocrinology: Basic and Clinical Principles* (P. M. Conn and S. Melmed, eds.), Humana Press Inc., Totowa, NJ.

tems. The presence of an appropriate receptor therefore defines the population of target cells for a given hormone and provides a molecular mechanism by which the hormone elicits its biologic actions. These hormone receptor proteins are the focus of this chapter. Section 2. will consider general concepts of receptor action, including receptor structure, interaction with the hormone ligand, activation of cellular effector systems, and receptor regulation. Sections 3. and 4. will then examine the major families of hormone receptors, grouped with respect to their structures and signaling properties, in greater detail, using specific examples that illustrate the general features of each family. Throughout the chapter, special attention will be paid to endocrinopathies that result from known alterations in hormone receptor structure or function.

2. GENERAL ASPECTS OF RECEPTOR ACTION

2.1. Receptors as Mediators of Endocrine Signals

The concept that hormone action is mediated by receptors is most often attributed to the work of Langley on the actions of nicotine and curare on the neuromuscular junction (Langley, 1906). Langley referred to the target for these compounds as the "receptive substance," and postulated that "it receives the stimulus, and by transmitting it, causes contraction," a clear description of the role of receptors in mediating the actions of signaling molecules. Of course, Langley could not know the nature of these receptive substances, suggesting only that they were "radicals of the protoplasmic molecule." Indeed, despite a wealth of physiological evidence in support of the receptor concept, firm biochemical evidence for the existence of specific receptors was not forthcoming until radiolabeled hormones became available. For hormones unable to traverse the cellular membrane, such as the polypeptide hormones, specific binding sites could be demonstrated, but their membrane association and low abundance precluded their characterization for many years. Only with the advent of molecular cloning techniques was it possible to establish firmly the structures of the hormone receptors and to show that these proteins could, in effect, convert a nontarget cell into a target cell by conferring to the cell the ability to bind to and, in some cases, appropriately respond to the corresponding hormone.

A second key event in the development of the receptor concept was the demonstration by Sutherland (1972) that cAMP could mediate the intracellular effects of many different hormones, establishing the notion of "second messengers," and providing a cogent molecular explanation of how hormones and hormone receptors might elicit their widespread effects on cellular activity. The notion that many different signaling molecules, working through distinct receptors, could stimulate a common intracellular signaling pathway, together with the subsequent discovery of additional effector enzymes and intracellular second messengers, provided a rationale explanation for the tremendous diversity in cellular responses to hormones.

At about the time that second messenger systems were being discovered, different concepts were evolving on the mechanism of action of the small lipophilic steroid hormones. Radiolabeled steroids, such as estrogen, were synthesized by Jensen and others, and found to accumulate preferentially in known target organs for the hormone (Jensen and Jacobson, 1962). Specific steroid binding proteins were subsequently identified, and the important finding that binding of agonists and antagonists to

these receptors correlated with their biological activity provided evidence that they were direct mediators of steroid action. These steroid receptors were shown to be soluble intracellular proteins, differentiating them from the membrane-associated receptors for the polypeptide hormones and facilitating their early purification, beginning with the identification of the estrogen receptor by Toft and Gorski (1966). The findings that the steroid receptors associated with chromatin in the cell nucleus, and that steroid hormones affected RNA and protein synthesis, provided the basis for models of direct genomic actions of the hormone–receptor complex that we now know to be correct.

2.2. Membrane-Associated vs Intracellular Receptors

The hormone receptors are commonly subdivided, based on their structures and mechanism of action, into those that span the cellular membrane and act to transduce an extracellular signal into an intracellular response (the cell-surface receptors), and those that reside within the cell and act as direct regulators of gene expression (the intracellular receptors). The unique cellular localization and mode of action of these two receptor classes are illustrated in Fig. 1.

The membrane-associated receptors are an extremely diverse group of signaling molecules. Their common feature is the presence of one or more hydrophobic domains that span the cell membrane and anchor the receptor at the cell surface. Extracellular sequences often participate in hormone binding, whereas intracellular sequences generally either have direct enzymatic function, or associate with one or more intermediary or effector proteins. The functional cell-surface hormone receptor is often composed of multiple protein subunits that may play a role in hormone binding, signaling, or both activities. It is clear that the receptors for structurally and functionally diverse hormones can be closely related to one another, most commonly within their intracellular domains. Thus, a limited number of basic signaling strategies are used repetitively by a very large number of receptor proteins, defining distinct receptor families that will be considered in Section 3.

As discussed earlier, the intracellular receptors for the steroid hormones were the first to be biochemically purified. Following the molecular

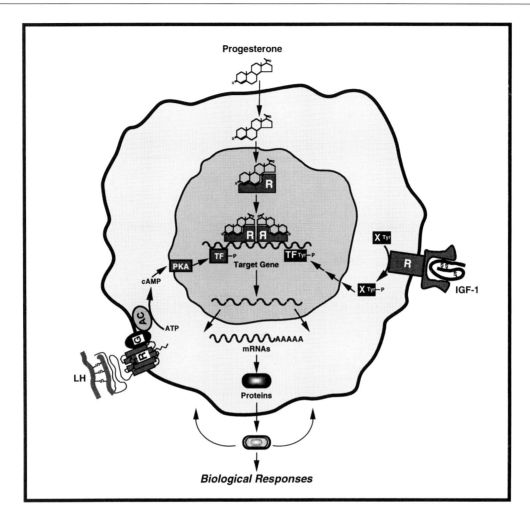

Fig. 1. Hormonal signaling by cell-surface and intracellular receptors. The receptors for the water-soluble polypeptide hormones, LH, and IGF-1 are integral membrane proteins located at the cell surface. They bind the hormone-utilizing extracellular sequences, and transduce a signal by the generation of second messengers, cAMP for the LH receptor, and tyrosine-phosphorylated substrates for the IGF-1 receptor. Although effects on gene expression are indicated, direct effects on cellular proteins, for example, ion channels, are also observed. In contrast, the receptor for the lipophilic steroid hormone progesterone resides in the cell nucleus. It binds the hormone, and becomes activated and capable of directly modulating target gene transcription. Tf = transcription factor; R = receptor molecule.

cloning of the receptors for all of the classic steroid hormones (Evans, 1988), it became clear that these receptors comprise a family of highly related proteins consisting of distinct structural domains. The highly conserved central DNA-binding domain is composed of two zinc-finger motifs, and it is flanked by amino-terminal sequences that are important for activation of target gene transcription and by carboxyl-terminal sequences that are necessary for hormone binding. The subsequent identification of the thyroid hormone, retinoic acid, and vitamin D receptors places them into this nuclear receptor superfamily, along with an expanding number of "orphan receptors" that either act in a ligand-independent fashion or for which appropriate ligands have not yet been identified. Not all intracellular receptors are structurally related to the steroid hormone receptors, prime examples being the nitric oxide (NO) and aryl-hydrocarbon receptors. Although this chapter includes a discussion of both the membrane-associated and intracellular receptors, the focus will be on the former group, in that the intracellular steroid hormone receptors are covered in substantial detail in Chapter 4 in this volume.

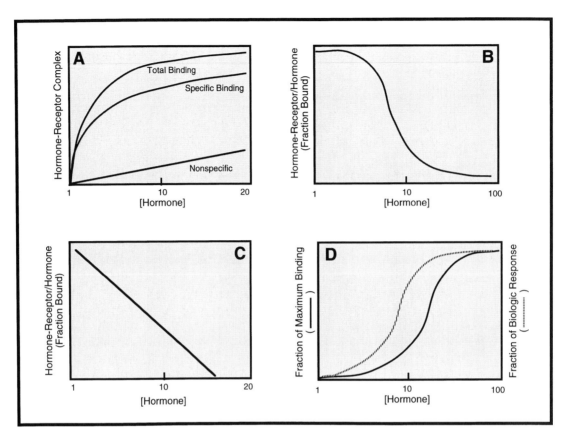

Fig. 2. Measurement of hormone-receptor interactions by binding analysis. Panel **A** indicates saturable binding to a target cell preparation as the concentration of radiolabeled hormone is increased. Panel **B** illustrates a competition or displacement experiment in which the binding of a radiolabeled tracer to the receptor is competed as excess unlabeled hormone is added. Panel **C** represents the Scatchard linear transformation of this binding data, from which receptor number and affinity for the hormone can be determined. Panel **D** shows the consequence of spare receptors. The biological response is fully activated when only a fraction of the receptors are occupied by hormone. See text for details.

2.3. Measurement of Receptor–Ligand Interaction

Hormone receptors are most commonly detected and measured using direct binding assays. This requires a labeled ligand, usually a radiolabeled hormone, such as a tritiated steroid or iodinated peptide, a source of the receptor being analyzed, typically tissue extracts, cells, or cell membranes, and a physical means of separating the bound hormone from that which is unbound, commonly centrifugation or filtration. As shown in Fig. 2A, when increasing amounts of a labeled polypeptide hormone are added to a constant amount of a cell preparation, the fraction of hormone bound to the cell surface increases and eventually approaches a maximum. In addition to specific binding to its cell-surface receptor, the hormone can bind nonspecifi-

cally to other cellular constituents or to the reaction vessel, and this component is commonly measured by performing the binding reaction in the presence of a large excess of unlabeled hormone, to ensure complete displacement of the labeled hormone from specific sites. Specific binding is then established by subtracting the nonspecific binding from the total binding.

In a useful variation of this assay, a competition binding experiment, a constant, small amount of the labeled hormone is mixed with cells or cell membranes in the presence of increasing concentrations of unlabeled hormone. A typical competition or displacement curve resulting from this type of experiment is shown in Fig. 2B. The binding that remains at high hormone concentrations represents the nonspecific binding, and the hormone concentration at which 50% of the radiolabeled tracer is displaced approximates the affinity constant of the receptor for the its ligand, as described below.

The interaction of the hormone and its receptor can be described by the equation H + R → [HR], where H is the free hormone, R the free receptor, and HR the hormone–receptor complex. Binding is assumed to be reversible, and the steady-state dissociation constant $K_d = [H][R]/[HR]$ provides a measure of the affinity of the receptor for its ligand. The total amount of receptor can be described as that which is free plus that which is liganded ($[R_T] = [R] + [HR]$), and the two equations together can be written in the form $[HR] = [R_T][H]/[H] + K_d$. When [HR] is plotted as a function of [H], the hyperbolic plot shown in Fig. 2A is obtained. The previous equation can be rearranged to the form $[HR]/[H] = [R_T]/[H] + K_d$, and when [HR]/[H] is plotted as a function of log[H], the sigmoidal curve shown in Fig. 2B is obtained. Scatchard (1947) described a commonly used linear rearrangement of this relationship, $[HR]/[H] = 1/K_d[HR] + R_T/K_d$, and as shown in Fig. 2C, the plot of [HR]/[H] as a function of [HR] provides the total receptor number, R_T as the intercept with the abscissa, and the dissociation constant, K_d, is derived from the slope, which is $-1/K_d$. The linear relationship shown in Fig. 2C becomes curvilinear when multiple binding sites with differing affinities are present or when cooperative binding interactions occur.

Most commonly, the K_d values for hormone receptors are near the physiological concentration of the relevant hormone, meaning that fluctuations in the hormone level can elicit both positive and negative responses with respect to receptor activation. However, in many cases, it has been shown experimentally that occupancy of only a small fraction of the cell-surface receptors is needed to elicit a maximal biological response. The term "spare receptors" has evolved to describe this phenomenon, which is illustrated in terms of binding and activation curves in Fig. 2D. The ability of a small fraction of occupied receptors to stimulate a biologic response fully points to the tremendous amplification potential of the enzyme effectors that act downstream of the hormone receptors. Spare receptors may allow a response to be kinetically favorable even at very low hormone concentrations.

2.4. Cellular Signal Transduction Themes

Hormones most commonly initiate a cascade of signaling events in their target cell, ultimately leading to an appropriate biologic response. These cascades are referred to as signal transduction pathways, and although they are extremely diverse with respect to the specific molecules involved, they do have several common features. In many cases, the initial activation of the hormone receptor or receptor-associated effector system results in the formation of either soluble second messengers or activated secondary signaling molecules. These signaling molecules then commonly initiate cascades of protein phosphorylation or dephosphorylation that can be extraordinarily complex. This in turn results in changes in gene expression or alterations in protein activity, eliciting the ultimate biologic response. Chapter 3 provides a comprehensive treatment of this topic, and therefore only a few key points necessary for the subsequent discussion of hormone receptors and their actions are introduced in this section.

The first second messenger to be described was cAMP, and the pathways leading to the generation of cAMP and to the subsequent initiation of protein phosphorylation events are among the best understood (Krebs, 1993). Hormone receptors that signal through a cAMP second messenger are coupled to a G-protein that, in turn, modulates the activity of the enzyme adenylate cyclase, resulting in changes in intracellular cAMP levels. The G-proteins are a large family of GTP-binding proteins that are heterotrimeric, consisting of α, β, and γ subunits, and serve to stimulate or repress the activity of multiple cellular effector enzymes (Gilman, 1981). A cycle of GTP binding and hydrolysis to GDP controls the activity of these proteins, as discussed in the following chapter. Stimulatory (G_s) and inhibitory (G_i) proteins, activated in a receptor-dependent fashion, are able to activate or repress, respectively, the enzyme adenylate cyclase, providing for both positive and negative regulation of the cAMP second messenger. cAMP simulates protein kinase A (PKA) by binding to its regulatory subunits, and causing the dissociation and activation of its catalytic subunit. Subsequent phosphorylation of target proteins, including ion channels and transcription factors by PKA, results in appropriate alterations in cellular function.

In a similar manner, additional effector systems can be regulated by G-proteins. Many hormones exert their actions by utilizing inositol phosphates, diacylglycerol, and calcium as second messengers (Berridge, 1993). This pathway can be initiated through receptor activation of a G_q protein, leading to

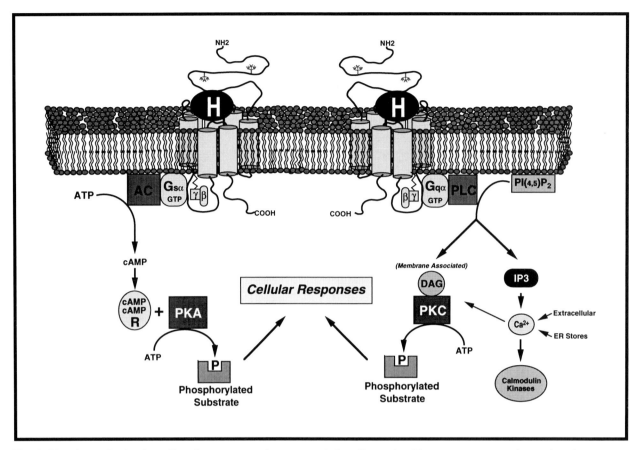

Fig. 3. Signal transduction by cell-surface receptors that are coupled to G-proteins. Two seven-transmembrane domain receptors coupled to different G-proteins (G$_s$ and G$_q$) are shown. Activation of G$_s$ leads to stimulation of the effector enzyme adenylate cyclase and the production of a cAMP second messenger, causing the activation of PKA and the initiation of potential phosphorylation cascades. Activation of G$_q$ leads to stimulation of the effector enzyme phospholipase C-β and the production of IP$_3$ and DAG second messengers, one effect of which is to activate PKC and initiate a potential phosphorylation cascade.

the stimulation of the enzyme phospholipase C, which hydrolyzes the breakdown of phosphatidylinositol 4,5-bisphosphate to diacylglycerol (DAG) and inositol triphosphate (IP$_3$). DAG activates protein kinase C (PKC) at the plasma membrane, whereas IP$_3$ releases calcium from endoplasmic reticulum stores through their interaction with a specific receptor. Among other actions, calcium can interact with its binding protein calmodulin to activate calcium/calmodulin-dependent protein kinases, and it is a coactivator for many of the isoforms of PKC as well. Thus, in this pathway, multiple protein kinases are activated and can propagate the signal through their phosphorylation of diverse target proteins. Key aspects of the G-protein-mediated cAMP, and IP$_3$/calcium signaling pathways are outlined in Fig. 3.

Perhaps the best understood signaling pathway, after that involving the G-protein-coupled receptors,

is the pathway utilized by receptors that have tyrosine kinase activity or that associate with proteins having tyrosine kinase activity. Many hormone and growth factor receptors have cytoplasmic domains with intrinsic protein tyrosine kinase activity. On hormone binding, the receptor rapidly forms a dimer, and the cytoplasmic kinase domain is activated, leading to auto- or trans-phosphorylation of the receptor. Phosphorylation of the receptor allows the subsequent binding of a broad repertoire of cellular proteins that have an SH2 (Src homology 2) domain that specifically recognizes tyrosine phosphorylation sites on the receptor (Pawson, 1995). Some of these SH2 domain proteins are direct substrates for phosphorylation by the receptor, and can serve as effector molecules in transducing the signal. Examples of substrates include the phosphatidylinositol-3-kinase regulatory subunit, the Src family protein kinases, the protein tyrosine phosphatase Syp, and phospholipase C (integrating the tyrosine kinase and G-protein-coupled signaling pathways). Other SH2 domain protein act simply as molecular adapters; they bind to the phosphorylated receptor and also associate with additional cellular proteins, commonly through a protein interaction domain referred to as the SH3 (Src homology 3) domain. Examples include Grb2, Nck, and Crk, which bind to a variety of hormone receptors. Several proteins, including the adapter Shc and the docking protein insulin receptor substrate (IRS)-1, utilize a novel phoso-tyrosine-binding (PTB) domain that recognizes an Asn-Pro-x-pTyr motif in target receptors. Yet other adapter and effector proteins in this signaling pathway contain pleckstrin homology (PH) domains, which may play a role in tethering these proteins at the plasma membrane. Adapter proteins mediate a broad spectrum of responses, but a common and well-characterized response leads to the activation of the small GTP-binding protein Ras. Ras activation initiates a kinase cascade (the mitogen-activated protein [MAP] kinase cascade), beginning with the phosphorylation of the Raf protein, that eventually results in the phosphorylation and activation of a variety of nuclear factors able to alter gene expression in the target cell.

Other hormone receptors lack intrinsic kinase activity, but instead associate with proteins that are tyrosine kinases. This is the case for most of the cytokine receptor superfamily proteins (Ihle and Kerr, 1995). Association of the activated receptor with a member of the Janus kinase family of protein kinases (Jaks or Tyks) leads to receptor phosphorylation on tyrosine residues. The phosphorylated receptor can then interact with SH2 domain adapter proteins as described above, leading to the activation of signaling pathways, such as the Ras-Raf-MAP kinase pathway. In addition, the Jak kinases can phosphorylate one or more members of a family of signaling molecules termed the signal transducer and activator of transcription (Stat) proteins, rendering the Stat proteins competent to bind to DNA and directly regulate the transcription of target genes. The Ras-Raf-MAP kinase, phospholipid, and Jak-Stat pathways of hormone receptor signaling through tyrosine kinases are illustrated in the diagram in Fig. 4.

2.5. Mechanisms of Receptor Regulation

It is clear that mechanisms must exist to regulate the levels of, or activity of, cell-surface receptors,

allowing for modulation or termination of the response to the hormone. In some cases, the biosynthesis of receptors is tightly regulated, so that additional receptors are generated when they are required. For example, the low-density lipoprotein receptor gene is activated by a protein that acts as both a sterol sensor and transcription factor, resulting in enhanced production of the receptor when sterol levels are low. In other cases, the degradation of receptors, and their corresponding ligands, is tightly regulated. Many hormones that act on cell-surface receptors are internalized through the process of receptor-mediated endocytosis, which is shown in Fig. 5A. The hormone–receptor complex is internalized into clathrin-coated vesicles that are acidified and lose their clathrin coat to form endosomes, where the low pH often results in hormone–receptor dissociation. The ligand is most commonly degraded in lysosomes, effectively removing the signal from the extracellular environment. The receptor typically has one of two fates; recycling to the cell surface, where it is again available to interact productively with hormone (for example, the insulin receptor), or degradation in the lysosome (for example, the epidermal growth factor receptor). In either case, internalization effectively reduces the number of cell-surface receptors, and the process is therefore a mechanism utilized to downregulate cell-surface receptors.

A second common mode of regulation targets the ability of cell-surface receptors to bind the hormone or subsequently to transduce a signal. The best-studied example of this is agonist-induced desensitization of the G-protein-coupled β-adrenergic receptor. In the continual presence of the agonist epinephrine, the cAMP signal is attenuated, although the receptor continues to bind epinephrine. Desensitization is a reversible process, and its is mediated by phosphorylation of the receptor on cytoplasmic serine and threonine residues. Some of this phosphorylation is catalyzed by protein-kinase A, which is activated in response to the epinephrine-induced cAMP signal and acts in a feedback manner to downregulate the signaling pathway. Because activated PKA has the ability to phosphorylate many receptors, potentially attenuating their activity, this phenomenon is referred to as heterologous desensitization. The agonist-occupied β-adrenergic receptor is also phosphorylated by a very specific cellular kinase called β-adrenergic receptor kinase (βARK). Because

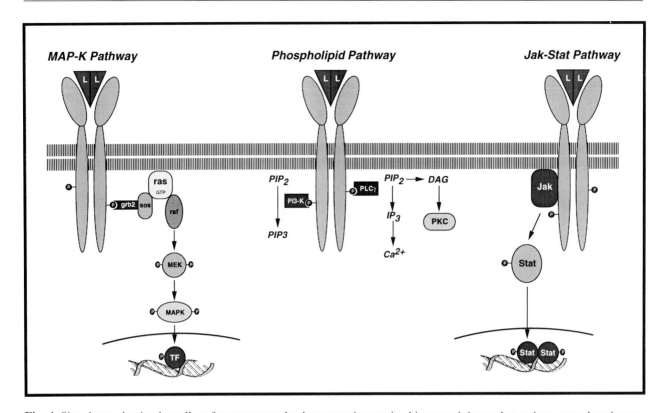

Fig. 4. Signal transduction by cell-surface receptors that have protein tyrosine kinase activity or that activate cytoplasmic protein tyrosine kinases. On the left is a typical receptor protein tyrosine kinase. Hormone binding induces receptor dimerization and auto- or cross-phosphorylation on tyrosine residues. This creates binding sites for adapter proteins, such as Grb2, or for effector enzymes as discussed in the text, often leading to the initiation of tyrosine phosphorylation cascades. The middle segment indicates that effector enzymes involved in phospholipid metabolism are also activated by the receptor protein tyrosine kinase pathway. On the right is a typical cytokine receptor superfamily protein that lacks intrinsic tyrosine kinase activity. In response to hormone binding and subunit dimerization, these receptors recruit cytoplasmic protein tyrosine kinases, such as the Jak kinase shown. One of several subsequent pathways leads to the activation, dimerization, and translocation to the nucleus of the Stat proteins, which are able to regulate target gene transcription directly.

this kinase targets only the β-adrenergic receptor, this phenomenon is referred to as homologous desensitization. The phosphorylated β-adrenergic receptor is unable to couple efficiently to its G-protein, resulting in the observed attenuation of the signal. In addition, several phosphorylated receptors, including the β-adrenergic receptor, bind proteins of the arrestin family, which serve to further suppress the signal by promoting uncoupling of the receptor and its G-protein. A rhodopsin kinase as well as multiple additional β-adrenergic receptor kinases have been identified (Lefkowitz, 1993). These kinases are broadly expressed and likely to play an important role in the desensitization of many hormonal responses mediated by G-protein-coupled receptors. Some of the regulatory processes involved in receptor desensitization are outlined in Fig. 5B. Desensitization is a major fac-

tor controlling the efficacy of action of many therapeutic agents that target G-protein-coupled receptors, such as the β-adrenergic receptor.

3. CELL-SURFACE RECEPTORS

3.1. Receptors with Tyrosine Kinase Activity

The protein tyrosine kinase receptors are found in all multicellular organisms and mediate the actions of a broad spectrum of hormones and growth factors on cell growth, metabolism, and differentiation. They are type I transmembrane proteins, having an external amino-terminus and a single membrane-spanning domain. The extracellular ligand binding domains of these receptors are quite distinctive, but one or more of a variety of recognizable structural motifs appear in

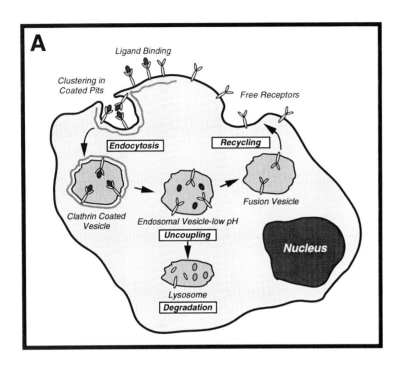

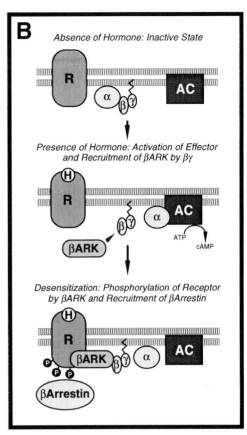

Fig. 5. Mechanisms for the regulation of cell-surface receptors. Panel **A** illustrates the process of receptor-mediated endocytosis. Following ligand binding, receptors rapidly move into coated pits and are internalized by endocytosis. The resulting clathrin-coated vesicles are acidified in an endosomal compartment, leading to dissociation of the ligand from the receptor. Vesicular sorting leads to a segregation of the ligand into vesicles that will fuse with primary lysosomes, resulting in the degradation or utilization of the ligand. The receptor can either be degraded, as often occurs for signaling receptors, such as the EGF and PDGF receptors, or can be recycled to the cell surface, as often occurs for transport receptors, such as the LDL (cholesterol uptake) and transferrin (iron uptake) receptors. Panel **B** shows steps involved in desensitization of the β-adrenergic receptor. In the continual presence of hormone, the G-protein βγ subunits recruit the β-adrenergic receptor kinase to the membrane, leading to specific phosphorylation of the receptor and an attenuation of signaling. The phosphorylated receptor is recognized by a β-arrestin, further suppressing the signaling pathway. The pathway shown is homologous desensitization. As discussed in the text, heterologous desensitization involving receptor phosphorylation by PKA also occurs. Panel B after Lefkowitz (1993).

most of the ligand-binding domains. These domains include cysteine-rich regions, leucine-rich regions, immunoglobulin-related domains, fibronectin type II repeats, and epidermal growth factor (EGF)-like repeats, among others. For the most part, the precise roles of these extracellular domains in hormone recognition have not been well established. The cytoplasmic catalytic domain of these receptors is much more highly conserved, and a number of amino acid residues critical to its enzymatic function are absolutely conserved. Based on the crystallographic structures of several soluble protein kinases as well as the insulin receptor tyrosine kinase domain, it appears

that the receptor protein tyrosine kinase catalytic domains are likely to consist of two lobes, one that binds Mg^{2+}/ATP utilizing a GXGXXG motif and the other that forms the actual catalytic loop. In some receptors in this family, the tyrosine kinase catalytic domain is interrupted by a spacer region.

The receptor protein tyrosine kinases can be subdivided into several families, based largely on their structural characteristics. Examples of some of the major subfamilies, by one recent classification (van der Geer et al., 1994), include the platelet-derived growth factor (PDGF) receptor subfamily, the fibroblast growth factor (FGF) receptor subfamily,

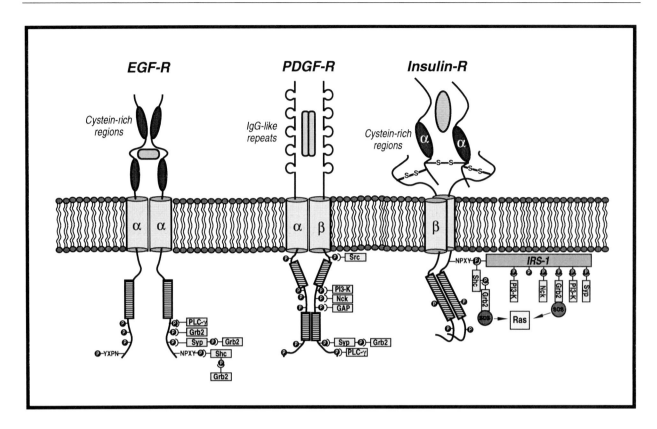

Fig. 6. Structural features and signaling properties of representative cell-surface receptors with protein tyrosine kinase activity. The receptors shown are the EGF, PDGF, and insulin receptors. Unique domains found in the extracellular regions of these receptors includes cysteine-rich repeats and immunoglobulin-like repeats as shown. The activated EGF receptor forms a homodimer, although it can also heterodimerize with several EGFR-related receptors. The activated PDGF receptor is shown as a heterodimer of α and β subunits, although the two subunits also form homodimers. The insulin receptor is synthesized as an αβ heterotetramer as discussed in the text. Autophosphorylation sites on these receptors are indicated, along with the repertoire of SH2 domain or PTB domain adapter and effector proteins that bind these sites. Most adapter and effector proteins bind directly to the phosphorylated EGF and PDGF receptors, whereas the insulin receptor utilizes a docking protein, such as IRS-1 to recruit adapter and effector proteins. The phosphorylation sites and adapter and effector interactions are not meant to be comprehensive, but they are representative. After Schlessinger and Ullrich (1992), Pawson (1995), and Myers and White (1995).

the insulin receptor subfamily, the EGF receptor subfamily, the nerve growth factor (NGF) receptor subfamily, the hepatocyte growth factor (HGF) receptor subfamily, and a series of additional receptors for which ligands have not yet been identified. Fig. 6 shows examples of the structural features of three of the best-characterized and representative receptor protein tyrosine kinases, the EGF, PDGF, and insulin receptors. The insulin receptor and the related IGF-1 receptor are unique in that the mature receptor is a heterotetramer consisting of two extracellular α subunits and two membrane-spanning β subunits linked by disulfide bonds. The α and β subunits are derived from the proteolytic processing of a single precursor protein.

The receptors in this superfamily all exhibit a hormone-dependent dimerization that is crucial for subsequent signal transduction. Although it is believed that ligand binding induces a conformational change in the extracellular domain leading to dimerization, the mechanism of this is not known. Some ligands for these receptors are themselves dimers (for example, PDGF), whereas others are monomers (for example, EGF). Although in most cases it is not known whether binding of a single hormone molecule will elicit dimerization or whether the binding of two hormone molecules is required, there is evidence to suggest that the binding of a single hormone molecule may be sufficient to induce the dimerization of many receptors. This, in turn, leads to auto- or trans-phosphorylation of the receptor within its cytoplasmic domain and the subsequent recruitment of substrates having affinity for the tyrosine-phosphorylated receptor, as described in the previous section on signal transduction.

Signal propagation by the prototypic EGF, PDGF, and insulin receptors is considered in greater detail in the schematic diagrams in Fig. 6, which depict some of the key effector and adapter proteins that interact with the phosphorylated receptors. The PDGF receptor interacts with a wide range of effectors, including PLC-γ, the p85 regulatory subunit of PI-3-kinase, and the Src kinase, as well as a number of adapter proteins, including Crk, Nck, Grb2, and Shc. The EGF receptor shares these interactions, with the possible exception of PI-3 kinase p85. In contrast, the insulin receptor cytoplasmic domain utilizes a somewhat different strategy, binding to IRS-1 or IRS-2, very large proteins that have been termed docking proteins. The insulin receptor phosphorylates the IRS proteins at multiple tyrosine residues, creating binding sites for the recruitment of many of the same effector and adapter molecules discussed above. These same docking proteins are likely to mediate the actions of additional receptors, including some cytokine receptors. Recent evidence also suggests that the Stat proteins, described in greater detail in a subsequent section, can bind to protein tyrosine kinase receptors, including the EGF receptor. Such examples of "crosstalk" between receptor signaling systems are becoming increasingly common.

The physiological functions of many of the receptors in the tyrosine protein kinase family have been explored through gene disruption approaches in mice, or by the identification of naturally occurring mutations in these receptors in animal models or in people. With respect to naturally occurring mutations, it should be realized that many of the receptor tyrosine kinases were initially discovered as transduced retroviral oncogenes that represent mutated, truncated, or inappropriately expressed versions of their cellular counterparts (Carbone and Levine, 1990). Although a complete discussion of the physiological functions of receptor tyrosine protein kinases is beyond the scope of this chapter, a few examples relating to the model receptors discussed in this section (EGF, PDGF, and insulin receptors) will be considered briefly here.

The EGF receptor played a key role in defining the relationship of cellular signaling pathways to retrovirus-induced cellular transformation and oncogene-sis. A truncated and transduced form of the EGF receptor represents one of two oncogenes (v-erbB) of the avian erythroblastosis virus, and the highly related Neu tyrosine kinase receptor (also referred to as c-erbB-2) is mutated or amplified in a wide variety of human cancers. Thus, inappropriate activation of the signaling pathways mediated by these tyrosine kinase receptors can lead to cell transformation and tumori-genesis. An inactivating mutation of the α subunit of the PDGF receptor has been characterized as a spontaneous mutation in mice, the *patch* mutation. This recessive lethal mutation has a variety of phenotypes in heterozygotes that affect neural-crest-derived cells, implicating PDGF and its receptor as critical for normal crest development. The insulin receptor is subject to mutation in patients with insulin resistance, and this has led to the identification of many different types of mutations that affect the synthesis or function of this receptor tyrosine kinase. These mutations are associated with type A insulin resistance, leprachaunism, and lipoatrophic diabetes. Interestingly, the mutations that reside within the tyrosine kinase domain of the insulin receptor can be mapped onto the recently solved crystallographic structure of this domain, and many of these mutations appear likely to destabilize hydrophobic packing within the kinase domain.

3.2. Receptors That Are Protein Phosphatases

A large number of protein tyrosine phosphatases have been identified by molecular cloning, and their structures suggest that at least seven of these are transmembrane proteins with the potential to act as ligand-regulated phosphatases (Fischer et al., 1991). They are distinct from the serine and threonine protein phosphatases, and might be expected to participate in cellular signal transduction by countering the activities of the receptor protein tyrosine kinases. Despite the striking similarity of these transmembrane protein tyrosine phosphatases to receptors, distinct ligands that might activate these proteins have not been identified. Some of these proteins have extracellular domains that include regions resembling segments of fibronectin or neural cell-adhesion molecule (NCAM), suggesting that the transmembrane protein tyrosine phosphatases might be involved in signaling in response to direct cell–cell communication or cell–matrix interaction.

The best characterized of the potential receptor protein tyrosine phosphatases is the leukocyte common antigen CD45. It consists of an external segment that is cysteine-rich and resembles a ligand-binding motif, a single transmembrane domain, and two tandem cytoplasmic protein tyrosine phosphatase domains. Multiple forms of CD45 arise through alternative RNA processing mechanisms, and these are differentially glycosylated and expressed on distinct subsets of lymphocytes. CD45 is known to be essential for antigen-stimulated proliferation of T-lymphocytes and for thymic development, but its exact role in signaling by the T-cell receptor remains enigmatic. Recent studies indicate that two members of the Src family of cytoplasmic protein tyrosine kinases, p56-Lck and p59-Fyn, are likely to be physiological substrates for the CD45 tyrosine phosphatase.

3.3. Receptors with Serine and Threonine Kinase Activity

Receptors in this family were identified relatively recently, beginning with the expression cloning of the activin type II receptor (Mathews, 1994). Activin is a protein hormone in the transforming growth factor-β (TGF-β) superfamily, and this superfamily includes such hormones as Mullerian inhibiting substance (MIS), the bone morphogenic proteins (BMPs), and nonmammalian homologs, such as *Drosophila* decapentaplegic (*dpp*) and *Xenopus* Vg-1. Receptor nomenclature has been based on crosslinking studies with TGF-β that revealed three distinct protein species designated type I, II, and III receptors. The type III receptor is a large proteoglycan that is thought to play a role in the storage or clearance of TGF-β, or to facilitate delivery of the hormone to the signaling receptors, whereas the type I and type II receptors are both known to be involved in signaling.

The initial cloning of a type II activin receptor revealed a transmembrane protein with a relatively short extracellular domain and a cytoplasmic domain predicted to be a protein serine or threonine kinase. This type II activin receptor was found to be related to two putative orphan receptor serine or threonine kinases found previously in *C. elegans (daf-1)* and in maize (*ZmPK1*). The related type II TGF-β receptor has been cloned, and subsequent biochemical studies confirm that the activin and TGF-β receptors are specific for serine and threonine phosphorylation, and that the type II subunit alone has high-affinity ligand-binding capacity. Additional type II receptors,

including putative mammalian BMP and MIS receptors as well as a second *C. elegans* receptor (*daf-4*), have recently been identified.

Subsequent low-stringency screening approaches have resulted in the identification of additional related receptors that have been designated as type I receptors by several criteria. First, these proteins have the ability to form type I affinity-labeled complexes as first described for the TGF-β receptors. Second, the type I receptors alone are unable to bind ligand, and they require a coexpressed type II receptor to interact with ligand. Last, the type I receptors are structurally distinct from the type II receptors, and they have a cytoplasmic juxtamembrane domain that has a conserved amino acid motif (GSGSG) termed the GS domain within a larger serine-threonine-rich region that is that to be a target of receptor phosphorylation. A family of at least six mammalian type I receptors has been identified, and these receptors appear promiscuous with respect to their type II-dependent interaction with ligand, in that several of the type I receptors are able to mediate the formation of type I complexes in response to either activin or TGF-β. The structures of the type I and type II serine and threonine kinase receptors are schematically shown in Fig. 7A.

Based largely on work with the type I and type II TGF-β receptors (Wrana et al., 1994), it is thought that the two receptor subunits form a noncovalent heteromeric complex, and that both type I and type II subunits are required for receptor signaling. It is not certain whether formation of the heteromeric complex, which is likely to be a heterotetramer, requires the presence of ligand. In a current model for TGF-β signaling, the type II receptor is proposed to be a constitutively active kinase that recruits the type I receptor in a ligand-dependent fashion and phosphorylates the type I receptor within the GS domain, leading to activation of the type I receptor and subsequent signal transduction. This model is depicted in Fig. 7B.

Unlike the related receptor tyrosine kinases, little is known about signaling events downstream of the serine or threonine kinase receptors. If phosphorylation of the GS domain is a key event in signaling, this might act either to create appropriate docking sites for the association of signaling molecules, as described for the tyrosine kinase receptors, or to regulate the kinase activity of the type I receptor for substrates. One approach that has been used to look for

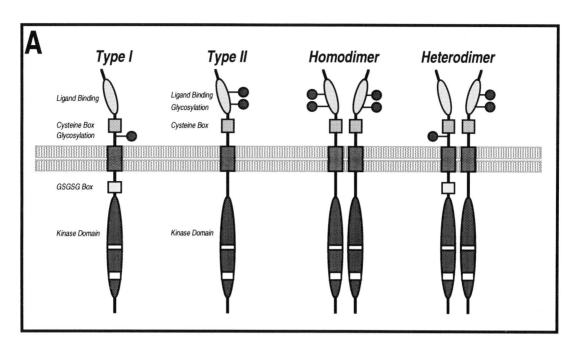

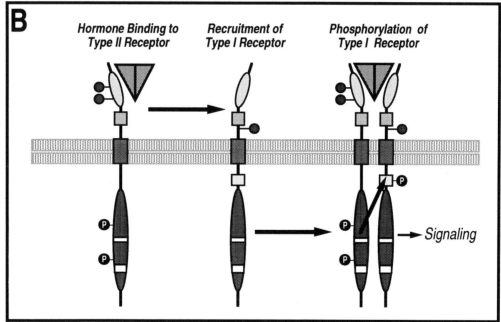

Fig. 7. Structural features and potential signaling mechanism of cell-surface receptors with protein serine and threonine kinase activity. Panel **A** shows in schematic fashion the structural features of the type I and type II receptors for hormones including TGF-β and activin. The predominant structural difference is the conserved GS box (GSGSG within a serine-threonine-rich region) unique to the type I receptors. Two forms of receptor interactions are known to occur, leading to the formation of type II homodimers or type I–type II heterodimers as indicated. The actual composition of the heteromer may be that of a tetramer. Panel **B** is a model for activation and signaling based on studies with the TGF-β receptors. The type II receptor, which is constitutively phosphorylated, is able to bind the hormone, leading to a recruitment of type I receptor to form the active heterodimer. The type II receptor is proposed to phosphorylate the type I receptor within the GS box, leading to activation. The substrates or effectors interacting with this receptor family are largely unknown. Panel **B** after Wrana et al. (1994).

potential substrates is two-hybrid screening in yeast, and this has resulted in the identification of the small immunophilin FKBP-12 as a protein interacting with the cytoplasmic domain of the type I receptors. This interaction is weakened if a mutant type I receptor cytoplasmic domain with a substitution in the ATP-binding site that eliminates signal transduction is utilized for the protein interaction assays. Another recent report has identified a protein that specifically interacts with the type II TGF-β receptor cytoplasmic domain as a novel WD-domain (a protein interaction domain) protein. This association is lost in kinase-defective mutants of the type II TGF-β receptor, and is not observed for the related type II activin receptor, suggesting that the type II receptor may have signaling roles in addition to the crossphosphorylation of the type I receptor. The importance of these or other interacting proteins in signaling by the serine and threonine kinase family of receptors remains to be established.

Although the ligands of the TGF-β superfamily have been extensively studied through genetic approaches, little information is available from the analysis of induced or naturally occurring mutations in the receptors for these hormones. Aspects of the function of the activin and TGF-β receptors have been examined through the use of dominant-negative receptor mutations, and by receptor overexpression or disruption in transgenic animals. A dominant-negative form of the activin IIB receptor, expressed in *Xenopus* embryos, causes a failure of mesoderm formation and arrests development prior to gastrulation, indicating an important role of activin signaling during early development. The type II activin receptor gene has been disrupted in transgenic mice, and these mice generally survive to adulthood, although they have suppressed follicle-stimulating hormone levels and deficiencies in reproductive performance. Importantly, the defects in these mice are much less severe than those in mice lacking the activins themselves, which die shortly after birth. These combined results suggest that activin may signal through receptors other than the type II activin receptor in early embryonic development. Very recently, inactivating mutations in the type II TGF-β receptor have been reported in human colon cancer cell lines with microsatellite instability, suggesting that these cells may proliferate by escaping the inhibitory effects of TGF-β on epithelial cell growth.

3.4. Receptors That Associate with Signaling Subunits

Many well-characterized transmembrane receptors lack apparent enzymatic functions, such as kinase or phosphatase domains, within their cytoplasmic regions, and their modes of signal transduction were unknown until quite recently. This family includes the receptors for the interleukins, interferons, erythropoietin, granulocyte-macrophage colony-stimulating factor, growth hormone, and prolactin, among others, and is known as the cytokine receptor superfamily. The functional receptors include single chains (growth hormone, prolactin, erythropoietin), ligand-specific chains that interact with a common shared chain (interleukins-2, 3, and 6 [IL-2, IL-3, and IL-6]), and multiple unique chains (interferons). Although these receptors all lack tyrosine kinase activity, conserved membrane-proximal regions of their cytoplasmic domains mediate interaction with one or more cytoplasmic protein tyrosine kinases, the Janus kinases, or Jaks (Ihle and Kerr, 1995). These kinases, including Jak1, Jak2, Jak3, and Tyk2, have amino-terminal homology domains of unknown function, and two carboxyl-terminal kinase domains, although the first of these lacks critical residues necessary for catalytic activity and is inactive. The Jak kinases are tyrosine phosphorylated and activated following ligand binding to the cytokine receptors, and this requires an association of the Jak kinases with two conserved membrane-proximal motifs in the receptor referred to as box 1 and box 2. It is thought that receptor dimerization brings the associated Jak kinases into close proximity, and allows cross-phosphorylation and activation to occur. Thus, two Jak kinases associate in the same manner as two cytoplasmic kinase domains of the receptor tyrosine protein kinases associate. In addition to Jak kinase phosphorylation, the activation process is associated with phosphorylation of the receptor itself on specific tyrosine residues.

The pathway from Jak kinase activation to changes in target cell gene expression was completed through the analysis of proteins mediating the transcriptional responses to interferon, a family of proteins now known as the Stat proteins (Darnell et al., 1994). The Stat proteins are activated by tyrosine phosphorylation and subsequently form dimers, translocate to the nucleus, and bind to specific DNA elements (originally γ interferon activation sequences, or GAS elements) near target genes to regulate transcription. Stat proteins include a highly conserved SH2 domain as well as an SH3-related domain in the carboxyl-terminal regions, in addition to a conserved carboxyl-terminal tyrosine critical for regulating their activity. At least six Stat proteins have been identified, and it appears that these serve as the link between Jak kinase activation and cellular transcriptional responses. It is thought that the Jak kinases selectively phosphorylate and activate the Stat proteins.

It is clear that different receptors in the cytokine receptor superfamily preferentially associate with one or more Jak kinases and subsequently preferentially activate one or more Stat proteins, but the mechanisms of specificity are largely unknown. It also seems likely that the Jak-Stat pathway is not the only one involved in signaling by these receptors. Jak-induced phosphorylation of the erythropoietin and IL-3 receptors generates sites for the binding of adapter molecules, such as Shc, leading to association of a Grb2 adapter, binding of Sos, and the activation of Ras and Raf, as described for receptors with direct tyrosine kinase activity. Other cytokines, such as IL-2, activate Src family kinases, whereas phosphorylation of many of the cytokine receptors leads to the binding of a hematopoietic cell phosphatase (HCP) through its SH2 domain, which is believed to act to suppress receptor activity.

Because the cytokine receptor superfamily is large and the receptors utilize diverse signaling mechanisms, it is informative to consider one example focused on the endocrine system in greater detail. One of the best-studied receptors in this class is the growth hormone receptor. It is representative of the single-chain class of cytokine receptors, and has the two pairs of conserved cysteines in the extracellular domain that are a hallmark of this family. Interestingly, two receptor chains bind to a single growth hormone molecule at distinct sites on the hormone, and thus a single ligand catalyzes receptor dimerization and subsequent signal transduction, as shown in Fig. 8A. This has been demonstrated by determination of the crystallographic structure of the extracellular domain of the growth hormone receptor complexed with growth hormone. Site 1 on growth hormone must be occupied prior to occupancy of site 2. At high concentrations of hormone, saturation of all receptors by binding to site 1 on growth hormone is predicted to inhibit receptor dimerization and the subsequent biological response. This has been experimentally demonstrated for a hybrid growth hormone-cytokine receptor, as shown

in Fig. 8A, and may represent an additional mode of receptor regulation. The growth hormone receptor is somewhat unique in that the extracellular domain of the receptor also functions as a soluble serum-binding protein for growth hormone. The extracellular domain is released from the mature receptor by proteolysis in some species, whereas it is encoded by a distinct mRNA generated by alternative RNA processing in other species.

The activated growth hormone receptor associates with the Jak2 kinase, leading to the phosphorylation and activation of Stat1 as well as Stat3. In addition, the MAP kinase pathway is also activated by growth hormone, presumably through the interaction of an adapter protein, such as Shc with the phosphorylated growth hormone receptor, or with Jak2 itself, leading to the activation of the Ras and Raf pathway as described for protein tyrosine kinase receptors. These pathways of growth hormone signal transduction are shown in Fig. 8B. Additional roles of the phospholipase C and PKC pathways in growth hormone action have also been suggested, pointing out the complexity of signaling systems operative in response to a single hormonal stimulus.

The growth hormone receptor is also a good example of the potential involvement of receptors within this superfamily in endocrine disease. Mutations in the growth hormone receptor/binding protein are responsible for the growth hormone resistance observed in Laron-type dwarfism, in which serum growth hormone is elevated in association with classical symptoms of growth hormone deficiency, including reduced levels of insulin growth factor (IGF)-1 and short stature. More than a dozen distinct mutations in the receptor have been found, and nearly all are in the extracellular domain and result in gross alterations in receptor structure, generally through premature termination of translation. An interesting growth hormone receptor mutation occurs in the sex-linked dwarf (SLD) chicken, in which an invariant amino acid within a conserved cytoplasmic membrane proximal sequence found in nearly all class I cytokine receptors, the WSXWS motif, is altered, perhaps affecting Jak kinase interaction with the receptor.

3.5. Receptors Coupled to G-Proteins

The G-protein-coupled receptors comprise the largest known family of cell-surface hormone receptors. Hundreds of these receptors have already been

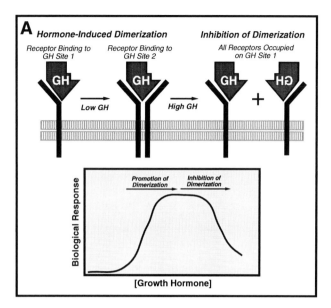 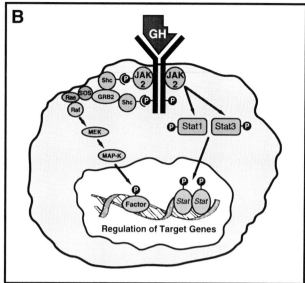

Fig. 8. Hormone-induced dimerization and signaling by the growth hormone receptor, a member of the cytokine receptor super-family. Panel **A** illustrates dimerization of the growth hormone receptor by a single molecule of growth hormone. The receptor first binds site 1 on growth hormone, allowing interaction at site 2 and leading to dimerization. The two distinct sites on growth hormone are bound by very similar domains within the two receptor chains. At high growth hormone concentrations, full occupancy of all receptors at site 1 is expected to occlude interaction at site 2, inhibiting formation of the dimer. In a model system utilizing the growth hormone receptor extracellular domain and a cytokine receptor signaling domain, this leads to an inhibition of the biologic response at high hormone amounts as indicated in the lower part of panel A. Panel **B** indicates two major signal-ing pathways activated by the growth hormone receptor. Association with the tyrosine kinase Jak2 leads to receptor phosphory-lation, and activation of Stat proteins, including Stat1 and Stat3, that stimulate target gene transcription. SH2-domain adapter proteins, such as Shc, can mediate interaction of the growth hormone receptor and/or Jak2 with Grb2, leading to the eventual acti-vation of Ras and Raf and the stimulation of the MAP kinase mitogenic pathway. Panel A after Fuh et al. (1992).

cloned and characterized. Their common features are seven hydrophobic potential membrane-spanning domains and the ability to stimulate the exchange of bound GDP for GTP on associated G-protein α subunits in response to agonist binding. As indicated in Fig. 9A, the G-protein-coupled receptor superfamily can be divided into several major families that share significant sequence simi-larities. The three predominant mammalian families are family A (receptors related to rhodopsin and the β_2-adrenergic receptor), family B (receptors related to the calcitonin and parathyroid hormone recep-tors), and family C (receptors related to the metabotropic glutamate receptors). Further subdivi-sions into groups are indicated in the figure, as are families D–F of nonmammalian receptors. Family A is by far the largest family of G-protein-coupled receptors, and its prototypes, rhodopsin and the β_2-adrenergic receptor, are among the best-character-ized receptors. Therefore, much of what is known about the structure, function, and regulation of G-

protein-coupled receptors in general comes from studies of these model proteins.

The major structural features of a model G-protein-coupled receptor, the β_2-adrenergic recep-tor, are shown in Fig. 9B. The extracellular domain is relatively short, although for some family A receptors, those for the glycoprotein hormones FSH, LH, and TSH, this domain is more than 300 amino acids in length. There are typically several sites for asparagine-linked glycosylation within the extracel-lular domain. The seven membrane-spanning domains follow, creating three extracellular loops and three cytoplasmic loops that can be quite vari-able in length among different receptors. The car-boxyl-terminal cytoplasmic domain is typically short and is often associated with the plasma mem-brane through palmitoylation of a conserved cys-teine residue. As discussed in an earlier section, phosphorylation plays an important role in the regu-lation of receptor activity, and potential sites for phosphorylation by PKA as well as the specific

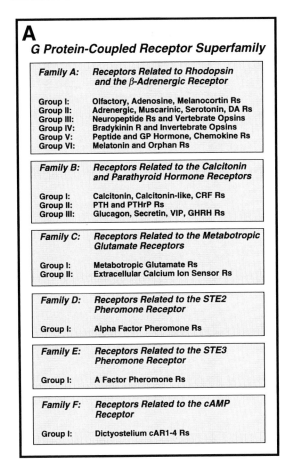

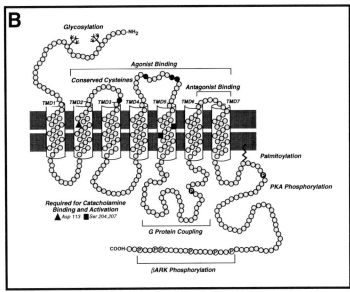

Fig. 9. Classification and basic architecture of cell-surface receptors that couple to G-proteins. Panel **A** lists the major families and groups of G-protein-coupled receptors. The mammalian receptors are confined to families A, B, and C. Family A is the largest and includes the diverse oderant receptors as well as prototypic G-protein-coupled receptors, such as rhodopsin and the β-adrenergic receptor. Panel **B** shows a schematic structure of one of the most extensively characterized G-protein-coupled receptors, the β-adrenergic receptor. Major structural features are indicated and are expanded on in the text. Panel **A** after Kolakowski (1994), and the GCRDb data base, maintained by LF Kolakowski at http://receptor.mgh.harvard.edu. GCRDBHOME.html. Panel **B** after Dohlman et al. (1991).

β-adrenergic receptor kinase are found within the third cytoplasmic domain and the carboxyl-terminal tail of the receptor.

Mutagenesis has been extensively applied to elucidate features of the β$_2$-adrenergic receptor important for ligand interaction and for subsequent G-protein coupling. A strategy that has been particularly useful for the analysis of the G-protein-coupled receptors has been the generation of chimeras between two homologous receptors with distinct ligand-binding or signaling properties. Such chimeras between the β$_2$-adrenergic and α$_1$-adrenergic receptors have implicated the transmembrane domains and associated extracellular loops in specific agonist binding, and have shown that transmembrane domain seven is par-

ticularly important in specifying antagonist binding. Similar experiments to examine signaling through the stimulation (β$_2$-adrenergic receptor) or inhibition (α$_1$-adrenergic receptor) of adenylate cyclase by G$_s$ and G$_i$, respectively, led to the conclusion that the regions between transmembrane domains five and six, including the third cytoplasmic loop, were particularly important in determining G-protein recognition. Additional mutagenesis has indicated that the carboxyl-terminal domain of the receptor, a major site of potential phosphorylation, is particularly important for desensitization, and that several conserved residues are critical for catacholamine binding and activation, including an aspartic acid residue in transmembrane domain two, and two serine residues in transmembrane domain five of the β_2-adrenergic receptor.

In general, much of what has been learned from model receptors, such as the β_2-adrenergic receptor, has been applicable to additional G-protein-coupled receptors. The basic membrane topology of the β-adrenergic receptor, discerned through proteolysis and antibody epitope mapping studies, holds for other members of the superfamily that have been examined. There are differences in ligand-binding determinants, and in general, receptors that interact with small molecules utilize the transmembrane domain segments more extensively for binding, whereas receptors that interact with larger peptides or proteins make greater use of the amino-terminal and extracellular loops. An extreme example of this is ligand recognition by the glycoprotein hormone receptors, where the large amino-terminal extracellular domain, expressed independently of the transmembrane domains, has the ability to bind the ligand with normal affinity. The mechanisms by which ligand binding leads to an ability of the receptor to productively interact with a G-protein are largely unknown, but molecular modeling of these receptors based on the structure of bacteriorhodopsin and the altered properties of mutant receptors is beginning to shed light on the potential conformational changes that accompany activation. As additional members of this family are characterized, novel modes of receptor activation are also being observed. For example, thrombin proteolytically cleaves its G-protein-coupled receptor in the extracellular domain, revealing a new amino-terminus that acts like a ligand to mediate activation of the receptor.

Tremendous diversity is a hallmark of the G-protein-coupled receptor superfamily. Many of the neurotransmitter and peptide hormone receptors are encoded by multiple genes that produce related, yet distinct receptors. For example, five distinct somatostatin receptors have been characterized. These are expressed with unique, but overlapping tissue and cell specificity, and they are able to mediate signaling through several different G-proteins. An extreme example of this is represented by the olfactory oderant receptors, a family that already numbers more than 100. Other receptors are produced from a single gene, but alternative RNA processing results in the generation of multiple receptor isoforms, either produced in specific tissues or able to couple differentially to G-protein-mediated signaling pathways. For example, the dopamine D2 receptor exists as two splice variants expressed in unique tissue-specific patterns, whereas the pituitary adenylate cyclase activating polypeptide (PACAP) receptor exists as five splice variants that differ in their ability to activate adenylate cyclase vs phospholipase C effectors.

Given the diversity of the G-protein-coupled receptors, it is perhaps not surprising that many endocrinopathies can be attributed to mutations in specific G-protein-coupled receptors. This connection first became apparent through the analysis of the G-proteins these receptors interact with, when it was demonstrated that mutations that constitutively activate $G\alpha_s$ by inactivating its intrinsic GTPase function were causative in acromegaly in association with pituitary adenoma (a late somatic mutation confined to the pituitary gland) as well as in McCune-Albright disease (an earlier somatic mutation affecting many endocrine systems). Subsequently, mutations in many G-protein-coupled receptors have been identified, both in human diseases and in animal models of human disease. These represent both loss of function and gain of function mutations in the targeted G-protein-coupled receptors. For example, inactivating mutations of the calcium-sensing receptor cause familial hypocalciuric hypercalcemia in the heterozygous state and neonatal severe hyperparathyroidism in the homozygous state, whereas an activating mutation in this same receptor causes a dominant form of hypocalcemia. In some cases, analysis of these mutations, which generally have a known phenotype, has revealed much about important structural features of these receptors. For example, more than 50 different mutations of the vasopressin V2 receptor in patients with nephrogenic diabetes insipidus have been found, providing a wealth of information on residues essential for hormone binding or activation of this receptor. Representative examples of G-protein-coupled receptors involved in disease are listed in Fig. 10.

3.6. Receptors with Guanylyl Cyclase Activity

As their name implies, the receptors in this small family have cytoplasmic domains that possess guanylyl cyclase (GC) activity, promoting the production of a cGMP second messenger. They are distinct from, but related to, the soluble GCs (Drewett and Garbers, 1994). They are single-chain

Diseases Caused by Mutations in G Protein-Coupled Receptors

Condition	Receptor	Inheritance	Δ Function
Retinitis Pigmentosa	Rhodopsin	AD/AR	Loss
Nephrogenic Diabetes Insipidus	Vasopressin V2	X-linked	Loss
Isolated Glucocorticoid Deficiency	ACTH	AR	Loss
Color Blindness	Red/Green Opsins	X-linked	Loss
Familial Precocious Puberty	LH	AD (male)	Gain
Familial Hypercalcemia	Ca^{2+} Sensing	AD	Loss
Neonatal Severe Parathyroidism	Ca^{2+} Sensing	AR	Loss
Dominant Form Hypocalcemia	Ca^{2+} Sensing	AD	Gain
Congenital Hyperthyroidism	TSH	AD	Gain
Resistance to Thyroid Hormone	TSH	AR (comp het)	Loss
Hyperfunctioning Thyroid Adenoma	TSH	Somatic	Gain
Metaphyseal Chondrodysplasia	PTH-PTHrP	Somatic	Gain
Hirschsprung's Disease	Endothelin-B	Multigenic	Loss
Coat Color Alteration (*E* locus, mice)	MSH	AD/AR	Loss & Gain
Dwarfism (*little* locus, mice)	GHRH	AR	Loss

Fig. 10. Diseases caused by mutations in G-protein-coupled receptors. All are human conditions with the exception of the final two entries, which refer to the mouse. AD = autosomal dominant, AR = autosomal recessive inheritance. Loss of function refers to inactivating mutations of the receptor, and gain of function to activating mutations. Abbreviations for G-protein-coupled receptors, ACTH = adrenocorticotropic hormone, LH = luteinizing hormone, TSH = thyroid-stimulating hormone, PTH-PTHrP = parathyroid hormone and parathyroid hormone-related peptide, MSH = melanocyte-stimulating hormone, GHRH = growth hormone-releasing hormone, FSH = follicle-stimulating hormone.

transmembrane proteins with an extracellular ligand-binding domain, a membrane proximal cytoplasmic domain that resembles a protein kinase domain, but is catalytically inactive, and the carboxyl-terminal GC domain. The first members of this receptor family to be characterized were the sperm receptors for egg peptides from sea urchins (resact and speract) with sperm-stimulatory properties. Subsequently, a number of homologous proteins have been identified in mammalian systems. Currently, there are six cloned transmembrane GCs. GC-A, B, and C all represent receptors for natriuretic peptides or heat-stable enterotoxins. The GC-A receptor binds atrial natriuretic peptide (ANP) as well as the related BNP, GC-B binds the natriuretic peptide CNP, and GC-C binds heat-stable enterotoxin and probably binds the novel peptide guanylin. GC-D is expressed in olfactory sensory neurons, whereas GC-E and GC-F are expressed within the eye. These latter three remain orphan receptors with no known ligand, and suggest a subfamily of GC receptors restricted to sensory tissues.

Although they are not cell-surface receptors, it is worth noting in this section that the soluble forms of GC, which are α-β heterodimers, serve as the target for the signaling molecule NO, leading to the formation of a cGMP second messenger. A bound heme confers sensitivity to NO in these proteins. At least one form of the β subunit, $β_2$, has a consensus isoprenylation sequence near its carboxyl-terminus, raising the possibility that some of the presumed soluble forms of GC may actually be membrane-associated. Thus, members of the GC family have functions as both membrane-associated and intracellular receptors for diverse signaling molecules.

The GC-A receptor gene has been disrupted in mice, and this results in a chronic elevation in blood pressure that is independent of salt intake, suggesting that alterations in GC-A function might explain some salt-resistant forms of essential hypertension in humans. Because disruption of the ANP gene in mice does not produce this phenotype, other ligands for the GC-A receptor, such as BNP, may be involved in this regulatory pathway, and conversely, ANP may regulate natriuresis through a receptor other than GC-A.

3.7. Ligand-Gated Ion Channels

The ligand-gated ion channels mediate the rapid actions of a variety of neurotransmitters by creating a ligand-regulated pore through which ions can flow down their electrochemical gradients (Unwin, 1993). There are two major functional families of these channels. The acetylcholine, serotonin, and glutamate-gated ion channels allow the passage of cations at excitatory synapses, whereas the glycine and aminobutyric acid (GABA)-gated ion channels allow the passage of anions at inhibitory synapses. At the amino acid sequence level, the acetylcholine, serotonin, GABA, and glycine-gated channel subunits are homologous, whereas the glutamate-gated channels are larger and are distinct in sequence. The glutamate-gated channels can be divided based on agonist selectivity into the α-amino-3-hydroxy-5-methyl-4-isoxazole proprionic acid (AMPA), N-methyl-D-aspartate (NMDA), and kainate types.

The ligand-gated channels are multisubunit proteins, with an $\alpha_2\beta\delta\gamma$ pentameric composition in the case of the acetylcholine receptor. Each subunit has four presumed transmembrane domains, both the amino- and carboxyl-termini are extracellular, and most subunits are thought to be glycosylated. There is a large cytoplasmic loop between the third and fourth transmembrane domains that is a site for phosphorylation in some of the receptor subunits. Transmembrane domain 2 is thought to contribute most strongly to forming the actual pore, and there are several highly conserved amino acid residues within this domain, including charged residues thought to be important for cation or anion transport. Most of the structural studies of this family have been performed using the acetylcholine receptor. This receptor binds two molecules of acetylcholine, one to each α subunit of the pentamer, inducing a conformational change that results in a transient increase in permeability to Na$^+$ and K$^+$. On prolonged exposure to an agonist, this channel desensitizes, probably as a result of a major conformational change in the pentamer. The large multisubunit receptor complex can be visualized with electron microscopy at remarkable resolution and appears as a channel that extends a tubular pore into the synaptic cleft.

Mutations in several of these ligand-gated ion channel subunits have been found in human neurological diseases, including mutation of the α_1 subunit of the glycine receptor in hyperekplexia (or startle syndrome) and mutation of the acetylcholine receptor ϵ subunit in slow-channel syndrome. The mouse mutation *spastic*, a model for congenital myoclonus (a hyperexcitability disorder), results from a mutation of the glycine receptor β subunit.

3.8. Transport Receptors

A significant number of cell-surface receptors may not have classical signaling functions, but rather serve to transport substances into the cell. These include the receptors for transferrin, low-density lipoproteins (LDL), asialoglycoproteins, mannose-6-phosphate, and other plasma proteins. These receptors bind their ligand, cluster into coated pits, and are rapidly endocytosed into endosomal or lysosomal vesicles where the ligand can be dissociated and utilized, and the receptor either degraded or recycled back to the cell surface, as described in an earlier section. Several of these receptors have proven to be important models for investigating the cell biology of cell-surface receptor trafficking. Two receptors that exemplify this family of transport proteins, the LDL receptor and the mannose-6-phosphate/IGF-2 receptor, are discussed below.

The LDL receptor extracellular domain consists of a cysteine-rich and negatively charged ligand-binding region, an EGF precursor homology domain, and a juxtamembrane domain rich in O-linked glycosylation sites (Brown and Goldstein, 1986). The cytoplasmic domain is short and has no obvious signaling features, but is critical for clustering the receptor into coated pits for subsequent endocytosis and eventual lysosomal hydrolysis of the cholesterol esters of LDL to generate cellular stores of cholesterol. The importance of this receptor in the transport of LDL is underscored by the finding of many different defects in the LDL receptor in patients with the disease familial hypercholesterolemia, in which plasma levels of cholesterol are highly elevated. These mutations affect nearly all aspects of receptor function, including synthesis, transport, binding, and internalization of the receptor.

The mannose-6-phosphate (M-6-P)/IGF-2 receptor is referred to as a multifunctional protein because it is known to bind at least two ligands utilizing distinct sites on the extracellular domain of the receptor (Kornfield, 1992). The receptor is a large protein of 275 kDa, more than 90% of which is extracellular. Fifteen conserved repeat sequences of ~150 amino acids, each with 8 conserved cysteines and 16–38% overall identity, constitute the large extracellular domain of the receptor, whereas the cytoplasmic domain is small and includes multiple potential phosphorylation sites. The receptor binds proteins containing M-6-P and is important for both the sorting of newly synthesized lysosomal enzymes and for the endocytosis of extracellular lysosomal enzymes. A second M-6-P receptor, the cation-dependent receptor, is a 46-kDa protein that has a extracellular domain that is a single copy of the conserved repeat sequence of the larger M-6-P/IGF-2 receptor, and it is important for the sorting of newly synthesized lysosomal proteins. Although IGF-2 binds to the M-6-P/IGF-2 receptor with high affinity at a site distinct from the M-6-P-binding site, the role of this receptor in IGF-2 signaling remains uncertain, and it has been suggested that IGF-2 may instead act through the IGF-1 receptor, a member of the protein tyrosine kinase receptor family. The M-6-P/IGF-2 receptor gene has been disrupted in mice through a natural deletion of the chromosomal region in which it resides, the T-maternal effect (*Tme*) mutation. Homozygous mutant mice die at about embryonic d 15 and exhibit defects in lysosomal protein targeting, developmental abnormalities, and increased size. These developmental defects are likely to results from IGF-2 overexpression, since they are not observed in mice lacking both IGF-2 and the M-6-P/IGF-2 receptor. An additional feature of interest regarding the M-6-P/IGF-2 receptor is that the gene encoding this receptor is subject to genomic imprinting effects, and only the maternal allele is expressed.

4. INTRACELLULAR RECEPTORS

4.1. The Steroid, Thyroid, and Retinoid Hormone Receptors

The receptors in this superfamily are structurally and functionally distinct from the cell-surface receptors, in that they are located either in the cytoplasm or nucleus, where they bind hydrophobic ligands that are able to diffuse passively through the plasma membrane of the cell. In response to hormone binding, these receptors undergo a conformation change and become competent to bind to specific DNA elements that act as hormone-dependent enhancers of gene expression, presumably through the direct or co-factor-mediated interaction of the receptors with components of the basal transcriptional apparatus. The steroid hormone receptors are considered in greater detail in Chapter 4 within this volume, and the intent of this section is to contrast briefly the structure and function of the intracellular receptors with the cell-surface receptors, rather than to review this class of receptors comprehensively.

The nuclear receptor superfamily includes the receptors for the classical steroid hormones, such as estrogens progestins, androgens and glucocorticoids, the receptors for thyroid hormones, retinoids and vitamin D, and a large number of orphan receptors that share basic features of the superfamily, but that have no known activating ligand (Evans, 1988). These proteins all have a distinct and common domain structure, shown schematically in Fig. 11A. The defining feature of these proteins is the presence of a highly conserved DNA-binding domain (DBD) that includes two zinc fingers of the Cys-4 type. Sequences within this domain, particularly those near the end of the first zinc finger and the beginning of the second zinc finger, are important for determining the DNA-binding specificity of each receptor. These receptors bind to specific DNA elements near target genes termed hormone response elements (HREs), which are usually either direct or inverted repeats of a 6-bp core consensus sequence, separated by a variable-length spacer, the combination of which is unique for each receptor class. Sequences within the DBD and the adjacent carboxyl-terminal domain are also required for nuclear localization of the receptor and for dimerization. The receptors bind to HREs either as monomers (some orphan receptors, such as NGF-1b), homodimers (steroid receptors, such as the glucocorticoid [GR] and estrogen [ER] receptors), or heterodimers (the thyroid hormone [TR], retinoic acid [RAR], and vitamin D [VDR] receptors) (Glass, 1994). In the latter class, the retinoid-X-receptor (RXR) serves as a common heterodimerization partner. These modes of DNA binding are illustrated in Fig. 11B. There is a region of highly variable length and sequence amino-

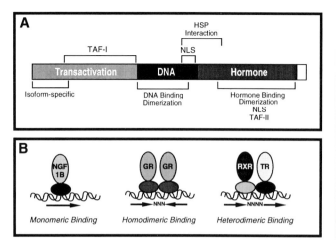

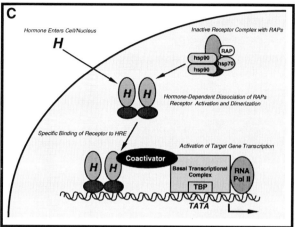

Fig. 11. Structural features and mechanism of action of intracellular receptors for steroid, thyroid, and retinoid hormones. Panel **A** illustrates the general features of the nuclear receptor superfamily proteins. The predominant domains are the DNA-binding domain, the hormone-binding domain, and the transactivation domains TAF-1 and TAF-2, as discussed in the text. Panel **B** indicates three potential modes of DNA binding. Some orphan receptors bind DNA in a monomeric form, steroid receptors bind DNA as homodimers, and thyroid, retinoid, and vitamin D receptors bind DNA as heterodimers with the partner RXR. The orientation and spacing of core motifs (indicated by arrows) in the binding sites are also indicated. Panel **C** is a generic model for signal transduction by the steroid hormones. The unliganded receptor can be either cytoplasmic or nuclear, and is found in a complex with receptor-associated proteins, such as hsp90. Hormone binding leads to the dissociation of hsp90 and the formation of receptor dimers competent to bind to DNA. Binding of the receptor at hormone-response elements alters target gene transcription through interactions with the basal transcriptional complex that are likely to be mediated by coactivator proteins that are for the most part uncharacterized. Panel **B** after Glass (1994).

terminal to the DBD, and in many receptors, this region includes a domain important for transcriptional activation, termed TAF-1. The carboxyl-terminal region of the receptor includes the specific hormone-binding domain (HBD), as well as a second transactivation domain, TAF-2, and regions necessary for dimerization.

In the absence of hormone, the steroid, thyroid, and retinoid receptors are thought to be localized predominantly in the nucleus. An exception is the GR, which appears to be predominantly cytoplasmic, presumably because the nuclear localization signal is masked in the unliganded protein. Unliganded steroid receptors, including the GR, progesterone receptor (PR), ER, and androgen receptor (AR), associate with a variety of cellular proteins thought to be important in the folding and maturation of the receptor. The most ubiquitous of these is the heat-shock protein hsp90, which strongly associates with the steroid receptors and dissociates following ligand binding. In the case of the GR, associated hsp90 may be necessary for hormone binding. A second heat-shock protein, hsp70, associates with some receptors (PR and GR), whereas immunophilin p59 appears to bind to

most steroid receptors, perhaps in an hsp90-dependent fashion. In general, the roles of these receptor-associated proteins remain to be established. A model depicting the dissociation of receptor-associated proteins on hormone binding, the dimerization of the receptor and its binding to DNA, and the regulation of target gene transcription by the hormone-activated receptor is presented in Fig. 11C.

There appear to be mechanisms by which some of the steroid receptors can be activated in a ligand-independent fashion (O'Malley et al., 1991). Stimulators of cellular kinase activity (cAMP) or inhibitors of cellular phosphatase activity (okadaic acid) can activate some of the steroid receptors in the absence of any steroid ligand. For example, the PR, ER, and VDR can all be activated by the neurotransmitter dopamine in a manner that does not involve binding to the receptor, whereas the ER can be activated by a variety of polypeptide growth factors. In other cases, ligand-independent activation is not observed. Although the pathways mediating this activation are not established, it seems likely that receptor phosphorylation is involved. The steroid receptors are phosphoproteins and some receptors, such as the PR, are inducibly phosphorylated upon ligand binding, although the kinases involved are not known. Thus, ligand independent activation of these receptors may provide an important mechanism of crosstalk between the steroid receptor pathway and other cellular signal transduction pathways involving kinase cascades.

The steroid receptors play critical roles in endocrine communication, and it is therefore not surprising that receptor mutations are associated with a range of endocrine disorders. Resistance to thyroid hormone can involve mutation or deletion of the thyroid hormone receptor β gene, whereas familial glucocorticoid resistance can be caused by deletions or point mutations in the GR gene. Hypocalcemic vitamin D-resistant rickets results from mutations in the VDR that can affect hormone binding, DNA binding, or nuclear translocation of the receptor. More than 100 distinct mutations in the AR have been found in patients with androgen insensitivity syndromes. Only one example of mutation of the ER gene in a man with estrogen resistance has been reported, whereas no mutations of the PR in the human are known. Although these latter findings might imply lethality of ER or PR mutations, disruption of these genes in mice results in animals that live to adulthood, although they have impaired reproductive function. Similar gene targeting approaches are being widely applied to investigate the physiologic roles of other nuclear receptor superfamily members, such as the multiple forms of the RARs.

4.2. The Arylhydrocarbon Receptor

Arylhydrocarbons (Ahs) include 2,3,7,8-tetrachlorodibenzo -*p*-dioxin (TCDD) and related dioxinlike environmental pollutants, such as the polychlorinated biphenyls (PCBs), as well as compounds, such as indolo[3,2-b]carbazole, that are generated naturally through the digestion of plant metabolites. These toxic, carcinogenic, and highly persistent compounds act through specific binding to a soluble intracellular receptor, the Ah receptor, also known as the dioxin receptor, to modulate gene expression. It is not clear if the Ah receptor's primary function is in defense against these foreign chemicals, but there are no known endogenous ligands for this receptor, and target genes for Ah receptor regulation include enzymes that metabolize these foreign chemicals to forms that can be excreted. There is substan-

tial variation in responses to TCDD in inbred strains of mice owing to polymorphisms at the Ah receptor locus, but the extent of polymorphism at this locus in the human population is unknown.

The molecular cloning of the Ah receptor revealed it to be a ligand-activated transcription factor (Swanson and Bradfield, 1993). Although it has a similar mode of action to the steroid, thyroid, and retinoid receptors described in the previous section, its structure is not consistent with it being a member of the steroid receptor superfamily. The Ah receptor is a 90-kDa protein. At the amino-terminus is a basic helix-loop-helix (HLH) domain, a motif found in many DNA-binding transcription factors. This is followed by the ligand-binding domain (as determined by photoaffinity labeling of this region), and a long carboxyl-terminal domain that includes a glutamine-rich sequence characteristic of the activation regions of many transcription factors. Although the Ah receptor is not related to the steroid receptor superfamily, it is related in structure to two *Drosophila* proteins, *Sim* (single-minded) and *Per* (a circadian rhythm protein), as well as to the mammalian protein Ah receptor nuclear translocator (ARNT). These four proteins share a structural domain that includes the basic HLH region (except in *Per*) as well as two 51 amino acid repeats called the A-B repeats. The entire domain is now referred to as the PAAS domain, derived from the names of the four proteins. The structure of the Ah receptor and other PAAS domain proteins is shown in Fig. 12A.

The ARNT protein was isolated based on its ability to rescue a cell line defective in Ah receptor signaling. It does not bind dioxins, but instead is suggested to act as a heterodimerization partner for the Ah receptor, much as RXR acts as a heterodimerization partner for TR and RAR. Basic HLH domains are known to mediate dimerization of other transcription factors, and are likely to serve this role in the Ah receptor and ARNT. The unliganded Ah receptor is found in the cytoplasm and associates with hsp90, much like the steroid receptors. Following ligand binding, hsp90 dissociates, the receptor translocates to the nucleus, and binds to ARNT to form the heterodimer. The Ah receptor–ARNT complex binds to selective DNA elements known as xenobiotic response elements (XREs) or dioxin response elements (DREs) to regulate target gene transcription. A model for arylhydrocarbon receptor action is illustrated in Fig. 12B.

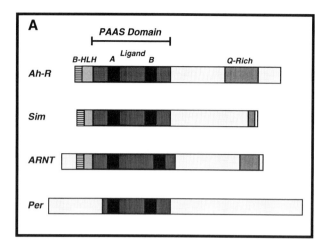
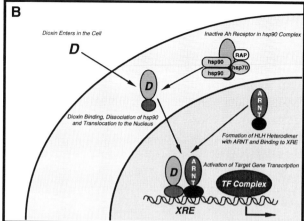

Fig. 12. Structural features and mechanism of action of the intracellular receptor for arylhydrocarbons. Panel **A** compares the structure of the Ah receptor with the ARNT and the *Drosophila* proteins *Sim* and *Per*, as described in the text. The conserved PAAS domain common to these proteins is indicated, as is the basic HLH dimerization and DNA-binding domain at the amino-terminus. Panel **B** is a model for signaling by the environmental contaminant dioxin through the Ah receptor. Dioxin causes the receptor to dissociate from associated proteins, including hsp90, and to translocate to the nucleus, where it forms a heterodimer with the ARNT protein able to bind to the XRE to regulate target gene transcription. After Burbach et al., (1992); and Bock (1993).

5. SUMMARY

In assessing the structure and function of hormone receptors, several interesting issues emerge. It is clear that a fairly limited number of general strategies have been utilized repeatedly to generate the tremendous diversity of cellular responses to hormonal stimuli that are observed. Thus, superfamilies and families of receptors that have hundreds of members often represent subtle variations on a general structural or functional theme, such as tyrosine kinase activation, G-protein-coupling, or DNA binding. This knowledge is extremely useful for identifying novel receptors, based on conserved structural features, and for attempting to understand the mechanism of action of novel receptors once they are isolated. At a second level, aspects of receptor function, such as heterodimerization with multiple partners or generation of multiple isoforms through alternative RNA processing, further contribute to diversity. It is also apparent that substantial functional diversity can be generated at the level of the signal transduction cascades that receptors utilize. For example, coupling of a receptor to different G-proteins, leading to the activation of distinct effectors, or interaction of a receptor with different adapter proteins, leading to the activation of distinct kinases, may occur in a tissue or cell-spe-

cific fashion or in a developmentally regulated manner, generating dissimilar signaling responses to a single receptor.

In most of the examples considered in this chapter, our knowledge of the signaling pathways from hormone–receptor interaction to biological response are still at best rudimentary. Despite tremendous progress in isolating receptors, in deciphering signal transduction cascades, and in unraveling the intricacies of gene transcription, there are relatively few examples where a complete response pathway has been elucidated, and perhaps no example where the complexities of the interaction of multiple signaling pathways in generating an appropriate cellular response is fully appreciated. It seems certain that substantial progress is needed to characterize better the signaling processes that are already known, and to uncover the novel receptor activation and signal transduction pathways that surely await discovery.

An important outcome of the quest to understand the actions of hormone receptors has been a recognition of the critical role that receptors play in cellular and organismal homeostasis, and of the consequences of aberrant receptor function in endocrine diseases. The number of specific diseases or disorders associated with gain of function, loss of function, or alteration of function mutations in hormone receptors has increased dramatically in the last five years. This knowledge has already had immediate application in the diagnosis of endocrine disease, and is likely to have eventual application in the rational design of therapeutic strategies for the prevention or treatment of these diseases. Finally, receptor biology provides a focal point for the scientific investigation of many of the critical outstanding questions in biology, including the control of cell proliferation, cell death, and cell differentiation, the coordinated interaction of cells during the development of a multicellular organism, and the generation of appropriate cellular responses to environmental and sensory stimuli. Further understanding of receptor-mediated signal transduction promises to contribute greatly to these fundamentally important issues.

REFERENCES

Berridge MJ. Inositol triphosphate and calcium signaling. *Nature* 1993; 361:315.

Bock KW. Aryl hydrocarbon or dioxin receptor: biologic and toxic responses. *Rev Physiol Biochem Pharmacol* 1993; 125:1.

Brown MS, Goldstein JL. A receptor-mediated pathway for cholesterol homeostasis. *Science* 1986; 232:34.

Burbach KM, Poland A, Bradfield CA. Cloning of the Ah-receptor cDNA reveals a distinctive ligand-activated transcription factor. *Proc Natl Acad Sci USA* 1992; 89:8185.

Carbone M, Levine A. Oncogenes, antioncogenes, and the regulation of cell growth. *Trends Endocrinol Metab* 1990; 1:248.

Darnell JE Jr, Kerr IM, Stark GR. Jak-STAT pathways and transcriptional activation in response to INFs and other extracellular signaling proteins. *Science* 1994; 265:1415.

Dohlman HG, Thorner J, Caron MG, Lefkowitz RJ. Model systems for the study of seven-transmembrane-segment receptors. *Ann Rev Biochem* 1991; 60:653.

Drewett JG, Garbers DL. The family of guanylyl cyclase receptors and their ligands. *Endoc Rev* 1994; 15:135.

Evans RM. The steroid and thyroid hormone receptor superfamily. *Science* 1988; 240:889.

Fischer EH, Charbonneau H, Tonks NK. Protein tyrosine phosphatases: a diverse family of intracellular and transmembrane enzymes. *Science* 1991; 253:401.

Fuh G, Cunningham BC, Fukunaga R, Nagata S, Goeddel DV, Wells JA. Rational design of potent antagonists to the human growth hormone receptor. *Science* 1992; 256:1677.

Gilman AG. G proteins; transducers of receptor-generated signals. *Ann Rev Biochem* 1987; 56:615.

Glass CK. Differential recognition of target genes by nuclear receptor monomers, dimers and heterodimers. *Endoc Rev* 1994; 15:391.

Ihle JN, Kerr IM, Jaks and stats in signaling by the cytokine receptor superfamily. *Trends Genetics* 1995; 11:69

Jensen EV, Jacobson HI. Basic guide to the mechanism of estrogen action. *Rec Prog Hormone Res* 1962; 18:387.

Kolakowski LF. GCRDb: a G-protein-coupled receptor database. *Receptors and Channels* 1994; 2:1.

Krebs EG. Protein phosphorylation and celular regulation. *Bioscience Reports* 1993; 13:127.

Langley JN. On nerve endings and on special excitable substances in cells. *Proc Royal Soc Lond* 1906; 78:170.

Lefkowitz RJ. G protein-coupled receptor kinases. *Cell* 1993; 74:409.

Mathews LS. Activin receptors and cellular signaling by the receptor serine kinase family. *Endoc Rev* 1994; 15:310.

Myers MG Jr, White MF. New frontiers in insulin receptor substrate signaling. *Trends Endocrinol Metab* 1995; 6:209.

O'Malley BW, Schrader WT, Mani S, Smith C, Weigel NL, Conneely OM, Clark JH. An alternative ligand-independent pathway for activation of steroid receptors. *Rec Prog Hormone Res* 1995; 50:333.

Pawson T. Protein modules and signaling networks. *Nature* 1995; 373:573.

Scatchard G. The attraction of proteins for small molecules and ions. *Ann NY Acad Sci* 1949; 51:660.

Schlessinger J, Ullrich A. Growth factor signaling by receptor tyrosine kinases. *Neuron* 1992; 9:383.

Sutherland EW. Studies on the mechanism of hormone action. *Science* 1972; 177:401.

Swanson HI, Bradfield CA. The Ah receptor: genetics, structure and function. *Pharmacogenetics* 1993; 3:213.

Toft D, Gorski J. A receptor molecule for estrogens: isolation from the rat uterus and preliminary characterization. *Proc Natl Acad Sci USA* 1966; 55:1574.

Unwin N. Neurotransmiter action: opening of ligand-gated ion channels. *Neuron* 1993; 10 (Suppl):31.

van der Geer P, Hunter T, Lindberg RA. Receptor protein-tyrosine kinases and their signal transduction pathways. *Ann Rev Cell Biol* 1994; 10:251

Wrana JL, Attisano L, Wieser R, Ventura F, Massagué J. Mechanism of activation of the TGF-β receptor. *Nature* 1994; 370:341.

SELECTED READINGS

Gammeltoft S, Kahn CR. Hormone signaling via membrane receptors. In: DeGroot LJ, ed. *Endocrinology*. Philadelphia: Saunders, 1995:17.

Kornfield S. Structure and function of the mannose-6-phosphate/insulin-like growth factor II receptors. *Ann Rev Biochem* 1992; 61:307.

Mayo KE, Park-Sarge O-K. Molecular biology of endocrine receptors in the ovary. In: Findlay JK, ed. *Molecular Biology of the Female Reproductive System*. San Diego: Academic 1994:153.

3 Second Messenger Systems and Signal Transduction Mechanisms

Eliot R. Spindel, MD, PhD

CONTENTS

1. INTRODUCTION

1.1. Signal Transduction: from Hormones to Action

Hormones are secreted, reach their target, and bind to a receptor. The interaction of the hormone with the receptor produces an initial signal that through a series of steps, results in the final hormone action. How does the binding of a hormone to a receptor result in a cellular action? For example, in times of stress, epinephrine is secreted by the adrenal glands, is bound by receptors in skeletal muscle, and results in the hydrolysis of glycogen and the secretion of glucose. Signal transduction is the series of steps and signals that links the receptor binding of epinephrine to the hydrolysis of glycogen. Signal transduction can be simple or complex. There can be only one or two steps between receptor and effect, or

From: *Endocrinology: Basic and Clinical Principles* (P. M. Conn and S. Melmed, eds.), Humana Press Inc., Totowa, NJ.

multiple steps. Common themes, however, are specificity of action and control; the hormone produces just the desired action and that action can be precisely regulated. The multiple steps that are involved in signal transduction pathways allow for precise regulation, modulation, and a wide dynamic range.

There are two major mechanisms of signal transduction. These are transmission of signals by small molecules that diffuse through the cells and transmission of signals by phosphorylation of proteins. The diffusible small molecules that are used for signaling are known as second messengers. Examples of second messengers are cAMP, calcium (Ca^{2+}) and inositol (1,4,5)triphosphate (IP3). Equally important is the transmission of hormonal signals by phosphorylation. Hormone-induced phosphorylation of proteins is a key way to activate or inactivate protein action. For example, the interaction of epidermal growth factor (EGF) with its receptor stimulates the phosphorylation of a tyrosine residue in the EGF receptor. This in turn triggers the phosphorylation of other proteins in sequence, finally resulting in the phosphorylation of a transcription factor and increased gene expression. Enzymes that phosphorylate are called kinases. Balancing kinases are enzymes that remove phosphate groups from proteins, and these are called phosphatases. In a typical signal transduction pathway, second messengers and phosphorylation mechanisms are both used. For example, cAMP transmits its message by activating a kinase (cAMP-dependent protein kinase A, or simply protein kinase A, PKA).

Some hormones produce effects without a membrane receptor. The best examples of these are the steroid hormones, which bind to a cytoplasmic receptor and the receptor then translocates to the nucleus to produce its desired effects. Even these actions are, however, modified by the actions of kinases and phosphatases. Steroid receptors are discussed in detail in Chapter 4.

Nature and evolution are parsimonious. Mechanisms that evolved for the regulation of yeast and for regulation of development and nervous function are also used for signaling in endocrine systems. Fundamental discoveries about the growth of yeast, development of drosophila, regulation of cancerous growth, and neurotransmission in the brain have led to fundamental discoveries of endocrine mechanisms of signal transduction. Therefore, similar receptors and pathways underlie signaling by neurotransmitters and by hormones. Similarly, growth and differentiation factors trigger cell growth and development by similar mechanisms, as do hormones. Thus, signal transduction is a major unifying area among endocrinology, cell biology, and neuroscience.

1.2. A Brief Overview of Signal Transduction Mechanisms

One approach to classifying signal transduction mechanisms is as a function of the structure of the hormone receptor. Thus, while both thyroid stimulatory hormone (TSH) and growth hormone are both pituitary hormones, the TSH receptor is a seven-transmembrane G-protein-coupled receptor linked to cAMP, and the growth hormone receptor is a single-transmembrane receptor kinase linked to receptors. The fact that both hormones are pituitary hormones tells nothing about the signal transduction mechanism. In contrast, knowledge of the receptor structure involved gives some information regarding the potential mechanisms of signal transduction and the potential mediators involved. Complicating matters however, hormones can have multiple receptors often with different signal transduction mechanisms. A good example of this is somatostatin, which at last count had five different receptor subtypes. For neurotransmitters, there is even more diversity involved. Glutamate has four groups of receptors, including both seven-transmembrane and four-transmembrane receptors.

The major classes of membrane receptors are seven-transmembrane (7TM), single-transmembrane, and four-transmembrane (4TM) receptors. Within each of these classes of receptors, there are multiple signal transduction mechanisms, but certain unifying concepts emerge. The 7TM receptors are G-protein-linked, and initial signaling is conducted by the activated G-protein subunits. The single-TM receptors convey initial signals via phosphorylation events (sometimes direct, sometimes induced by receptor dimerization) and the 4TM receptors are usually ion channels.

As discussed in greater detail below, the 7TM receptors are linked to G-proteins. G-proteins are composed of three subunits, and binding of the ligand to the receptor–G-protein complex causes disassociation of the G-protein. The disassociated subunit then acts to stimulate or inhibit second messenger formation. Thus, 7TM receptors signal through second messengers, such as cAMP, IP3, and/or calcium. Examples of G-protein-linked hormones are parathyroid hormone (PTH), thyrotropin-releasing hormone (TRH), TSH, glucagon, and somatostatin. The 4TM receptors are typically ligand-gated ion channels. Binding of the ligand to the receptor opens an ion channel, allowing cellular entry of Na or Ca. Examples of the 4TM receptors are the nicotinic receptors, the AMPA and kainate glutamate receptors, and the serotonin type 3 receptor. The single-TM receptors form the most diverse class of hormone receptors, including both single and multisubunit structures. These receptors signal through endogenous enzymatic activity or by activating an associated protein that contains endogenous enzymatic activity.

1.3. Hormone Action—the End Result of Signal Transduction

After hormone binding, there are multiple signaling steps until the hormone action is achieved.

Hormones often have multiple actions, so there must be branch points within the signal transduction cascade and the ability to regulate these multiple branches independently. This need for multiple, independently controlled effects is one reason why signal transduction pathways are so diverse and complicated. End effects of the signal transduction cascade fall into three general groups: enzyme activation, membrane effects, and activation of gene transcription. These individual actions are covered in more detail in the specific hormone chapters, but it is important to understand the general concepts of how signals link to the final action.

The classic example of hormone-induced enzyme activation is epinephrine-induced glycogenolysis in which binding of epinephrine to its receptor (β_2-adrenergic receptor) stimulates formation of cAMP, which activates a kinase (cAMP-dependent PKA). PKA then phosphorylates the enzyme phosphorylase kinase, which in turn phosphorylates glycogen phosphorylase, which is the enzyme that liberates glucose from glycogen. Phosphorylation is the most common mechanism by which hormonally induced signal transduction activates enzymes.

One example of membrane action is cAMP regulation of the cystic fibrosis transmembrane conductance regulator (CFTR), which is a chloride channel that opens in response to PKA-mediated phosphorylation. Another important example of a membrane effect is insulin-induced glucose transport, in which insulin increases glucose transport by inducing a redistribution of the Glut4 glucose transporter from intracellular stores to the membrane.

Hormone-induced gene transcription is mediated by hormone activation of transcription factors or DNA-binding proteins. For steroid hormones and the thyroid hormones, the hormone receptor itself is a DNA-binding protein. How these hormones interact with nuclear receptors to stimulate gene transcription is discussed in Chapter 4. As might be predicted from the preceding paragraphs, membrane-bound receptors stimulate gene transcription through phosphorylation of nuclear-binding proteins. Typically, these factors are only active when properly phosphorylated. Transcription factor phosphorylation can be mediated by hormone-activated kinases, such as PKA-induced phosphorylation of the cAMP-responsive transcription factor CREB. This is discussed in greater detail below. Growth hormone or prolactin stimulate, gene transcription

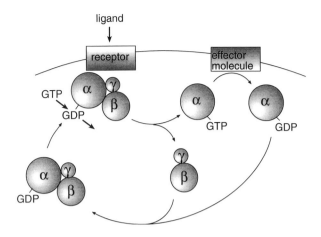

Fig. 1. The G-protein cycle.

by a series of steps leading to phosphorylation of the Stat transcription factors, which then bind and transactivate DNA.

2. SIGNALING THROUGH G-PROTEIN-LINKED RECEPTORS

2.1. Overview of G-Proteins

As described in Chapter 2, the 7TM receptors signal through G-proteins. The G-proteins are composed of three subunits: α, β, and γ. The α subunit is capable of binding and hydrolyzing guanosine triphosphate (GTP) to guanosine diphosphate (GDP). As shown in Fig. 1, the trimeric G-protein with one molecule of GDP bound to the α subunit binds to the unliganded receptor. Binding of ligand to the receptor causes a conformational shift, such that GDP disassociates from the α subunit and GTP is bound in its place. The binding of GTP produces a conformational shift in the α subunit, causing its disassociation into a $\beta\gamma$ dimer and an activated α subunit. Signaling is achieved by the activated α subunit binding to an effector molecule. Specificity of hormonal signaling is achieved by different α subunits coupling to different effector molecules. The α subunit remains activated until the bound GTP is hydrolyzed to GDP. On hydrolysis of GTP to GDP, the α subunit reassociates with the $\beta\gamma$ subunit and returns to the receptor to continue the cycle. The α subunit contains intrinsic GTPase activity (hence the name G-proteins), and how long the α subunit stays activated is a function of the activity of the GTPase activity of the α subunit. Until recently, it was thought that only the α subunit signaled, but it is now appreciated that the $\beta\gamma$ dimer also has a signaling role.

There are multiple subtypes of the α, β, and γ subunits. The subtypes form different families of the G-proteins. Most important are the subtypes of the α subunits, since they regulate the effector molecules that the G-protein activates. The major families of the G-proteins are G_s, G_i, and G_q. Specificity of hormone action is achieved because only specific G-proteins (composed of the proper subunits) will couple to specific hormone receptors and because the free βγ dimer and the activated α subunit subtypes will couple only to specific effector molecules. The G_s family couples to and increases adenylyl cyclase activity, and also opens membrane K^+ channels; the G_i family couples to and inhibits adenylyl cyclase, opens membrane K^+ channels, and closes membrane Ca^{2+} channels; and the G_q family activates phospholipase C-β to increase IP3, diacylglycerol (DAG), and intracellular Ca^{2+}. The signaling of these three families is discussed further below.

In addition to the trimeric G-proteins discussed above, there is also a class of small G-proteins, consisting of single subunits, of which Ras, Rho, and Rac are important members. These proteins also hydrolyze GTP and play a role in coupling tyrosine kinase receptors to effector molecules.

2.2. Hormonal Signaling Mediated by G_s

Hormones that signal through G_s to activate adenylate cyclase and increase cAMP represent the first signaling pathway as described by the pioneering work of Sutherland (1972) in the initial discovery of cAMP. Elucidation of this pathway led to Nobel prizes for the discovery of cAMP and for the discovery of G-proteins. Examples of hormones that signal through this pathway are TSH, luteinizing hormone (LH), follicle-stimulating hormone (FSH), adrenocorticotropic hormone (ACTH), epinephrine, and glucagon, among others. Signaling in this pathway is outlined in Fig. 2. As described above, the binding of hormone to the receptor–G_s complex results in the active α subunit binding to an effector molecule, in this case adenylate cyclase. Adenylate cyclase is a single-chain membrane glycoprotein of mol wt 115–150 Kda. The molecule itself has two hydrophobic domains, each with six transmembrane segments. Binding of the activated α subunit of G_s results in catalyzing the formation of cAMP from ATP. Eight different isoforms of adenylate cyclase have been described to date. These isoforms differ in their distribution and regulation by other factors, such as calmodulin, βγ subunits, and

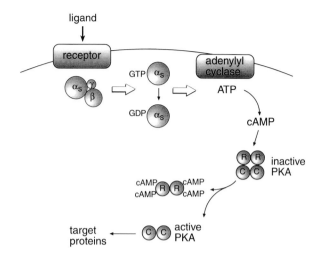

Fig. 2. Signaling by G_s.

specificity for α subunit subtypes. Next cAMP binds to and activates the cAMP-dependent PKA. PKA is a serine/threonine kinase that phosphorylates proteins with the recognition site Arg-Arg-X-(Ser or Thr)-X, where X is usually hydrophobic. PKA is a heterotetramer composed of two regulatory and two catalytic subunits. The regulatory subunits suppress the activity of the catalytic subunits. The binding of cAMP to the regulatory subunits causes their disassociation from the catalytic subunits, allowing PKA to phosphorylate its targets. There are a number of PKA subtypes, but the key difference reflects the type I regulatory subunit (RI) vs the type II (RII) subunits in which the RI subunit will disassociate from PKA at a lower concentration of cAMP than will the RII subunit.

PKA phosphorylates multiple targets, including enzymes, channels, receptors, and transcription factors. Enzymes can be activated or inhibited by the resulting phosphorylation at Ser/Thr residues. The example of regulation of glycogen phosphorylase was discussed above. An example of a PKA-regulated channel is the CFTR chloride channel that requires phosphorylation by PKA for chloride movement. PKA phosphorylates 7TM receptors as part of the mechanism of receptor desensitization.

Major discoveries in the last five years have begun to explain hormonal regulation of gene transcription. These discoveries have included the identification of DNA-binding proteins (transcription factors) whose ability to activate gene transcription is stimulated by cAMP. The basic concept is that cAMP activates PKA, which phosphorylates a transcription factor. The transcription factor then stimu-

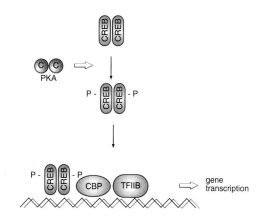

Fig. 3. The role of CREB in regulating gene transcription.

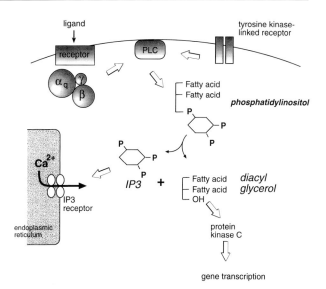

Fig. 4. Signaling by G_q.

lates transcription of the target gene. Several classes of cAMP-activated transcription factors have been characterized. These include CREB, CREM, and ATF-1. Probably the most is known about is CREB, and it will be used as an example (Fig. 3). CREB is a 341 amino acid protein with two primary domains, a DNA-binding domain and a transactivation domain. The DNA-binding domain binds to specific DNA sequences in the target genes that are activated by cAMP. When CREB is phosphorylated, its transactivation domain binds to a coactivator protein, CREB-binding protein (CBP). This positions CBP next to the basal transcription complex, potentially allowing interaction with TFIIB to activate transcription. Defects in CBP lead to mental retardation in a disease called Rubinstein-Taybi Syndrome (RTS), one of the first diseases discovered that is caused by defects in transcription factors.

2.3. Hormonal Signaling Mediated by G_i

Hormonal signaling through 7TM receptors linked to G_i is similar to that linked to G_s, except $G\alpha_i$ inhibits adenylyl cyclase rather than stimulating it as does $G\alpha_s$. Thus, adenylyl cyclase activity represents a balance between stimulation by $G\alpha_s$ and inhibition by $G\alpha_i$. $G\alpha_i$ also couples to calcium channels (inhibitory) and potassium channels (stimulatory). Receptors that couple to G_i include somatostatin, enkephalin, and the α_2-adrenergic receptor, among others.

2.4. Hormonal Signaling Mediated by G_q

Hormonal signaling through 7TM receptors linked to G_q proceeds by activation of phospholipase C-β. Examples of hormones that bind to G_q include TRH, gastrin-releasing peptide (GRP), GnRH,

angiotensin II, substance P, cholecystokinin (CCK), and PTH. Binding of hormone to its receptor leads to formation of active $G\alpha_q$ or $G\alpha_{12}$, which then activates phospholipase C (PLC) to hydrolyze phosphoinositides (Fig. 4) to form two second messengers, IP_3 and DAG. IP_3 diffuses within the cell to bind to specific receptors on the endoplasmic reticulum. The IP_3 receptor is a calcium channel, and the interaction of IP_3 with its receptor opens the channel and allows calcium to flow from the endoplasmic reticulum into the cytoplasm, thus increasing free cytosolic calcium levels. The IP_3 receptor is composed of four large subunits ($\approx$310 Kda) that each bind a single molecule of IP_3. The binding of IP_3 to the subunits opens the channels and also desensitizes the receptor to binding additional IP_3. Thus, IP_3 leads to increased Ca^{2+}, which is the next step in signaling. Calcium is returned to the endoplasmic reticulum by ATP-dependent Ca^{2+} pumps (SERCA). Thapsigargin is a drug that blocks the SERCA, thus resulting in transient high intracellular Ca^{2+} levels, but it also depletes Ca^{2+} levels in the ER making it a convenient tool to study IP_3-dependent Ca^{2+} release. In excitable cells, a similar mechanism triggers calcium release from internal stores, except here calcium directly triggers additional Ca^{2+} release from the ER via the ryanodine receptor. Depolarization opens voltage-sensitive Ca^{2+} channels on the cell membranes, allowing influx of Ca^{2+}. This calcium then binds to the ryanodine receptor (very similar to the IP_3 receptor, except the ryanodine receptor is gated by Ca^{2+})

and allows Ca^{2+} efflux from the ER. The ryanodine receptor also allows Ca^{2+} efflux from the sarcoplasmic reticulum in muscle.

Calcium is a major intracellular second messenger, and its levels are tightly regulated by calcium pumps in the endoplasmic reticulum (SERCA), calcium pumps in the membrane plasma membrane Ca^{2+}–Mg^{2+} ATPase (PMCA), voltage-gated calcium channels, and ligand-gated calcium channels. Resting cell Ca^{2+} is 100 nM, far lower than the 2-mM levels that occur extracellularly. Thus, there is ample room to increase intracellular Ca^{2+} rapidly. Increased intracellular Ca^{2+} signals primarily by binding to proteins and causing a conformational shift, which activates their function. Examples include Ca^{2+} binding to troponin in muscle cells to stimulate contraction and Ca^{2+} binding to calmodulin. The Ca^{2+}–calmodulin complex then binds to a variety of kinases. There are two general classes of Ca^{2+}–calmodulin kinases, dedicated, i.e., with only a specific substrate, and multifunctional, with many substrates. Examples of dedicated CAM kinases are myosin light-chain kinase and phosphorylase kinase. The multifunctional CAM kinases can phosphorylate transcription factors to effect gene transcription. For example, CAM kinase can phosphorylate CREB, which provides a mechanism for crosstalk between receptors linked to G_s and G_q.

The other second messenger of the PLC pathway is DAG. The primary action of DAG is to activate protein kinase C (PKC), a serine-threonine kinase. PKC modifies enzymatic activity by phosphorylation of target enzymes, and like PKA, PKC can modify gene transcription by regulating phosphorylation of transcription factors. PKC is activated by the class of compounds known as phorbol esters, which were originally described for their ability to promote tumor growth. One phorbol ester that potently stimulates PKC activity is 12-*O*-tetradecanoylphorbol-13-acetate (TPA or PMA). It was initially shown that TPA could activate gene transcription though a DNA sequence element known as the AP-1 binding site. Isolation of the transcription factors that bound to AP-1 led to the isolation of jun and fos which bind to the AP-1 site as hetero or homodimers to regulate transcription. Thus, hormones that signal through G_q regulate gene transcription through DAG, which activates PKC, leading to phosphorylation of jun and fos. PKC, like PKA, can also regulate receptor activity by directly phosphorylating ion channels and 7TM receptors.

3. SIGNALING THROUGH RECEPTORS LINKED TO TYROSINE KINASE OR SERINE/THREONINE KINASES

In recent years, our understanding of signaling pathways that involve cascades of kinases has greatly increased. These pathways can be divided into those that commence with a tyrosine phosphorylation event and those that commence with a serine/threonine phosphorylation event. These pathways are similar in that they are a series of protein-binding and/or phosphorylation events. There are two primary mechanism by which the binding of hormone to its receptor causes signal propagation. In the first mechanism, hormone binding triggers receptor autophosphorylation via an intrinsic receptor kinase. Receptor phosphorylation then allows binding of a special class of proteins called SH2 domain proteins, which specifically bind to phosphotyrosines. The EGF receptor uses this pathway. In the second mechanism, hormone binding triggers a receptor conformational change that stimulates binding of a second protein to the receptor. One important way in which hormone binding to the receptor triggers conformational change is by causing receptor dimerization. Examples of this are the GH and Prl receptors. These are discussed in greater detail below.

3.1. Signaling Through Receptors with Intrinsic Tyrosine Kinase Activity (EGF, Insulin, IGF-1)

Hormones and growth factors that signal through receptors with intrinsic tyrosine kinase activity include the EGF receptor, the PDGF receptor, and the insulin receptor. Binding of ligand to the receptor stimulates the receptor's intrinsic tyrosine kinase, resulting in autophosphorylation (i.e., the receptor phosphorylates itself), which then induces binding of the next signaling protein or effector protein. Within this category, there are differences depending on receptor structure. Prototype signaling mechanisms are discussed below.

3.1.1. EGF Receptor Signaling

The EGF receptor is a single TM receptor that binds EGF as a monomer. EGF binding causes a change of conformation that induces dimerization with a second EGF–EGF receptor complex. Dimerization of the EGF–receptor complexes activates the EGF receptor's intrinsic tyrosine kinase, and each receptor in the dimer transphosphorylates the other receptor at multi-

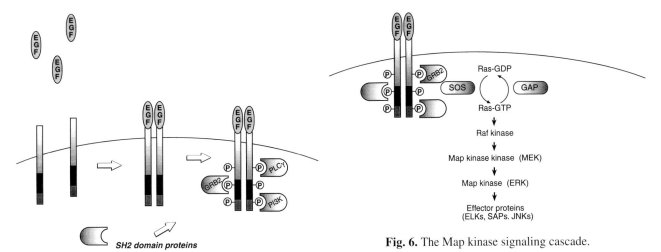

Fig. 6. The Map kinase signaling cascade.

Fig. 5. Signaling by the EGF receptor.

ple tyrosine residues. These phosphotyrosines then serve as docking sites for SH2 domain proteins. SH2 domains are conserved regions of approx 100 amino acids that serve to target proteins to phosphotyrosines. Depending on the amino acids adjacent to the phosphotyrosine, different SH2 domain proteins will have different affinities for the phosphotyrosine residue. Thus, depending on which tyrosine residues are phosphorylated, and the sequences surrounding those tyrosines, different proteins will dock on the ligand-activated receptor. This provides specificity of effector action and the ability for multiple proteins to dock on a single receptor. The binding of the SH2 domain protein to the receptor propagates signals by a number of mechanisms including:

1. It brings an effector molecule to the membrane where it is next to its target molecule;
2. Binding triggers a conformational change that can activate endogenous enzymatic activity in the SH2 proteins (e.g., kinase activity); and
3. Binding can position the SH2 protein so it can be phosphorylated and activated.

The EGF receptor employs these mechanisms as follows.

As shown in Fig. 5, the binding of EGF to its receptor activates the MAP kinase pathway, phospholipase C γ, phosphotidyl 3-kinase, and transcription factors. Many growth factors use pathways similar to EGF, so it is important to consider the multiple pathways of EGF signal transduction. As previously described,

Ras is a small G-protein with GTPase-like activity. When the EGF receptor is phosphorylated, a complex of the SH2 domain protein (growth factor receptor-binding protein 2) GRB2 and guanine nucleotide-releasing protein (GNRP, also known as "son of sevenless" or SOS because of its homology to the *drosophila* protein) bind to the EGF receptor (Fig. 6). This brings GNRP close to the membrane and in close proximity to Ras, which is anchored in the membrane. GNRP then converts ras-GDP into the active ras-GTP form. Ras-GTP then activates Raf kinase, which activates MAP kinase, which activates MAP kinase, which phosphorylates the final effector proteins that regulate growth or cellular metabolism. There are in fact a number of parallel MAP kinase pathways with different MAP kinases and MAP kinase kinases. Other MAP kinase pathways include MEK kinase, which is equivalent to MAP kinase kinase, and ERK, which is equivalent to MAP kinase. Transcriptional targets for ERK include the ELK and SAP transcription factors. One important MAP kinase subtype is Jun kinase (JNK), which activates the Jun transcription factors. Specificity of these pathways comes in part from the initial SH2 docking protein that binds to the tyrosine kinase pathways and also from multiple inputs from other proteins.

The second major signaling pathway of tyrosine kinase receptors, such as the EGF receptor, is through activation of PLCγ. Although PLCβ is activate by Gα$_q$, PLCγ is an SH2 domain protein. Thus, when EGF stimulates phosphorylation of the EGF receptor, PLCγ through its SH2 domains binds to phosphotyrosines in the EGF receptor. This serves two purposes. First, it brings PLCγ close to the

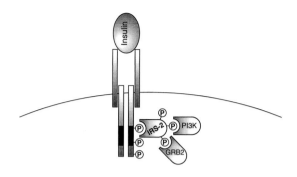

Fig. 7. Signaling by the insulin receptor.

membrane adjacent to phosphatidylinositols, and second, it allows the EGF receptor to phosphorylate PLCγ. Phosphorylation activates PLCγ, resulting in hydrolysis of phosphatidylinositol to IP3 and DAG. Thus, tyrosine kinase-linked receptors, like G_q-linked receptors, also signal through IP_3 and DAG. The third major pathway by which the EGF receptor signals is by activation of other enzymes, such as phosphoinositol 3-kinase, which generates phosphoinositols other than IP_3 (e.g., 1,3,4,5 phosphoinositol) which also likely have important signaling roles. The EGF receptor can also directly activate by phosphorylation nuclear transcription factors such as the interferon-γ stimulated gene factor.

The EGF receptor has been discussed in depth because it serves as a model for most other tyrosine kinase receptors. The key concept is that ligand binding induces autophosphorylation and SH2 proteins then bind to phosphotyrosines to activate multiple signaling mechanisms. Specificity is achieved in that different SH2 proteins recognize different phosphotyrosines.

3.1.2. Signaling by the Insulin and Insulin-Like Growth Factor Receptors

The signal transduction mechanism employed by the insulin receptor is a variation of that employed by the EGF receptor (Fig. 7). Binding of insulin to the insulin receptor (a heterotetramer composed of two α subunits and two β subunits), like binding of EGF to its receptor, triggers receptor autophosphorylation. However, the insulin receptor does not signal by directly binding SH2 domain proteins. Rather ligand-induced receptor autophosphorylation stimulates binding of a bridging protein called insulin receptor substrate-1 (IRS-1). IRS-1 binds to the insulin receptor and is phosphorylated, and then multiple SH2 proteins bind in turn to IRS-1. Just as EGF-induced

signaling depends on which SH2 domain proteins bind to the EGF receptor, insulin signaling depends on which SH2 proteins bind to IRS-1. Examples of proteins that bind to IRS-1 include GRB2 and Pl3 kinase. The second messengers produced by the action of Pl3 kinase then likely play a role in activating glucose transport into the cell via activation of GLUT4. IRS-1 does not bind to the insulin receptor via SH2 domains. The exact nature of the domains that mediate IRS-1 binding is still being worked out, but tentatively, two domains called the PTB and PID domains have been identified in IRS-1. The PTB domain also occurs in IRS-2 and several other signaling molecules.

3.2. Signaling Through Receptors That Signal Through Ligand-Induced Binding of Tyrosine Kinases (GH, Prl).

The growth hormone and prolactin receptors belong to a large superfamily of receptors that include the cytokine receptors for IL-2, IL-3, IL-4, IL-5, IL-6, IL-7, IL-9, IL-11, IL-12, erythropoietin, granulocyte-macrophage colony stimulating factor (GM-CSF), IFN-β, IFN-γ, and ciliary neurotrophic factor (CNTF). Many of these receptors are heterodimers consisting of an α-ligand binding subunit. and a β-signaling subunit. However, the GH and Prl receptors have single subunits that contain both the ligand-binding and signaling domains. The receptors in this family lack intrinsic tyrosine kinase activity. Instead, these receptors associate with kinases belonging to the JAK kinase family. Ligand binding to the receptor induces receptor dimerization bringing two JAK kinases in close apposition, which results in the activation of the associated JAK kinases by reciprocal phosphorylation (Fig. 8). The JAK kinases then phosphorylate target proteins, and signaling commences. The name JAK kinase is short for Janus kinase where Janus is the ancient Roman god of gates and doorways who is depicted with two faces, one looking outward and one looking inward (it has also been claimed that JAK stands for "**J**ust **A**nother **K**inase"). There is a family of JAK kinases and different receptors associate with different kinases. At the present, time four members of the family have been described, Jak1, Jak2, Jak3, and tyk2. The different kinases phosphorylate different targets to achieve signaling specificity. For example, the Prl and GH receptor bind Jak2, the IL-2 and IL-4 receptors bind Jak 1 and Jak3 kinases and the IFN receptors bind tyk2.

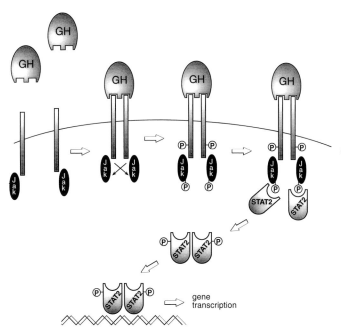

Fig. 9. Formation of NO.

Fig. 8. Signaling by the GH receptor.

The activated JAK kinases phosphorylate the Stat (**S**ignal **t**ransduction and **a**ctivation of **t**ranscription) proteins among others. Six *Stat proteins* have been described to date, though there are likely more members of this important gene family. Stat proteins contain an SH2 domain and a single conserved tyrosine residue that is phosphorylated in response to ligand binding. Phosphorylation of Stat results in Stat proteins binding to DNA as homodimers or as heterodimers with other Stats or with unrelated proteins to stimulate transcription (Fig. 8). For example, IFN-α stimulates gene transcription by activation of Stat1 and Stat2, which heterodimerize and bind to DNA. Similarly, CNTF or IL-6 results in binding of Stat1 and Stat3 heterodimers to DNA. A key question remaining to be clarified is how exact signal specificity is achieved. There are more receptors and ligands than JAK kinases and Stats. Specificity may reside in the time-course of activation (reflecting the balance between kinases and phosphatases), which Stats are activated, phosphorylation status of other proteins, and the binding of other transcriptional regulators elsewhere in the gene.

3.3. Signaling Through Receptors with Intrinsic Serine/Threonine Kinase Activity (Activin, Inhibit, TGF-β)

A relatively newly described signaling pathway is used by receptors with intrinsic serine/threonine kinase activity. These receptors include the activin, inhibin, and TGF-β receptors. Relatively little is yet known about this pathway, though it is appears for the TGF-β receptor that binding likely stimulates polymerization of four receptor subunits with resulting autophosphorylation of the heteromeric receptor complex. The downstream targets of the receptors are still being determined.

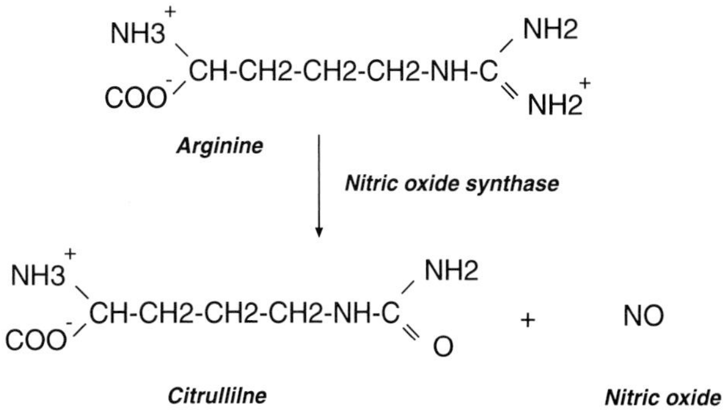

4. SIGNALING THROUGH NITRIC OXIDE (NO) AND THROUGH RECEPTORS LINKED TO GUANYLATE CYCLASE

4.1. Signaling Through Nitric Oxide (NO) and Soluble Guanylate Cyclase

The role of NO as a signaling molecule has only recently been appreciated. Knowledge of this signaling pathway arose in part from the discovery that NO is the active metabolite of nitroglycerin and other nitrates used for vasodilation. NO is synthesized by the oxidation of the amidine nitrogen of arginine through the actions of the enzyme NO synthase (NOS) (Fig. 9). The study of the role of NO has been greatly facilitated by substituted arginine analogs, such as L-NAM, which act as potent NOS inhibitors. Because NO has a short half-life, is not stored, and is released immediately on synthesis, NO release reflects regulation of NOS. There are three major forms of NOS. An inducible form present in macrophage, a brain-specific form, and a endothelium-specific form. The brain and endothelial forms are activated by calcium and calcium–calmodulin complexes. The primary signaling mechanism of NO appears to be through cGMP. NO binds specifically to a soluble guanylate cyclase to stimulate the formation of cGMP. cGMP in turns activates ion channels and activates a cGMP-activated protein kinase (PKG), which can then activate enzymes and signal similarly to PKC and PKA. The soluble guanylate cyclase, which acts as the NO receptor, is a heterodimer of M_r 151,000. However, activation of guanylate cyclase likely does not explain all of NO's actions, and other NO signal transduction mechanisms remain to be determined. NO likely plays an important role in signaling by sensory neurotransmission mediated by neuropeptides, such as substance P, VIP, and somatostatin, that increase intracellular calcium.

4.2. Hormones That Signal Through Membrane Bound Guanylate Cyclase (Natriuretic Peptides)

The action of the atrial natriuretic peptides are mediated by a membrane-bound form of guanylate cyclase. There are three natriuretic peptides; ANP, BNP and CNP. ANP and BNP bind to guanylate cyclase A (GC-A) and CNP binds to guanylate cyclase B (GC-B). There is a third natriuretic peptide receptor that binds all three peptides. This receptor has been thought to be primarily a clearance receptor, but recent studies suggest it may also have independent signal transduction properties. GC-A and GC-B are single transmembrane domain receptors with an extracellular ligand-binding domain, a transmembrane domain, and an intracellular catalytic (guanylate cyclase) domain. Binding of natriuretic peptide to GC-A or GC-B activates the receptor's guanylate cyclase activity, thus stimulating the formation of cGMP. cGMP then signals as discussed above. A third type of membrane-bound guanylate cyclase (GC-C) has also been described in the GI tract and kidney. The endogenous ligand of this cyclase may be the small peptide guanylin.

5. CROSSTALK BETWEEN SIGNALING SYSTEMS

As might be imagined given the complexity and multiplicity of the signaling systems described in this chapter, there is considerable opportunity for crosstalk between signal transduction systems. Although signaling systems in this chapter have been discussed as if isolated, it is important to realize in the cell that there is abundant crossactivation. For example, multiple hormones can activate the same

kinases, and the same kinase can in turn phosphorylate targets in more than one signaling pathway. Thus, signal transduction should not be considered a linear pathway, but rather a network of activation, and signaling events represents the summation of activation. Equally important is the time-course of activation as reflected by the half-life of second messengers and the balance between phosphorylation and dephosphorylation.

6. DISEASES ASSOCIATED WITH ALTERED SIGNAL TRANSDUCTION

As might be expected given the diverse mechanisms and multiple effector molecules, there are a number of disease entities associated with signal transduction. Doubtless many more remain to be described.

6.1. Oncogenes

Given the relation between signal transduction and growth, it is not surprising that mutations in signal transduction molecules can lead to unregulated growth and tumorigenesis. Genes that when mutated can cause transformation are called oncogenes (the normal unmutated gene is a protooncogene). Alterations in receptor structure can lead to constitutive activation and constant stimulation of the signaling cascaded. Example of this include the neu oncogene, a point mutation of the EGF receptor, which leads to rat neuroblastoma and the trk oncogene, a truncation of the NGF receptor, which occurs in human colon carcinomas. Mutations of the transcription factors jun and fos result in oncogenes carried by avian and murine retroviruses. Similarly, other avian retroviruses carry mutated forms of the tyrosine kinases ras and src.

6.2. Alteration of G-Protein Function

6.2.1. PERTUSSIS AND CHOLERA TOXIN

These two toxins of major clinical importance achieve their actions in part by interacting with G-protein α subunits. Cholera toxin causes ADP ribosylation of the α subunit of G_a. This has the effect of inhibiting the α subunits GTPase activity, thus "locking" the subunit in its active GTP-bound conformation, which increases its ability to activate adenylyl cyclase and results in increased levels of cAMP. Increased levels of cAMP in the intestinal epithelial cells causes fluid secretion throughout the intestinal tract and the massive diarrhea that characterizes cholera. Pertussis toxin causes the ADP ribosylation of the α subunit of G_i. This results in uncoupling of the G-protein from the receptor, and leads to constitutive activation of adenylyl cyclase and increased levels of cAMP.

6.2.2. TYPE 1 PSEUDOHYPOPARATHYROIDISM

Type 1 pseudohypoparathyroidism, also known as Albright's hereditary osteodystrophy (AHO), is a genetic disorder caused by defects in $G\alpha_s$. AHO is characterized by a distinctive phenotype of short stature, round face, obesity, shortened metacarpals, and subcutaneous ossification. In examining kindreds of type 1 pseudohypoparathyroidism, multiple defects in $G\alpha_s$ have been described. These include point mutations, frame shifts, and splicing mutations, which all produce decreased levels of $G\alpha_s$. This results in decreased responsiveness to PTH, which signals through G_s and hence the appearance of apparent hypoparathyroidism. As would be expected given that G_s mediates signaling for multiple other hormones, patients with pseudohypoparathyroidism exhibit multiple hormone resistance, and a variety of cell types have lowered levels of adenylyl cyclase. As well as the hallmark symptoms associated with PTH resistance, patients with AHO also frequently exhibit hypothyroidism and hypogonadism. Pseudohypoparathyroidism is discussed further in Chapter 20.

6.3. Alterations in cAMP-Induced Gene Transcription Rubinstein-Taybi Syndrome

RTS is a well-defined syndrome with facial abnormalities, broad thumbs, broad big toes, and mental retardation. It has recently been discovered that RTS is caused by genetic defects in CREB-binding protein. Kindreds of RTS have chromosomal breakpoints, microdeletions, or point mutations in the CPB gene. The disease occurs in patients heterozygous for the mutation. Because CPB mediates the ability of cAMP and CREB to stimulate gene transcription, mutations in CPB will interfere with a large number of target genes. How this results in the specific syndrome remains to be determined.

6.4. Alterations in cGMP Signaling (Heat Stable Enterotoxin)

Some strains of pathogenic bacteria produce a heat-stable enterotoxin. These toxins are a major cause of diarrhea in humans and animals, and are a major cause of infant mortality in developing countries. They typically present as a watery diarrhea without fever. These toxins act by binding to the membrane-bound forms of guanylate cyclase to increase cGMP. The increased cGMP appears to cause the diarrhea. There are two forms of heat-stable enterotoxin, STa and STb. STa binds to guanylate cyclase type C (GC-C), which is found in the intestinal mucosa. The exact mechanism by which STa activates guanylate cyclase remains to be determined. Some of the effects of STa may also be mediated by cGMP activation of PKA.

REFERENCES

Sutherland EW. Studies on the mechanism of hormone action. *Science* 1972; 177:401.

SELECTED READINGS

Berridge MJ, Irvine RF. Inositol phosphates and cell signaling. *Nature* 1989; 341:197.

Collins FS. Cystic fibrosis: Molecular biology and therapeutic implications. *Science* 1992; 256:774.

Drewett JG, Garbers DL. The family of guanylate cyclase receptors and their ligands. *Endocrin Rev* 1994; 15,135.

Gilman AG. G proteins and regulation of adenylyl cyclase. *JAMA* 1989; 262:1819.

Heldin C-H. Dimerization of cell surface receptors in signal transduction. *Cell* 1995; 80:213.

Myers MG Jr., White MF. New frontiers in insulin receptor signaling. *Trends Endocrinol Metab* 1995; 6:209.

Neer EJ. Heterotrimeric G proteins: organizers of transmembrane signals. *Cell* 1995; 80:249.

Petrij F, Giles RH, Dauwerese HG, et al. Rubinstein-Taybi syndrome caused by mutations in the transcriptional co-activator CBP.

Reuveny E, Slesinger PA, Inglese J, et al. Activation of the cloned muscarinic potassium channel by G protein βY subunits. *Nature* 1994; 370:143.

Schindler C, Darnell JE. Transcriptional responses to polypeptide ligands: The Jak-Stat pathway. *Annu Rev Biochem* 1995; 64:621.

Schlessinger J, Ullrich A. Growth factor signaling by receptor tyrosine kinases. *Neuron* 1992; 9:383.

Sutherland EW. Studies on the mechanism of hormone action. *Science* 1972; 177:401.

4   Steroid Hormones

Jonathan Lindzey, PhD, and Kenneth S. Korach, PhD

1. INTRODUCTION

Steroids are lipophilic molecules used as chemical messengers by organisms ranging in complexity from water mold to humans. In vertebrates, steroids act on a wide range of tissues and influence many aspects of biology, including sexual differentiation, reproductive physiology, osmoregulation, and intermediate metabolism. Major sites of steroid synthesis and secretion include the ovaries, testes, adrenals, and placenta. Based on the distance of a target site from the site of synthesis and secretion, steroid hormones can be classified as either endocrine (distant target tissue), paracrine (neighboring cells), or autocrine (same cell) factors. When secreted into the environment, steroids can also act as pheromones by conveying information to other organisms.

Owing to the pervasive effects of steroids in vertebrate biology, a number of pathological states can occur because of problems related to steroid hormone action (*see* Section 4.). These disease states include cancer, steroid insensitivity, and abnormal

From: *Endocrinology: Basic and Clinical Principles* (P. M. Conn and S. Melmed, eds.), Humana Press Inc., Totowa, NJ.

steroid synthesis. The purpose of this chapter is to provide an overview of steroid synthesis, steroid hormone effects in normal physiology, molecular and biochemical mechanisms of action of steroid hormones, and pathological states related to steroid hormone action.

2. STEROID HORMONE SYNTHESIS

Steroid hormones are lipid molecules derived from a common cholesterol precursor (Cholestane, C27). There are four major classes of steroids: progestins, androgens, estrogens, and corticoids, which contain 21, 19, 18, and 21 carbons, respectively. Steroid hormones are synthesized by dehydrogenases and cytochrome P450 enzymes, which catalyze hydroxylation and dehydroxylation-oxidation reactions. Eukaryotic cytochromes P450 are membrane-bound enzymes expressed in either the inner mitochondrial or endoplasmic reticulum membranes of steroid-synthesizing tissues. A common and important rate-limiting step for the synthesis of all steroid hormones is the cleavage of the side chain from cholesterol (C27) to yield pregnenolone (C21), the common branch point for synthesis of

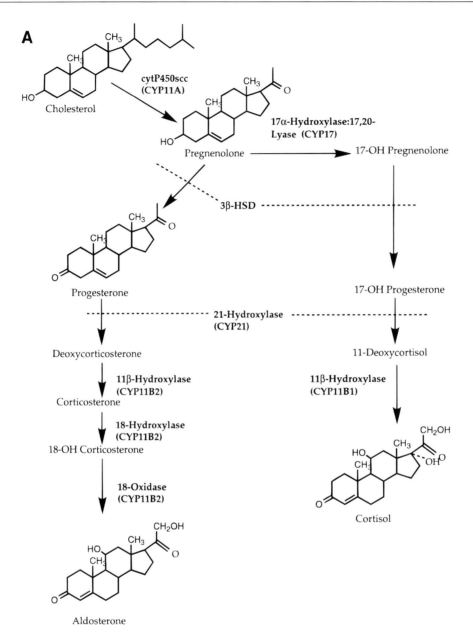

Fig. 1. (A) Synthetic pathways and structures of the major progestins and corticoids found in humans. Major enzymes involved in the synthesis are in boldface. **(B)** Synthetic pathways and structures of the major androgens and estrogens found in humans. Major enzymes involved in the synthesis are in boldface.

progestins, corticoids, androgens, and, hence, estrogens (Fig. 1).

In vertebrates, the synthesis and secretion of steroid hormones are regulated by trophic hormones from the anterior pituitary, such as follicle stimulating hormone (FSH), luteinizing hormone (LH), and adrenocorticotrophic hormone (ACTH). Mineralocorticoids are also regulated by ion con-

centrations and circulating levels of angiotensin II. Common regulatory mechanisms for steroid synthesis and release are feedback loops in which elevated circulating levels of steroids suppress production of trophic hormones by acting at specific sites in the brain and the anterior pituitary. The complex interplay between different components of the hypothalamic–pituitary–gonad/adrenal axes is an important

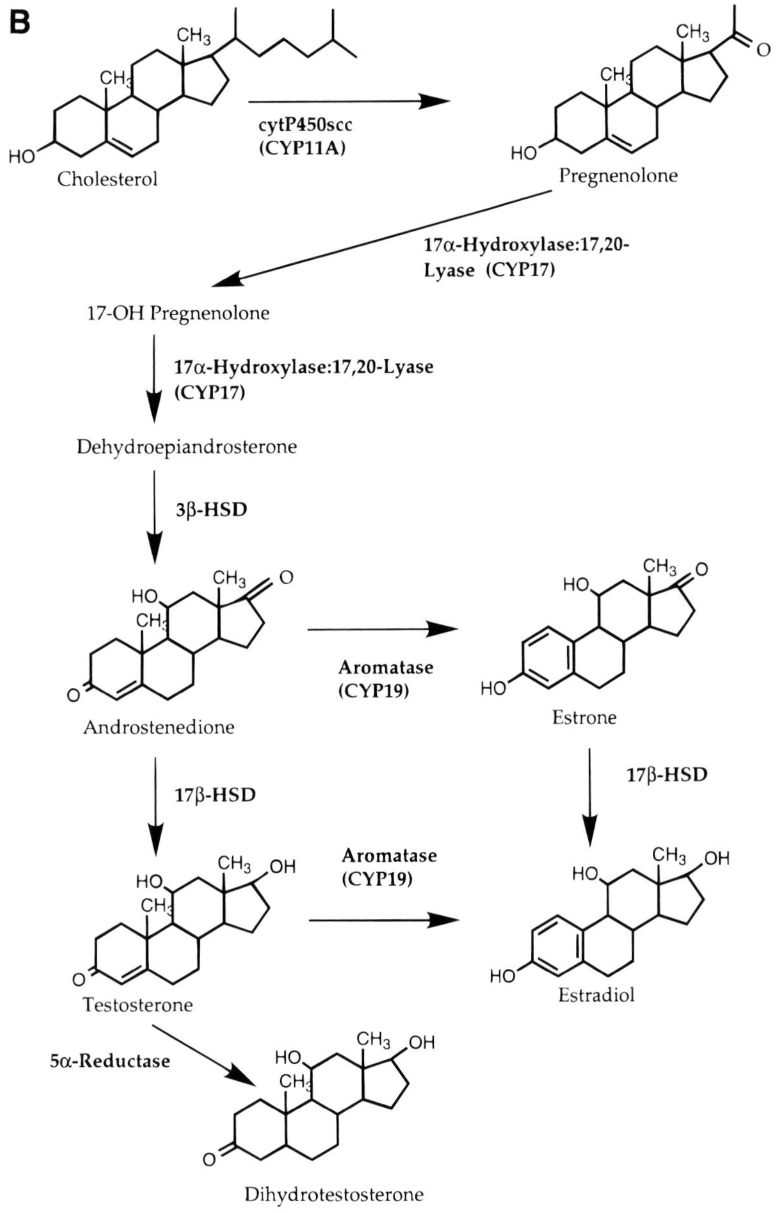

Fig. 1. *Continued*

feature of endocrine physiology that will be discussed in Section 5.

2.1. Progesterone Synthesis

Pregnenolone serves as a principal precursor to all the other steroid hormones synthesized by the ovary, testes, or adrenals. It appears that the rate-limiting step for progesterone synthesis is side-chain cleavage of cholesterol by P450scc. Pregnenolone is then converted to progesterone by 3 β-hydroxysteroid dehydrogenase (3β-HSD). Thus, deficiencies in

either P450scc or 3β-HSD have profound effects on synthesis of all steroids.

In the ovary, progesterone is produced at all stages of follicular development as an intermediate for androgen and estrogen synthesis, but becomes a primary secretory product during the periovulatory and postovulatory (luteal) phases. Synthesis of progesterone is under the control of FSH during early stages of folliculogenesis and, following acquisition of LH receptors, becomes sensitive to LH later in the ovarian cycle. In addition, the placenta secretes high levels of progesterone during pregnancy, although a different isozyme of 3β-HSD is involved in the synthesis.

2.2. Androgen Synthesis

Androgens are synthesized and secreted primarily by the Leydig cells of the testes, thecal cells of the ovary, and cells in the reticularis region of the adrenals. In most tetrapod vertebrates, testosterone (T) is the dominant circulating androgen. Testicular synthesis and secretion of T are stimulated by circulating LH, which upregulates the amount of 17α-hydroxylase: 17,20-lyase, a rate-limiting enzyme for conversion of C21 to C19 steroids. Once taken up by target tissues, T can be reduced by 5α-reductase to yield a more active androgen metabolite, 5α-dihydrotestosterone (DHT). T and androstenedione can also be converted into estrogens, such as 17β-estradiol (E_2) or estrone, through a process termed aromatization. Aromatization is carried out by a cytochrome P450 aromatase enzyme, which is expressed in the granulosa cells of the ovary, Leydig cells of the testes, and many other tissues, including the placenta, brain, pituitary, liver, and adipose tissue. Indeed, many of the effects of circulating testosterone are owing to conversion to either 5α-DHT or E_2 within target tissues.

2.3. Estrogen Synthesis

Estrogens and progestins are synthesized and secreted primarily by maturing follicles, corpora lutea of ovaries, and the placenta during pregnancy. The predominant estrogen secreted is E_2, and the predominant progestin is progesterone (P). The profile of estrogen synthesis changes during the course of folliculogenesis and follows a well-conserved, "two-cell" pattern where, under the influence of LH, the thecal cells synthesize and secrete androstenedione and T, which diffuses across the basement membrane and are subsequently aromatized to estrone and E_2, respectively, by the granulosa cells. The levels of aromatase and, hence, estrogens produced in the granulosa cells are under the control of fsh during midfollicular phases. Later in the cycle, the follicle/corpora lutea express greater numbers of LH receptors, and LH begins to regulate E_2 production. During pregnancy, the placenta utilizes androgen precursors from the fetal adrenal gland and secretes large amounts of E_2. In addition, in male vertebrates, many target tissues, such as pituitary

cells and hypothalamic neurons, convert circulating T into E_2.

2.4. Corticoid Synthesis

Corticoids are divided into gluco- and mineralocorticoid hormones. The predominant human glucocorticoid, cortisol, is synthesized in the zona fasiculata of the adrenal cortex. Synthesis of cortisol involves hydroxylations of progesterone at the 17α, 21 (CYP21) and 11β (CYP11B1) positions. Cortisol synthesis is under the control of an anterior pituitary hormone, ACTH, and a feedback mechanism in which elevated cortisol suppresses release of ACTH (*see* Section 5).

The dominant human mineralocorticoid is aldosterone, which is produced in the zona glomerulosa of the adrenal. Synthesis of aldosterone involves synthesis of corticosterone and subsequent hydroxylation and oxidation at C18 to yield aldosterone. Synthesis of aldosterone is regulated by levels of potassium and the effects of alterations in sodium and blood volume on levels of angiotensin II (*see* Section 5).

3. MECHANISMS OF STEROID HORMONE ACTION

Steroid effects are typically slow in relation to the rapid time-courses for effects of second messenger-mediated peptide hormones. This is owing both to the signal amplification inherent to second messenger cascades and to the slower changes in gene transcription and translation exerted by steroids (genomic effects). Early experiments confirmed these paths of steroid action by utilizing protein and RNA synthesis inhibitors, such as cycloheximide and actinomycin D, respectively. Though most characterized steroid effects are mediated via nuclear receptors and genomic pathways, there are examples of very rapid, "nongenomic" effects of steroids that appear to be possible only by membrane-mediated effects. Although this is an exciting new area of research, our discussion will focus on the well-characterized "genomic" mechanisms of action.

3.1. Genomic Mechanisms of Steroid Action

The basic genomic mechanisms of action of steroids hold relatively constant across different target tissues and different classes of steroid hormones. In the absence of hormone, estrogen (ER), androgen (AR), and progesterone (PR) receptors

Table 1
SREs

Type of response element	Sequence	Gene	Species
Estrogen	GGTCAcagTGACC	vitA2	*Xenopus*
	GGTCAcggTGGCC	PS2	Human
	GG*T*CAnnnTGA*C*C	Consensus	
Androgen	AGAACAgcaAGTGCT	PSA	Human
Progesterone	AGTACGtgaTGTTCT	C(3)	Rat
Glucocorticoid	AGA/G*A*CAnnnTG*T*A/CCC/T	Consensus	
Mineralocorticoid			

Sequences of some characterized response elements for ERs vs ARs, PRs, and corticoid receptors. Also shown are consensus sequences for these two classes. Italicized nucleotides demonstrate potential sites for mutation that can convert one class of SREs to another.

are principally localized in the nucleus, whereas glucocorticoid receptors (GR) are located in the cytoplasm. Current dogma holds that steroid hormones move passively from the circulation and interstitial spaces across cell membranes, and bind to and activate nuclear steroid receptor (SR) proteins. The activated SR–ligand complex then binds to specific DNA sequences, termed steroid response elements (SREs), which are associated with promoter regions that regulate transcription of genes (Fig. 2). SRs bind to DNA as homodimers, and the binding of the activated SR–ligand complexes to an SRE is thought to position the activated SRs so that transactivation domains of the SRs interact with proteins comprising the transcriptional complex bound to a promoter and, hence, stimulate or inhibit rates of transcription.

SREs are a family of highly related DNA palindromic repeats. The estrogen, COUP factor, thyroid hormone, and retinoic acid receptors share highly homologous consensus response elements, whereas GR, AR, PR, and mineralocorticoid (MR) share very similar and, in some cases, identical elements. The high degree of homology between and within these two groups of SREs is also reflected in the high degree of homology between protein sequences of the DNA-binding domains (DBDs) of the various receptors. This would seem to create a problem with specificity of hormone action, but as seen in Table 1, mutation of two nucleotides is sufficient to alter a consensus estrogen response element (ERE) into a consensus androgen response element (ARE). In addition, as other nonconsensus elements are charac-

terized, more light is shed on the nature of SR-specific interactions with the genome.

The different classes of steroid hormones are all present in the circulation, and their respective levels vary with the different physiological states of the organism. In addition many target cells express multiple classes of SRs. This presents the organism with the problem of how to activate a specific gene by a specific steroid hormone. Specificity of steroid hormone-activated gene expression lies in:

1. Hormone-specific binding by the receptor;
2. DNA-specific binding exhibited by the different types of steroid receptors; and
3. Control of access of steroid receptors to genes through differential organization of chromatin in the many different target cells and tissues.

Many of the hormone-insensitivity syndromes stem from mutations that alter steroid- or DNA-binding characteristics of the SR.

As a whole, steroid hormone receptors are a highly conserved group of "ligand-dependent," nuclear transcription factors. SRs are modular in nature and can be broken down into different functional domains, such as transactivating domains, DBD, and steroid binding domain (SBD). Between the different classes of SR, AR, PR, ER, GR, and MR, the DBD is the most highly conserved region followed by the steroid-binding domains and then the amino-terminal transactivating domain. The following discussion of different functional domains focuses on the ER, but many of the characteristics hold true for other SR types.

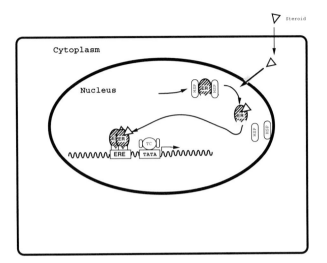

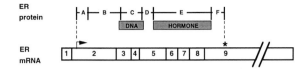

Fig. 3. ER protein and gene structure. Depicted are the different domains of the ER protein and the exons that correspond to these domains. DBD and SBD domains are designated. Transactivation functions are localized within domains B and E.

Fig. 2. Mechanisms of steroid action. Estrogen diffuses across the cell membrane and binds to ER, causing dissociation of heat-shock proteins and allowing the activated ligand–ER complex to bind an ERE. Activation domains of the ER interact with components of the transcriptional machinery to alter gene activity.

3.2. Structure of the ER Gene and Protein

The ER is coded for by a gene that contains nine exons. The ER protein has been divided into six domains that are termed A/B, C, D, E, and F domains. These domains have been found to possess the following functions: transcriptional activation function (A/B, E), DNA binding (C), steroid binding (E), nuclear localization (D), and dimerization (E) (Fig. 3). The modular nature of the different functional domains and the interdependency of these domains mean that splice variants of SR mRNAs can produce altered proteins that behave in appreciably different fashions from the full-length SR. The importance of these variants in normal physiology is still under investigation, but splice variants may play a role in disease states, such as the progression from steroid-dependent to steroid-independent cancer (*see* Section 4).

3.2.1. SBD

The SBD (domain E) of the ER consists of approx 250 amino acids and is coded for by exons 5–9. It forms a large hydrophobic pocket that exhibits specific, high-affinity binding for estradiol (Kd ~ 0.1 nM). Binding of estrogens to this region results in transcriptional activation or suppression of target genes. Based on studies in which removal of the SBD results in a constitutively active or "ligand-indepen-

dent" ER, it is possible that the SBD functions as a repressor of a transcriptional activation function that would normally be constitutively active. Indeed, a constitutively active exon 5 splice variant of ER was recently detected in some human breast cancers.

3.2.2. DBD

The DBD exhibits specific binding for sequences of DNA termed estrogen response elements (EREs). This region is highly conserved and contains two "zinc-finger" motifs, each of which contains cysteine residues that bind zinc. The first zinc finger dictates sequence-specific interactions with DNA, whereas the second appears to dictate the spacing requirements between the arms of the palindrome. These fingers are critical for DNA binding, but the surrounding amino acids also influence binding. The canonical element is a palindrome inverted repeat (GGTCAnnnTGACC), although deviations from this consensus sequence are quite common (*see* Table 1). Binding of the ER–ligand complex to an ERE sequence positions the ligand-activated ER where it can interact with the basal transcription complexes and influence the rate of gene transcription.

3.2.3. Transcription Activation Functions

The ER contains two regions known to possess transcriptional activation functions, AF1 and AF2, that are located in the A/B and E domains, respectively. Depending on the cell type and target genes, AF1 and AF2 can act independently or in concert. For instance, removal of AF1 has no effect on E_2 induction of a reporter construct containing the vitellogenin ERE, whereas the same AF1-deficient ER has only 20% of wild-type induction of a PS2-ERE. As mentioned earlier, removal of the SBD (containing AF2) can lead to a constitutively active ER. Interestingly, this constitutive activity may require phosphorylation and activation by second messengers. Studies using AF1 and AF2 truncated ER have demonstrated AF1 responds to growth factors that act via second messengers, such as cAMP, whereas AF2 is E_2(ligand)-dependent. Thus, the ER is actually a nuclear transcription factor that responds to both steroid and second messenger signaling pathways. "Ligand-independent" or second messenger activation of transcriptional activity has also been demonstrated for AR and PR, suggesting this may be an important and conserved mechanism for physiological activation of steroid receptors.

3.2.4. DIMERIZATION

Most data indicate that SRs act as homodimers, although some data suggest possible effects by SR monomers. The region of the protein responsible for dimerization of the mouse ER overlaps with steroid-binding function and spans amino acids 501–522. These amino acids form an amphipathic, helical structure with an imperfect heptad repeat of hydrophobic amino acids reminiscent of the leucine zippers found in the JUN/FOS and CREB families of transcription factors. Mutations of amino acids in this hydrophobic stretch have proven that this area is critical for dimerization, steroid binding, and hence, transactivation. The dimerization function is critical for the effects of SR homodimers, but may also play a role in the formation of heterodimers between SR and other transcription factors with similar dimerization domains, such as JUN/FOS. The potential for such crosstalk between steroid and second messenger pathways is an exciting area of research.

3.2.5. NUCLEAR LOCALIZATION SIGNAL (NLS)

SRs and many other transcription factors possess a segment of amino acids that targets the proteins to the cell nucleus. These stretches of amino acids tend to be basic and have been termed the NLS. It appears the NLS is located between amino acids 250 and 270 of the ER, a region that shares homology with the nuclear localization domains of the GR and PR.

4. STEROIDS AND DEVELOPMENT

Scientists have known for years that *in utero* and neonatal exposure to steroids are critical for sexual differentiation of the brain and peripheral reproductive structures. A guiding concept for the study of developmental actions of steroid effects is the organization-activation hypothesis. Stated simply, prenatal or neonatal exposure to steroid hormones organizes or alters differentiation of the phenotypes, such that hormonal exposure in adulthood is more likely to activate a particular response. A corollary of this rule is that the initial exposures must fall within certain critical periods of sensitivity. These critical periods typically occur during fetal and neonatal stages and puberty.

Steroids affect development of organs and tissues through both induction and inhibition of growth. Inhibition occurs via active cell death, a process termed apoptosis. Apoptosis is an active process requiring protein synthesis, and resulting in chromatin condensation, degradation of chromatin in a characteristic "ladder" pattern, and development of apoptotic bodies.

4.1. Stromal–Mesenchymal Interactions

A recurring theme in development of steroid-dependent glandular tissues is the importance of stromal-mesenchymal tissue induction. In this scheme, the fate of undifferentiated epithelium is determined by the underlying mesenchyme with which it comes into contact. For instance, undifferentiated epithelium combined with prostatic or integumental mesenchyme develops a phenotype dictated by the type of mesenchyme. In the case of hormone-directed morphogenesis, such as in the prostate or breast, hormonal influences on the glandular epithelium can occur either directly on epithelial cells or indirectly via inductive influences of the mesenchyme. Recent experiments demonstrate that epithelium can also influence the underlying mesenchyme, indicating a bidirectional epithelial–mesenchymal interaction.

4.2. Secondary Sex Structures

In the developing mammalian embryo, gonadal sex is determined by genotype. In turn, the embryonic gonads secrete hormones that when coupled with maternal hormones, determine the early hormonal milieu to which secondary sex structures are exposed and, hence, dictate development of male or female phenotype. Dogma holds that mammals possess a default system such that embryos develop a female phenotype in the absence of any gonadal steroid hormones. In males, as the developing testes begin to develop sex cords, the testes secrete mullerian inhibiting substance (MIS) and testosterone. The MIS induces ipsilateral regression of the mullerian ducts, which prevents development of mullerian derivatives, such as the uterus and fallopian tubes. Elevated T stimulates development of Wolffian derivatives, such as epididymis, vas deferens, and seminal vesicles. Differentiation of external genitalia and accessory glands (such as the prostate) from the genital tubercle, scrotal folds, and urogenital sinus requires 5α-DHT. This is illustrated by 5α-reductase-deficient males who have normal Wolffian derivatives, but have feminized external genitalia despite the presence of normal levels of T (*see* Section 6).

Although it is true that external genitalia and internal reproductive structures of genotypic females are grossly feminized without the influence of gonadal steroids, it is clear that steroid effects are needed for complete and functional differentiation of some structures, such as the uterus and breast. For instance, transgenic mice lacking functional estrogen receptor (ERKO) possess uteri that contain all the normal tissue types and structures, but are hypoplastic. In addition, exposure to estrogens and progestins is required for differentiation of the nipple and mesenchyme surrounding the epithelium of breast tissue. Estrogen and progesterone also increase alveolar formation and branching of mammary ducts.

4.3. Sex Behavior and Sexual Dimorphisms of the Brain

Sex behavior in most adult vertebrates is dependent on (1) organizational effects of hormones early in development and (2) activational effects of circulating steroids in the adult. In many species, *in utero* and neonatal hormone exposures alter adult patterns of sex behaviors. Historically, this observation led to the assumption that at some organizational level, the brains of males and females must be morphologically or functionally distinct in order to favor female- or male-typical behaviors. In the case of the rat, sexually dimorphic nuclei (SDN) have been located in the central nervous system. Male rats possess an enlarged SDN present in the medial preoptic area of the hypothalamus and an SDN in the spinal cord. The development of these nuclei and subsequent function in adult males are androgen-dependent; androgen ablation during early critical periods of differentiation leads to smaller, female-typical nuclei and also decreases in male-typical copulatory behavior. In rats, the effects of testicular T on SDNs appear to be predominantly through aromitization to E_2; treatment with E_2 mimics T effects and use of an aro-

matase inhibitor can prevent masculinization of SDN by circulating T. Similar steroid-dependent dimorphisms are found in the central nervous sytems of gerbils, voles, song birds, lizards, and fish. These dimorphisms may be present as differences in gross volume, cell number, cell size, dendritic arborization, and levels of expression of enzymes, neurotransmitters, neuropeptides, or receptors. Sexual dimorphisms in humans have also been reported in the anterior hypothalamus, preoptic area, and anterior commissure, although there are conflicting data in these studies. Thus, the presence of sexually dimorphic brain nuclei in humans and, in particular, their impact on sexually dimorphic behaviors in humans are controversial at this time.

4.4. Steroids and Bone

Bone cells express ER, AR, and PR, and the development and maintenance of bone structure is regulated by estrogens and androgens. Pubertal surges in estrogens and androgens initiate growth spurts, including long bone growth and, subsequently, cessation of bone growth through epiphyseal closure. In adults, E_2 maintains bone mass and mineralization. The importance of E_2 effects on bone growth and development is manifest in individuals lacking in E_2 action. For instance, a human male patient lacking functional ER exhibits continued bone growth, decreased bone density, and absence of epiphyseal closure (*see* Section 4.3.). In addition, absence of E_2 owing either to ovariectomy or menopause results in osteoporosis, whereas exogenous E_2 prevents this condition. Excess production of cortisol results in a loss of bone mass (osteopenia).

4.5. Steroids and Liver

Liver cells express ER and AR that regulate production of secreted proteins and steroid-metabolizing enzymes. In humans, the liver synthesizes and secretes into the bloodstream a plasma protein termed sex hormone-binding globulin (SHBG). This protein serves to sequester and prevent steroids from being metabolized and/or cleared from the bloodstream. SHBG binds DHT with high affinity (Kd ~ 0.5 nM) and T and E_2 with approx 5- and 15-fold lower affinity, respectively. Estrogens stimulate whereas androgens inhibit the synthesis and secretion of hepatic SHBG.

There are distinct sex differences in the profile of steroid metabolites excreted in urine. The basis of

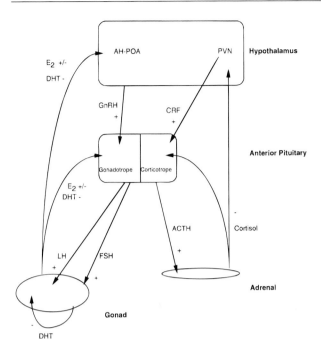

Fig. 4. Hypothalamic–pituitary–gonadal/adrenal axes. Depicted are the pathways and major trophic hormones involved in regulating the production of gonadal and adrenal steroids.

such sex differences results from sex differences in expression of metabolic-enzymes in the liver. For instance, the female liver expresses 15β-hydroxylase activity, whereas the male does not express this enzyme. In rats, these sex differences are regulated by what constitutes a hypothalamic–pituitary–hepatic axis in which neonatal androgens masculinize the growth hormone axis. In turn, the pattern of growth hormone secretion dictates a male or female profile of steroid metabolism. This is evident by the fact that pulsatile surges of GH (male-like pattern) or tonic, low-level GH infusions (female-like) into hypohysec-tomized rats produces a male- or female-typical pattern of enzyme expression and metabolism, respectively.

5. STEROIDS AND NORMAL PHYSIOLOGY

5.1. Hypothalamic–Pituitary–Gonadal Axes

Gonadal function is regulated by the pituitary gonadotropins (LH and FSH), which are regulated by the hypothalamic peptide, GnRH, steroids, and gonadal peptides (Fig. 4). GnRH is synthesized by small populations of neurons in the preoptic area,

anterior hypothalamus, and mediobasal hypothalamus, and released into the hypophysial portal system, which carries GnRH to the pituitary. GnRH stimulates synthesis and release of LH and FSH, which, in turn, regulate steroidogenesis and gametogenesis. Elevations in the circulating concentrations of gonadal steroids feed back on hypothalamic and pituitary sites to regulate gonadotropin synthesis and release. In addition to steroids, the gonads also secrete peptide hormones (activin and inhibin) that feed back on the pituitary to regulate gonadotropin synthesis and release.

GnRH secretion occurs as both an episodic, tonic pattern and a surge associated with ovulatory events in females. The tonic pattern of GnRH secretion occurs in a pulsatile fashion with a periodicity of approx 1 pulse/h. Steroids feed back on the GnRH pulse generator thought to be located in the medial basal hypothalamus to regulate tonic patterns of GnRH secretion. Regulation of the the ovulatory GnRH surge, however, appears to require input from the preoptic area/anterior hypothalamus regions. In addition, androgens and estrogens can feed back directly on pituitary gonadotropes to regulate cell growth, sensitivity to GnRH, and basal levels of gene expression of gonadotropins. A final level at which steroids feed back is on steroidogenic cells themselves. For instance, experiments indicate that androgens can downregulate LH-induced expression of steroids by Leydig cells. The feedback effects of steroids on these different levels constitute long-loop (gonad– hypothalamic), short loop (gonad–pituitary), and ultra short-loop (gonad–gonad) feedback circuits (Fig. 4).

5.1.1. Female Reproductive Cycles

Humans and most other female mammals are spontaneous ovulators where the cyclical buildup of estrogen triggers a "spontaneous" pulse of gonadotropin that results in ovulation independent of mating stimuli. However, in some species, females are reflex ovulators in which physical mating stimuli are responsible for triggering GnRH and gonadotropin surges that provide the proximate cues for ovulation. The discussion below discusses normal ovarian cycles in spontaneous ovulators.

As a follicle matures under the influence of basal levels of FSH, circulating levels of E_2 increase to a peak at or near ovulation. The increase in E_2 increases gonadotrope sensitivity to GnRH by upregulating

GnRH receptors and, at peak levels, triggers a GnRH surge that, in turn, produces an LH surge. This LH surge induces ovulation, formation of a corpora lutea from granulosa cells of the follicle, and synthesis and secretion of P and E_2. Over the course of the ovarian cycle, ovarian steroids exert control over GnRH and gonadotropins, maturation of follicles, preparation of the uterus for implantation, alterations in vaginal and cervical function, and behavior.

5.1.1.1. Feedback. Long-term ovariectomy of mice leads to a large increase in steady-state message for FSH and LH, whereas estrogen treatments reverse this effect. However, this is an oversimplification of the complex effects of ovarian steroids on feedback regulation of the hypothalamus and pituitary. Estrogen and progesterone appear to have biphasic effects where initial exposure to E_2 during the follicular phase results in (1) increased sensitivity of gonadotropes to GnRH and (2) a pulse of GnRH. Subsequent E_2 exposure inhibits gonadotropin levels. Similarly, following E_2 priming, the initial exposure to P results in increased sensitivity to GnRH followed by long-term inhibition. Indeed, elevated P associated with formation of the corpora lutea results in suppression of estrus cycles.

5.1.1.2. Effects of Estradiol and Progesterone on Accessory Sex Structures. As E_2 levels increase during the follicular phase, the luminal epithelium of the uterus undergoes a proliferative phase in preparation for implantation. During the initial phases (1–4 h), these changes include hyperemia and water imbibition followed by increases in DNA and protein synthesis, hyperplasia, and hypertrophy. An important effect of E_2 during this stage is the induction of synthesis of PR, which allows the uterus to respond to elevated progesterone. During luteal phases, elevated P completes the preparation of the endometrium for implantation of the blastocyst by increasing vascularization and thickening the mucosal layer of the epithelium. In the absence of implantation, the corpora lutea degenerates, serum P levels drop, and the endometrium degenerates. The hypothalamic–pituitary–gonadal axis is then freed from P suppression to resume another round of folliculogenesis.

Mammary gland function is regulated by the coordinated actions of estradiol, progesterone, and prolactin. Estradiol promotes lobuloalveolar development by acting directly on the mammary gland, and by stimulating prolactin synthesis and secretion by the anterior pituitary. Estradiol-stimulated increases in PRL also help prepare the glandular tissue for lactation. Progesterone promotes glandular development, but requires (1) the presence of pituitary hormones and (2) priming with E_2, which upregulates levels of PR. Although P and E_2 help prepare the glandular tissue for lactation, these two hormones also suppress lactation until parturition and expulsion of the placenta cause an abrupt drop in E_2 and P.

5.1.1.3. Puberty. Critical stages of sex determination and sexual differentiation occur *in utero* and early in neonatal life. However, terminal differentiation of sexually dimorphic structures and the onset of reproductive fertility occur during puberty. In humans, the onset of puberty is marked by an increase in tonic, pulsatile GnRH release, and increased secretion of LH and FSH. In the female, increased gonadotropin levels initiate waves of folliculogenesis, and associated increases in E_2 and androgens. As levels of E_2 increase, terminal differentiation of the breasts begins and females undergo a growth spurt. As E_2 levels increase over the course of puberty, E_2 induces epiphyseal closure and cessation of the growth spurt. Exposure to increasing levels of E_2 results in an initial proliferation of the endometrium followed by the first menses (menarche) owing to a drop in E_2 at the end of a follicular wave. The inital ovulatory event takes place approx 1 yr following menarche, presumably because the mechanisms regulating a GnRH surge now respond to E_2-positive feedback. In the male, the pubertal onset of increased GnRH and gonadotropin synthesis and release is marked by testicular enlargment, and initiation of spermatogenesis and steroidogenesis. As levels of circulating T increase, penile enlargement, pubic hair growth, and growth spurts commence. In addition, the glandular epithelium of secretory glands, such as the seminal vesicle and prostate, undergo a proliferative phase and begin to produce secretory products that become components of the semen.

5.1.1.4. Effects of E_2 and P on Sexual Behavior. In many vertebrates, E_2 and P act to coordinate periods of maximum sexual receptivity with periods of maximum likelihood of fertilization. Thus, E_2 priming during follicular phases followed by a surge of P associated with ovulation and luteinization results in maximum receptivity at about the time of ovulation.

The effects of the estrus cycle on behavior can be re-created in ovariectomized females treated with E_2 followed by P. The E_2 treatment has a facilitatory effect alone, but is greatly augmented by subsequent P treatment. Based on lesion studies and intrahypothalamic implants of E_2 and P, the ventromedial hypothalamus appears to be the site of E_2 and P effects on receptive and proceptive behaviors in female mammals. One effect of E_2 is to upregulate PR in the ventromedial hypothalamus. The significance of E_2 and P in sexual behaviors of female humans is less profound than other mammals with a distinct behavioral estrus.

5.1.2. MALE REPRODUCTIVE CYCLES

Regulation of the male hypothalamic–pituitary–gonadal axis is a less dynamic process in which GnRH pulses are lower in magnitude and do not undergo surges like those associated with ovulation in females. In rodents, the male GnRH system cannot respond to exogenous E_2 with a surge, whereas in humans and monkeys, injections of exogenous E_2 result in a GnRH surge. Thus, the absence of a GnRH surge in male humans is owing to the absence of the estrogen buildup associated with folliculogenesis in females.

GnRH stimulates gonadotropes to synthesize and release FSH and LH, which act on spermatogenesis and steroidogenesis, respectively. LH elevates cAMP levels, which stimulates synthesis and secretion of T from the Leydig cells. Elevated T assists spermatogenesis and feedsback to downregulate GnRH levels and, hence, synthesis and release of gonadotropins. It appears that T may feed back both directly as an androgen and as an estrogen following aromatization. Since neither AR or ER has been detected in GnRH-secreting neurons, this feedback is indirect via AR- and ER- containing neurons that regulate function of GnRH neurons.

Sex behavior in most adult male vertebrates is dependent on elevated circulating levels of T. T acts on brain nuclei of the anterior hypothalamus/preoptic area to activate male-typical sex behaviors; lesions of these brain areas or castration results in a cessation of sex behaviors. Depending on the species, behavioral effects of androgens can be owing to both aromatization to E_2 and direct effects as T or DHT. T also acts on Sertoli cells, where it can maintain spermatogenesis, even in hypophysectomized males. Another important function is stimulation of accessory sex structures, such as the prostate and seminal vesicle. Circulating T is converted to 5α-DHT, which causes hypertrophy of secretory epithelium, increases in RNA and protein synthesis, and increased protein secretions. As adults, the continued functioning of these androgen-dependent responses relies on exposure to circulating T.

5.2. Hypothalamic–Pituitary–Adrenal Axis

Synthesis and secretion of glucocorticoids, such as cortisol, are stimulated by the pituitary hormone ACTH. The release of ACTH from corticotrophs is stimulated by a hypothalamic peptide, corticotrophin-releasing factor (CRF), produced by the paraventricular nucleus of the hypothalamus. Increased levels of cortisol act directly at the level of the corticotroph to reduce ACTH production and at the paraventricular nucleus of the hypothalamus to suppress CRF levels (Fig. 4). Thus, hypophysectomy leads to a decrease in cortisol, whereas adrenalectomy leads to an increase in ACTH that is reversed by cortisol treatment. Continuous ACTH secretion characteristic of chronic stress also leads to adrenal cortical hypertrophy, elevated glucocorticoid levels, and, in some cases, adrenal failure.

ACTH has a reduced trophic effect on the zona glomerulosa and aldosterone levels in mammals. Primary regulators of aldosterone synthesis and secretion include potassium (K^+), sodium (Na^+), blood volume, and angiotensin II. Elevated angiotensin II, K^+ loading, and low serum Na^+ levels, however, cause release of adrenal aldosterone, which promotes Na^+ recovery by the glomeruli. Conversely, Na^+ loading produces hypertension or circulatory expansion, and decreases levels of aldosterone.

Potassium appears to act directly at the level of the glomerulosa both in vivo and in vitro. Furthermore, K^+ loading appears to affect release of renin and synergizes with angiotensin II to increase release of aldosterone. Sodium depletion decreases blood volume, which stimulates the juxtaglomerular apparatus to secrete renin. In turn, renin acts on angiotensinogen to begin a cascade that eventually leads to elevated levels of angiotensin II and subsequent elevation of aldosterone. The elevated aldosterone promotes Na^+ retention, and elevates blood volume and arterial pressure, which, in turn, feeds back to decrease renin production.

5.2.1. CARBOHYDRATE METABOLISM

Adrenalectomy leads to reduced liver glycogen and low blood glucose, resulting from increased oxidation of glucose and decreased gluconeogenesis from protein. Conversely, administration of cortisol leads to a rise in blood sugar and an increase in liver glycogen stores. Glucagon also elevates glucose levels and promotes glycogen breakdown. Insulin, however, has opposite effects favoring lower blood sugar (decreased gluconeogenesis) and increased glycogen synthesis and storage.

5.2.2. STRESS RESPONSES

Stress can be induced by social interactions, physical stress, and physiological challenges. A classic stress response is increased secretion of glucocorticoids triggered by increased secretions of CRF and ACTH. Hormonal responses to stress can be very fast (minutes) and dissipate quickly, or in some cases, become chronic. In stressful situations, elevated glucocorticoids stimulate an adaptive rise in glucose levels from carbohydrate energy sources. The effects of long-term elevated glucocorticoid include suppression of hypothalamic–pituitary–gonadal function and suppression of the immune system.

Elevated glucocorticoids suppress production of GnRH by hypothalamic neurons, and consequently, alter gonadotropin and steroid synthesis and gametogenesis. Glucocorticoids also directly affect gonadotrope function by suppressing basal and second messenger-induced synthesis, and release of gonadotropins. At the level of the gonad, glucocorticoids also suppress gonadotropin and second messenger-stimulated steroid synthesis. Thus, the suppressive effects of elevated glucocorticoids on reproduction are exerted at all levels of the hypothalamic–pituitary–gonadal axis.

Glucocorticoids play a role in the apoptotic events leading to differentiation of the immune system and regulation of the immune system in adults. Apoptosis is an active process of programmed cell death in which a series of programmed events lead to the death of a cell. In the developing immune system, glucocorticoids induce apoptosis in autoreactive T-cells and unreacted B-cells. High levels of glucocorticoids can also lead to apoptosis of immune cells in the adult, and consequently, a compromised immune system and increased susceptibility to disease.

5.2.3. ELECTROLYTE BALANCE

Salt balance is achieved primarily by mineralocorticoids and neurohypophyseal peptides, such as arginine vasopressin or arginine vasotocin. Aldosterone,

the principal human mineralocorticoid, reduces Na^+ loss by enhancing resorption by the renal tubules of the kidney. Thus, adrenalectomy or deficiencies in adrenal steroid synthesis result in rapid decreases in blood Na^+ and circulatory collapse, unless Na^+ or exogenous aldosterone is provided.

6. STEROIDS AND PATHOPHYSIOLOGY

Steroid-related pathologies include nonheritable steroid-dependent cancers and heritable syndromes that affect the synthesis or function of steroids and their receptors, resulting in steroid-insensitivity syndromes. Even though the effects of steroids on steroid-dependent cancers are environmental and nonheritable, there are clearly genetic predispositions to develop such cancers. The heritable defects in steroid action are generally autosomal recessive diseases that lead to developmental anomalies with various degrees of severity (Table 2).

6.1. Cancer

A number of steroid-dependent and steroid-independent tumors occur in steroid target tissues, such as the uterus, breast, and prostate. In the case of prostate cancer, a clear link with androgens is provided by the fact that castrated males never develop prostate cancer. Furthermore, many prostate cancers exhibit a period of regression and remission following castration and antiandrogen treatment. Unfortunately, many of these cancers enter a steroid-independent stage, during which growth and metastases is independent of androgens or hormonal therapy.

A vital question is why prostate cancer becomes steroid-independent. Since normal proliferation and growth cycles are dependent on androgens, the question becomes: Why do these tumor cells lose their normal requirement for androgen stimulation? Two hypotheses seem viable: (1) splice variants result in a constitutively active variant AR that stimulates growth independent of androgens, and (2) key regulatory points in the cell cycle lose the requirement for androgen stimulation. These hypotheses remain to be tested in this and other steroid-independent tumors.

Breast cancer is often amenable to treatment with steroid antagonists as assessed clinically by assays for both ER and PR in mammary biopsies. The presence of receptor levels >10–15 fmole suggests the cancer is probably steroid-dependent and likely to respond to antihormone therapy. However, breast

Table 2
Steroid-Associated Defects

Defect	Phenotype
AR	XY—feminization of external genitalia, androgen-resistant
5α-Reductase	XY—feminization of external genitalia
ER	XX—mammary agenesis, normal Mullerian structures, elevated androgens and gonadotropins, polycystic ovaries Human XY—tall stature, open epiphyseal plate, elevated estrogens and gonadotropins
Aromatase	XX—mammary agenesis, ambiguous external genitalia, normal Mullerian structures, elevated androgens and gonadotropins, polycystic ovaries XY—phenotypes similar to those from ER defects, but responds to estrogen therapy
PR	XX—anovulatory, mammary agenesis, no lordosis XY—grossly normal
P450scc	XX—asteroidogenesis, hyponatremia, altered glucose metabolism, no pubertal changes XY—same as XX, external genitalia are feminized, Wolffian structures absent
3β-HSD	XX—similar to P450scc deficiency except some masculinization may be present XY—similar to P450scc deficiency
21-Hydroxylase	Inability to synthesize cortisol XX—increased androgens, ambiguous genitalia, masculinization, rapid postnatal somatic growth XY—increased androgens, rapid postnatal somatic growth

cancer can become estrogen-independent and unresponsive to antiestrogens, such as tamoxifen. Recent work characterized a constitutively active ER splice variant in some breast tumors that may provide one explanation of how cancers can progress to a steroid-independent state.

6.2. Androgen-Based Developmental Defects

A number of different types of androgen-based defects have been documented. These range from a defective 5α-reductase enzyme that occurs as a rare autosomal mutation to a defective AR resulting from mutations within the X-linked AR gene. In addition, alterations in steroidogenic enzymes earlier in the synthetic pathways can also result in developmental anomalies of androgen-dependent tissues. The phenotypic manifestations of these defects range from infertility in phenotypically normal males to complete feminization of external genitalia. In cases of enzymatic deficiencies, hormone therapy often ame-

liorates some of the symptoms, whereas those symptoms related to receptor defects are more resistant to hormone therapy.

6.2.1. 5α-Reductase Deficiency

Humans express two isozymes of 5α-reductase. Type 1 is expressed at low levels in peripheral tissues, whereas type 2 is expressed at high levels in male genital structures. In males, 5α-reductase-type 2 deficiencies result in varying degrees of ambiguity of the external genitalia ranging from hypospadias to complete feminization. Under the influence of elevated T, Wolffian derivatives, such as the epididymis and seminal vesicle, develop normally, whereas the external genitalia are feminized to varying degrees. In addition, Mullerian derivatives are absent owing to production of MIS by the testes. In extreme cases of feminization, this syndrome is often diagnosed at the age of puberty when a patient with female phenotype exhibits amenorrhea and/or some increased masculinization owing to the increased levels of T associated with puberty. Prior to puberty, these individuals are usually raised with female gender roles, but following pubertal changes in phenotype sometimes assume male gender roles.

6.2.2. Androgen Insensitivity Syndrome (AIS) and Testicular Feminized Males (TFM)

Androgen insensitivity actually presents itself as a spectrum of disorders ranging from complete external feminization to infertility in phenotypic males. A wide variety of AR receptor gene defects have been documented, ranging from point mutations that cause a premature stop codon in the Tfm mouse to a complete deletion of the AR gene in a human family. Known mutations within the human AR appear to cluster primarily within the DBD and SBD of the receptor. Generally, there is a reasonable correlation between the degree of feminization and the degree to which normal function of the AR is altered, as assessed by various in vitro assays. For instance, mutations that totally abolish steroid binding lead to profound feminization, whereas more subtle mutations effecting thermolability and steroid dissociation rates lead to less profound effects, such as infertility and hypospadia.

Fertility problems related to AR defects are resistant to therapy, whereas anomalies, such as mild hypospadia, can be treated by surgical correction. In cases of complete feminization, inguinal and labial testes are removed owing to increased incidences of testicular cancer. Although completely feminized XY individuals are infertile, they develop female gender roles and tend to maintain these roles throughout adulthood.

6.3. Estrogen-Based Developmental Defects

Until recently, no mutations in the aromatase or ER genes had been detected. Additionally, ER mRNA had been detected during very early embryonic stages using reverse transcriptase-polymerase chain reaction (RT-PCR). Thus, it was suspected that estrogen is critical for development of a viable embryo and that mutations of either of the above-mentioned genes would be lethal. Recent findings, however, have documented aromatase deficiency and estrogen insensitivity (ER defects) in adult humans. In addition, a transgenic mouse line in which the ER gene has been disrupted (ERKO mouse) demonstrates that embryos can develop in the absence of functional ER. Although these data suggest that estrogens may not be critical for embryonic survival, a number of phenotypic abnormalities occur owing to these gene mutations.

6.3.1. Aromatase Deficiency

Mutations in the aromatase enzyme lead to alterations in phenotypes in both males and females. A male homozygous for defective aromarase exhibited tall stature, incomplete epiphyseal closure, continued linear bone growth, and osteoporosis. Circulating androgens and gonadotropin levels were increased, but gross sexual phenotype was normal. In an aromatase deficient female, the individual presented with ambiguous genitalia at birth, but normal internal Mullerian structures by subsequent laparoscopic examination. At puberty, the individual possessed the following symptoms: absence of breast development (mammary agenesis), primary amenhorrea, elevated gonadotropins, elevated androgens, and polycystic ovaries. Estrogen treatment alleviated many of these symptoms. The masculinization is the result of a lack of conversion of C19 steroids to estrogens and, hence, excess circulating androgens.

6.3.2. ER Mutations

Recent work documented a normally masculinized, human male with clinical symptoms very similar to the aromatase deficient male: tall stature, incomplete epiphyseal closure, osteoporosis, decreased sperm viability, and elevated T and gonadotropins. Estrogen levels were also elevated, and the patient exhibited no response to E_2 therapy. Molecular analysis revealed a point mutation that created a premature stop codon in the ER gene, resulting in a truncated mutant form of the receptor protein.

The female ERKO mouse shows a number of interesting phenotypes, incuding reduced uterine development, absent uterine responsiveness to E_2, mammary agenesis, hemorrhagic cystic ovaries, anovulation, elevated gonadotropins, and elevated T and E_2. Male ERKO mice exhibit normal gross phenotype, but are infertile as a result of reduced intromissions, reduced sperm counts, and decreased sperm motility. The gross sexual phenotype of the external genitalia and internal androgen-dependent structures appears normal with the exception of testicular dysmorphogenesis and reduced testis size.

6.4. Progesterone-Based Developmental Defects

Defects in progesterone synthesis can arise because of mutations in P450scc and 3β-HSD. However, owing to the pivotal position of progesterone in the synthetic pathways leading to other steroids, the consequences of absence of progesterone synthesis are clouded by the absence of other important steroids. Thus, consequences of defects in progesterone action may be more easily elucidated from cases involving a defective PR. To this end, a PR knockout mouse (PRKO) was recently developed and characterized. Female PRKO mice were anovulatory, possessed underdeveloped mammary glands, and did not display lordosis behavior. However, estrogen treatments did cause uterine enlargement, hyperplasia, and edema, indicating a functional ER system. The male PRKO was fertile and grossly normal, except for an underdeveloped preputial gland.

6.5. Corticoid-Based Developmental Defects

Congenital adrenal hyperplasia is a heritable disorder in which the adrenal does not synthesize cortisol effectively. The inability to synthesize cortisol can result from defects in any of the enzymes involved in synthesis of cortisol from cholesterol. As a consequence of these disorders, feedback inhibition of the pituitary is absent, and high levels of ACTH are secreted, resulting in hypertrophy of the adrenal and, depending on the affected enzyme, high levels of precursors for cortisol synthesis. A large buildup of cortisol precursors can result in synthesis of excess androgens and subsequent masculinization of females.

Deficiency in cholesterol desmolase (P450scc) leads to a deficiency in all steroid hormones and a syndrome referred to as congenital lipoid adrenal hyperplasia. Deficiency in 3β-hydroxysteroid dehydrogenase also leads to a disorder in which synthesis of corticoids and sex steroids is deficient in adrenals and gonads. These disorders are characterized by an inability to produce cortisol and aldosterone, and hence, a reduced ability to regulate glucose metabolism, an inability to conserve salt, and severe hyponatremia. In males, the absence of sex steroids results in feminized external genitalia, whereas secretion of MIS by inguinal testes leads to regression of Mullerian derviatives. Females with P450scc deficiencies are normal in appearance at birth, but do not undergo pubertal changes. Females with 3β-HSD deficiencies may show some masculinization of external genitalia owing to secretion of dehydroepiandrosterone, a weak androgen. Typically, treatment of these disorders involves replacement with gluco- and mineralocorticoid hormones followed by sex steroid therapy near pubertal age.

The most common form of adrenal hyperplasia is the result of deficiency in 21-hydroxylase. The resulting inability to synthesize cortisol leads to a buildup of precursors and subsequent conversion to T. Clinically, females often present with ambiguous genitalia, irregular menstrual cycles, and some virilization. Both sexes undergo rapid somatic growth (postnatal), accelerated skeletal growth, and early closure of epiphyseal plates. Some patients also have defects in the ability to synthesize aldosterone, resulting in a "salt-wasting" form of the disease.

If diagnosed prenatally via genotyping of biopsy samples, dexamethasone treatment of the mother can suppress excess production of androgens by the fetal adrenal cortex and, thus, reduce masculinization of female offspring. Neonatal screening for 21-hydroxylase can be accomplished by assaying for 17-hydroxyprogesterone. This may be useful in preventing deaths related to salt-wasting forms of 21-hydroxylase deficiency.

7. SUMMARY

Steroid hormones are synthesized and secreted by the ovary, testis, adrenal, and placenta. Most documented steroid effects occur through binding to specific intracellular receptor proteins, which regulate gene transcription in target tissues. Steroids are critical for sexual differentiation of different target organs and, in the adult, are important regulators of many aspects of normal physiology. Thus, alterations in either the synthesis of steroid hormones and steroid receptor proteins or mutations in the receptor can result in profound clinical pathologies. Steroid-dependent tumors can become steroid-independent by somatic mutations in receptor genes and alternate splicing of mRNAs. Heritable deficiencies in steroid synthesis or receptor action often lead to permanent alterations in differentiation of adult phenotype and, hence, altered function in the adult. Recent advances in molecular endocrinology have allowed scientists to begin to elucidate the molecular mechanisms by which steroid hormones regulate normal physiology and pathophysiology.

SUGGESTED READING

Clark JH, Markarevich BM. Actions of ovarian steroid hormones. In: Knobil E, Neil J, eds. *The Physiology of Reproduction*, vol. 1. New York: Raven, 1988:675.

Clark JH, Peck EJ, eds. *Female Sex Steroids:Receptors and Function*, New York: Springer-Verlag, 1979.

Coffey DS. Androgen action and the sex accessory tissues. In: Knobil E, Neil J, eds. *The Physiology of Reproduction*, vol. 1. New York: Raven, 1988:1081.

Couse JF, Curtis SW, Washburn TF, et al. Analysis of transcription and estrogen insensitivity in the female mouse after targeted disruption of the estrogen receptor gene. *Mol. Endocrinol.* 1995; 9(11):1441.

Fink G. Gonadotropin secretion and its control. In: Knobil E, Neil J, eds. *The Physiology of Reproduction*. vol. 1. New York: Raven, 1988:1349.

George FW, Wilson JD. Sex determination and differentiation. In: Knobil E, Neil J, eds. *The Physiology of Reproduction*, vol. 1. New York: Raven, 1988:3.

Green S, Chambon P. The oestrogen receptor: from Perception to Mechanism. In: Parker MG, ed. *Nuclear Hormone Receptors: Molecular Mechanisms, Cellular Functions. Clinical Abnormalities*. San Diego: Academic, 1991:15.

Issacs JT. Role of androgens in prostate cancer. In: Litwack G, ed. *Vitamins and Hormones*, vol. 49. San Diego: Academic, 1994:433.

Jordan CV, ed. *Estrogen/Antiestrogen Action and Breast Cancer Therapy*. Madison: University of Wisconsin Press, 1986.

Lindzey J, Kumar MJ, Grossman M, Young C, Tindall, DJ. Molecular mechanisms of androgen action. In: Litwack G, ed. *Vitamins and Hormones*, vol. 49. San Diego: Academic, 1994:383.

Lubahn DB, Moyer JS, Golding TS, Couse JF, Korach KS, Smithies O. Alteration of reproductive function but not prenatal sexual development after insertional disruption of the mouse estrogen receptor gene. *Proc Nat Acad Sci USA* 1993; 90:11162.

Mougdil VK, ed. *Molecular Mechanism of Steroid Hormone Action: Recent Advances*. New York: Walter de Gruyter, 1985.

Parker MG, ed. *Nuclear Hormone Receptors: Molecular Mechanisms, Cellular Functions. Clinical Abnormalities*. San Diego: Academic, 1991.

Sluyser M. Mutations in the estrogen receptor gene. *Hum Mutat* 1995; 6:97.

Smith EP, Boyd J, Frank GR, Takahashi H, Cophen RM, Specker B, Williams TC, Lubahn DB, Korach KS. Estrogen resistance caused by a mutation in the estrogen-receptor gene in a man. *N Engl J Med* 1994; 331:1056.

White PC. Genetic diseases of steroid metabolism. In: Litwack G, ed. *Vitamins and Hormones*, vol. 49. San Diego: Academic, 1994:131.

5 Hormone Actions in the Brain

Bruce S. McEwen, PhD

CONTENTS

1. INTRODUCTION

The central nervous system responds to circulating hormones of the gonads, adrenals, and thyroid gland, as well as being the master controller of endocrine function through the autonomic nervous system and via the hypothalamus and pituitary gland. The actions of hormones on the brain play important roles during early development in the process of sexual differentiation and in actions of thyroid hormone. Circulating hormones are also important chemical signals during adult life in regulating reproductive behavior as well as food, water, and mineral homeostasis and diurnally related neural events involving food intake and cognitive function. Hormones also play an important role as mediators of the impact of stress and the aging process on the brain.

Hormone actions on the brain involve the same cellular and molecular mechanisms of action that

From: *Endocrinology: Basic and Clinical Principles* (P. M. Conn and S. Melmed, eds.), Humana Press Inc., Totowa, NJ.

take place in all hormone target tissues, although there are some important specializations of these mechanisms that allow circulating hormones to work in concert with endogneous neurotransmitters in influencing structural plasticity of synapses and dendrites. Of recent interest are the "neurosteroids," hormones produced within the brain itself, and the related "neuroactive steroids," steroids that act on cell-surface receptors, such as the GABAa-benzodiazepine receptor. There are also actions of circulating hormones on neuropeptide gene expression that have influences on neurotransmission and neuroendocrine function.

This chapter provides an overview of the effects of steroid and thyroid hormone from the cellular and molecular level to the level of integrated neural and neuroendocrine function. It provides a glimpse into the surprising structural plasticity of the adult as well as developing brain, and the important signaling role played by circulating hormones in such plasticity. Finally, the implications of the role hormones play in pathophysiology of some disease processes are considered.

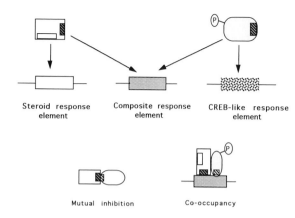

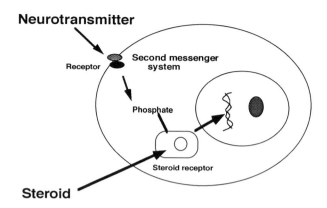

Fig. 1. Steroid hormones act on target genes by attaching to steroid response elements that are usually found in the promotor region. They also can act via composite response elements, along with actions of other DNA-binding proteins, such as members of the CREB family. CREB-like DNA-binding proteins are regulated in their activity by phosphorylation and dephosphorylation related to the activation of second messenger systems.

Fig. 2. Steroid hormones work on at least some target neural cells in cooperation with second messenger activation of the steroid receptor via phosphorylation mechanisms. The second messenger activation of the steroid receptor is sufficient to cause the steroid recetor to bind to DNA response elements and regulate gene expression.

2. CELLULAR AND MOLECULAR MECHANISMS OF HORMONE ACTION

2.1. Actions That Converge on the Genome

Hormones act via a variety of cellular mechanisms involving receptors on cell surfaces or inside cells. Cell-surface receptors respond to protein and polypeptide hormones, as well as small molecules, such as epinephrine, and these receptor either open ion channels or transmit messages across the cell membrane via second messenger systems that act by regulating the phosphorylation of target proteins inside of cells. The target proteins are themselves important cellular consititutents, such as membrane or intracellular receptors, G-proteins, ion channels, enzymes, or DNA-binding proteins that regulate gene expression. Steroid hormones and thyroid hormone enter cells and interact with "hormone responsive elements, HRE" via intracellular protein receptors (*see* Chapters 4 and 19). HREs are nucleotide sequences associated with hormone-regulated genes, in their promotor regions. The hormone receptors bind to the HREs and thereby alter the rate of transcription of the particular gene (see Fig. 1). DNA-binding proteins that regulate gene transcription are called "transacting factors." The presence of HREs upstream of the promotor regions of a gene is indicative of regulation of that gene by hormones, although the absence of the typical HREs does not

necessarily rule out hormonal regulation for reasons that are explained below.

Second messengers affect gene expression by altering the phosphorylation state of proteins that bind to DNA in a manner similar to steroid and thyroid hormone receptors. The CREB family of transacting factors is regulated by phosphorylation via a cAMP-dependent protein kinase (*See* Chapter 3). Transacting factors exist for which phosphorylation is controlled by calcium-calmodulin protein kinases or by protein kinase C, which is stimulated by diacylglycerol, a product of phospholipase C cleavage of inositol phospholipids.

Steroid hormone receptors can be activated via second messenger systems. Dopamine has been shown to activate progesterone receptors, and result in nuclear translocation and gene activation even in the absence of progesterone. This mechanism appears to participate in the regulation of sexual behavior in the female rat (*see* Fig. 2).

Many of the transactivators described above work together, sometimes in concert, and sometimes in competition to regulate different genes. HREs represent one kind of nucleotide sequence capable of responding to transacting factors. As noted in Fig. 1, analogous sites for CREB and other transacting factors have been identified, and there are also so-called composite response elements that require several transacting factors for activity. These are different from the simple response elements and HREs referred to above. Depending on the gene being reg-

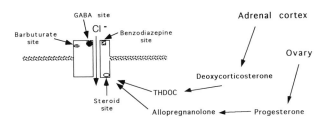

Modulated ion channel

Fig. 3. Neuroactive steroids bind to the GABAa receptor, which gates a chloride channel. Together with benzodiazepines, barbiturates, and GABA itself, the neuroactive steroid facilitates opening of the ion channel. The neuroactive steroids, such as tetrahydrodeoxycorticosterone (THDOC) and allopregnenolone, are A-ring-reduced metabolites of deoxycorticosterone and progesterone, respectively.

ulated, the binding of both a steroid hormone receptor and another transactivator may stimulate or may inhibit transcription. As represented in Figure 1, transactivators also interact with each other directly, resulting in mutual inhibition by removing themselves from the ability to bind to DNA, or resulting in what is called "tethering" as a means of increasing or decreasing the binding affinity to DNA.

2.2. Steroid Actions at the Cell Surface

Steroid hormones are also capable of an entirely different mode of action via cell-surface receptors that affect membrane excitability. In the early history of the study of steroid hormone action, such interactions were recognized in the pioneering work of Selye (1941) on anesthetic effects of progesterone and progesterone derivatives. Many decades later, progesterone metabolites, as well as metabolites of desoxycorticosterone, were recognized to bind to sites on the chloride channel of the GABAa receptor and positively regulate chloride flux through the channel. (*see* Fig. 3). Such effects may be involved in the normal stress response, as well during the estrous cycle, because natural metabolites with high affinity for the GABAa receptor are produced after stress and at the time of the proestrus peak of progesterone. Anxiolytic and antiepileptic effects appear to result from these interactions in vivo.

In addition to affecting the GABAa receptor, there are known interactions of progesterone with the calcium ion mobilizing systems of spermatozoa and oocytes, and with membrane receptors that regulate dopamine and luteinizing hormone-releasing hormone (LHRH) release in brain. There are also actions of estradiol via non-*N*-methyl-D-aspartate receptor (NMDA) receptors in cerebellum, cortex, and hippocampus that facilitate excitatory effects of glutamate. Two other endogenous steroids, pregnenolone sulfate and dehydroepiandrosterone sulfate (DHAS), affect the excitatory activity of NMDA receptors and influence calcium channel activity. They are also reported to be enhancers of memory retention in mice.

DHA and DHAS (Fig. 4) occur in the blood, and their levels decline with increasing age and during a number of pathophysiological conditions. These two steroids are also known to have enhancing effects on the immune system, and they protect from viral infections and interfere with immunosuppressive effects of such glucocorticoids. In many respects, DHA behaves like a glucocorticoid antagonist, yet no receptor mechanism has been elucidated for its actions.

2.3. Neurosteroids and Neuroactive Steroids

Pregnenolone sulfate and DHAs are examples of "neurosteroids," steroids that are generated by neural tissue following the side-chain cleavage of cholesterol. Progesterone is also generated as a "neurosteroid" (*see* Fig. 4). The capacity of the brain to produce its own steroids had been a mystery until recently, when it was been shown that one of these neurosteroids, progesterone, is an important factor in the growth of Schwann cells and formation of myelin. Thus, the production of endogenous steroids by the brain may play a local signaling role in neuronal development, differentiation, or survival.

3. CIRCULATING HORMONES AS MEDIATORS OF CHANGE IN ADULT BRAIN

How do these diverse mechanisms of steroid hormone action in brain regulate physiological processes? One of the most important roles of circulating hormones is to coordinate cellular and organ responses during cyclic processes, such as reproduction and daily sleep–waking activity, by synchronizing neural activity and behavior with processes throughout the body. Circulating hormones complement the actions of neural connections and release of neurotransmitters, in that, whereas neural actions are rapid, hormone actions have longer-lasting influences

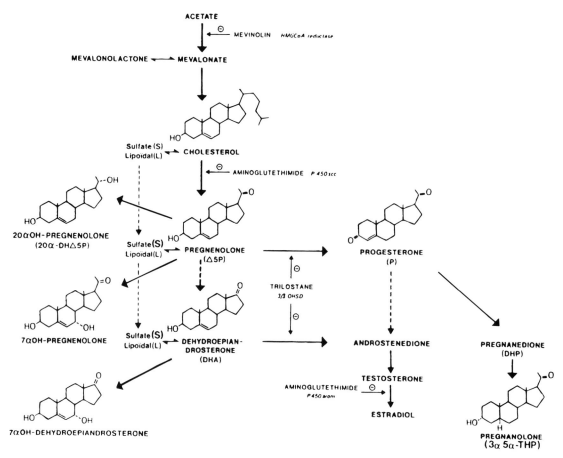

Fig. 4. Biosynthesis/metabolism of so-called neurosteroids in the Central Nervous System. The conversion Δ5P to DHA is postulated, but not demonstrated. Δ5PS and DHAS inhibit, and 3α5α-THP potentiates GABAa receptor function. Full arrows indicate demonstrated pathways; dotted arrows indicate possible pathways. Metabolic inhibitors of enzymes are indicated by 0. From Baulieu and Robel (1990) by permission.

and can affect tissues independently of whether they are innervated, providing they have hormone receptors. Gonadal hormones act both in the brain and peripherally to coordinate the timing of mating with the optimal chance for pregnancy, and adrenal hormones play a key role both peripherally and centrally in coordinating energy metabolism with food-seeking behavior and cognitive alertness. Adrenocortical steroids also play an important role in maintaining water and mineral homeostasis and do so, in part, through actions on ingestive behaviors.

3.1. Cyclic Events Associated with Ovarian Function and Reproductive Behavior

The capacity for reproduction is usually tied to cycles—seasonal in some species, monthly in humans and primates, and on the order of a few days in rats and mice. The ovarian cycle of the female is the key

for successful reproduction; for the rat, synchronizing the time of ovulation with the time of behavioral sexual receptivity and preparation of the reproductive tract for pregnancy is the function of circulating estradiol and progesterone. In males, actions of testosterone may be seasonal or more or less continuous.

Although many aspects of reproduction have been intensively investigated by endocrinologists, reproductive behavior has been the province of behavioral scientists, that is, until the past two decades, when behavioral neuroscience has emerged and moved ever closer to the cellular, molecular, anatomical and neurophysiological aspects of neuroscience as well as to cellular and molecular endocrinology. And studies of lordosis behavior in the female rat have been particularly useful in elucidating brain mechanisms underlying reproductive behavior. This is because there is a well-localized hypothalamic

Table 1
Estrogen Effects In Vivo on Structure and Neurochemistry of
Ventromedial Nucleus of Female Rat

Parameter	Time frame
Cell nuclear volume increases	Rapid, several hours
Nucleolar volume increases	Rapid, several hours
More ribosomal RNA and rough RER	Rapid, several hours
Increased synaptic density	Delayed, 12–48 h
Induction of gene products	Delayed, 12–48 h
Progestin receptors	
Oxytocin receptors	
Preproenkephalin mRNA	
Nitric oxide synthase	
Isozyme of protein kinase C	

These changes underlie the activation of the lordosis response, which is controlled by the VMN in the female rat.

region, the ventromedial nuclei, that responds to ovarian hormones and regulates the behavioral response. The mechanisms by which hormones affect lordosis behavior are believed to have some relevance to the actions of androgens on the male brain for the control of male sexual behavior.

In the female rat, the 4–5 d estrous cycle is tightly coupled to the diurnal clock, and increasing levels of estradiol during the initial phase of the cycle serve to amplify a diurnal peak of luteinizing hormone (LH) secretion, so that on the afternoon of proestrus, this peak becomes the LH surge, which is the immediate stimulus for ovulation. The LH surge also stimulates a surge of ovarian progesterone release; the progesterone synergizes with the prior secretion of estradiol to trigger neural mechanisms subserving the mating response of the female rat, namely, lordosis behavior. Lordosis behavior is primed by estradiol acting in various neural sites, principally the ventromedial nuclei (VMN) of the hypothalamus, and a number of neurotransmitter systems are believed to be involved. Estradiol priming acts via genomic receptors in the cell nuclei of VMN neurons to induce a number of fundamental changes in these cells, as summarized in Table 1. These changes illustrate types of cellular responses that may characterize the response of other neuronal systems to circulating hormones of the adrenals, gonads, and thyroid gland, and they also provide clues regarding the control mechanism that governs sexual behavior in the female rat.

The VMN is not the only brain region to show cyclic changes with ovarian function. Estradiol and progesterone regulate cyclic synaptogenesis in the CA1 region of the hippocampus, and this process involves a complex interaction between circulating ovarian steroids and endogenous neurotransmitters, particularly excitatory amino acids and GABA. Blockade of NMDA receptors during estrogen treatment prevents synapse induction, indicating that excitatory neurotransmission is vital to synapse formation. On the other hand, downregulation of the induced synapses involves progestin receptors, as indicated by the ability of the intracellular progestin receptor antagonist, Ru486, to prevent the natural down-regulation of synapses that occurs in the 24 h between the day of proestrus and the day of estrus. The role of these cyclic changes in hippocampus, a brain region involved in memory and spatial orientation, may be to provide enhanced capacity for spatial or other information processing at the time of ovulation and mating.

3.2. Coordination of Food-Seeking, Metabolism, Salt Intake, and Cognition

Sodium homeostasis, blood pressure regulation, circadian rhythmicity, energy metabolism, and locomotor activity are physiological processes that are regulated by circulating adrenal steroids. Both mineralocorticoids, such as aldosterone, and glucocorticoids are involved, and they produce their effects in large part through two types of intracellular receptors, Type I and Type II. Type I receptors, otherwise known as mineralocorticoid receptors, are high-affinity receptors for aldosterone and for glucocorticoids; whereas Type II receptors, otherwise known as glucocorticoid receptors, have a low affinity for aldosterone and a moderately high affinity for glucocorticods. In discussing the involvement of adrenal steroids, we will refer to evidence generated for the involvement of Type I and Type II receptors from the use of specific receptor agonists or antagonists.

3.2.1. SODIUM APPETITE

The effects of mineralocorticoids on sodium intake are biphasic, with adrenalectomized rats displaying an avid appetite for sodium that is owing in part to increased angiotensin II activity acting on the brain as the consequences of renal sodium loss resulting from the removal of the adrenal steroids. Mineralocorticoid administration that returns steroid levels to the normal physiological range decreases the appetite for sodium by restoring sodium balance and by normalizing angiotensin activity. However, going beyond the physiological range, administration of either aldosterone or deoxycorticosterone to adrenalectomized rats at pharmacological doses will cause a mineralocorticoid-induced sodium intake. This appetite is induced independently of brain angiotensin and is similar to that seen in adrenal intact rats given pharmacological doses of mineralocorticoids. In addition, adrenally intact rats that are depleted of sodium by various natural or pharmacological treatments also express a sodium appetite, and this sodium appetite occurs through the synergistic interaction between aldosterone and the central renin-angiotensin system. When the Type I receptor antagonist, RU28318, is infused into the cerebral ventricles, the synergistic interaction with brain angiotensin is blocked and sodium appetite is suppressed. Other neuropeptides, particularly oxytocin and tachykinins, play a role in the neural regulation of salt appetite as inhibitors.

3.2.2. BLOOD PRESSURE

Mineralocorticoid infusion into the cerebral ventricles or deoxycorticosterone given systemically increases blood pressure, whereas glucocorticoid infusion has the opposite effect. Type I receptors promote increased blood pressure, in that the hypertension is reversed, and basal blood pressure is decreased, by the central infusion of the Type I receptor antagonist RU28318. In contrast, Type II receptors promote decreased blood pressure.

3.2.3. CIRCADIAN BEHAVIORS AND FOOD INTAKE

The adrenal steroids are secreted in a circadian pattern, and this secretion helps to coordinate daily activities, such as sleep–wake cycles, ingestive, and locomotor behavior. Prior to waking and the beginning of the daily cycle of eating and drinking, plasma adrenocorticotrophic hormone (ACTH) and corticosterone levels reach their diurnal peak. This daily rise in corticosterone occurs at a time when energy stores are low; and it helps promote both gluconeogenesis as well as appetite for food. Therefore, the rise in glucocorticoids precedes, and may act as a signal for, feeding. This is best demonstrated in food-restricted animals where the peak of circadian corticosterone precedes the time of restricted food availability and schedule-induced behaviors, such as wheel running and polydipsia (see Section 3.2.4). These schedule-induced behaviors are attenuated by adrenalectomy and return with adrenal steroid replacement. The best studied of these behaviors is food intake.

An important aspect of adrenal steroid action in normal physiology is its ability to activate food intake and specific hunger for carbohydrates at the time of waking during the diurnal rest–activity cycle in animals having normal body weight. Both mineralocorticoids and glucocorticoids modulate food intake by interaction with multiple neurotransmitter systems that include the α-adrenergic system, neuropeptide Y (NPY), and galanin. When administered systemically or directly into the paraventricular nucleus, low levels of corticosterone and aldosterone facilitate food intake and ingestive behavior, but higher levels of corticosterone suppress food intake and reduce body weight, although such inhibitory effects are replaced by stimulatory ones when there has been food deprivation and body weight loss, with a depletion of endogenous energy reserves.

Type I adrenal steroid receptors are implicated in the stimulatory effects of aldosterone and low doses of corticosterone on food intake, whereas Type II receptors are implicated in the inhibitory effects of high levels of corticosterone as well as of synthetic steroids, like dexamethasone and RU28362, on food intake. Type I receptors have been found in low levels in the hypothalamus along with Type II receptors, although Type I receptors are more plentiful in other brain areas, especially the hippocampus, where their relatioship to control of food intake is unknown.

3.2.4. FOOD INTAKE AND OBESITY

High levels of glucocorticoids suppress food intake and reduce body weight, except when endogenous energy reserves have already been depleted by prior food deprivation and body weight loss. In animal models of inherited obesity, treatment with the Type II receptor antagonist, RU38486, is effective (as is adrenalectomy) in preventing the onset of obesity. Increased food intake and body weight, leading to obesity, occur naturally in several strains of rats and mice. Obesity can also be produced experimentally by lesions of the paraventricular and ventromedial nuclei of the hypothalamus. Both natural and lesion-induced obesity are dependent to a very large degree on the presence of circulating adrenal steroids, and obesity can be attenuated by adrenalectomy. Genetically obese mice and rats show enhanced basal secretion of ACTH and corticosterone, as well as enhanced sensitivity to glucocorticoid effects on target tissues. Furthermore, Type II receptors are prominent in these effects.

3.2.5. "Food-Shift" Effect

In addition to obesity, the other striking connection between glucocorticoids and food intake is the "food-shift" effect, in which the adrenal steroids play an important role in synchronizing food intake with food availability. When food is available for restricted periods, an anticipatory elevation of glucocorticoids occurs along with a shift in body temperature; this shift is independent of the suprachiasmatic nucleus or ventromedial nucleus, and blinding or constant light do not prevent it. Thus, the cycle of fasting and eating appears to be a more potent synchronizer of the hypothalamo-pituitary-adrenal (HPA) axis than the light-dark cycle and may involve a neural timing system lying outside of the suprachiasmatic nucleus (SCN) clock.

Although the hypothalamus is most directly implicated in glucocorticoid actions on food intake, the anticipation of food availability and whether or not food actually becomes available appears to involve information passing through the hippocampal formation. This is because rats with damage to the fornix or ablation of the hippocampus fail to show elevations of plasma corticosterone when eating is blocked or during the initial phase of extinction of lever response for food reward.

3.2.6. Schedule-Induced Behaviors

Both food and water deprivation lead to increased corticosterone secretion, particularly in anticipation of access to food and water or when there is a high level of uncertainty regarding its availability. The consummatory act leads to a reduction in glucocorticoid levels, sometimes in conjunction with a biphasic elevation. Neither salt hunger nor water deprivation is as potent synchronizer of HPA activity as food deprivation.

Related to the food-shift effect described above are the schedule-induced behaviors. The mesolimbic dopamine system is involved in schedule-induced polydipsia. Moreover, adrenal steroids appear to control this behavior negatively, in that it is elevated by adrenalectomy. Furthermore, adrenal steroids are part of a negative feedback loop, and adrenal steroid levels are elevated in rats that have acquired this behavior, but glucocorticoid secretion is reduced during the actual behavior. The negative feedback loop between adrenal steroids and schedule-induced behavior is consistent with decreased glucocorticoid secretion as a result of consummatory behaviors in rats that are food-deprived and show elevated, anticipatory glucocorticoid levels. Such a link to expectation takes us back to another brain structure, namely, the hippocampus. As noted above in discussing the "food-shift" effect, there is evidence in these latter situations that the hippocampus plays a role in the recognition that expectations are violated or met.

3.2.7. Locomotor Activity

There is a diurnal rhythm of food intake and locomotor activity that is synchronized in part by adrenocortical secretions. Adrenalectomy decreases spontaneous exploratory activity in rats, and corticosterone restores this activity. Hippocampal lesions increase locomotor activity, and these effects are also reduced by chemical adrenalectomy with metyrapone, indicating that the hippocampus is an inhibitor of locomotor activity and not the primary site of action of glucocorticoids to facilitate locomotion. However, as we have noted above, the hippocampus may be involved in timing of motor events and matching them to the appropriate cues.

In addition to the hippocampus, the nigrostriatal system is involved in the synchronization of locomotor activity, and neuropeptides, such as enkephalin and substance P, appear to be implicated, since enkephalin and substance P administration into both ventral tegmentum and nucleus accumbens stimulates locomotor activity. Glucocorticoids elevate preproenkephalin and neurokinin A mRNA, and there is evidence for a diurnal rhythm of neuropeptide mRNA and enkephalin release.

Spontaneous locomotor activity in rats predicts their propensity to self-administer amphetamine and cocaine, and drug self-administration is at least partially dependent on adrenal steroids.

3.2.8. SLEEP

Adrenal steroids have been shown to influence sleep in humans and in experimental animals, and the diurnal rhythm of glucocorticoid secretion involves a peak at the end of the sleeping period. In humans, glucocorticoids, as well as ACTH infusions, produce a reduction in total time in rapid eye movement (REM) sleep. Moreover, glucocorticoids tend to increase intermittent wakefulness yet the natural glucocorticoid, cortisol, increases slow-wave sleep time, whereas synthetic glucocorticoids and ACTH infusions do not do so. Addison's disease patients respond poorly to ACTH infusions and show less reduction in REM sleep time than normal subjects receiving ACTH, whereas Cushing's disease patients, having excess adrenal steroid secretion, have much reduced levels of total sleep and REM sleep. In studies with an antagonist of Type I receptors, potassium canrenoate, the reduction of increased slow-wave sleep by cortisol was antagonized, whereas the cortisol effect to reduce REM sleep duration was not blocked by canrenoate, suggesting that it might be mediated by Type II receptors.

3.2.9. NEURONAL EXCITABILITY AND LONG-TERM POTENTIATION (LTP)

Adrenal steroids modulate excitability of hippocampal neurons in a biphasic manner, with Type I receptors enhancing excitability and Type II receptors inhibiting it. These effects are manifested in the excitability that relates to LTP, a possible model of processes involved in learning and memory. The biphasic modulation of excitability and LTP is consistent with information on animal and human cognitive function, in which high levels of glucocorticoids impair hippocampally related cognitive processes, whereas low to moderate levels may be associated with the coordination of cognitive function in the diurnal cycle and thereby also associated with the cognitive dysfunction that accompanies jet lag.

4. IMPACT OF STRESSFUL EXPERIENCE ON THE BRAIN

An important function of circulating hormones is to mediate responses to external challenges that are frequently stressful to the organism. Natural disasters, transportation accidents, military combat, rape, physical trauma, and stressful life events, such as job loss, divorce, and death of a loved one, are all occurrences that are not cyclic and that produce a huge impact on those who experience them.

One of the main roles of hormonal responses to stressful situations is to protect the organism from further damage, although at the same time, there are circumstances in which the same hormones exacerbate damage (*See* Fig. 5). The secretion of adrenaline and adrenocortical hormones is the most general hormonal feature of the stress response. Whereas adrenaline secretion is a rapid reaction and involved in the "fight-or-flight" reaction, the role of adrenal steroids is as a second line of defense, helping to restore and repair systems and also preventing the primary reactions, such as adrenaline secretion, from gaining the upper hand. Both inflammation and primary immune responses are examples of rapid reactions to insults to the body, and glucocorticoids contain and "counterregulate" these actions.

Neurochemical systems in the brain follow a similar pattern, i.e., a primary response to stressors and "counterregulation" by glucocorticoids (*see* Fig. 5). The production and secretion of corticotrophin releasing factor (CRF) is a primary response mechanism to stressors, leading to behavioral activation and to the secretion of ACTH and glucocorticoids, as well as immunosuppressive effects. Glucocorticoid secretion counterregulates part of this system, particularly the hypothalamic production of CRF, and it keeps this part of the corticotrophin-releasing hormone (CRH) system in check. Likewise, noradrenaline (NA) is released from the locus cerulus system in response to arousing and stressful stimuli, and repeated stress induces a progressively greater capacity to produce and release NA, because it induces the rate-limiting biosynthetic enzyme, tyrosine hydroxylase. Glucocorticoids keep this system in check by inhibiting release of catecholamines and by reducing the postsynaptic response to released NA via a suppression of the adenylate cyclase response to NA.

Like the noradrenergic system, the serotonergic system is turned on by stressful events. Glucocorticoids facilitate the synthesis of serotonin, but glucocorticoid feedback counterregulates the 5HT1A receptors in hippocampus. However, it also upregulates the 5HT2 receptor in cerebral cortex. The

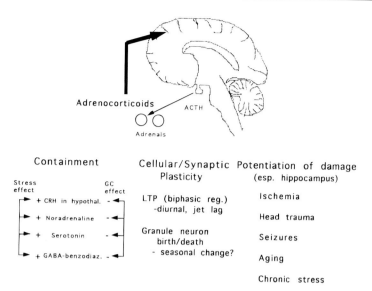

Fig. 5. Adrenal steroids exert paradoxical effects on the brain. On the one hand, they protect the brain by counterregulating neurochemical responses set in motion by stressful events, such as the release of CRH, noradrenaline, serotonin, and excitatory amino acids. On the other hand, they exacerbate damage produced by insults, such as ischemia, head trauma, and seizures, and they participate in neuronal loss during aging and as a result of chronic stress.

response of the brain to serotonin is thus modulated in different brain regions, and there is also regional modulation by glucocorticoids of the responses to CRF and NA. For example, there are a number of groups of neurons making CRH outside of the hypothalamus that are not counterregulated by glucocorticoids. Likewise, the counterregulation of cyclic AMP production and adenylate cyclase activity is more pronounced in the cerebral cortex than in the hippocampus.

Glucocorticoid actions on neurochemical systems involve more than counterregulation. We have noted that acute actions of corticosteroids facilitate the stress-induced activity of the serotonergic system and also potentiate the activity of GABAa-benzodiazepine receptors. Both of these effects may be produced by nongenomic actions of steroids. Although it is not known how glucocorticoids activate serotonin formation, metabolites of deoxycorticosterone, a steroid release by the adrenal cortex during stress, activate GABAa-benzodiazepine receptors, as shown in Fig. 3.

The actions of glucocorticoids on neurochemical systems modulate their arousal and excitation, and prevent any of them from overresponding to stressful stimuli. The protective role of adrenal steroids in relation to behavioral consequences of stress may be related to the finding that adrenalectomy enhances the development of learned helplessness in rats in

response to inescapable shock. Learned helplessness is a putative animal model of depressive illness, and depression may thus be regarded as a failure of normal adapation in the face of stressful experiences.

5. STEROID HORMONES REGULATE NEURONAL MORPHOLOGY AND NEURONAL SURVIVAL

One of the most surprising aspects of steroid hormone action in the adult brain is their influence on synaptic and dendritic morphology, and neurogenesis and neuronal survival. Estrogen-induced synaptogenesis (*see* Section 3.1.) is a cyclic event detected in both the hippocampus and ventromedial hypothalamus during the estrous cycle of the female rat. Androgen induction of synapse formation and enlargement of neuronal processes have been found in the spinal nucleus of the bulbocavernosus, which innervates the penis. Adrenal steroids, on the other hand, are involved in somewhat paradoxical effects on neuronal survival and morphology in the hippocampus (*see* Fig. 6).

Type I adrenal steroid receptors also play an important role in stabilizing the neuronal population of the dentate gyrus, since adrenalectomy has been found to cause the death of granule neurons, and aldosterone replacement of adrenalectomized rats blocks this neuronal death. When adrenalectomy stimulates granule neuron death, it also accelerates

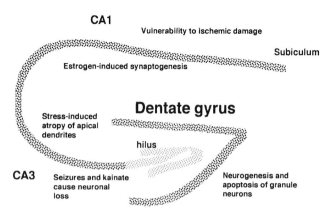

Fig. 6. Plasticity and vulnerability of the hippocampus. Cross-section of the hippocampal formation showing the location of dentate gyrus, hilus, and Ammons horn areas CA1 and CA3, as well as subiculum. Events are indicated involving plasticity of the hippocampus in which sex and stress hormones are involved.

the process of neurogenesis in the dentate gyrus of the adult rats, and new granule neurons are born. The functional significance of the neuronal birth and death in the dentate gyrus of the adult rat is presently obscure, but it is conceivable that it is part of a seasonal or even diurnal mechanism by which neuronal number is changed.

The actions of adrenal steroids on dentate gyrus granule neurons are but one example of hormone effects on neuronal morphology. Yet another example of morphological plasticity is the damaging effect of adrenal steroids on hippocampal pyramidal neurons. Loss of pyramidal neurons in the hippocampus was first described during aging in the rat. The loss could be attenuated by adrenalectomy in midlife, and glucocorticoid treatment for 12 wk caused pyramidal neuron loss in the hippocampal formation of young adult rats. Prolonged social stress was later shown to produce hippocampal neuronal loss in vervet monkeys and tree shrews, and it has been tempting to conclude that stress-induced secretion of glucocorticoids is to blame (*see* Fig. 6).

However, the probable mechanism for hippocampal neuronal loss is a good deal more complicated. This was first indicated by the finding that neuronal damage produced by the excitotoxin, kainic acid, was potentiated by endogenous and exogenous glucocorticoids. Likewise, ischemic damage to the hippocampus, which also involves excitatory amino acids, is potentiated by glucocorticoids, and excitotoxic effects on hippocampal neurons in cell culture

are exacerbated by glucocorticoids in the medium acting via Type II glucocorticoid receptors.

There are also important regional differences within the hippocampal formation, namely, that ischemic damage is worse in CA1 pyramidal neurons and subiculum, whereas age- and stress-related damage is more pronounced in the CA3 pyramidal layer (*see* Fig. 6). One difference between these two regions is that the CA3 neurons receive the mossy fiber input from the dentate gyrus as well as a direct perforant pathway input from the entorhinal cortex, wheras CA1 neurons do not receive the Schaeffer collateral input from the CA3 neurons.

The CA3 neurons are known to be very susceptible to seizure-induced damage. CA3 neurons also respond to several weeks of repeated restraint stress or to repeated injections of corticosterone by showing atrophy of the apical dendrites of the long-shaft pyramidal neurons. This atrophy does not occur in the basal dendrites, and there is no indication of neuronal death. The stress-induced atrophy can be blocked by several types of treatments:

1. Interference with release and action of excitatory amino acids by phenytoin;
2. Enhancement of serotonin reuptake by tianeptine, an atypical tricyclic antidepressant drug; and
3. Inhibition of adrenal steroid synthesis in response to stress.

The atrophy of dendrites of CA3 pyramidal neurons may represent the first stage of the degenerative process, or, alternatively, it may represent an adaptive mechanism that is intended to protect the CA3 neurons from overstimulation. Further research is needed to distinguish between these possibilities, but it is clear that the hippocampus is a vulnerable brain structure, and that permanent damage can result from severe and prolonged stress, as well as from seizures and ischemia.

6. CIRCULATING HORMONES AND DEVELOPMENTAL TRAJECTORIES

Developmental actions of hormones are qualitatively different from the reversible and cyclic actions, in that they are permanent, and they set the stage for the susceptibility and responsivity of the mature organism to hormones and other regulatory agents. Here developmental actions of thyroid hormone, testosterone, and of adrenal steroids, as well as early stressful experience, will be described.

6.1. Thyroid Hormone

Thyroid hormone action early in life plays a key role in determining the normal timing of neural development. Both the excess and the insufficiency of thyroid hormone during early development leads to abnormalities in brain structure that are particularly evident in the basal forebrain and hippocampus. Insufficiency of thyroid hormone during this same time, or even later in postnatal life, was reported to decrease neuronal number in the CA1 pyramidal cell layer of the hippocampus, but not in the CA3 region. The dendritic and glial morphology of the hippocampus and basal forebrain has so far not been investigated in relation to postnatal hypothyroidism, but one would predict opposite effects to those seen after developmentally induced hyperthyroidism. This is because transient excess of thyroid hormone on days 1 and 4 of postnatal life in rats caused hypertrophied development of pyramidal neurons of the CA3 region of hippocampus, and of astroglial cells within the hippocampus and basal forebrain. The basal forebrain cholinergic system was also permanently increased by transient postnatal hyperthyroidism. In contrast to the newborn brain, hyperthyroidism in adulthood causes different changes, namely, a reduction in dendritic spine density in the CA1 region of the hippocampus.

6.2. Sexual Differentiation

In sexual differentiation of the brain, reproductive tract, and secondary sex characteristics, the presence or absence of testosterone determines two distinctly different patterns of development.

6.2.1. THE BASIC PLAN AND ITS VARIANTS

Sexual differentiation is an event in which "nurture" triumphs over "nature," in that testosterone can turn a genetic female into a phenotypic male. In mammals, the principal role of the Y chromosome is to determine that the presumptive gonad differentiates into a testis, whereas the presence of two X chromosomes means that ovaries will develop. The testes then secrete testosterone during a specific period of embryonic or neonatal life, whereas the ovary does not secrete any hormones during this time. As a result of the actions of testosterone on a variety of tissues, including the brain, the masculine phenotype becomes differentiated.

Various plans exist in the animal kingdom. Insects, such as the fruit fly, undergo sexual differentiation as a "cell autonomous" event, meaning that

there are no hormonal signals, and embryos made up as mosaics of male and female cells will show the expression of male and female phenotypes next to one another in the same organism. In fish, such as the Wrasse, the death of the male in a colony triggers the selection of one of the females to differentiate into a male; thus, there is no such thing as a genetic determination of sex in the Wrasse, but, rather, a socially determined control mechanism. Marsupials follow the mammalian plan for the most part, but certain traits, such as the pouch of the female and scrotum of the male, differentiate independently of testosterone, almost as if they were directly programmed by the X and Y chromosomes, respectively. Finally, birds generally have the opposite pattern of sex chromosomes from the mammals, namely, that the male is homozygous (WW), whereas the female is heterozygous (WZ). Thus, the female becomes different from the basic male pattern owing to the secretion of gonadal hormones during early development.

There are three phases of testosterone secretion during early life in the developing human male: a testosterone peak at midgestation (12–20 wk), which masculinizes the reproductive tract and probably also the hypothalamus; a second testosterone surge within the first year after birth, which may act on the developing cerebral hemispheres; and a third testosterone elevation at the time of puberty. In the rat, the first two peaks are fused into one, since the rat is born in an immature state; however, there are important distinctions between what happens prenatally and postnatally.

6.2.2. BRAIN SEXUAL DIFFERENTIATION

How do we know that the brain undergoes sexual differentiation? Until the late 1960s, the brain was not regarded as different between males and females. Then a landmark paper was published by Geoffrey Raisman and Pauline Field (1971) showing morphological sex differences using the electron microscope that are developmentally programmed by testosterone early in postnatal life. This study opened the floodgates of studies at the light microscopic and neurochemical level that established numerous sex differences in brains of rats, songbirds, and other species, including humans. One of the earliest examples of a morphological sex difference at the light microscopic levels for mammals was the finding of the sexually dimorphic nucleus of the preoptic areas, whereas sex differences were described in vocal control areas of the songbird brain. Another important example concerns the sexual dimorphism of the spinal nucleus of the bulbocavernosus muscle, which innervates the penis and is present only in males. The retention of this nucleus during early development is promoted by the presence of androgens, which promote survival of the muscle and of the motor neurons that innervate them; an important question is whether the androgen is acting on the muscle, on the motor neurons, or on both.

6.2.3. MECHANISMS OF NEURAL SEXUAL DIFFERENTIATION

Brain sex differences arise through the developmental actions of testosterone (or its metabolite, estradiol) on developing neuronal systems via intracellular androgen and estrogen receptors. During pre- or early postnatal development, depending on the species, these receptors are expressed permanently in hypothalamus, preoptic area, and pituitary, and transiently in cerebral cortex and hippocampus. What cellular events do these receptors control that lead to the structural sex differences (see Fig. 7)? Neuronal migration and survival are among the processes influenced by hormones that give rise to morphological sex differences, and the actions of testosterone to promote a larger sexually dimorphic nucleus of the preoptic area and larger nucleus of the bulbocarvernosus of the spinal cord involve promoting the survival of neurons born before the expression of gonadal steroid receptors.

Hormones also promote differentiation of specific programs of response of neuronal systems when they are mature. For example, progestin receptor induction by estradiol is reduced in male rats by developmental actions of testosterone at birth, and blockade of aromatization of testosterone in neonatal male rats allows female-like progestin receptor induction as well as estrogen and progestin activation of female sexual (lordosis) behavior. Moreover, the ability of estradiol to induced cyclic synaptogenesis in the ventromedial hypothalamus of the adult female rat is suppressed early in life by the defeminizing actions of testosterone in the male. The same thing is true for estrogen induction of synapses in hippocampus. In this case, blockade or aromatizing enzymes at birth renders the male hippocampus more sensitive to the synapse-inducing effects of estradiol in adult life. The hippocampus expresses both estrogen receptors and aromatizing enzymes transiently during neonatal life, and the actions of testosterone or estradiol during this period causes spatial navigation to develop in a male-like manner.

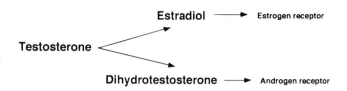

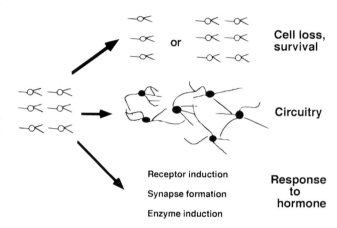

Fig. 7. Testosterone promotes sexual differentiation by acting as a prohormone, which is converted either into dihydrotestosterone and acts via androgen receptors or to estradiol and acts via estrogen receptors. Mechanisms at the cellular level for sexual differentiation of the brain include hormone actions to promote neuronal survival or cell loss; actions that alter the circuitry and patterns of connectivity between nerve cells; and actions that result in male and female brain cells that respond qualitatively or quantitatively in different ways to the actions of circulating hormones during adult life.

6.2.4. SEX DIFFERENCES IN THE HUMAN BRAIN

In humans, as in the rat, nuclei in the hypothalamus are larger in men than in women. On the other hand, the size of segments of the corpus callosum and the anterior commissure, both of which connect the two cerebral hemispheres, are greater in women than in men, on the average; this feature correlates with, and may eventually help to explain, the greater ability of women to overcome congenital defects or brain damage to one cerebral hemisphere by using the other cerebral hemisphere to compensate.

Because brain sex differences have been detected in the human species as differences in size of cell groupings, or "nuclei" at the hypothalamic level as well as in the size and shape of the corpus callosum and anterior commissure, this leads to the conclusion that the process of sexual differentiation may well operate on the human brain much as it does in lower mammalian species. However, it is not clear whether the midgestation testosterone peak or the postnatal testosterone elevation is responsible for producing these sex differences.

6.2.5. FUNCTIONAL IMPLICATIONS OF BRAIN SEX DIFFERENCES

Although many of the structural sex differences in the brain are not tied to known functions, some of the morphological sex differences have clear and specific functional correlates. In songbirds, the size of brain nuclei that control the production of song is larger in males than in females in accordance with the greater and more complex song production by males. In rats and other species, the male has a spinal motor control nucleus that innervates the penis; as noted, this nucleus is absent in females.

In our own species, it is difficult to specify the behavioral or neurological traits that are associated with the morphological sex differences. Play behavior of children has been studied with regard to boy–girl differences in energy level and choice of play styles and toys, by analogy with studies in rhesus monkeys and rats showing that males engage in more "rough and tumble" play. However, attribution of sex differences in behavior to developmental hormonal influences is virtually impossible owing to the many social factors that contribute to play behavior in children. A more objective end point has been spatial learning, as in the mental rotation of figures test, and we have noted above that, in rats, development of a male-like spatial orientation is dependent on the developmental actions of testosterone acting via estradiol and affecting the hippocampus, among other brain regions. For spatial performance in humans, men outperform women significantly on mental rotation of figures. However, just as there is overlap in brain morphological traits between men and women, so is there overlap in test scores on the mental rotation test, so that sex differences in mean measures should not obscure the fact that there is much overlap between the sexes. Nevertheless, there are some data showing a developmental endocrine influence on this test. In the adrenogenital syndrome (AGS), genetic females with an enzyme defect in adrenal steroid production produce androgens that masculinize the fetus; normally the masculinized genitalia of AGS girls is surgically corrected at birth, and these individuals are raised as girls. Nevertheless, there are clear-cut data showing a mean performance by AGS girls on men-

tal rotation of figures tests that approximates that of normal males.

6.3. Stress Effects on the Developing Brain

Prenatal stress of a pregnant mother rat by restraint or unpredictable shock produces offspring with a hyperactive adrenocortical stress response, whereas postnatal handling of rat pups (i.e., removing them from their mother for 15 min/d) results in animals that have a less reactive adrenocortical stress response. Rats with a highly reactive adrenocortical stress response tend to be more likely to self-administer drugs, such as amphetamine and cocaine; in addition, their cognitive function associated with the hippocampus appears to age more rapidly. On the other hand, rats with a less reactive adrenocortical stress response show slower rates of aging of the hippocampus and hippocampus-dependent cognitive function. It is unclear what hormonal mechanism may be responsible for these effects. For handling, corticosterone administration to lactating mothers produces offspring that resemble neonatally handled rats in having less reactive adrenocortical stress responses. Handling may work by increasing serotonergic activity and 5HT2 receptors, leading to elevated adrenal steroid receptors levels in hippocampus.

7. EMERGING CONCEPTS LINKING NEURAL ACTIONS OF HORMONE TO FUNCTION

In attempting to summarize the specific information concerning the major types of hormone effects on the brain, we can make some generalizations that pertain more generally to the plasticity of the brain in response to the environment.

First, the brain changes all the time, in adult life and not just during early development, and these changes involve remodeling of synaptic connections. For example, we have seen that there are the reversible and cyclic changes—during the 4–5 d estrous cycle of the female rat—in synaptogenesis in hypothalamus and hippocampus that are controlled by estradiol and progesterone. There are also irreversible changes, such as those produced by stress on the hippocampus, or the increased neurogenesis and cell death of dentate gyrus granule neurons following adrenalectomy. These structural changes, together with reversible induction and downregulation of neurotransmitter and peptide systems and their receptors by hormones and by other agents, are some examples from the realm of hormone action that illustrate the dynamic nature of the adult brain.

Second, many of these actions of circulating hormones on brain structure and chemistry differ across developmental stage as well as among brain regions. As an example of developmentally programmed differences, we have noted that estrogen actions during early postnatal development mediate the effects of testosterone on brain sexual differentiation, and that one of the consequences of sexual differentation of the rat hypothalamus is the reprogramming of how the adult hypothalamus will respond to estradiol in adult life. We have noted that in males, the ability of estradiol to induce progesterone receptors or to elicit synapse formation in the adult hypothalamus is markedly suppressed compared to the female. As an example of brain regional differences in hormone action, we have noted the protective action of adrenal steroids on dentate gyrus neurons, in which they block programmed cell death while suppressing neurogenesis, whereas neighboring hippocampal pyramidal neurons show neither neurogenesis nor apoptosis in response to adrenalectomy, but are in fact made more vulnerable to excitotoxic damage by elevated circulating glucocorticoids. However, both dentate gyrus granule neurons and hippocampal pyramidal neurons have adrenal steroid receptors, and thus one cannot predict what effect the relevant hormone will have simply on the basis of what hormone receptors are present.

Third, developmental effects often bias or determine an adult response. It has already been noted how the process of sexual differentiation suppresses the ability of the adult male hypothalamus to respond to estradiol in showing progesterone receptor induction and synaptogenesis. Sexual differentiation also confers on the male nervous system the ability to respond to hormones in adult life, for example, by promoting the survival and differentiation of the motor neurons of the spinal nucleus that innervates the penis. Another illustration is how developmental hyperthyroidism alters not only basal forebrain and hippocampal morphology, but also compromises the efficiency of radial maze learning in adult life. Some strains of mice appear to be born in a thyroid-deficient state, so that neonatal treatment with thyroid hormone actually improves spatial learning ability.

Fourth, hormones participate in the expression of individual as well as group differences. The thyroid

hormone example cited above shows, in principle, how deviations in normal thyroid hormone levels during early development can help to determine not only morphology, but also learning ability on an individual basis. Likewise, the effects of prenatal stress and postnatal handling have shown long-term influences on emotionality as well as the rate at which the hippocampus ages. There is evidence in infrahuman primates that prenatal stress can lead to impairments in motor coordination and attention span, and that adrenal steroids may participate in these effects. Finally, sex hormones play a major role in determination of sex (i.e., group) differences in brain structure, neurochemistry, and certain features of behavior, and there is the intriguing possiblity that sexual orientation—which can be regarded as an individual trait, but also as a subgroup of human sexual behavior—may also involve a combination of hormonal, genetic, and experiential factors.

Finally, hormone actions on the brain are relevant to pathophysiological processes and diseases in humans and, in particular, to nervous and mental disorders. There are disorders associated with cyclic events, including catamenial epilepsy, premenstrual tension, and jet lag. Sex differences play a significant role in the occurrence of diseases. In addition to the higher frequency of cardiovascular disease in men compared to premenopausal women, males also have more frequent developmental learning disorders, and mental disorders differ in occurrence between the sexes according to type, anxiety disorders and depression being more common in women, whereas substance abuse and antisocial behavior are more prevalent in men. An important message is that men and women must be studied separately as far as actions of psychotropic drugs, including antidepressants, as well as antipsychotics and benzodiazepines are concerned. This is because differences in circulating hormone levels, as well as intrinsic, developmentally programmed sex differences in brain structure and function bias the mechanisms by which these pharmaceutical agents act on the brain. Also stress is a factor in exacerbating symptoms of a number of diseases, such as atherosclerosis, asthma, diabetes, gastrointestinal disorders, and resistance to viral infections and metastasis of tumors. In addition stress hormones play a paradoxical role, as we have seen, as both protectors against and mediators of some of these disorders. However, it is not always clear what aspects of stressful experience contribute to the pathophysiological process, and it is likely that both chronic and acute stress are involved. For example, chronic stress appears to facilitate development of atherosclerotic plaques, whereas acute stress may precipitate myocardial infarction.

8. CONCLUSION

This chapter has provided glimpses into specific mechanisms for sex, stress, and thyroid hormone actions on diverse neurochemical mechanisms and structural changes in brain, with interactions occurring between development and later effects on the mature brain. One important generalization is that hormones mediate the effects of experiences in mediating expression of individual differences, and they do so at least in part by regulating the expression of genes. As we have seen, some of these genetic traits that are regulated by hormones may contribute to the vulnerability of the individual to develop a disease. However attractive as this notion may be, future studies must offer specific evidence for specific mechanisms by which hormones affect normal brain function, as well as affecting mechanisms by which the endocrine system participates in the development of pathological states.

REFERENCES

Baulieu EE, Robel P. Neurosteroids: A new brain function? *J Steroid Biochem Mole Biol* 1990; 37:395.

Raisman G, Field P. Sexual dimorphism in the preoptic area of the rat. *Science* 1971; 173:731.

SELECTED READINGS

Adkins-Regan E. Early organizational effects of hormones. In: Adler N, ed. *Neuroendocrinology of Reproduction*. New York: Plenum, 1981:159.

Allen L, Hines M, Shryne J, Gorski R. Two sexually dimorphic cell groups in the human brain. *J Neurosci* 1989; 9:497.

Becker J, Breedlove SM, Crews D, eds. *Behavioral Endocrinology*. Cambridge: MIT Press, 1992.

Cameron HA, Gould E. The control of neuronal birth and death. In: Shaw C, ed. *Receptor Dynamics in Neural Development*. Boca Raton FL: CRC, 1996:141.

Dellu F, Mayo W, Vallee M, LeMoal M, Simon H. Reactivity to novelty during youth as a predictive factor of cognitive impairment in the elderly: a longitudinal study in rats. *Brain Res* 1994; 653:51.

Forger NG, Breedlove SM. Steroid influences on a mammalian neuromuscular system. *Seminar Neurosci* 1991; 3:459.

Gould E, Woolley C, McEwen BS. The hippocampal formation: morphological changes induced by thyroid, gonadal and adrenal hormones. *Psychoneuroendocrinology* 1991; 16:67.

Hodgkin J. Sex determination and generation of sexually dimorphic nervous systems. *Neuron* 1991; 6:177.

Joels M, DeKloet ER. Control of neuronal excitability by corticosteroid hormones. *TINS* 1992; 15:25.

Kimura D. Sex differences in the brain. *Sci Ame* 1992; 267:119.

Kow LM, Mobbs CV, Pfaff DW, Roles of second-messenger systems and neuronal activity in the regulation of lordosis by neurotransmitters, neuropeptides and estrogen: A review. *Neurosci Biobehav Rev* 1993; 18:251.

Landfield P. Modulation of brain aging correlates by long-term alterations of adrenal steroids and neurally-active peptides. *Prog Brain Res* 1987; 72:279.

Marinelli M, Piazza PV, Deroche V, Maccari S, LeMoal M, Simon H. Corticosterone circadian secretion differentially facilitates dopamine-mediated psychomotor effect of cocaine and morphine. *J. Neurosci* 1994; 14:2724.

McEwen BS. Non-genomic and genomic effects of steroids on neural activity. *Trends in Pharm Sci* 1991; 112:141.

McEwen BS. Ovarian steroids have diverse effects on brain structure and function. In: Berg G, Hammar M, eds. *The Modern Management of the Menopause*. New York; Parthenon, 1994:269.

McEwen BS. Stress and neuroendocrine function: Individual differences and mechanisms leading to disease. In: Wolkowitz OM, Rothschild T, eds. *Psychoneuroendocrinology for the Clinician*. Washington, DC: American Psychiatric Press, 1996, in press.

McEwen BS, Sapolsky RM. Stress and cognitive function. *Curr Opinion Neurobiol* 1995; 5:205.

McEwen BS, Sakai RR, Spencer RL. Adrenal steroid effects on the brain: versatile hormones with good and bad effects. In: Schulkin J, ed. *Hormonally-Induced Changes in Mind and Brain*. San Diego: Academic, 1993:157.

McEwen BS, Albeck D, Cameron H, Chao HM, Gould E, Hastings N, Kuroda Y, Luine VN, Magarinos A-M, McKittrick CM, Orchinik M, Pavlides C, Vaher P, Watanabe Y, Weiland N. Stress and the brain: A paradoxical role for adrenal steroids. In: Litwack GD, ed. *Vitamins and Hormones*. San Diego: Academic, 1995:371.

McEwen BS, Gould E, Orchinik M, Weiland NG, Woolley CS. Oestrogens and the structural and functional plasticity of neurons: implications for memory, ageing and neurodegenerative processes. In: Goode J, ed. Ciba Foundation Symposium #191 The Non-reproductive Actions of Sex Steroids, London: CIBA Foundation, 1995:52.

Meaney MJ, Tannenbaum B, Francis D, Bhatnagar S, Shanks N, Viau V, O'Donnell D, Plotsky PM. Early environmental programming hypothalamic-pituitary-adrenal responses to stress. *Semin Neurosci* 1994; 6:247.

Nottebohm F, Arnold AP. Sexual dimorphism in vocal control areas of the songbird brain. *Science* 1976; 194:211.

Paul SM, Purdy RH. Neuroactive steroids. *FASEB J* 1992; 6:2311.

Pfaff DW. *Estrogens and Brain Function*. New York: Springer-Verlag, 1980.

Sapolsky R. *Stress, the Aging Brain and the Mechanisms of Neuron Death* Cambridge: MIT Press, 1992.

Selye H. The anaesthetic effect of steroid hormones. *Proc Soc Exp Biol Med* 1941; 46:116.

Shaw G, Renfree MB, Short RV. Primary genetic control of sexual differentiation in marsupials. *Aust J Zool* 1990; 37:443.

Williams CL, Meck WH. The organizational effects of gonadal steroids on sexually dimorphic spatial ability. *Psychoneuroendocrinology* 1991; 16:155.

Witelson S. Hand and sex differences in the isthmus and genu of the human corpus callosum. *Brain* 1989; 112:799.

6

Peptide Growth Factors

Peter Rotwein, MD

CONTENTS

1. OVERVIEW AND GENERAL PRINCIPLES OF GROWTH FACTOR BIOLOGY

1.1. Introduction

Growth factors are secreted proteins that exert multiple effects on cell growth, metabolism, differentiation, and on the growth and development of organisms as diverse as flies, worms, frogs, and humans. Although the term growth factor was used initially to describe secreted substances that enhanced cell division, this phrase now includes peptides that stimulate or inhibit the progression of cells through mitosis, as well as proteins that act principally to regulate cellular differentiation. To accomplish these and other biological actions, growth factors activate specific cellular receptors. Receptors are modular proteins that can bind growth factors with high affinity and can transmit the information generated by binding into changes in cellular biochemistry. Growth factors also interact with other cell-associated or secreted binding proteins. In general, binding proteins do not mediate biological effects directly, but modulate growth factor availability. The interactions among these three components to regulate growth factor action are schematized in Fig. 1.

From: *Endocrinology: Basic and Clinical Principles* (P. M. Conn and S. Melmed, eds.), Humana Press Inc., Totowa, NJ.

In the last several decades, there has been an explosive increase in knowledge about growth factor biology. This has included the characterization of many growth factors, their receptors, and binding proteins. The structural information derived from the determination of the amino acid sequences of these components and results of studies of biological function have led to the classification of growth factors into several discrete families. The information explosion has become accelerated by the advent of molecular cloning in the early 1980s and by the ability to produce pure recombinant growth factors through molecular biological techniques. Table 1 lists the names of major growth factor families and provides an abbreviation for each class.

1.2. General Principles of Growth Factor Action

1.2.1. HORMONES, GROWTH FACTORS, AND CYTOKINES: LOCAL VS SYSTEMIC EFFECTS

As summarized throughout this volume, many hormones also regulate the growth and development of cells and tissues, and thus could be classified as growth factors. In general, hormones are substances that are produced in specialized organs, termed glands, are secreted into the blood stream, and act at locations distant from their sites of synthesis. Although this endocrine mode of action is shared by

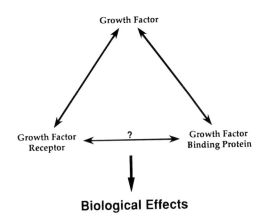

Fig. 1. Interactions among growth factors, their receptors, and binding proteins mediate growth factor action.

Table 1
Major Growth Factor Families

Name	Abbreviation	No. of members
Epidermal growth factor	EGF	>10
Fibroblast growth factor	FGF	9
Insulin-like growth factor	IGF	2
Nerve growth factor	NGF	4
Platelet-derived growth factor	PDGF	2
Transforming growth factor-β	TGF-β	~24

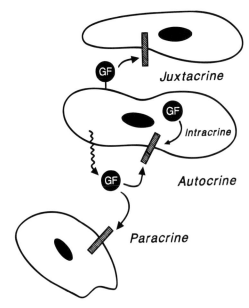

Fig. 2. Cellular actions of growth factors: autocrine, paracrine, juxtacrine, and intracrine pathways.

some growth factors (e.g., insulin-like growth factor [IGF], platelet-derived growth factor [PDGF], transforming growth factor-β [TGF-β] families), fundamental differences exist between these two classes of proteins. Unlike hormones, growth factors are produced by many tissues in the body and, thus, are not exclusively found in specific glands. Growth factors also employ modes of action that distinguish them from hormones. These include paracrine, autocrine, and juxtacrine effects (*see* Fig. 2). A paracrine mode of action occurs when a growth factor that is secreted by one cell has effects on adjacent cells. A juxtacrine mode of action is similar, although the growth factor is bound to the cell membrane or extracellular matrix. Autocrine actions include biological effects that are mediated by a growth factor on its cell of origin after its secretion into the extracellular environment. A variation on this theme has been termed intracrine and

was first described for an oncogenic variant of PDGF termed *v-sis*. Intracrine actions occur in the cell of origin prior to growth factor secretion. These modes of action are diagrammed in Fig. 2.

Cytokines are secreted proteins produced principally by macrophages, lymphocytes, and precursors of blood cells that act to regulate the function of the immune and hematopoietic systems. These proteins are very similar to traditional growth factors in their modes of action and are described in Chapter 8.

1.2.2. Growth Factor Receptors and Signaling Pathways

As noted earlier, the effects of growth factors are mediated by specific receptors. Growth factor receptors are transmembrane proteins that consist of three domains: an extracellular region that binds the growth factor with high affinity, a membrane-spanning segment, and an intracellular domain that directly mediates the biological effects of the growth factor. Despite the diversity of growth factors and receptors characterized to date, these proteins share several structural features. All growth factor receptors function as ligand-activated intracellular enzymes. With the exception of receptors for the TGF-β family, all receptors studied to date show tyrosine kinase activity. Receptors for TGF-β and related molecules phosphorylate substrates on serine and threonine residues rather than tyrosine.

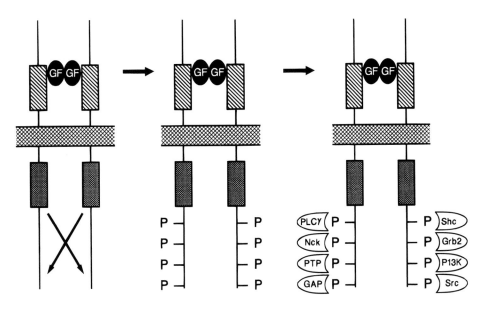

Fig. 3. Signal transduction by growth factor receptors. **Left** panel—binding of a growth factor to the extracellular part of its receptor induces receptor dimerization and activates the receptor kinase. **Center** panel—ligand-activated tyrosine phosphorylation of the receptor occurs by transphosphorylation. **Right** panel—intracellular substrates with SH2 domains bind to phosphorylated tyrosine residues of the activated receptor. The extracellular ligand-binding domain of the receptor and the intracellular tyrosine kinase domain are depicted by boxes.

Intensive investigation in the field of signal transduction has revealed a general pathway of growth factor receptor activation and action (Fig. 3). The binding of a growth factor to the extracellular domain of its receptor first leads to receptor dimerization or oligomerization. Dimerization of the receptor occurs either because the growth factor itself is a dimer and binds to two receptors (e.g., PDGF, TGF-β, nerve growth factor [NGF]), because a growth factor monomer has two binding sites for its receptor (e.g., epidermal growth factor [EGF]), or because the receptor is a preformed dimer (e.g., IGF-1, insulin). The conformational changes induced by ligand binding then activate the intracellular kinase domain of the receptor, leading first to phosphorylation of the receptor itself by a transphosphorylation mechanism and then to the phosphorylation of other substrates. Autophosphorylation, particularly on tyrosine residues, creates a series of docking sites for other intracellular proteins that contain segments termed SH2 domains, for their similarity with a region of 100 amino acids first identified in the cellular oncogene *c-src*. Different proteins containing SH2 domains bind to distinct docking sites based both on recognition of a phosphorylated tyrosine in the receptor and on the sequence of amino acids adjacent to this modified tyrosine. Recently, another

class of phosphotyrosine-binding sites distinct from SH2 domains has been identified, although it is functionally equivalent to SH2 domains in mediating the interaction between a phosphorylated amino acid and a signaling protein. Thus, activated growth factor receptors with many phosphorylated tyrosines in different amino acid contexts become the focal point for the transient aggregation of many SH2-containing proteins (Fig. 3). These proteins include a variety of intermediates in signal transduction pathways, with the ultimate effect being an amplification of the initial signal induced upon growth factor binding to its receptor. For example, the activated PDGF receptor binds a series of adapter molecules (Shc, Nck, Grb2), enzymes (PI3 kinase regulatory subunit, phospholipase C gamma [PLCγ] protein tyrosine phosphatase 1D [PTPID], *c-src*), and other proteins, which together participate in the pleiotropic biological effects of PDGF (*see* Chapter 3 for a more detailed description of signal transduction pathways). Analogous pathways are stimulated by other growth factor receptors.

1.2.3. NUCLEAR ACTIONS OF GROWTH FACTORS

The long-term changes in cellular economy induced by growth factors are secondary to alterations in gene expression. From the perspective of the growth factor receptor, these changes are but one outcome of the multiple signaling pathways induced after the assembly of proteins on the activated receptor. For example, the binding of the adapter molecule Grb2 to a phosphorylated tyrosine of an activated growth factor receptor brings this protein and its partner, termed Son-of-Sevenless (SOS), a guanine nucleotide exchange protein, to the cell membrane. SOS can then physically associate with the membrane-bound signaling intermediate, c-*ras*, leading to ras activation through stimulation of its GTP-bound form. This step sets into motion a series of enzymatic reactions, which lead to the phosphorylation and activation of a family of serine-threonine protein kinases, the mitogen-activated (MAP) or extracellular receptor (ERK) kinases (*see* Chapter 3 for further details). MAP kinases in turn phosphorylate and activate many cytoplasmic and nuclear proteins, including the transcriptional activator, ternary complex factor (TCF), which stimulates expression of the gene encoding c-*fos*. This pathway reflects a primary response to growth factors, since it is dependent on a series of protein–protein interactions and enzymatic steps that do not require new synthesis of cellular proteins. The protein c-*fos* combines with c-*jun* as components of the transcription factor AP1, which in turn regulates the activity of a variety of genes. Thus, gene expression and protein biosynthesis are altered after growth factor signaling is stimulated.

A related pathway mediated by activated growth factor receptors leads to the stimulation of another member of the MAP kinase family termed c-*jun* N-terminal kinase (JNK, also known as stress-activated protein kinase or SAPK). JNK/SAPK phosphorylates c-*jun* on two serine residues that are critical for its activation as a transcription factor. Thus, both c-*jun* and c-*fos* are induced through growth factor-stimulated signaling pathways.

Stat transcription factors (for signal transducers and activators of transcription) represent additional nuclear mediators of growth factor action. Stats were identified originally as transcription factors induced by the cytokines, interferon α and γ, but recently have been shown to be activated by other cytokines, by certain hormones, and by growth factors (*see* Chapter 8 for further details). These proteins comprise an expanding gene family that currently contains at least six members. Stats are located in the cytoplasm until they become phosphorylated on tyrosine residues after growth factor receptor activation. The phosphoryla-

Table 2
General Principles of Growth Factor Biology

Growth factors are secreted peptides that exert major effects on cell growth, differentiation, and metabolism, and on the growth and development of the whole organism.

Growth factors can be grouped into families that share structural and functional features

Growth factor action is mediated by interactions with cellular receptors and with cell-associated or secreted binding proteins

Growth factor receptors are transmembrane proteins that function as ligand-activated protein kinases; changes in phosphorylation of intracellular substrates regulate signaling pathways that ultimately transmit the biological effects of growth factors

Abnormalities in growth factors or their receptors contribute to disorders of growth, development, and differentiation

tion of Stats promotes their dimerization and nuclear translocation, and their activation as DNA-binding proteins and transcriptional regulators. The diversity of Stats provides another mechanism whereby growth factors can have pleiotropic effects on gene expression. In addition to the well-characterized steps leading to induction of c-*fos*, c-*jun*, and Stats, signaling pathways activated by growth factors regulate many other transcription factors.

1.3. Summary

Peptide growth factors are multifunctional proteins that exert diverse biological effects through interactions with cellular receptors that function as ligand-activated intracellular enzymes. The enzymatic pathways that are initiated by the binding of a growth factor to its receptor lead to long-term changes in gene expression and protein biosynthesis that alter a cell's phenotype, and have profound effects on growth and development in the whole animal. Table 2 summarizes some of the general features of growth factor biology. Specific issues pertinent to individual growth factor families are described in the following sections.

2. INDIVIDUAL GROWTH FACTORS

2.1. EGF Family

2.1.1. INTRODUCTION

EGF was the second growth factor to be identified (NGF was first). In 1962, purified EGF was shown to induce precocious eyelid opening and incisor eruption in neonatal mice. Since that initial purification, several members of the EGF family of ligands have been characterized (Table 3), and four structurally related receptors have been cloned that mediate their biological effects. Both ligands and receptors are expressed in multiple tissues.

2.1.2. STRUCTURE OF EGF AND RELATED MOLECULES

EGF is a 53 amino acid single-chain peptide with three intrachain disulfide bonds. It is a conserved protein (37/53 residues are identical between mouse and human EGF) that is synthesized as a large precursor of 1217 amino acids. In addition to EGF itself, the precursor protein contains eight additional segments with structural homology to EGF, a hydrophobic transmembrane domain, and a short intracellular carboxyl-terminal tail. The mechanisms regulating processing of the precursor are not known, and a discrete function for membrane-bound EGF has not been documented.

TGF-α, a 50 amino acid protein that is 44% identical to EGF, was initially identified as a tumor-derived factor responsible in part for confering the transformed phenotype to cultured cells. TGF-α also is synthesized as a membrane-bound precursor. Removal of its amino-terminal segment generates a biologically active membrane-associated protein that can signal adjacent cells by binding to the EGF receptor (juxtacrine mode of action, as described earlier). It is not known if membrane-bound and secreted TGF-α have different biological effects.

Amphiregulin, heparin-binding EGF, crypto, and betacellulin are EGF-related proteins characterized from tumor-derived cell lines. Heparin-binding EGF has been shown to be a potent mitogen, acting through the EGF receptor, and amphiregulin can both inhibit and promote cell growth, depending on the cell line studied. Surprisingly, the membrane-bound precursor of heparin-binding EGF serves as a receptor for the B subunit of diphtheria toxin, and thus is the mediator of toxin entry into cells. Other physiological roles for heparin-binding EGF and amphiregulin have not been described. Similarly, the functions of crypto and betacellulin are unknown.

Pox virus growth factors also are structurally similarity to EGF. Cells infected with vaccinia virus secrete a 77 amino acid protein, vaccinia virus growth factor (VGF), that is 37% identical to EGF,

Table 3
EGF Family

Name	Abbreviation
Epidermal growth factor	EGF
Transforming growth factor α	TGFα
Amphiregulin	AP
Heparin-binding epidermal growth factor	HB-EGF
Betacellulin	
Crypto	
Vaccinia virus growth factor	VGF
Heregulin subfamily	
Heregulin/neu-differentiation factor	HRG/NDF
Glial growth factor	GGF
Acetylcholine receptor-inducing activity	ARIA
Sensory and motor neuron-derived factor	SMDF

and can bind to and activate the EGFR. The role of these factors in viral infection or replication is not known.

Heregulins or neu-differentiation factors are recent additions to the EGF family. These proteins are derived from alternatively spliced products of a single gene, and are composed of various combinations of several structural domains, including a kringle-like region (such as is found in blood clotting proteins), an immunoglobulin-like-segment, an EGF-related domain, a transmembrane region, and a cytoplasmic segment. To date, several members of this subfamily have been characterized and their cDNAs have been cloned based on distinct biological effects (Table 3). From studies using recombinant heregulin components, receptor binding appears to be determined primarily by the EGF-like domain of these proteins.

2.1.3. EGF RECEPTORS

There are four structurally related EGF receptors: EGF receptor (EGFR), ErbB2, ErbB3, and ErbB4 (Fig. 4). Binding studies have shown that the EGFR binds EGF, TGF-α, and heparin-binding EGF, and that ErbB3 and ErbB4 bind heregulins. As seen with other growth factor receptors, ligand binding first induces receptor dimerization, and this is followed by kinase activation, leading to autophosphorylation by a transphosphorylation mechanism. Recent

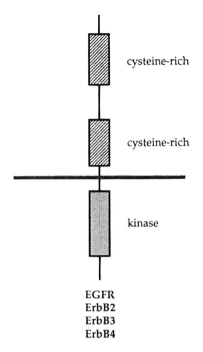

Fig. 4. EGFR and related receptors. Two cysteine-rich segments in the extracellular region and the intracellular tyrosine kinase domain are indicated by boxes.

studies indicate that receptor heterodimers may form, thus extending the diversity of signaling pathways mediated by these receptors. For example, binding of EGF to the EGFR leads to tyrosine phosphorylation of ErbB2 in cells also expressing the latter receptor, even though EGF cannot bind to the extracellular domain of ErbB2. Similarly, heregulins do not stimulate the tyrosine phosphorylation of ErbB2 unless ErbB3 or ErbB4 are expressed in the same cell. By contrast, heregulins can bind to cells just expressing ErbB3 or ErbB4. In addition, in some cell types, EGF treatment activates PI3 kinase, even though the intracellular domain of the EGFR lacks a binding site for the SH2 domain of the PI3 kinase regulatory subunit, p85. Since ErbB3 contains a PI3 kinase docking site, which becomes phosphorylated on treatment of EGF, it has been proposed that ErbB3 is a substrate for the EGFR kinase domain. Surprisingly, the intracellular region of ErbB3 does not contain a functional tyrosine kinase. A major role for ErbB3 thus may be as a docking protein for intracellular signaling molecules containing SH2 domains. Such crosstalk between receptors of the EGF family thus adds the potential to increase the range of biological

responses initiated by a given ligand on binding to its receptor, depending on what other members of the receptor family are expressed in the same cell or tissue or at the same developmental stage.

One initial additional surprising feature of the EGFR is its potential function as an accomplice in the process by which *Salmonella typhimurium* invades the intestinal epithelium. *Salmonella* invasion is associated with activation of the receptor as indicated by its tyrosine phosphorylation and by increases in intracellular calcium. The mechanism by which *Salmonella* uses the EGF receptor is not known.

2.1.4. BIOLOGICAL EFFECTS

The precise physiological roles of the EGF family of growth factors in growth and development remain unsolved questions, despite the plethora of actions attributed to these proteins. Attempts to address these issues by genetic approaches have begun to yield intriguing results, however, with studies in invertebrates being most compelling. In the nematode *Caenorhabditis elegans*, an EGF analog is encoded by the lin-3 gene. Complete disruption of lin-3 is lethal, and diminished expression leads to developmental defects in induction of the vulva. The lin-3 protein binds to a homolog of the EGFR, termed let-23. Decreased expression of the receptor also affects vulval development. Signal transduction through let-23 requires an adapter protein with SH2 domains, sem-5, whose mammalian homolog is Grb2, and a *ras* homolog, let-60. Each of these proteins also is critical for vulval development.

A genetic approach in mammalian species also has yielded intriguing insights into functions of the EGF family. These experiments have taken advantage of the power of gene disruption in mice through targeted replacement in embryonic stem cells. Ablation of the TGF-α gene demonstrated that this protein was required for hair growth, but was dispensable for most other aspects of normal growth and development. In the absence of TGF-α, whiskers and fur showed pronounced waviness that was secondary to a variety of abnormalities in the hair follicles. Deficiencies in eye development, including open eyelids at birth, also were seen in some mice, but other physiological parameters, including wound healing, were normal.

In contrast to the modest developmental problems caused by TGF-α deficiency, disruption of the EGFR led to multiple severe abnormalities. Depending on the mouse strain, receptor-deficient embryos died during early gestation because of degeneration of the inner cell mass (which would eventually become the fetus) or during midgestation secondary to placental deficiency. In other genetic backgrounds, some mutant mice survived until the early postnatal period, but showed reduced growth compared with normal littermates. Abnormalities were found in the skin, hair follicles, eyes, brain, liver, gastrointestinal tract, kidney, and other tissues. These results indicate that the EGFR and EGF signaling play a critical role in embryogenesis and in the development of many organs and tissues. The nature of the strain-specific modifiers that modulate these effects is not known. Analogous studies have not been reported yet for other EGF-related receptors or for their ligands.

2.1.5. Therapeutic Uses

A major current application for EGF is to induce the shedding of wool, and it is used as an alternative to shearing sheep.

2.2. Fibroblast Growth Factor (FGF) Family

2.2.1. Introduction

FGFs comprise a family of heparin-binding growth factors with diverse effects on development, wound healing, angiogenesis, and other biological processes. The term FGF was initially applied to two factors, acidic FGF (now FGF-1) and basic FGF (FGF-2), that were isolated from brain and pituitary based on the ability of these proteins to stimulate DNA synthesis in fibroblasts. The FGF family of ligands now contains nine members (Table 4) and includes keratinocyte growth factor (KGF or FGF-7), and the products of several oncogenes (*int-2* is FGF-3, *hst-1* and *hst-2* are FGF-4 and FGF-6, respectively). Their actions are mediated by interactions with transmembrane FGF receptors and with heparin sulfate proteoglycans (HSPGs). FGF receptors also comprise a multicomponent family that consists of four related genes termed FGFR1–4. Multiple receptor isoforms are produced by alternative RNA splicing.

2.2.2. Structure of FGFs

The nine known FGFs show structural similarities in a core region that is required for binding to FGF receptors. FGF-1 and 2 are both highly conserved 155 amino acid proteins that are 55% identical to each other. Both proteins lack classical amino-terminal signal sequences for directing protein secretion.

Table 4
FGF Family

Current abbreviation	Old name and abbreviations
FGF-1	Acidic FGF (aFGF)
FGF-2	Basic FGF (bFGF)
FGF-3	Integration site-2 (int-2)
FGF-4	Human stomach tumor-1 (hst-1)
	Kaposi sarcoma FGF (k-FGF)
FGF-5	—
FGF-6	Human stomach tumor-2 (hst-2)
FGF-7	Keratinocyte growth factor (KGF)
FGF-8	—
FGF-9	—

Despite considerable investigation, how these proteins reach the extracellular environment remains an unsolved problem. FGF-2 mRNA also can be translated beginning with upstream CUG codons, leading to variants with extended amino-termini. The functions of these variants are unknown. The FGF-3 precursor also exhibits alternative translation initiation, although this protein contains a signal peptide, as do FGF-4–8. Like FGF-1 and 2, FGF-9 lacks a signal peptide, and its mechanism of secretion is similarly unknown.

2.2.3. FGF Receptors and Binding Proteins

The FGF receptors (FGFRs) are protein products of four related genes. They function as ligand-activated tyrosine protein kinases with different specificities for the nine FGF ligands. Receptor diversity results from various combinations of alternative RNA splicing that have been defined for the FGFR1 and FGFR2 genes. The extracellular domains of FGFRs are composed of two or three immunoglobulin (Ig)-like motifs, followed by a single transmembrane region and an intracellular tyrosine kinase domain that is split into two parts by a kinase insert region (Fig. 5). The intracytoplasmic domain also contains juxtamembrane and carboxyl-terminal segments. The latter region is relatively divergent in sequence among FGFRs and may be responsible for interactions with cellular substrates that are specific to each receptor. PDGF receptors have a similar organization, although they contain five Ig-like repeats in their extracellular portions.

FGFR1 and 2 exist in both transmembrane and secreted forms (Fig. 5). Transmembrane versions of

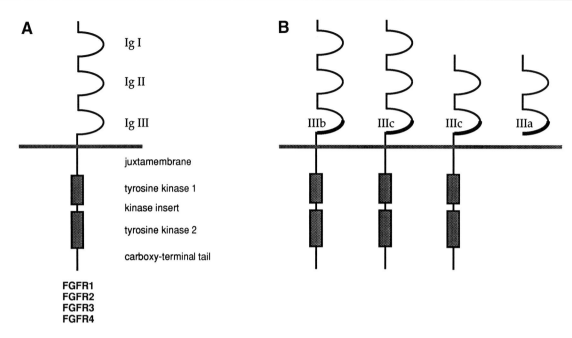

Fig. 5. (A) Schematic of FGF receptors. Various domains are labeled. **(B)** Alternative RNA splicing of the FGFR1 gene regulates the synthesis of multiple receptor isoforms. Receptors with two or three immunoglobulin (Ig) domains and with different exons encoding the carboxy-terminal part of Ig domain III are illustrated. Additional receptor isoforms with minor variations on these patterns have been described.

FGFR1 contain three Ig domains or lack domain I. The absence of Ig region I does not alter binding to FGF-1 or 2. Binding affinity can be modified depending on which of three alternatively spliced exons is used to code for the carboxyl-terminal half of the third Ig domain. Receptors using segment IIIb bind FGF-1 with higher affinity than FGF-2, whereas receptors containing region IIIc bind both growth factors equally. Receptors containing segment IIIa are secreted and may function as FGF-binding proteins. Additional minor receptor variants have been characterized that do not affect ligand binding.

FGFR2 also has multiple isoforms that are generated in a matter analogous to FGFR1. The receptor for KGF (FGF-7) is the splicing variant for FGFR2 that contains the IIIb segment encoding the carboxyl-terminal half of Ig domain 3. Only single receptor isoforms have been identified to date for FGFR3 and FGFR4.

The expression of different FGFRs and splicing variants are regulated in both tissue-specific and developmentally specific ways. In addition, several receptor isoforms have been shown to be coexpressed in the same tissues. This receptor diversity provides one mechanism for regulating FGF action in different tissues and at different developmental stages.

In addition to the FGFRs described above, FGFs also bind with lower affinity to HSPGs. These interactions are essential for high-affinity binding to FGFRs. Other HSPGs in the extracellular matrix serve as storage pools for FGFs.

Binding to FGFRs leads to rapid receptor dimerization and to autophosphorylation by a transphosphorylation mechanism. Since FGFs do not form dimers and are not bivalent ligands, the mechanism of receptor dimerization has been unclear. One hypothesis for the role of cell-surface HSPGs is to provide the equivalent of a dimerization interface for FGFs by binding several growth factor molecules simultaneously. This would allow the FGF–HSPG complex to interact with several receptor molecules at the same time and thus stimulate receptor oligomerization. Experimental evidence for this idea has been demonstrated recently for the interaction of FGF-1 with FGFR2.

2.2.4. BIOLOGICAL AND CLINICAL EFFECTS

Recent studies have underscored the critical roles of different members of the FGF family in growth, development, and morphogenesis in many different

Table 5
Human FGF Receptor Mutations

Syndrome	Phenotype	Receptor	Mutation
Pfeiffer	Craniosynostosis; abnormal great toes and thumbs; occ syndactyly	FGFR1	Linker between Ig II and III
Crouzon	Craniosynostosis	FGFR2	Ig IIIc
Jackson-Weiss	Craniosynostosis; syndactyly	FGFR2	Ig IIIc
Apert	Craniosynostosis; severe syndactyly	FGFR2	Linker between Ig II and III
Acondroplasia	Shortening of limbs	FGFR3	Transmembrane domain
Thanatophoric dysplasia	Severe shortening of limbs; abnormalities in vertebrae, ribs, skull	FGFR3	Linker between Ig II and III, carboxy-terminal tail (type I); tyr. kinase domain (type II)

species. Experiments employing dominant negative receptors have demonstrated a requirement for FGF signaling in the induction and patterning of mesoderm that occur early in the development of the frog, *Xenopus laevis*. FGF action is needed for induction of a subset of mesodermal cell types, particularly skeletal muscle. FGF also may collaborate with activins (members of the TGF-β family) in induction of the notochord. Several FGFs and FGF receptor subtypes have been cloned from *Xenopus* and are expressed in the early embryo.

A role for FGF in limb development has been defined in the chick embryo. Implantation of beads soaked in either FGF-1, FGF-2, or FGF-4 into the flank of an early embryo caused the appearance of an extra limb bud and led to the formation of a completely normal supernumerary limb. Although the molecular mechanisms of this phenomenon have not been established, it is likely that this concentrated source of FGF mimics the normal situation by enhancing local cell proliferation, and also by stimulating the expression of several other factors that control limb patterning and morphogenesis.

Several FGFs have been shown to play important roles in mouse development, as assessed by targeted gene disruptions. FGF-3 deficiency caused abnormalities in formation of the tail and inner ear. The absence of FGF-5 led to mice with abnormally long hair, implying a key role for this growth factor in

regulation of the hair growth cycle. A homozygous knockout of FGF-4 gene expression was a lethal abnormality. Embryos developed minimally after implantation into the uterus. This defect was not seen in heterozygotes.

Defects in FGFRs also cause developmental anomalies in mice and in humans. Targeted disruption of the FGFR1 gene in mice led to early embryonic death. Nullizygous embryos died before midgestation, soon after the onset of gastrulation, and had multiple defects in mesodermal derivatives. Heterozygotes developed normally.

In humans heterozygous mutations in FGFR1, FGFR2, and FGFR3 are associated with craniosynostosis syndromes and with chondrodysplasias (Table 5). Point mutations in the extracellular domains of either FGFR1 or FGFR2 cause Pfeiffer syndrome, a disorder consisting of craniosynostosis (abnormal development and premature fusion of the cranial sutures), with flattening of the midface, abnormalities in the great toes and thumbs, and occasionally syndactyly (cutaneous and bony fusion of the digits) affecting other fingers and toes. The same mutations in FGFR2 are seen in Crouzon syndrome. In this developmental disorder, the patients have craniosynostosis, but normal hands and feet. The missense mutations in both syndromes cause amino acid changes in the carboxyl-terminal portion of the variable third Ig domain, segment IIIc, of the FGFR2 gene. A different mutation in the same segment of the receptor is present in Jackson-Weiss syndrome, another craniosynostosis associated with syndactyly, and amino acid substitutions in the linker portion of FGFR2 between Ig domains 2 and 3 have been identified in Apert syndrome, a malformation consisting of craniosynostosis and severe syndactyly of the hands and feet.

Two distinct skeletal dysplasias are linked to mutations in FGFR3. Achondroplasia, a common form of dwarfism caused by shortening of the limbs, is associated with heterozygous mutations in the transmembrane domain. Thanatophoric dysplasia, a lethal autosomal dominant skeletal disorder with diverse abnormalities in the long bones, vertebral bodies, and ribs is linked to mutations in several different regions of FGFR3.

These clinical genetic observations indicate that FGFRs play a critical role in skeletal formation during human embryogenesis, and point to the existence of potentially complicated patterns of ligand binding and signal transduction by these receptors during development. Further insights into the roles of FGF signaling pathways in cranial and limb morphogenesis can be anticipated once these mutations are engineered into mouse embryos via targeted gene replacement.

2.2.5. POTENTIAL DIAGNOSTIC AND THERAPEUTIC USES

The potential application of the FGFs in wound healing has been under active investigation. Because FGFs are potent angiogenesis factors and angiogenesis is required to support actively growing tumors, their measurement has been considered as a diagnostic marker for aggressive cancers. In addition, based on the linkage between mutations in FGFR genes and skeletal dysplasias, it should be possible to develop DNA-based tests for *in utero* diagnosis of these severe disorders.

2.3. IGF Family

2.3.1. INTRODUCTION

IGF-1 and IGF-2 are a pair of single-chain peptides with diverse effects on growth, differentiation, and intermediary metabolism. These proteins were discovered through three parallel lines of research. IGF-1 was identified as a growth hormone-dependent serum growth factor, IGF-1 and IGF-2 were discovered as serum factors with insulin-like metabolic actions, and IGF-2 was purified by virtue

of its properties as an autocrine growth-promoting substance. With insulin and the more distantly related hormone relaxin, the IGFs comprise the insulin-IGF family. IGF action is mediated by binding to two distinct cell-surface receptors, the IGF insulin receptor IR and IGF-IIR, and by interactions with six secreted IGF-binding proteins (IGFBPs).

2.3.2. STRUCTURE OF IGF-1 AND IGF-2

IGF-1 is a 70 amino acid single-chain peptide with three intrachain disulfide bonds. The protein is composed of four contiguous domains termed B, C, A, and D. The B and A domains are homologous to the B and A chains of insulin, and the two proteins have similar three-dimensional structures. IGF-1 is a highly conserved protein: 65/70 residues are identical among seven mammalian species, and the human and trout proteins are 80% identical. In mammals, IGF-1 is synthesized as two large precursors (IGF-1A and IGF-1B) with carboxyl-terminal extensions termed E domains. The different E domains are derived from distinct exons of the IGF-1 gene by alternative RNA splicing. The functions of these precursor proteins are unknown, and the mechanisms of proteolytic processing leading to the mature 70 residue IGF-1 molecule have not been defined.

IGF-2 is a 67 amino acid protein that is structurally similar to IGF-1 and insulin. Human IGF-1 and IGF-2 are nearly 80% identical in amino acid sequence. IGF-2 also is highly conserved: 61/67 residues are identical among six mammalian species; and human and trout proteins are 76% identical. Like IGF-1, IGF-2 is synthesized as a precursor with a carboxyl-terminal E domain. The mechanisms of proteolytic processing to generate mature IGF-2 also are unknown, and the function of the conserved E domain has not been determined.

2.3.3. IGF RECEPTORS

There are two IGF receptors. The IGF-IR is a ligand-activated tyrosine protein kinase that is structurally related to the insulin receptor. It can bind IGF-1 and IGF-2 with high affinity and mediates biological effects of both growth factors. The IGF-2R is a multifunctional protein that lacks intrinsic tyrosine kinase activity. Its role in ligand-activated signaling is controversial. The protein also is known as the cation-independent mannose 6-phosphate receptor, and plays a key role in the transport and targeting of lysosomal enzymes. It binds IGF-2, but not IGF-1 under physiological conditions.

2.3.4. THE IGF-1 RECEPTOR

The IGF-IR is a heterotetramer composed of two α and two β chains (Fig. 6). The protein is produced as a single polypeptide precursor that is modified and cleaved into α and β subunits during its biosynthesis. Two disulfide-linked αβ half-receptors are joined through disulfide bonds to form the mature holoreceptor. Thus, unlike other growth factor receptors, the IGF-IR is a preformed dimer. The insulin receptor (IR) has a similar structure and receptor hybrids have been described consisting of an αβ dimers from the IR and IGF-IR.

Like other tyrosine kinase receptors, the IGF-IR is activated by ligand binding to the extracellular domain. Ligand binding triggers kinase activation and receptor autophosphorylation by a transphosphorylation mechanism. The activated receptor kinase also phosphorylates a 185-kDa substrate, termed insulin receptor substrate-1 (IRS-1). This protein was first characterized as a key intermediate in signaling by the IR receptor, and functions as an adapter for proteins containing SH2 domains. IRS-1 contains multiple potential tyrosine phosphorylation sites, and several serve as docking sites for signaling intermediates, such as Grb2, Nck, the PI3 kinase regulatory subunit, and others. Thus, by analogy with other growth factor receptors, the IGF-IR and IR activate several signal transduction pathways through intermediates containing SH2 domains, but do so by using the adapter IRS-1. The recent identification of the related protein, IRS-2, offers the potential for further amplification and diversification of signaling through these receptors.

2.3.5. IGF-2 RECEPTOR

The IGF-IIR is an approx 230-kDa glycoprotein that spans the cell membrane once (Fig. 6). The large extracellular domain of the IGF-IIR is composed of 15 structurally related motifs of approx 150 amino acids each. Each motif also is related to a single similar element found in the extracellular part of the other lysosomal targeting receptor, the cation-dependent mannose 6-phosphate receptor; this latter protein does not bind IGF-2. The IGF-IIR binds several other glycoproteins, including thyroglobulin and the latent form of TGF-β. The binding of latent TGF-β may be important for growth factor activation.

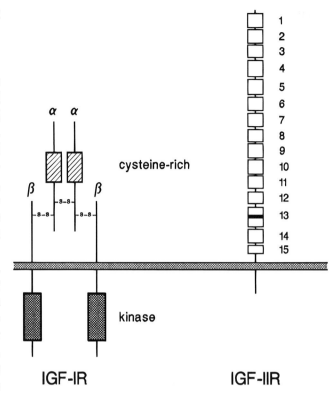

Fig. 6. Schematic of the IGF-1 and IGF-2 receptors. Cysteine-rich ligand-binding domains in the extracellular part and the tyrosine kinase domain in the intracellular part of the IGF-IR are depicted by boxes. The 15 extracellular repeating motifs of the IGF-IIR also are indicated by boxes.

The IGF-IIR is involved in the internalization and clearance of IGF-2 although studies in tissue-culture systems indicate that ligand-receptor interactions also may initiate a signal transduction pathway. It has been proposed that the heterotrimeric G-protein, Gi2, couples the activated IGF-IIR to a variety of biological responses. At present, this intriguing hypothesis has not been proven.

2.3.6. IGF-BINDING PROTEINS

IGFs present in the blood and in other biological fluids are bound to IGFBPs. Six structurally related IGFBPs have been characterized and comprise a family of secreted proteins varying in length from 216–289 amino acids with cysteine-rich amino- and carboxyl-terminal domains. IGFBPs are modulators of IGF action (Table 6). IGFBP3, in conjunction with another protein, termed acid labile subunit, is primarily responsible for maintaining a reservoir of IGFs in the circulation. Other IGFBPs found in the bloodstream, including IGFBP1, IGFBP2, and IGFBP4,

Table 6
IGF-Binding Proteins

Binding protein	Potential functions	Binds to cell surface or extracellular matrix	Activity modified by proteolysis
1	Minor serum carrier; potentiates/inhibits IGF action	Yes	No
2	Minor serum carrier; potentiates/inhibits IGF action	No	Yes
3	Major serum carrier; potentiates/inhibits IGF action	Yes	Yes
4	Inhibits IGF action	No	Yes
5	Potentiates/inhibits IGF action	Yes	Yes
6	Potentiates/inhibits IGF action?	No	Possibly

can cross endothelial barriers, and thus may transport IGFs from the circulation to peripheral tissues. Several IGFBPs are found in the extracellular environments of many tissues, and may regulate IGF accessibility to receptors and/or provide a local storage depot. These local functions of IGFBPs may be modulated by interactions with the extracellular matrix and with the cell surface. In addition, local levels of several IGFBPs are modified through specific proteolysis. Thus, the dynamic interactions between IGFs and their binding proteins regulate IGF availability and, ultimately, IGF action.

2.3.7. BIOLOGICAL EFFECTS

2.3.7.1. Growth The major in vivo actions of both IGFs are to regulate somatic growth. Growth hormone (GH)-deficient humans or animals have low circulating IGF-1 levels, and IGF-1 administration will enhance somatic growth even in the absence of GH. In addition, the accelerated growth seen in conditions causing GH excess is correlated with elevated IGF-1 levels.

2.3.8. DEVELOPMENT

Although IGF-1 has been characterized primarily as a postnatal growth factor regulated principally by GH, it also plays a key role in somatic growth and in tissue maturation during fetal development. As demonstrated through gene targeting experiments, IGF-1-deficient mice were small at birth, and exhib-

ited variable defects in skeletal muscle, skin, and bone maturation. These mice also grew poorly after birth. A similar degree of growth impairment was seen during fetal development in IGF-2 deficient mice, although these mice grew at a normal rate after birth and were otherwise normal. Thus, in mice, IGF-2 is principally a fetal growth factor, whereas IGF-1 regulates somatic growth throughout life. These gene targeting studies also provided the first indication that the activity of the IGF-2 gene was controlled by genomic imprinting. Imprinting is an epigenetic modification that controls the expression of individual genes depending on the parental chromosome of origin. Through unknown mechanisms, the IGF-2 gene is expressed from the paternally derived chromosome in most tissues.

A "knockout" of IGF-IR expression also caused dramatic growth impairment in mice. IGF-IR-deficient mice were smaller than IGF-I-deficient animals, and exhibited more pronounced deficits in muscle, skin, and bone. Most mice lacking the IGF-IR died within minutes of birth because of an inability to expand their lungs secondary to severe muscle hypoplasia. Neither IGF-1 nor the IGF-IR genes are imprinted, and heterozygous mice are essentially normal.

The IGF-IIR gene is also imprinted in mice. In contrast to IGF-2 the IGF-IIR gene is expressed primarily from the maternally derived chromosome. This idea was initially formulated through analysis of a mouse mutation, termed T-maternal effect (Tme), and has been confirmed through targeted

IGF-IIR deficiency. Mice with a targeted disruption of the IGF-IIR gene were large at birth and had increased levels of circulating IGF-2, indicating a role for the IGF-IIR in removing IGF-II from the circulation. IGF-IIR-deficient mice died in the perinatal period secondary to major cardiac abnormalities, and it is of interest that the heart is the organ with the highest levels of IGF-IIR expression in the fetus. Potentially these high levels of IGF-IIR normally modulate IGF-2 action in the developing heart. In the absence of receptors, cardiac overgrowth and heart failure ensue, and these abnormalities may be secondary to excessive local actions of IGF-2.

The roles of individual IGFBPs in growth and development have not been examined in detail. Mice lacking IGFBP2 have been generated and are reported to be normal, but knockouts of other IGFBP genes have not been established. It is likely that several IGFBPs share identical functions; thus, deficiency of multiple IGFBPs may be required to reveal developmentally significant abnormalities.

2.3.9. OTHER ACTIONS

Other biological effects include acute insulin-like actions on glucose metabolism, and the stimulation of the survival, proliferation, and/or differentiation of a wide variety of cell types.

2.3.10. THERAPEUTIC USES

One potential application for IGF-1 is in the treatment of GH-insensitivity syndromes (formerly Laron-type dwarfism). In these disorders, GH action is defective, and IGF-1 levels in blood are reduced. In several subjects with this syndrome, IGF-1 administration enhanced somatic growth.

IGF-1 treatment also may be effective in patients with diabetes associated with insulin resistance, although the acute glucose lowering actions of IGF-1 are only approx 7% of those of insulin in normal individuals. Unlike insulin, IGF-1 action is buffered by IGFBPs, leading not only to diminished acute effects, but also to prolonged activity. Initial success has been reported in patients with extreme insulin resistance and in diabetic subjects with mutations in the insulin receptor.

IGF-1 treatment also appears to be effective in initial studies in patients with acute renal failure. Administration is associated with improved glomerular filtration rate and renal blood flow, and may enhance renal growth. IGF-1 also has been reported to be beneficial in patients with the neurodegenerative disorder, amyotrophic lateral sclerosis, although the mechanisms are unknown. Other potential uses for IGF-1 and IGFBPs are in wound healing. IGF-1 also may be beneficial in combination with growth hormone to spare protein loss in conditions associated with tissue catabolism, such as severe burns and major surgery.

2.4. NGF Family

2.4.1. INTRODUCTION

NGF was the first growth factor to be characterized. Its discovery was based on the observation that a diffusible factor, initially identified in a sarcoma cell line, stimulated enlargement of the peripheral sensory nervous system and the sympathetic ganglia. Later studies demonstrated that NGF was critical for survival of sensory and sympathetic neurons. There are currently four members of the NGF or neurotrophin family. These proteins exert diverse effects on the survival of different components of the nervous system by activating three related neurotrophic receptors, TrkA, TrkB, and TrkC, and by binding to a low affinity NGF receptor (NGFR).

2.4.2. STRUCTURE OF NGF AND RELATED MOLECULES

Human NGF is a 120 amino acids protein with three intrachain disulfide bonds. It is synthesized as a precursor with an amino-terminal extension. The structures of the other three neurotrophins are similar. Brain-derived neurotrophic factor (BDNF), and neurotrophins 3 and 4/5 (NT3, NT4/5) are secreted proteins of 118–130 residues with three intrachain disulfide bonds. The four neurotrophic factors are approx 50–60% identical in amino acid sequence. All four proteins bind to their receptors as homodimers.

2.4.3. NEUROTROPHIN RECEPTORS

The high-affinity neurotrophin receptors or Trk family of tyrosine protein kinases was identified initially through studies of an oncogene found in colon cancer. A gene rearrangement resulted in the fusion of a then novel tyrosine kinase with tropomyosin. Analysis of the cellular proto-oncogene led to the characterization of a receptor-like molecule, TrkA, whose tissue distribution correlated with the known distribution of NGE-responsive neurons. Other studies identified two additional members of this family,

TrkB and TrkC (Fig. 7). These proteins are structurally related and share approx 80% amino acid identity in their intracellular tyrosine kinase domains, but are less similar in the extracellular ligand-binding segments. Like other growth factor receptors, the Trks are activated by ligand binding to their extracellular domain, which leads to receptor dimerization, kinase activation, and transphosphorylation of sites within the intracytoplasmic region. The phosphorylated tyrosines then serve as docking sites for intracellular proteins with SH2 domains. There are distinct specificities for ligand binding. NGF binds to TrkA, BDNF and NT4/5 to TrkB, and NT3 to TrkC and TrkB.

In addition to the Trks, a structurally distinct lower-affinity NGFR also has been described. This protein, also known as p75, is capable of binding all four neurotrophins. Ligand binding has not been linked directly to signal transduction.

2.4.4. Biological Effects

The key role of NGF was first shown when injected neutralizing antibodies led to the elimination of the peripheral sympathetic nervous system in newborn rats. Subsequent studies indicated that peripheral target tissues synthesized neurotrophic peptides that maintained neuronal survival and promoted innervation. These observations led to the concept of "target-derived neurotrophic factor." Recent gene disruption studies in mice have validated this hypothesis, and have defined specific and essential functions for most of the neurotrophins and their receptors. Homozygous mutation of TrkA resulted in the nearly complete loss of peripheral sympathetic neurons, and the disappearance of distinct populations of pain- and temperature-sensitive neurons. This lethal mutation caused alterations that were similar to those seen after treatment of newborn rodents with NGF antibodies.

TrkB knockout mice had a marked deficiency in cranial and spinal sensory neurons, and loss of some cranial and spinal motor neurons. The sensory deficits were similar, but more severe than those seen with homozygous deficiency of either BDNF or NT4/5, indicating that both neurotrophins are ligands of TrkB, at least in sensory neurons. TrkB deficiency also was lethal.

A null mutation for TrkC was lethal and caused loss of proprioceptive neurons in the spinal chord and innervating the muscle spindle. These neurons mediate awareness of limb position. Spinal proprioceptive neurons also were diminished in NT3-deficient mice.

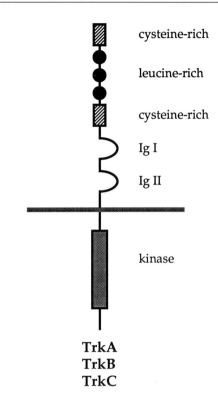

Fig. 7. Trks A, B, and C encode receptors for neurotrophins. Various domains are labeled.

Ablation of the low-affinity NGFR led to defects in a portion of the peripheral sensory nervous system responsible for sensing changes in skin temperature. The mice were otherwise viable. The sympathetic nervous system was normal in these animals.

Although marked abnormalities were observed throughout the spinal chord and peripheral nervous system in Trk-deficient and neurotrophin-deficient mice, minimal changes were seen in the central nervous system (CNS), despite the widespread distribution of TrkB and TrkC in the CNS. This may reflect functional redundancy of neurotrophin signaling in the CNS or the requirement for other collaborating neurotrophic molecules, such as ciliary neurotrophic factor, a member of the cytokine-hematopoietic family of growth and differentiation factors, or others. Future studies should address these questions.

2.4.5. Therapeutic Uses

There are presently no compelling data linking abnormalities in neurotrophins or their receptors with any neurological diseases. Nevertheless pharmacological treatment with these agents, either alone or in concert with other growth factors, may prove beneficial in treating neurodegenerative disorders.

2.5. PDGF Family

2.5.1. INTRODUCTION

PDGF was discovered as a substance released from the α granules of platelets that was responsible for much of the effect of serum on the proliferation of cells in culture. It was purified from platelets as a highly basic 30-kDa dimeric protein. Purified PDGF was found to consist of two related disulfide-bonded proteins, PDGF-A and PDGF-B chains, that are products of separate genes. PDGF binds to two cell-surface receptors, PDGFR-α and PDGFR-β, that also are structurally related. The growth factors and their receptors are widely distributed.

2.5.2. STRUCTURE OF PDGF

Mature PDGF-A and -B chains are 109 amino acids in length and are 60% identical. Eight cysteine residues are completely conserved between the two proteins. Both growth factors are synthesized as pre-cursors that undergo posttranslational processing to yield mature glycoproteins. The B-chain is homologous to *v-cis*, the transforming protein of simian sarcoma virus. All three combinations of growth factor dimers have been isolated from tissues: AA, AB, and BB. The AA and AB isoforms are secreted efficiently from cells; a significant fraction of BB is retained intracellularly by a basic stretch of amino acids near the carboxyl-terminus. In addition to platelet α granules, PDGF has been isolated from macrophages and from smooth muscle cells from the aorta. It also is secreted from cultured vascular endothelial cells, although levels are higher than are found in freshly isolated blood vessels.

2.5.3. PDGF RECEPTORS

The two PDGF receptors (PDGRs) are ligand-activated tyrosine protein kinases. The receptors are composed of an extracellular region that contains five immunoglobulin-like domains, a transmembrane segment, and an intracellular region with a tyrosine kinase domain that is split by a kinase insert of approximate 100 amino acids (Fig. 8). The binding of PDGF to the extracellular region of the receptor induces receptor dimerization. Both homo- and heterodimers can form, depending on the ligand and the relative receptor abundance. PDGFR-β homodimers bind only PDGF BB; PDGFR-α homodimers bind all three ligand iso-

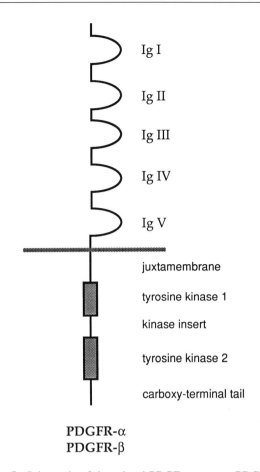

Fig. 8. Schematic of the related PDGF receptors, PDGFRα and PDGFRβ. Different domains are labeled.

forms: AA, AB, and BB; and PDGFR-α β heterodimers bind PDGF BB and AB. As described earlier, ligand binding triggers the receptor kinase, leading to autophosphorylation by a transphosphorylation mechanism. As with other growth factors, tyrosine phosphorylation creates docking sites for signal transduction molecules that contain SH2 domains.

2.5.4. BIOLOGICAL EFFECTS

2.5.4.1. Wound Healing One of the major actions of PDGF is in wound healing. Tissue injury leads to the rapid release of abundant PDGF AB by degranulating platelets. Other acute sources include activated macrophages and activated endothelial cells. Later in the history of a wound, keratinocytes also are induced to produce PDGF. PDGF acts in several ways during wound healing. It is chemotactic for smooth muscle cells, fibroblasts, neutrophils, and monocytes, and stimulates macrophage activation. It acts as a vaso-constrictor, thus assisting in the closure of damaged blood vessels. It also is a potent mitogen for fibroblasts and smooth muscle cells, and together with other growth factors, it stimulates the proliferative response of these cell types. PDGF induces expression of fibronectin, of some types of collagen, and of collagenase, and these substances participate in the tissue remodeling that occurs during wound healing.

2.5.5. ATHEROSCLEROSIS

The actions of PDGF that follow injury to the intima of blood vessels are similar to those occurring after a wound and contribute to the pathophysiology of atherosclerosis. Release of PDGF by aggregating platelets will trigger the same spectrum of biological responses that is seen in a wound, and these effects are involved in the proliferative changes that are associated with atherosclerotic plaques.

2.5.6. DEVELOPMENT

A mutation in each PDGFR is associated with major developmental anomalies in mice. The PDGFR-α gene is absent as part of a large chromosomal deletion in the Patch mouse. Most homozygotes die in midgestation and show poor development of many mesodermal derivatives, including cartilage and the dermal layer of the skin. The remaining embryos die during late gestation, and have defects in the thyroid, thymus, cardiac outflow track, and in other tissues. A targeted mutation in the PDGFR-β gene also is lethal when homozygous. These mice do not survive birth. Death is accompanied by hemorrhage, and by maldevelopment of the kidneys, with near absence of mesengial cells. A similar phenotype is seen in mice with a homozygous null mutation in the PDGF B-chain gene. These results are consistent with PDGF BB being the sole ligand for the β receptor.

2.5.7. THERAPEUTIC USES

Exogenous PDGF accelerates the healing of incisional wounds in experimental animals, and has been shown to enhance the closure of chronic pressure ulcers in human studies. In several wound healing models, PDGF is most active when used in combination with other growth factors.

2.6. TGF-β Family

2.6.1. INTRODUCTION

TGF-β is a dimeric protein of 25 kDa. In mammals, three isoforms have been described, TGF-β1, TGF-β2, and TGF-β3. These proteins are prototypi-

Table 7
TGF-β Family

TGF-β
    TGF-β1, β2, β3, β4, β5

Inhibins and activins
    Inhibin $\alpha\beta$A, $\alpha\beta$B
    Activin AA, AB, BB

Bone morphogenetic proteins (BMP)
    BMP 2, 3, 4, 5, 6, 7, 8
    Vg1
    Growth-differentiation factors 1, 3 (GDF 1, 3)
    Dorsalin
    Nodal

MIS

GDNF

cal members of a large family of growth factors with diverse biological effects in many different species. TGF-β and related proteins control aspects of development, differentiation, and determination, regulate immune function and the response to inflammation, and play pivotal roles in reproduction. TGF-β action is controlled by interactions with several classes of receptors, and with cell-associated and extracellular binding proteins. Two classes of high-affinity TGF-β receptors have been defined. Both Type I and type II receptors are ligand-activated serine-threonine protein kinases. A Type III receptor modulates binding to Type I and Type II receptors, but lacks signaling properties.

2.6.2. STRUCTURE OF TGF-B AND RELATED PROTEINS

The TGF-β superfamily contains at least 24 members in vertebrates (Table 7); several homologs exist in invertebrates as well. These proteins are all synthesized as larger precursors with amino-terminal extensions. Proteolytic cleavage releases the mature protein, which in its biologically active form is a homo- or heterodimer. Amino acid sequence similarity among family members is confined to the mature 110–140 residue growth factor. Members of the TGF-β family share seven nearly invariant cysteine residues. Six cysteines are involved in the formation of intrachain disulfide bonds, which link the protein into a rigid structure termed a "cysteine knot," as initially defined in the crystal structure of TGF-β2. The seventh cysteine forms the disulfide bridge that

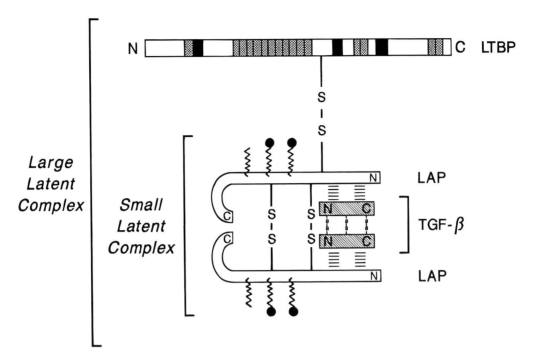

Fig. 9. TGF-β is found in latent complexes. Small latent complexes contain LAP, a glycoprotein derived from the TGF-β precursor (carbohydrates are indicated by squiggles and mannose 6-phosphate residues by black circles). TGF-β and LAP associate through noncovalent interactions as depicted by the short parallel horizontal lines. Large latent complexes additionally contain LTBP. LTBP also is a glycoprotein and consists of several domains, including cysteine-rich sequences (black boxes) and motifs related to EGF (stippled boxes).

binds two monomers into the TGF-β dimer. Surprisingly, the crystal structure of the TGF-β monomer is very similar to that of PDGF and NGF, even though these proteins share little amino acid similarity. All three growth factors contain the cysteine knot motif and have nearly superimposable three-dimensional structures.

2.6.3. TGF-β

Five structurally related TGF-β molecules have been characterized. TGF-β1, TGF-β2, and TGF-β3 were isolated from mammalian tissues, TGF-β4 from the chicken, and TGF-β5 from *Xenopus laevis*. The mature proteins are 64–82% identical. Mammalian TGF-β monomers are 112 amino acids in length and contain nine cysteines. They are synthesized as precursors of approx 350–400 residues, and are secreted as latent complexes of approx 100 kDa. Latent complexes consist of the mature TGF-β dimer noncovalently associated with a dimer of the precursor protein, which is termed latency associated peptide (LAP). This small latent complex is unable to bind to TGF-β receptors. A larger latent complex also has

been described. It consists additionally of a 125–160 kDa cysteine-rich glycoprotein known as latent TGF-β-binding protein (LTBP) (*see* Fig. 9). Activation of the latent complex offers one mechanism for regulating growth factor availability. Although the precise pathway of activation has not been elucidated, it appears to involve proteolysis at the cell surface. LAP is a glycoprotein and several of its sugar side chains contain mannose 6-phosphate residues. The IGF-IIR can bind the latent TGF-β complex through these sugar residues, and this binding appears essential for activation in tissue-culture cells. Activation also requires proteases. Latent complexes have not been described for other members of the TGF-β family.

2.6.4. INHIBINS AND ACTIVINS

Inhibins were identified as proteins found in ovarian follicular fluid that inhibited pituitary secretion of follicle-stimulating hormone (FSH). The two inhibins are heterodimers between a common α subunit and one of two β subunits, βA and βB. Activins were characterized as stimulators of FSH secretion, and are composed of dimers of inhibin β chains.

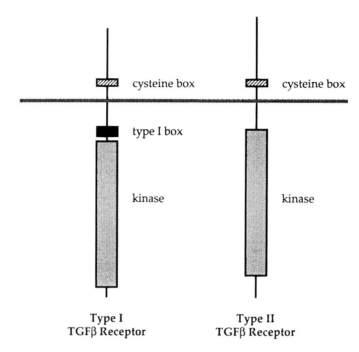

Fig. 10. Structure of Type I and Type II TGF-β receptors. Different domains are labeled.

Three isoforms have been isolated: AA, AB, and BB. Inhibins and activins are functional antagonists.

2.6.5. Bone Morphogenetic Proteins (BMPs)

Seven BMPs, BMP2–8, have been characterized. These proteins are dimers of molecular wt 26–31 kDa. BMPs were identified initially by their ability to induce cartilage and bone. BMP2 and BMP4 are closely related in sequence to each other and to the *Drosophila* protein *decapentaplegic (dpp)*. *Dpp* plays essential roles in morphogenesis and in bodily patterning in the fly. Perhaps surprisingly, human BMP4 can rescue some of the defects that occur in *dpp* mutants, indicating that the two proteins are functionally related.

BMP5–8 are 74–91% identical to one another, and are similar in structure to another *Drosophila* protein, *60A*, whose function is unknown. Additional proteins that are related to the BMPs include vegetal 1 (Vg1), growth-differentiation factors 1 and 3 (GDF-1, GDF-3; GDF-3 is also known as vegetal-related 2 Vgr2), dorsalin, and nodal. Together this grouping is termed DVR, for *dpp* and Vg1-related. Vg1 was identified as a *Xenopus laevis* factor that can induce dorsal mesoderm formation during early development. Nodal was identified through analysis of a mouse mutation in which mesoderm formation was dis-

rupted. The roles of the GDFs and dorsalin have not been defined.

2.6.6. Mullerian Inhibitory Substance

MIS was characterized as a factor secreted by male mammalian embryos that caused regression of the Mullerian duct, which otherwise would develop into the oviducts, uterus, and upper one-third of the vagina. It is a disulfide-linked dimer that is secreted as a dimeric precursor of approx 140 kDa. MIS is distantly related in sequence to TGF-β (approx 30% amino acid identity).

2.6.7. Glial-derived Neurotrophic Growth Factor

GDNF was isolated through its ability to promote survival and differentiation of dopaminergic neurons. It is < 25% identical to other members of the TGF-β family.

2.6.8. TGF-b Receptors

TGF-β binds to three major cell-surface proteins that were initially termed Type I, Type II, and Type III, based on approximate mol wt of 53, 70–85, and >200 kDa. Several cDNAs encoding each class of receptor were subsequently cloned. Type I and Type II receptors are structurally related (Fig. 10). Both are composed of extracellular ligand-binding regions of 102–196 amino acids containing a short cysteine-rich box, single transmembrane segment, and an intracytoplasmic region of approx 400–500 residues. The intracellular portion contains a kinase domain that will phosphorylate itself and exogenous substrates on serine and threonine residues. Structurally related receptors have been identified by their ability to bind to activins or BMPs.

Evidence has accumulated demonstrating that Type I and Type II proteins interact to create functional signaling receptors. Type I receptors will bind TGF-β only when coexpressed with Type II receptors. Binding specificity appears to be determined by the Type II receptor, since the same Type I protein will bind either activin or TGF-β, depending on the coexpressed Type II receptor. In addition, the signaling properties of Type II receptors can be modified depending on the Type I receptor that is available. Thus, the interaction of different heteromeric receptor complexes can lead to distinct biological effects initiated by the same ligand.

2.6.9. Type III Receptors and TGF-β Binding Proteins

The Type III receptor, called betaglycan, is a transmembrane proteoglycan with a protein core mole wt of 130 kDa. A secreted version has been identified in the extracellular matrix. Betaglycan is structurally related to endoglin, a transmembrane glycoprotein composed of two disulfide-linked 95-kDa subunits; endoglin has been shown to bind TGF-β1 and TGF-β3. Both proteins consist of large extracellular domains, a single transmembrane segment, and a short intracytoplasmic region. One role for betaglycan is in presenting TGF-β to Type II receptors. Betaglycan and endoglin also may function in the storage and clearance of TGF-β. No comparable Type III receptors have been identified yet for activins, BMPs, or other members of the TGF-β family.

Other TGF-β binding proteins include LTBP, described earlier, and follistatin, a widely distributed, secreted glycoprotein that binds activin and inhibits its actions. In addition, α_2-macroglobulin, a serum protein, binds both mature TGF-β and activin, and may play a role in growth factor clearance from the circulation.

2.6.10. Biological Effects

As noted earlier, members of the TGF-β family exert diverse biological effects. The actions of activins, inhibins, and MIS are described in other chapters. This section will outline some of the functions of other members of this growth factor family.

2.6.11. Development

Genetic studies indicate major roles for several TGF-—related proteins in early development. The *Drosophila* protein *dpp* is essential for normal dorsoventral patterning, for development of the gastrointestinal tract, and for other aspects of cell lineage determination. In the nematode *C elegans*, homologs of Type I and Type II receptors (daf-1 and daf-4, respectively) control a signal transduction pathway that is required for formation of a special larval stage (dauer larva) when population density exceeds food supply. The ligands for these receptors have not been defined. During the early development of the frog, *Xenopus laevis*, Vg1, activins, and BMPs exert striking effects on the formation and patterning of mesoderm. Similarly, in mice, mutations in the protein nodal disrupt normal mesoderm formation.

Mutations in the BMP5 gene also cause marked developmental abnormalities, including alterations in the size, shape, and number of skeletal components and a diminution in the size of the external ear. It is likely that other BMPs play analogous roles in skeletal development.

TGF-β1 also is important in mouse development. A targeted disruption of the TGF-β1 gene leads to neonatal death secondary to cardiac abnormalities. This phenotype is seen only in progeny of TGF-β1-deficient mothers, because transplacental passage of TGF-β1 and absorption of TGF-β1 in mother's milk normally compensate for the lack of growth factor production by the nullizygous fetus and infant.

2.6.13. Control of Inflammation and the Response to Tissue Injury

Mice born from heterozygous mothers with a homozygous null mutation in the TGF-β1 gene have no morphological abnormalities at birth, but die soon after weaning (age 2–3 week) of multiple organ failure secondary to massive infiltration of inflammatory cells. This result potentially reflects the bivalent actions of TGF-β in inflammation and repair of tissue injury. Normally after an injury, TGF-β1, released by platelets, is strongly chemotactic for neutrophils, monocytes, T-lymphocytes, and fibroblasts. Monocytes and T-cells are then stimulated to produce other growth factors and cytokines, and fibroblasts are induced to enhance production of extracellular matrix proteins. Additional TGF-β also is synthesized by these cells. This TGF-β then down regulates these processes by inhibiting the functions of inflammatory cells once they have been activated. The normal result is cessation of the inflammatory response as the wound heals. This last step does not occur in TGF-β1-deficient mice once the source of maternal TGF-β has dissipated, and massive inflammation persists.

Excessive production of TGF-β as part of the response to inflammation also can enhance tissue fibrosis and contribute to a variety of fibrotic disorders, including glomerulopathies, liver cirrhosis, rheumatoid arthritis, and others. In experimental glomerulonephritis, neutralizing antibodies to TGF-β1 prevented the accumulation of extracellular matrix proteins and minimized fibrosis.

2.6.14. THERAPEUTIC USES

One major use of TGF-β is in wound healing. A single local treatment greatly accelerates wound repair in experimental animals. Topical TGF-β2 has clinical application in repair of retinal tears. Antagonists of TGF-β action also have potential as antifibrotic agents. In addition to the effectiveness of neutralizing antibodies, initial studies have been promising with soluble Type III receptors and with LAP.

2.7. Other Growth Factor Families

Many growth-promoting substances have been identified that do not fit into the framework of the families described in the previous sections. Several of these substances have not been characterized completely and/or exert their effects on a limited subset of tissue and cell types, and thus will not be reviewed here. Others have more diverse actions. Two examples are hepatocyte growth factor (HGF) and stem cell factor (SCF); their properties are summarized below.

HGF is a disulfide-linked heterodimer consisting of a 69-kDa α chain and a 34-kDa β chain that was characterized as a potent serum-derived stimulator of liver cell growth in tissue culture. HGF binds to and activates a heterodimeric tyrosine kinase receptor that is the cellular homolog of the *v-met* oncogene (*c-met*). This receptor has a wide tissue distribution, and HGF has been shown to exert proliferative effects on multiple cell types. Its specific roles in liver regeneration and in other tissues have not been defined.

SCF is the ligand for a tyrosine kinase receptor that is the cellular homolog of the *v-kit* oncogene (*c-kit*). This receptor is structurally related to the PDGFRs, and is composed of an extracellular domain with five immunoglobulin-like motifs, a transmembrane region, and an intracellular tyrosine kinase domain that is split by a kinase insert. Different mutations in SCF (the steel locus) or in c-kit (the dominant white spotting or W locus) in mice cause multiple developmental anomalies, including alterations in coat color, anemia, and defective gonadal development. A heterozygous deletion of c-kit has been identified in humans with the piebald trait, which is characterized by a congenital white hair forelock and areas of depigmentation on the chest and extremities.

3. SUMMARY AND PERSPECTIVE

Peptide growth factors are multifunctional proteins that exert their diverse effects by activating transmembrane receptors. Their actions lead to both short-term alterations in cellular function and to long-term changes in the whole animal. As highlighted in this chapter, growth factors play critical individual and collaborative roles in many aspects of development in a wide variety of species, regulate somatic growth, influence tissue maturation and repair, and modulate intermediary metabolism throughout life. Only now is their potential for therapeutic use being investigated. Studies in the coming decade should lead to a further understanding of the importance of peptide growth factors in many areas of biology and medicine.

SELECTED READING
Growth Factors—General

Fantl WJ, Johnson DE, Williams LT. Signalling by receptor tyrosine kinases. *Annu Rev Biochem* 1993; 62:453.

Heldin C-H. Dimerization of cell surface receptors in signal transduction. *Cell* 1995; 80;213.

Karin M. Signal transduction from the cell surface to the nucleus through the phosphorylation of transcription factors. *Curr Opinion Cell Biol* 1994; 6:415.

EGF Family

Carpenter G. EGF: new tricks for an old growth factor. *Curr Opinion Cell Biol* 1993; 5:261.

Prigent SA, Lemoine NR. The type 1 (EGFR-related) family of growth factor receptors and their ligands. *Prog Growth Factor Res* 1992; 4:1.

FGF Family

Baird A. Fibroblast growth factors: activities and significance of non-neurotrophin neurotrophic growth factors. *Curr Opinion Neurobiol* 1994; 4:78.

Fernig DG, Gallagher JT. Fibroblast growth factors and their receptors: an information network controlling tissue growth, morphogenesis and repair. *Prog Growth Factor Res* 1994; 5:353.

IGF Family

Clemmons DR, Underwood LE. Uses of human insulin-like growth factor-I in clinical conditions. *J Clin Endocrinol Metab* 1994; 79:4.

Jones JI, Clemmons DR. Insulin-like growth factors and their binding proteins: biological actions. *Endocr Rev* 1995; 16:3.

NGF Family

Johnson J, Oppenheim R. Keeping track of changing neurotrophic theory. *Curr Biology* 1994; 4:662.

Saltiel AR, Decker SJ. Cellular mechanism of signal transduction for neurotrophins. *BioEssays* 1994; 16:405.

PDGF Family

Claesson-Welsh L. Platelet-derived growth factor receptor signals. *J Biol Chem* 1994;269:32023.

TGF-β Family

Border WA, Noble NA. Transforming growth factor β in tissue fibrosis. *New Engl J Med* 1994; 31:1286.

Kingsley DM. The TGF-β superfamily: new members, new receptors, and new genetic tests of function in different organisms. *Genes Dev* 1994; 8:133.

7 Prostaglandins and Leukotrienes

Locally Acting Agents

John A. McCracken, PhD

Contents

1. INTRODUCTION

This chapter is not intended for the prostaglandin (PG) specialist, but rather for those not familiar with the PG field. It will provide a brief overview of the biology of the eicosanoid family and how these local mediators may function in health and in disease. The term "eicosanoids" was coined to describe the broad group of compounds derived from C_{20} fatty acids, which, in turn, are derived from the essential dietary fatty acids. The predominant C_{20} fatty acid precursor for eicosanoid biosynthesis in most mammals is arachidonic acid (AA). The eicosanoids include the prostaglandins (PGs) and thromboxanes (TXs), the leukotrienes (LTs), the lipoxins (LPXs), and the hydroxyeicosanoic acids (HETEs). Since the biological activity of eicosanoids is rapidly destroyed both in tissues and in the circulation, it is likely that they act locally at the tissue and organ level, where they may regulate regional blood flow and other metabolic

activities. Moreover, their formation in various inflammatory sites indicates an important mediating role for these substances in diseased states. Indeed, eicosanoid inhibition by different classes of anti-inflammatory drugs underlines their importance in this regard. The chapter includes a brief historical background, together with a description of nomenclature, biosynthesis, and selected local actions of eicosanoids. For those requiring more detailed information, recent reviews and references on specific topics are included.

2. HISTORICAL BACKGROUND

The biological existence of PGs was established in the 1930s by the detection of smooth muscle contracting and vasodepressor activity in extracts of human and sheep seminal plasma. Ulf von Euler went on to demonstrate that these compounds were acidic lipids and the name "prostaglandins" was coined, because it was thought at the time that these acidic lipids emanated from the prostate gland, whereas we now know that the seminal vesicles are

From: *Endocrinology: Basic and Clinical Principles* (P. M. Conn and S. Melmed, eds.), Humana Press Inc., Totowa, NJ.

the main site of synthesis in the male reproductive system (*see* von Euler, 1988). It is not surprising that the biological activity of PGs was first detected in the male system, because they are present in microgram quantities in seminal plasma of many species including man, monkeys, and sheep. In contrast, PGs in other tissues are present in picogram or, at best, nanogram amounts. The function of PGs found in seminal plasma has not been fully documented, although a role has been suggested in contraction of the male accessory glands and the vas deferens. Also, it has been proposed that they assist in sperm transport by stimulating contraction of the female genital tract, the latter also being a major source of PG synthesis and action. Indeed, the most fully established physiological role of the PGs is that of $PGF_{2\alpha}$, a locally acting uterine luteolytic hormone in a number of mammalian species (*see* Section 6.7.).

Progress in identifying the chemical nature of the PGs was slow, partly because of World War II, and partly because the technology to detect these labile and elusive compounds was not available until the 1950s. Bergström and Sjovall (1957) using gas chromatography/mass spectrometry identified the structure of two different PGs, one of which they named PGE (found in the ethanolic fraction) and another named PGF (found in the phosphate fraction— spelled fosfate in Swedish), thus giving rise to the present nomenclature. A related product of AA metabolism that is a potent stimulator of platelet aggregation was discovered by Bengt Samuelsson and colleagues and named TX (Hamberg et al., 1975). Later a potent inhibitor of platelet aggregation derived from AA and formed in endothelium was discovered by John Vane and coworkers (Moncada and Vane, 1977; Sun et al., 1977), and named prostacyclin (PGI_2) because of its double-ring structure.

Shortly thereafter, Bengt Samuelsson and colleagues (Murphy et al., 1979) described a new class of AA metabolites from leukocytes, some of which have chemotactic properties and others of which increase vascular permeability. These substances were named LTs. They are produced from AA by the action of 5-lipoxygenase (5-LO). In some of the LTs, the amino acid cysteine is incorporated into the molecule to give rise to the sulfidopeptide LTs (*see* Section 4.3.). The LTs are considered to be involved in inflammatory processes where they most likely act synergistically with other mediators, such as histamine, bradykinin, and PGs, to produce the classical signs of inflamma-

tion described by Celsus, namely, redness (rubor), heat (calor), swelling (tumor), and pain (dolor). The involvement of both PGs and LTs in the inflammatory process is underlined by the effects of nonsteroidal anti-inflammatory drugs (NSAIDs), such as aspirin and indomethacin, which are potent inhibitors of PG biosynthesis via inhibition of cyclooxygenase (COX) activity. The NSAIDs, however, do not affect the lipoxygenase pathway responsible for LT biosynthesis. Indeed, because NSAIDs so efficiently block PG synthesis, these drugs most likely amplify LT synthesis by diverting AA into the lipoxygenase pathway. Thus in asthmatics, where LTs have been identified as major mediators of bronchoconstriction, the use of NSAIDs is contraindicated. On the other hand, corticosteroids have a potent inhibitory effect on phospholipase A_2 (PLA_2) activity, thus markedly reducing the availability of AA as a substrate for both the COX and the lipoxygenase pathways. As described later, corticosteroids also appear to inhibit the synthesis of the inducible form of the COX enzyme. Corticosteroids are thus the most useful therapeutic agents for asthmatics at present. However, drugs based on LT receptor antagonists and LT biosynthesis inhibitors are presently under development and may provide important alternatives to long-term corticosteroid therapy.

3. PG NOMENCLATURE

The major PGs of the two series are summarized below.

PGA_2 Dehydration product of PGE_2
PGB_2 Dehydration product of PGE_2
PGD_2 Abundant in neural tissues, sleep-inducing
PGE_2 Vasodilator, gastric cytoprotection
$PGF_{2\alpha}$ Vasoconstrictor, luteolysis and labor
PGG_2 Endoperoxide intermediate
PGH_2 Endoperoxide intermediate
PGI_2 Antiplatelet aggregation, vasodilator
TXA_2 Platelet aggregation, vasoconstrictor

3.1. Chemical Structure

The number of double bonds in the PG molecule is designated by a subscript, so that $PGF_{1\alpha}$ has one double bond in position 13:14 and $PGF_{2\alpha}$ has an a second double bond in position 5:6. $PGF_{3\alpha}$ has an a third double bond in position 17:18 (Fig. 1). In the case of PGF, the α designation indicates that the three hydroxyl groups are in the α orientation. The principal PG precursor in most species is AA, liberated

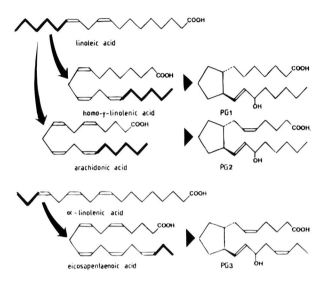

Fig. 1. Homo-γ-linolenic acid and AA are converted respectively into prostaglandins (PGs) of the 1 series (PG$_1$), exhibiting only one double bond, and into the 2 series (PG$_2$)—two double bonds. These polyunsaturated acids and their precursor, linoleic acid, are members of the biological family of ω-6 fatty acids, characterized by an end segment of 6 carbons (at the opposite end from the—COOH). Eicosapentaenoic acid, coming from the α-linolenic acid (ω-*3 family*), is converted to PG$_3$ (three double bonds). The characteristic end segment of ω-6 and ω-3 families are represented on this picture in thick lines (from Deby, 1988).

from phospholipids principally by phospholipase A$_2$, which gives rise to the two series of PGs. The one series of PGs is derived from homo-γ-linolenic acid which, in most species, is less abundant. Some species, especially when on diets rich in fish oils, produce the three series of PGs derived from eicosapentaenoic acid. It is suggested that the high consumption of fish oils by Eskimos has a protective effect on the cardiovascular system in the presence of a high-fat diet.

4. BIOSYNTHESIS

4.1. PGs

A simplified flow sheet of the major pathways of eicosanoid biosynthesis is shown in Fig. 2. Virtually all cells appear to have the capacity to synthesize PGs, the end product depending on the enzymes present that convert the endoperoxide intermediates to specific PGs. The initial step in PG biosynthesis is the formation of AA from phospholipid stores via the action of phosphlipase A$_2$ (PLA$_2$). The microsomal COX, which converts AA to the endoperoxide intermediates PGG$_2$

and PGH$_2$, is now known to exist in both a constitutive form (COX-1) and an inducible form (e.g., activated by serum or endotoxin), designated COX-2. The NSAIDs, such as aspirin or indomethacin, act mainly by inhibiting the activity of the COX enzymes (also known as PG syntheses). Indeed, recent studies indicate that different NSAIDs may have selective effects on the constitutive (COX-1) vs the inducible form (COX-2). Daniel Simmons and his coworkers (1993) have reviewed the evidence that glucocorticoids, which act primarily by blocking the phospholipase-mediated release of AA from phospholipids, also have a selective inhibitory effect by blocking the formation of the inducible form of COX (COX-2), thus contributing to the blockade of PG synthesis. Although it is well documented that PGs are an important component in acute inflammatory responses, it was observed that PGs of the E series may have certain modulating effects in some types of chronic inflammation, i.e., high tissue levels of PGEs may have anti-inflammatory effects. Robert Zurier (1988) and more recently Gerald Weissmann (1993), who have studied the role of PGs in inflammation for many years, suggest that the proposed anti-inflammatory action of PGE$_2$ in certain chronic inflammatory states may be mediated by its ability to generate cAMP. Because certain NSAIDs e.g., sodium salicylate, can alleviate inflammation without inhibiting PG synthesis, it has been proposed that PGs may be modulators rather than mediators of inflammation (Weissmann, 1993). Moreover, PGE has been shown to suppress adjuvant disease (Induced polyarthritis) in animal models and to inhibit neutrophil-mediated tissue injury (Zurier, 1988). Since the 5-LO is not inhibited by NSAIDs, leukotriene production may be potentially enhanced by diverting AA into the lipoxygenase pathway. In some instances, generation of leukotrienes can be inhibited by PGs, e.g., the production of LTB$_4$ by neutrophils (*see* Section 4.3), suggesting that there may be a subtle balance between COX and lipoxygenase pathways. It has been proposed that the administration of a combination of NSAIDs and long-acting PGE analogs could act synergistically in anti-inflammatory therapy (Weissmann, 1993).

4.2. Platelet-Activating Factor (PAF) (Alkyl-Acetyl-glycerophosphocholine)

PAF is derived from phosphatidylcholine as a product of PLA$_2$ action, although structurally it is not an eicosanoid. However, PAF is a potent platelet-aggregating substance that can operate without

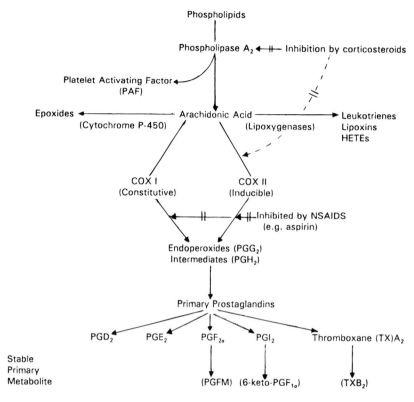

Fig. 2. Simplified pathway of eicosanoid biosynthesis.

adenosine 5'-diphosphate or TXA$_2$. Joseph O'Flaherty (1988) has reviewed the biosynthesis of PAF in various tissues, and concluded that PAF may act as both an intracellular and extracellular mediator. As well as acting as an intracellular mediator, PAF also appears to act in an autocrine fashion by binding to the parent cell receptors, thus initiating other second messenger signals. It appears to act in conjunction with endogenous eicosanoids with which it is often coformed during inflammatory states and allergic processes, such as asthma. PAF has also been suggested to play a local role during implantation of the embryo in the uterus, a process that also may involve PGs and other local mediators. A simplified chart showing the biosynthesis of PAF is shown in Fig. 3. In addition to the main PLA$_2$ pathway, the phospholipase C pathway is illustrated in the diagram to show that activation of this signal transduction mechanism may also generate AA for eicosanoid formation.

Recent studies by Elaine Tuomanen and colleagues (Cundell et al., 1995) indicate that virulent pneumococci utilize the PAF receptor to gain entry into host cells. This bacterium is a commensal in the human nasopharynx and is a major cause of sepsis, pneumo-

nia, and meningitis. Bacterial entry into endothelial cells is increased 20- to 40-fold following stimulation of PAF receptors by fibrin or tumor necrosis factor-alpha (TNF-α) and reversed by PAF receptor antagonists. It is suggested that bacterial cell-wall phosphatidylcholine is a cognate ligand for the PAF receptor and that bacterial attachment subverts the receptor (in the absence of signal transduction) to internalize the bacterium. These novel findings suggest that PAF receptor antagonists may be of therapeutic value, not only in blocking PAF bioactivity, but also by attenuating bacterial attachment, which leads to invasion of host cells.

4.3. LTs

Like the PGs, LTs are considered to be local mediators generated in the microenvironment and usually associated with inflammation. The LTs are generated from AA released from membrane phospholipids or from secretory granules of tissue cells, such as neutrophils or mast cells. The main enzyme in LT synthesis, 5-LO, requires activation by Ca^{2+} and translocation to a membrane-associated site. These requirements are in contrast to PG synthesis where

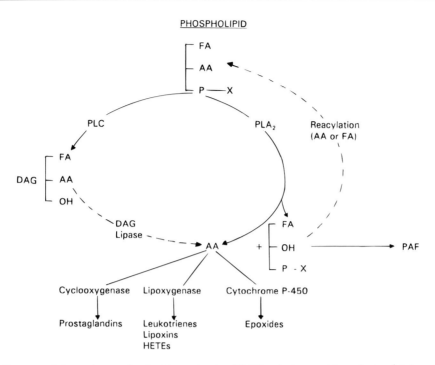

PHOSPHOLIPID

Fig. 3. Simplified diagram of the pathways for the biosynthesis of PAF and eicosanoid products of AA metabolism. Note that PLA$_2$ action forms both AA and PAF, whereas the action of PLC can form lesser amounts of AA indirectly from DAG via DAG lipase, e.g., during signal transduction.

COX does not require specific activation, but rather only the presence of substrate (AA). An additional regulatory component in LT biosynthesis is the existence of a 5-LO-activating protein (FLAP) thought to be essential for LT biosynthesis. Local synthesis of LTs is part of a cascade of events occurring during inflammation, which include the release of PGs, PAF, histamine, and other cellular mediators of this process. The LT pathway from AA involves the synthesis of LTA$_4$ via the 5-LO pathway (Fig. 4). LTA$_4$ is nonenzymatically converted to LTB$_4$ or into the sulfidopeptide leukotrienes LTC$_4$, LTD$_4$, and LTE$_4$. Human neutrophils have the selective capacity to synthesize LTB$_4$ and also appear to inactivate LTB$_4$, thus regulating its local activity, which includes chemotaxis and neutrophil adherence to endothelial cells. Eosinophils, on the other hand, generate only LTC$_4$ because they possess LTC$_4$ synthase, whereas monocytes generate both LTB$_4$ and LTC$_4$. Cells lacking the enzymes required to produce specific eicosanoids may utilize an intermediate provided by another cell type. For example, the transfer of PG endoperoxide intermediates from platelets to endothelial cells results in the formation of PGI$_2$, which has antiplatelet-aggregating activity. Erythrocytes lack

5-LO, but can convert LTA$_4$ to LTB$_4$. These cell–cell interactions illustrate the complexity of eicosanoid synthesis likely to occur, for example, in inflammatory processes. The three sulfidopeptide LTs (LTC$_4$, LTD$_4$, and LTE$_4$) constitute the slow-reacting substance of anaphylaxis, and they are implicated in the pathogenesis of asthma and other pulmonary conditions. Inhalation of LTD$_4$ and LTC$_4$ by humans is 1000 times more potent than histamine in causing airflow impairment at a fixed vital capacity, whereas LTE$_4$ is 10 times as potent as histamine. The involvement of LTs in anaphylaxis and asthma has prompted the synthesis of a number of LT-receptor antagonists, many of which are under clinical trials. Another approach is the development of LT biosynthesis inhibitors, which have no direct effect on the 5-LO enzyme itself, but bind with high affinity to FLAP, the expression of which is required for LT biosynthesis. The development of new LT-inhibiting drugs, including those binding to FLAP, has recently been reviewed by Anthony Ford-Hutchinson (1994). It is hoped that these LT antagonists and inhibitors will help to alleviate the clinical symptoms associated with asthma and other pulmonary conditions, thus providing an alternative to long-term corticosteroid therapy.

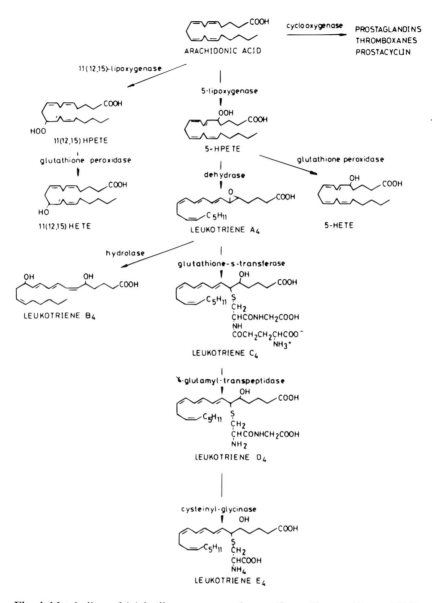

Fig. 4. Metabolism of AA by lipoxygenase pathways (from: Piper and Letts, 1988).

AA can also be converted via other lipoxygenase pathways to yield a series of HETE derivatives, including lipoxins and other HETEs (Fig. 2). These lipoxygenase products are considered to be associated with the immune system, as proposed by Jack Vanderhoek (1988), where they may play a role as endogenous immunosuppressive agents. For further reading on the biosynthesis and metabolism of LTs, the reader is directed to a minireview by Frank Austen and Roy Soberman (1988). AA also can be metabolized to epoxides by cytochrome P-450. The functional role of epoxides is only now being explored, but may include effects on intracel-

lular Ca^{2+} transport and on luteinizing hormone release.

Because eicosanoids are released from tissues as soon as they are formed, they are not stored within the cell. However, in the case of the male reproductive system, PGs accumulate in large amounts in the glandular secretions found in the lumen of the seminal vesicles. Most tissues metabolize PGs very rapidly via the 15-hydroxy-dehydrogenase/13:14 reductase complex, which is particularly abundant in lung tissue. In most species, one passage through the lungs can inactivate >90% of the biological activity of the primary PGs. The net effect is that although returning venous blood can contain considerable amounts of PGs (in the nanogram range), aortic blood is virtually devoid of PG activity (the levels may be as low as 0.1 pg/mL). Thus, PGs are regarded as locally acting agents, since their very potent biological activity has to be restricted by 15-hydroxydehydrogenases, both at the tissue level and in the vascular system by pulmonary metabolism and, to some extent, by metabolism in the liver and kidney.

4.4. Isoprostanes

In the past few years, Jackson Roberts and Jason Morrow (1994) have identified a novel series of PG-like compounds, termed F_2-isoprostanes, which are formed as products of lipid peroxidation of membrane phospholipids catalyzed by free radicals, i.e., independent of the COX pathway. One of the isoprostanes, 8-epi-$F_{2\alpha}$, has been identified as the most potent renal vasoconstricting substance ever discovered. The marked vasoconstrictor effect of this compound has been shown to be mediated by activation of TX receptors. Current work suggests that the overproduction of isoprostanes may play a causative role in the hepatorenal syndrome, defined as unexplained renal failure in the presence of severe liver disease. Thus, in addition to being markers of lipid peroxidation, it is likely that isoprostanes may be associated with the pathophysiology of oxidant stress, suggesting that antioxidant therapy may provide a new rationale for therapeutic intervention in certain diseased states.

5. EICOSANOID RECEPTORS

PGs, TXs, and LTs are considered to act locally via specific receptors located on the cell surface. However, the specificity of these receptors shows considerable overlap, so that responses to PGs within different tissues may vary or even have opposite actions. The nature and affinities of receptors for various PGs have been studied using radiolabeled ligands. In addition, biochemical studies have been conducted to examine the action of these compounds at the cellular level. PG receptors have also been characterized pharmacologically by comparing the potencies and responses of various PGs and their analogs in a variety of bioassay systems. Based on these findings, Robert Coleman and his colleagues (1994) have described a pharmacological classification in which each PG has its own receptor, some of which show subtypes. In the case of PGE, at least three subtypes have been assigned and designated EP1, EP2, and

EP3. Evidence has also accumulated that TXA_2 may have two receptor subtypes. On the other hand, binding studies, using ^{3}H-labeled $PGF_{2\alpha}$ have produced equivocal evidence for the existence of high- and low-affinity receptors for $PGF_{2\alpha}$. Based on the ability of PGF_2 to stimulate oxytocin secretion from the ovine corpus luteum, a known target tissue for $PGF_{2\alpha}$, Edward Custer and colleagues (1995) have provided in vivo evidence for the existence of functional high- and low-affinity states of the $PGF_{2\alpha}$ receptor. Presently, it is unclear whether these two affinity states are represented by a single protein, which may change its affinity from a high to a low state via activation of a G-protein, as has been demonstrated for the LTB_4 receptor in human myeloid cells (Slipetz et al., 1993). It is also possible that the product of a single gene could give rise to two types of receptors by alternative splicing or that each type of receptors could be encoded by two different genes. Alternatively, the differential response of the corpus luteum to low and high concentrations of $PGF_{2\alpha}$ could be mediated by a single-affinity $PGF_{2\alpha}$ receptor that exhibits a dose-dependent second messenger response to different concentrations of ligand (*see* Section 7.).

Shuh Narumiya (1995) has pioneered the cloning of the PG receptors, the first of which was TXA_2. This was accomplished by isolating and purifying it from human blood platelets, followed by cloning of the cDNA. These studies indicated that the TXA_2 receptor is a G-protein-coupled rhodopsin-type receptor with seven transmembrane domains. Because there is only a 10–20% homology with other rhodopsin-type receptors, it is proposed that TXA_2 and other prostanoids constitute a subfamily of the rhodopsin-type receptor superfamily. Based on this model, screening of mouse cDNA libraries revealed seven different prostanoid receptors. Three receptor subtypes of the PGE receptor were cloned and designated EP1, EP2, and EP3, thus confirming the above pharmacological classification. In addition to the receptors encoded by different genes, alternative splicing of the EP3 receptor transcript has yielded three isoforms of the receptor, which couple to various G-proteins and induce specific signaling systems (Fig. 5). Evidence is emerging that a fourth isoform of the EP3 receptor may also exist.

5.1. PG Transporter

Some years ago, John McCracken and colleagues (1972) showed that PGs diffuse rather slowly through the wall of the ovarian artery. However, in some

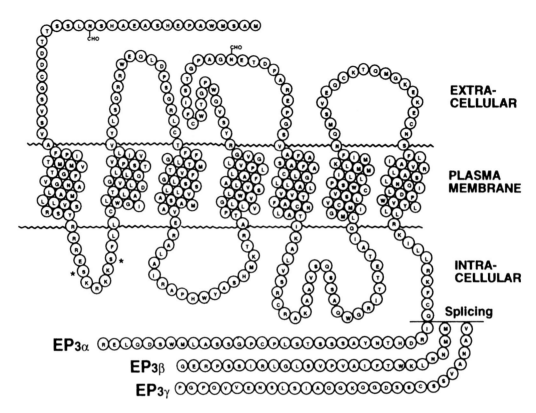

EXTRA-CELLULAR

PLASMA MEMBRANE

INTRA-CELLULAR

Splicing

EP3α

EP3β

EP3γ

Fig. 5. Seven-transmembrane-spanning model of the mouse EP3 isoforms showing alternative splicing for isoforms. Potential sites of N-linked glycosylation are indicated by CHO. Stars indicate potential phosphorylation sites for cAMP-dependent protein kinase (from: Negishi et al., 1995).

tissues, PG transport appears to be enhanced by a carrier-mediated transporter that has been identified in epithelial cells by Victor Schuster and colleagues as a protein with 12 transmembrane domains (*see* Kanai et al., 1995). Because the PG transporter appears to facilitate transport of PGs across cells membranes, it does not appear to be a receptor as such, particularly since it differs from the seven-transmembrane structure of the PG receptors. The PG transporter is thought to mediate the uptake and release of newly synthesized PGs from cells and to facilitate vectoral transport. Some PGs, such as PGI_2 and its metabolite, 6-keto-$PGF_{1\alpha}$, show very poor interaction with the PG-transporter, which may explain the much reduced metabolism of these compounds in the pulmonary circulation. The biological activity of other PGs present in venous blood is rapidly reduced by metabolism in one passage through the lungs, presumably because the PG transporter very efficiently allows access to the intracellular 15-hydroxy-dehydrogenases present in the lung parenchyma. This explanation is consistent with the finding that although PGI_2

is indeed a substrate for 15-hydroxy-dehydrogenase in cell free systems, it probably escapes metabolism in the lungs by virtue of its very weak interaction with the PG transporter. However, it should be emphasized that PGI_2 in vivo is intrinsically unstable, being transformed nonenzymatically to its inactive metabolite 6-keto-$PGF_{1\alpha}$ in about 20 sec. Thus it, is a "local hormone" rather than a circulating one, since arterial levels (about 3 pg/mL) are probably too low to have any systemic effect.

6. SELECTED EXAMPLES OF LOCAL ACTIONS OF EICOSANOIDS

6.1. Gastric Cytoprotection

PGE_2 appears to be an endogenous inhibitor of gastric acid secretion and to have a cytoprotective effect on the gastric mucosa. The ingestion of aspirin, indomethacin, and other NSAIDs that inhibit PG synthesis can cause severe damage to the gastric mucosa with formation of ulcers and gastric bleeding. That inhibition of PG synthesis leads to damage to the mucosa is demonstrated by the coadministration of NSAIDs and PGE_2, or one of its various analogs, which prevents mucosal damage. John Vane and R. M. Botting (1995) have evaluated the ability of several different NSAIDs to inhibit the two forms of COXs, COX-1 (constitutive) and COX-2 (inducible). The amino acid sequence of COX-2 shows a 60% homology with COX-1, but both enzymes have the same molecular wt of about 70 kDa and possess similar active sites for binding NSAIDs. Aspirin and indomethacin show greater inhibition of COX-1 (the predominant form in the gastric mucosa) than COX-2, which is consistent with the relative propensity among various NSAIDs to cause gastric ulceration. Thus, it may be possible to design NSAIDs, which have minimal effects on gastric COX-1, but which inhibit the COX-2 induced by inflammatory mediators in other tissues. Such drugs would permit safer oral administration for maximal systemic effects with minimal gastric side effects. An unusual example of local action of PGs on gastric function is provided by a species of Australian frog that incubates its eggs in the stomach. Extremely high levels of gastric PGE_2 during the incubation are thought to act locally to inhibit gastric acid secretion and to promote gastric mucus secretion, thus protecting the eggs against digestion in the stomach.

The local production of LTs may also play a role in gastric function, since ethanol-induced mucosal damage in the rat is accompanied by an increase in LTC_4. Moreover, nordihydroguaiaretic acid, a nonspecific lipoxygenase inhibitor, prevents ethanol-induced gastric mucosal damage and, at the same time, inhibits mucosal release of LTC_4. Thus, endogenous local production of PGE_2 has a protective effect on the stomach that is blocked by NSAIDs, whereas LTs appear to be local mediators of ethanol-induced damage to the gastric mucosa.

6.2. Local Action of PGs in Glaucoma

A biologically active substance was isolated from the iris and was found to increase during ocular inflammation. This substance, which caused a marked constriction of the pupil, was initially named irin. Subsequently the biological activity of irin was shown to be owing to PGs, principally $PGF_{2\alpha}$. This is consistent with previous findings that NSAIDs were effective in reducing inflammation in the eye. Paradoxically, it was found later that $PGF_{2\alpha}$ applied topically to the eye reduced intraocular pressure, suggesting a physiological role for PGs in regulating intraocular pressure. Johan Stjernschantz (1995) has pioneered the development of $PGF_{2\alpha}$ analogs for the treatment of glaucoma, which is characterized by a chronic increase in intraocular pressure. $PGF_{2\alpha}$ was found to reduce intraocular pressure not by increasing outflow via the trabecular meshwork or by reducing the production of aqueous humor, but rather by increasing the uveoscleral outflow of aqueous humor through the ciliary muscle. Although some modest side effects of daily topical application of $PGF_{2\alpha}$ analogs are observed, the dramatic and long-lasting reduction in intraocular pressure suggests that further the development of other $PGF_{2\alpha}$ analogs may provide a clinically useful treatment for glaucoma.

6.3. Local Effect of PGD_2 in Sleep Induction

For many years, Osamu Hayaishi and colleagues (1993) have studied the role of PGD_2 production in the preoptic area of the brain in relation to the induction of physiological sleep. They found that microinjection or infusion of PGD_2 in femtomolar concentrations into the preoptic area (an area considered to be the sleep center) or into the third ventricle of the rat or monkey was effective in inducing normal sleep. They went on to show that the specific activity of the enzyme that controls PGD_2 production in the brain, namely PGD_2 synthase, exhibits a circadian fluctuation that parallels the sleep/wake cycle. When PGD_2 synthase activity in the preoptic area was inhibited by the infusion of a specific inhibitor, namely selenium, sleep was inhibited. Such inhibition was reversed when the infusion of selenium into the preoptic area was stopped. They concluded that PGD_2 was produced and acted locally in the preoptic area of the brain as the physiological inducer of sleep.

6.4. Mediating Role of PGE_2 in Fever

Evidence has accumulated over several years that PGE_2 is a primary mediator of fever induced by bacterial pyrogens. Robert Skarnes and colleagues (1981) investigated the role of PGE_2 in endotoxin-induced fever in sheep. They showed that PGE_2, infused into the carotid artery of conscious sheep, caused a transient increase (10–20%) in blood pressure accompanied by a sustained (3 h) increase in core body temperature, which mimicked the effects seen during the first wave of fever induced by intravascular endotoxin. Subsequent experiments revealed that during the first phase of endotoxin-induced fever, a marked increase in both PGE_2 and $PGF_{2\alpha}$ occurred in the venous and arterial circulation. Intracarotid $PGF_{2\alpha}$ itself, however, did not exhibit the pyrogenic or pressor effects seen with intracarotid PGE_2. Further work showed that indomethacin blocked both the first and second phases of fever induced by endotoxin. Importantly, PGE_2 evoked both the pressor response and the first phase of fever during indomethacin blockade. They concluded that PGE_2, formed within the cranial vasculature, crosses the blood–brain barrier and acts on the thermoregulatory center in the hypothalamus to evoke the first phase of fever. However, since both first and second phases of fever are blocked by indomethacin, it appears that the presence of circulating levels of another AA metabolite may be responsible for the second phase (i.e., the phase associated with leukocyte pyrogen—interleukin-1).

Recent studies by Flavio Coceani and colleagues (1989), using the cat as a model, have confirmed the role of PGE_2 in the pathogenesis of fever induced by bacterial pyrogen. By means of a push–pull perfusion procedure, they demonstrated that iv endotoxin selectively caused an increase in PGE_2 in the anterior hypothalamic/preoptic region of the brain. The increase in PGE_2 production in these areas of the brain was consistent with the onset and progression of fever in their experimental model.

6.5. Pheromonal and Reproductive Function of PGs in Teleost Fish

Among the more unusual actions of PGs is their recently proposed role as pheromones in male Teleost fish. Peter Sorensen, and Frederick Goetz (1993) have investigated this phenomenon. $PGF_{2\alpha}$ and/or its metabolites are produced in large quantities in the ovaries of female Teleost fish, where they appear to act in a paracrine fashion by stimulating follicular rupture. In female Teleost fish, $PGF_{2\alpha}$ and/or metabolites secreted by the ovary pass into the systemic circulation and act centrally in the brain to elicit female spawning behavior. Apparently, relatively large amounts of PGF metabolites are released into the water during oviposition by the female fish and are detectable by the highly developed chemosensory system in the male fish. The male is thus "signaled" through a sensitive olfactory system to exhibit spawning behavior.

6.6. Local Action of PGs in the Uterus

Although PGs were first isolated and identified from secretions of the male reproductive tract, it was not long before they were also identified in the female

reproductive system, where they serve a number of important local functions. Key findings included the discovery that human menstrual fluid was a major source of PGs, particularly PGE_2 and $PGF_{2\alpha}$, and that the administration of $PGF_{2\alpha}$ into women during the luteal phase produced menstrual-like bleeding. Moreover, Joyce Eldering and coworkers (1993) have recently reported high production rates of several PGs (especially PGF) from endometrium of the rhesus monkey, primarily during the luteal phaase. These findings led to extensive studies on the role of PGs in normal menstruation and in abnormal conditions such as dysmenorrhea and menorrhagia. Marc Bygdeman and Viveca Lundstrom (1988) in Sweden have investigated the role of PGs in menstrual physiology. It is established that an overproduction of endometrial PGs explains the symptoms of dysmenorrhea in women. This conclusion is supported by the finding that a variety of NSAIDs alleviate the clinical symptoms of dysmenorrhea (uterine cramping) and menorrhagia (excessive blood loss). The effectiveness of different NSAIDs varies considerably owing to the fact that in addition to blocking COX activity in the uterus and, hence, PG production, some of these compounds (such as the fenamates) also act as PG receptor antagonists. Intrauterine devices (IUDs) stimulate the local production of endometrial PGs, which may mediate the mechanism of action of IUDs in preventing conception. In some individuals, the presence of an IUD results in an overproduction of PGs and the occurrence of dysfunctional bleeding which often can be controlled by NSAIDs.

6.7. Identification of $PGF_{2\alpha}$ as a Local Uterine Luteolytic Hormone

The occurrence of PGs in human menstrual fluid and their role in menstruation provided an important lead regarding the potential role of PGs in uterine physiology in mammals. Unlike primates, the presence of the uterus is essential for cyclic regression of the corpus luteum in many nonprimate species. John McCracken and coworkers (1972) investigated the role of uterine PGs in relation to cyclic regression of the corpus luteum using sheep with autotransplanted ovaries and/or uterus. The presence of a contiguous uterine horn was found to be a requirement for luteolysis in this species. This requirement was subsequently explained by the local uterine production and countercurrent transfer of $PGF_{2\alpha}$ from the uterine vein to the ovarian artery, the latter vessel being

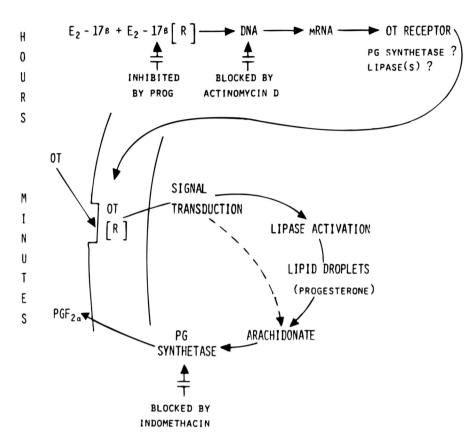

Fig. 6. A model for the endocrine control of $PGF_{2\alpha}$ synthesis in the endometrial cell of the sheep during luteolysis. *See text* for explanation (from McCracken et al., 1995).

highly contorted and adherent to the uterine vein. This mechanism allows $PGF_{2\alpha}$ secreted by the uterus to avoid metabolism in the pulmonary circulation, and to reach the adjacent ovary directly and, hence, cause luteolysis. Such a bypass mechanism from vein to artery allows the transfer of about 1% of the secreted amount of uterine $PGF_{2\alpha}$, which occurs as a series of episodic bursts during luteolysis. It is likely that similar countercurrent transfer mechanisms for PGs and other substances may occur where the appropriate vascular anatomy exists, for example, in the testicular vascular pedicle or in the kidney vasculature. Indeed, the transfer of tritiated water, krypton, and heat is reported to occur in the testicular vasculature. Also, steroids are known to be transferred within the ovarian vasculature of several species, including the human. Such a transfer mechanism may permit steroids and other substances to reach the ovary, the oviduct, and perhaps the uterus itself in a concentration greater than would be supplied via the systemic circulation (McCracken and Schramm, 1988).

7. A MODEL FOR THE ENDOCRINE CONTROL OF PULSATILE PGF2A SECRETION DURING LUTEOLYSIS IN THE SHEEP

The hormonal regulation of the uterine $PGF_{2\alpha}$ secretion, which initiates luteolysis in nonprimate species, has been studied extensively in the sheep, which offers a number of advantages as a model, e.g., the access to the uterine and ovarian circulation in sheep bearing a transplanted ovary and/or uterus. Early studies indicated control of uterine $PGF_{2\alpha}$ secretion by estrogen and progesterone. However, John McCracken and colleagues (1995) subsequently showed that these hormones acted indirectly by regulating the formation of oxytocin (OT) receptors in the endometrium, the site of uterine $PGF_{2\alpha}$ synthesis in sheep. A model for the cellular control of $PGF_{2\alpha}$ synthesis in the endometrium of the sheep is shown in Fig. 6. Estradiol-17β (E_2-17β) promotes the formation of endometrial OT receptors in 6–9 h

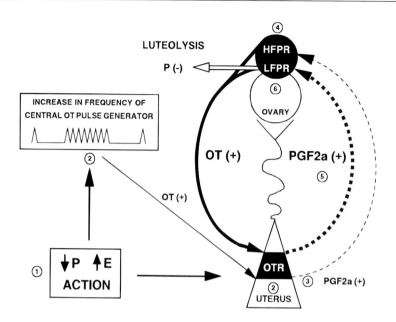

Fig. 7. A model for the neuroendocrine control of pulsatile $PGF_{2\alpha}$ secretion from the uterus during luteolysis in the sheep. *See text* for explanation of numbers in the model (from McCracken et al., 1995).

and may also increase PG synthetase and phospholipase levels. When OT receptors are present on the endometrial cell membrane, OT induces the immediate secretion of $PGF_{2\alpha}$. Signal transduction via the phosphatidylinositol-mediated increase in intracellular Ca^{2+} is thought to activate phospholipase A_2, resulting in liberation of AA from phospholipid stores. Some AA may also be generated from diacylglycerol via diacylglycerol lipase. Released AA is then rapidly converted to $PGF_{2\alpha}$ by PG synthetase (COX). Progesterone secreted during the luteal phase initially inhibits estrogen action and prevents the formation of endometrial OT receptors. During this period of inhibition, progesterone appears to increase lipid stores in the endometrial cells (the so-called priming effect of progesterone). Finally, progesterone action diminishes toward the end of the luteal phase via catalysis of its own receptor. Such a loss of progesterone action will facilitate the return of E_2-17β action with the consequent formation of endometrial OT receptors and hence the ability of OT to stimulate endometrial $PGF_{2\alpha}$ secretion. However, because of the progesterone priming effects, the amount of $PGF_{2\alpha}$ secreted in response to oxytocin is 50- to 100-fold greater than the response to OT before priming.

The model proposed in Fig. 6 explains the cellular regulation of $PGF_{2\alpha}$ synthesis via the induction of endometrial OT receptors, but it does not explain the role of circulating levels of OT. In the sheep and other ruminants, the regulation of blood levels of OT is complicated by the fact that in addition to the neurohypophysis, the corpus luteum is an ectopic site of OT synthesis. Recent work from our laboratory indicates that a finite store of OT exists in the corpus luteum. This supplemental source of OT reinforces periodic signals from the central OT pulse generator to amplify the magnitude of each luteolytic pulse of $PGF_{2\alpha}$ from the uterus. A model of the endocrine control of pulsatile secretion of $PGF_{2\alpha}$ from the uterus during luteolysis in the sheep is depicted in Fig. 7 (*See* numbers in model).

1. At the end of the cycle, loss of progesterone (P) action by catalysis of its receptor, both in the hypothalamus and in the uterus, results in returning estradiol-17β action;
2. Estradiol-17β (E) increases endometrial OT receptors (OTR) and causes intermittent increases in the frequency of the central OT pulse generator;
3. Low-level $PGF_{2\alpha}$ is generated by action of central OT on uterine OTR;

4. Low-level $PGF_{2\alpha}$ acts on the high-affinity $PGF_{2\alpha}$ receptor (HFPR) present on OT-containing luteal cells to stimulate OT secretion;

5. A high level of uterine $PGF_{2\alpha}$ secretion is now generated by luteal OT; and

6. High level of $PGF_{2\alpha}$ now has two effects via the low-affinity $PGF_{2\alpha}$ receptor (LFPR) in luteal cells. First, it stimulates additional luteal OT and second, it now depresses luteal P secretion (luteolysis).

The closed-loop positive feedback between the uterus (source of $PGF_{2\alpha}$) and the CL (source of OT) will continue until both types of $PGF_{2\alpha}$ receptors in the CL are desensitized, thus terminating each luteolytic pulse after 1 h. Additional luteolytic pulses will follow when luteal $PGF_{2\alpha}$ receptors and/or uterine OTR recover after 6–9 h, in time to respond to the next high frequency signal from the central OT pulse generator. A minimum of five luteolytic pulses of $PGF_{2\alpha}$ are necessary to complete functional luteolysis. Thus, in the sheep, in addition to the well-established interplay between ovarian steroids and the hypothalamic/anterior pituitary axis for the initiation of the ovarian cycle (via the gonadotrophins), there is now good evidence for an interplay between ovarian steroids and the hypothalamic/posterior pituitary axis for the termination of the reproductive cycle (via OT). In capsular form: the anterior pituitary hormones initiate the cycle, whereas a posterior pituitary hormone terminates the cycle. In species that do not synthesize OT in the ovary, it seems likely that OT secreted via the central OT pulse generator may alone be a sufficient stimulus for the generation of pulsatile luteolytic releases of uterine $PGF_{2\alpha}$ as in the mare and sow. Thus in sheep and other species, the uterus can be regarded as a transducer that, under appropriate hormonal conditions, converts neural signals into local hormonal signals from the uterus to cause luteolysis. Although the uterus is an abundant source of PGs in primates, the presence of the uterus is not required for luteolysis, since ovarian cyclicity is normal in hysterectomized subjects. However, many of the components present in the sheep utero-ovarian system are present within the primate ovary itself, namely small amounts of OT, OTR, $PGF_{2\alpha}$, $PGF_{2\alpha}$ receptors, and different luteal cell types, Thus, a local production and action of $PGF_{2\alpha}$ within the primate ovary itself could account

for luteolysis. However, this possibility is only now under investigation.

The endocrine control for the local production of $PGF_{2\alpha}$ in the endometrium at the time of luteolysis may also occur at the end of pregnancy during the induction of labor in a number of species. Current work by Anna-Riitta Fuchs and colleagues (1992) indicates an upregulation of OTR in the endometrium and in the placental membranes in the bovine feto-placental unit prior to the onset of labor. This upregulation of OTR is associated with the local formation of $PGF_{2\alpha}$ in these tissues. It is proposed that $PGF_{2\alpha}$, so formed, acts synergistically with low levels of OT on the myometrium to promote uterine contractions and the initiation of first-stage labor. The subsequent increase in maternal OT levels during the second or expulsive phase of labor is most likely owing to release of pituitary OT via the Ferguson Reflex. Another important local function of PGs during pregnancy is the maintenance of ductus arteriosus patency in the fetus. Kazuo and Momma (1988) investigated the role of PGE_2 in maintaining ductus patency. He concluded that PGE_2 is the prime agent in this respect. Moreover, the use of NSAIDs to effect ductus closure by inhibiting PGE_2 production remains a possible viable therapy in the newborn, especially in cases of fetal prematurity.

8. CONCLUSION

The foregoing selected examples of local action of eicosanoids were described to emphasize the diversity of function of these potent biological agents. Further examples of the diversity of action of eicosanoids may be obtained by referring to the References provided. Judging by the intense research efforts currently being extended in the eicosanoid field, it is clear that new information on the regulation and action of these biologically potent substances will continue to evolve. Moreover, their important pathophysiological roles in certain diseases give cause for optimism that the pharmacological control of their synthesis and action will be of considerable therapeutic value.

ACKNOWLEDGMENTS

Thanks are owed to Robert C. Skarnes and David Kupfer, as well as my associates Joyce A. Eldering and Edward E. Custer for critical evaluation of the text. I also wish to thank Merrilyn G. Nay for typing the manuscript.

REFERENCES

Austen KF, Soberman RJ. Biology of the leukotrienes. In: Levi R, Krell RD, eds. *Perspectives on Additional Areas for Research in Leukotrienes*, vol. 524. New York: Annals New York Academy of Sciences, 1988:xi.

Bergstrom S, Sjovall J. The isolation of prostaglandin. *Acta Chemica Scandanavica*, 1957; 11:1086.

Bygdeman M, Lundstrom V. Prostaglandins: biology and chemistry of prostaglandins and related eicosanoids. In: Curtis-Prior PB, ed. *Menstruation and Dysmenorrhoea*. London: Churchill Livingstone, 1988:490.

Coceani F, Bishai J, Lees J, Sirko S. Prostaglandin E$_2$ in the pathogenesis of pyrogen fever: validation of an intermediary role. *Adv Prosta Thromb Leuk Res*. 1989; 19:394.

Coleman RA, Smith WL, Narumiya S. International Union of Pharmacology classification of prostanoid receptors: properties, distribution and structure of receptors and their subtypes. *Pharmacol Rev* 1994; 46:205.

Cundell DR, Gerard NP, Gerard C, Idanpaan-Helkklla I, Tuomanen E. *Streptococcus pneumoniae* anchor to activated human cells by the receptor for platelet-activating factor. *Nature* 1995; 377:435.

Custer EE, Lamsa JC, Eldering JA, McCracken JA. Identification of functional high and low affinity states of the prostaglandin F$_{2\alpha}$ receptor in the ovine corpus luteum *in vivo* and their role in hormone pulsatility. *Endocrine* 1995; 3:761.

Deby C, Prostaglandins: biology and chemistry of prostaglandins and related compounds. In: Curtis-Prior PB, ed. *Metabolism of Fatty Acids, Precursors of Eicosanoids*. 1988:11.

Dennis EA, Krell RD. Summary: the enzymes, accessory proteins, and receptors of leukotriene metabolism and their inhibition and antagonism. *Adv Prosta Thromb Leuk Res*, 1994; 22:63

Eldering JA, Nay MG, Hoberg LM, Longcope C, McCracken JA. Hormonal regulation of endometrial prostaglandin F$_{2\alpha}$ production during luteal phase of the rhesus monkey. *Biol Reprod* 1993; 49:809.

Ford-Hutchinson AW. 5-Lipoxygenase activating protein and leukotriene C$_4$ synthase: therapeutic targets for inhibiting the leukotriene cascade. *Adv Prosta Thromb Leuk Res* 1994; 22:13.

Fuchs AR, Helmer H, Chang SM, Fields MJ. Concentration of oxytocin receptors in the placenta and fetal membranes of cows during pregnancy and labor. *J Reprod Fert*. 1992; 96:775.

Hamberg M, Svensson J, Samuelsson B. Thromboxanes: a new group of biologically active compounds derived from prostaglandin endoperoxides. *Proc Nat Acad Sci USA* 1975; 71:345.

Hayaishi O, Matsumura H, Urade Y. Prostaglandin D synthase is the key enzyme in the promotion of physiological sleep. *J Lipid Mediators* 1993; 6:429.

McCracken JA, Schramm W. Prostaglandins: biology and chemistry of prostaglandins and related eicosanoids. In: Curtis-Prior PB, ed. *Prostaglandins and Corpus Luteum Regression*, London: Churchill Livingstone, 1988:425.

McCracken JA, Custer EE, Lamsa JC, Robinson AG. The central oxytocin pulse generator: a pacemaker for luteolysis. *Adv Exp Med Biol* 1995; 395:133

McCracken JA et al. Prostaglandin F$_{2\alpha}$ identified as a luteolytic hormone in sheep. *Nature* 1972; 238:129.

Moncada S, Vane JR. Biochemical aspects of prostaglandins and thromboxanes. In: Kharasch N and Fried J, eds. *The Discov-ery of Prostacyclin—a Fresh Insight into Arachidonic Acid Metabolism*, New York: Academic Press, 1977:155.

Momma K. Prostaglandins: biology and chemistry of prostaglandins and related eicosanoids. In: Curtis-Prior PB, ed. *Ductus Arteriosus and Cardiovascular System in the Neonate*, London: Churchill Livingstone 1988:476.

Murphy RC, Hammarstrom S, Samuelsson B. Leukotriene C: a slow reacting substance (SRS) from murine mastocytoma cells. *Proc Nat Acad Sci USA* 1979; 76:4275.

Narumiya S. Structures, properties and distributions of prostanoid receptors. *Adv Prosta Thromb Leuk Res* 1995; 23:17.

Negishi M et al. Signal transduction of the isoforms of mouse prostaglandin E receptor EP3 subtype. *Adv Prosta Thromb Leuk Res* 1995; 23:255

O'Flaherty JT. Prostaglandins: biology and chemistry of prostaglandins and related eicosanoids. In: Curtis-Prior PB, ed. *Biochemical Interactions of Platelet-Activating Factor with Arachidonic Acid*. London: Churchill Livingstone, 1988:663.

Piper PF, Letts LG. Prostaglandins: biology and chemistry of prostaglandins and related compounds. In: Curtis-Prior PB, ed. *Biology of Leukotrienes*. 1988:616

Roberts LJ II, Morrow JD. Cellular generation, transport, and effects of eicosanoids. In: Goetzl EJ, Lewis RA, Rola-Pleszczynski M, eds. *Isoprostanes: Novel Markers of Endogenous Lipid Peroxidation and Potential Mediators of Oxidant Injury*, vol. 744. New York: Annals New York Academy of Sciences, 1994:237.

Simmons DL, Weilin X, Evett G, Merrill J, Robertson DL, Bradshaw WS. Drug inhibition and cellular regulation of prostaglandin G/H synthase isoenzyme 2, *J Lipid Mediators* 1993; 6:113.

Skarnes RC, Brown SK, Hull SS, McCracken JA. Role of prostaglandin E in the biphasic fever response to endotoxin, *J Exp Med* 1981; 154:1212.

Slipetz DM, Scoggan KA, Nicholson DW, Metters KM. Photo affinity labelling and radiation inactivation of the leukotriene B$_4$ receptor in human myeloid cells. *European J Pharmacol* 1993; 244:161.

Sorensen PW, Goetz FW. Pheromonal and reproductive function of F prostaglandins and their metabolites in teleost fish, *J Lipid Mediators* 1993; 6:385.

Stjernschantz J. Prostaglandins as ocular hypotensive agents; development of an analogue for glaucoma treatment. *Adv Prosta Thromb Leuk Res* 1995; 23:63.

Sun FF et al. Biochemical aspects of prostaglandins and thromboxanes. In: Kharasch N and Fried J, eds. *The Structure of Prostaglandin I$_2$*, New York: Academic Press, 1977:179.

Vanderhoek JV. Biology of the Leukotrienes. In: Levi R, Krell RD, eds. *Role of the 15-Lipoxygenase in the Immune System*, vol. 524. New York: Annals New York Academy of Sciences, 1988:240.

Vane Jr, Botting RM. A better understanding of anti-inflammatory drugs based on isoforms of cyclooxygenase (Cox-1 and Cox-2). *Adv Prosta Thromb Leuk Res* 1995; 23:41.

von Euler US. Prostaglandins: biology and chemistry of prostaglandins and related eicosanoids. In: Curtis-Prior PB, ed. *Biology of Prostanoids*. London: Churchill Livingstone, 1988:1.

Weissmann G. Prostaglandins as modulators rather then mediators of inflammation. *J Lipid Mediators* 1993; 6:275.

Zurier RB, Prostaglandins: biology and chemistry of prostaglandins and related eicosanoids. In: Curtis-Prior PB, ed. *Prostaglandins and Inflammation*. London: Churchill Livingstone, 1988:595.

8 Cytokines and Endocrine Function

Bryan L. Spangelo, PhD

CONTENTS

1. INTRODUCTION

Endocrine systems are influenced by a class of soluble mediators termed cytokines. These factors are glycoproteins ranging from 15,000–20,000 in molecular mass. Certain cytokines are also termed interleukins, denoting the importance of these proteins to the immune system. Interleukin-1 (IL-1) production by lymphocytes and monocytes affects inflammatory and cell-mediated immune responses. Although initially isolated from lymphocytes, many cytokines have been identified in other tissues. These proteins have a variety of functions depending on the tissue site of production. For example, IL-6 is a B-cell-differentiating and T-cell-activating cytokine. In addition, this protein enhances anterior pituitary hormone secretion and is produced within the anterior pituitary gland. This chapter will describe those cytokines that (1) affect endocrine functioning and (2) have sites of production within endocrine tissues. The cytokines most often associated with changes in endocrine function are IL-1, IL-2, IL-6, and tumor necrosis factor-α (TNF-α).

From: *Endocrinology: Basic and Clinical Principles* (P. M. Conn and S. Melmed, eds.), Humana Press Inc., Totowa, NJ.

2. CYTOKINE GENES

2.1. Structure and Amino Acid Sequence

2.1.1. IL-1, IL-2, IL-6 AND TNF-α

Table 1 illustrates the salient chemical features of IL-1, IL-2, IL-6, and TNF-α. The monokine IL-1 family actually consists of three members: IL-1α, IL-1β and IL-1ra (IL-1 receptor antagonist). IL-1α and IL-1β are 22% homologous in terms of the mature primary amino acid sequence. Both are synthesized as 31-kDa precursors and are processed to 17.5-kDa mol wt polypeptides. Neither IL-1α nor IL-1β are glycosylated, and with an isoelectric point of 5, IL-1α is often referred to as the acidic form of IL-1. The precursor forms of IL-1α and IL-1β do not contain a classical signal sequence directing their location to the lumen of the endoplasmic reticulum; thus, activated monocytes contain IL-1 in the plasma membrane and cytosol, but not in the endoplasmic reticulum. Precursor IL-1α is biologically active and can be presented on the cell surface. Precursor IL-1β is not biologically active and is usually processed by a specific protease (IL-1β-converting enzyme, ICE) and secreted as the mature, active IL-1β. Biologically active forms of IL-1α and IL-1β induce pyrogenic

115

Table 1
Cytokine Protein Size and Gene Location

| Cytokine | Amino Acids | | Glycosylation | Gene Location | Number of Exons |
	Precursor	Mature			
IL-1α	271	159	–	Chrom. 2	7
IL-1β	269	153	–	Chrom. 2	7
IL-2	153	133	+	Chrom. 4	4
IL-6	212	184	+	Chrom. 7	5
TNF-α	233	157	–	Chrom. 6	4

Data are presented for the human cytokines.

responses, T-cell and thymocyte activation, and the induction of other cytokines. The IL-1ra is synthesized with a signal sequence and is processed in the Golgi before secretion. This antagonist binds to IL-1 receptors with an affinity similar to those of IL-1α and IL-1β, but does not activate a second messenger system. All three IL-1 members exist as 12–14 antiparallel β-strands, resulting in barrel-shaped structures that are closed at one end.

IL-2 was first described as a lymphokine capable of increasing thymocyte and T-cell mitogenesis. Produced by antigen-stimulated helper T-cells, mature IL-2 consists of 133 amino acids and is glycosylated (*see* Table 1). This lymphokine contains six helical segments and one disulfide bridge (between cysteine residues 58 and 105). The cytokine IL-6 is a T-cell-activating and B-cell-differentiation factor of 26-kDa molecular mass. IL-6 is also a growth factor for plasmacytomas (transformed mature B-cells) and hybridomas (hybrids of transformed myelomas and normal B-cells), and can induce antibody production by normal B-cells. Because of variable glycosylation, IL-6 may range in molecular mass (21–28 kDa). Precursor IL-6 has 212 amino acids and a hydrophobic signal sequence of 28 amino acids (*see* Table 1). The removal of only four amino acids from the C-terminus of mature IL-6 results in a loss of biological activity. Mature TNF-α is a 157 amino acid polypeptide chain that was initially identified as cachectin. This cytokine can induce necrosis of certain tumors in vivo, is cytotoxic to a number of cell lines in vitro, and is responsible for the fever, weight loss, and acute-phase reaction often associated with neoplasia and infection. TNF-α is not glycosylated and exists as a trimetric molecule in circulation.

2.2. Regulation of Synthesis: Cis-Acting Domains and Trans-Acting Factors

Because of the diverse repertoire of activities attributed to cytokines, regulation of their gene expression is of paramount importance to homeostasis. In general terms, cytokine production is not constitutive, but is subject to a variety of inductive signals. In different lymphokine genes, the 5′-flanking regulatory regions range up to a few hundred base pairs from the transcription initiation site and possess limited homology. However, the 10-nucleotide sequence termed conserved lymphokine element 1 (CLE1) is found in the 5′-flanking region of several cytokine genes.

The IL-1α and IL-1β genes both contain seven exons. These two genes are differentially expressed, and although the IL-1α promoter does not contain the TATA and CAAT sequences, the IL-1β gene does contain these cis-regulatory elements. Thus, stimulated blood monocytes have a 40-fold increase in IL-1β mRNA, whereas the IL-1α mRNA is increased only two- to threefold. Both genes contain GC boxes (binding sites for the transcription factor Sp1) and glucocorticoid response elements (GRE) in their promoters and introns. A phorbol myristate acetate (PMA)-responsive enhancer is located upstream of the transcription start site in the IL-1β gene. In addition, endotoxin induction of IL-1α transcription utilizes nuclear factor IL-6-binding (NFIL-6) sites located distal and proximal to the transcriptional start site. A newly discovered cis-acting element, IL-1β-upstream nuclear factor 1 (IL-1β-UNF) is located in the distal endotoxin response region of the IL-1β gene; this enhancer binds a factor of 85–90 kDa. Intron 6 of the IL-1α gene has tandem repeats (46 bp) that contain recognition sequences for Sp1 as well as the GRE.

Induction of IL-2 gene expression requires around 300 bp located 5' of the transcription initiation site. In the human gene (four exons), three important DNA elements have been localized (sites A, D, and E). Different transcription factors recognize these sites. Thus, NFIL-2E specifically binds to positions –263 to –279 (site E). Transcriptional factor NFIL-2A recognizes both site A (–89 to –73) and site D (–255 to –217). Another site within the IL-2 gene (–206 to –195) is a target of the transcriptional factor NFκB following mitogenic stimulation. The human IL-6 gene consists of five exons (see Table 1). The 5'-promoter extends about 350 bp upstream of the transcriptional start site. This region contains activation protein 1 (AP-1) and NFκB-binding sites, as well as two GRE cis-acting elements and the traditional TATA box. Because increased intracellular cAMP produces enhanced gene expression, the IL-6 promoter also possesses a cAMP response element (CRE). The ability of IL-1 to increase IL-6 production may hinge on the presence of a 14-bp cis-acting element that binds NFIL-6. The TNF-α gene has four exons and contains NFκB, AP-1-, and Sp1-binding sites in the promoter region. Although human and mouse TNF-α promoter regions have multiple NFκB-binding sites, only the mouse binding sites function as endotoxin-inducible enhancers of transcription. Activation of NFκB does not necessarily lead to accumulation of TNF-α mRNA; however, an increase in this mRNA species is almost always preceded by NFκB activation.

3. CYTOKINE RECEPTOR GENES

3.1. Structure and Amino Acid Sequence

3.1.1. IL-1, IL-2, IL-6, AND TNF-α RECEPTORS

Two receptors for IL-1 have been characterized: Type I and Type II. The Type I receptor is present on nearly all cells, whereas while the Type II receptor is restricted in its distribution to mainly neutrophils, monocytes, and B-cells. Both receptors exist as single glycosylated proteins that span the plasma membrane only once. The extracellular ligand-binding domains have three immunoglobin (Ig)-like regions; deletion of any one of these regions in the Type I receptor results in diminished binding of IL-1. The human Type I receptor is 532 amino acids in length (80 kDa), whereas the Type II IL-1 receptor is smaller (372 amino acids; 60 kDa). The difference in size is owing the cytoplasmic portions of these molecules. Type I IL-1 receptor has a 213 amino acid cytoplasmic domain, whereas the Type II receptor possesses a cytoplasmic domain of only 29 amino acids. IL-1β has a higher affinity for the type II receptor, whereas IL-1α has a greater affinity for the Type I receptor. The affinity binding of IL-1ra is high for the Type I receptor and is in fact nearly irreversible. In addition, this interaction does not induce a response.

Mediation of biological responses to IL-1 requires the Type I receptor. This receptor occurs in very low copy number on most cells (100/cell); however, IL-1 binding to only 2–3% of these induces a response. The Type II IL-1 receptor does not transduce a signal and may function as a decoy receptor. Blocking antibodies against the Type II protein increase the IL-1 stimulation of cytokine production by monocytes. By increasing the cellular expression of the Type II receptor (or its circulating soluble form), the biological effects of IL-1 are potentially reduced. Thus, IL-4 inhibits IL-1 activation of monocytes by increasing the expression and release of the Type II receptor from these cells.

The IL-2 receptor system consists of three polypeptide chains: α, β, and γ. The IL-2 receptor β and α subunits are shared with other receptor systems (β is a subunit of the IL-15 receptor and γ is a subunit of the IL-4, lL-7, and IL-9 receptors). The cytoplasmic regions of the β and γ subunits are required for IL-2-induced biological effects, and heterodimerization of these two polypeptides chains is necessary for signal transduction. The α-chain has only a short cytoplasmic tail and probably does not contribute to signal transmission. However, this chain is necessary for high-affinity binding of IL-2 to the receptor complex. The IL-6 receptor is also a trimeric system composed of an α subunit (gp80) and a homodimer of the protein gp130. Regarding IL-2, the IL-6 receptor α-chain has a short cytoplasmic domain, binds IL-6, and does not transduce a signal. Signaling is triggered by the formation of gp130 homodimers. Thus, the IL-6–IL-6 receptor αchain complex interacts with gp130 and induces homodimerization of this protein by disulfide covalent bound formation. The gp130 protein is shared by several cytokine receptor complexes (e.g., ciliary neurotrophic factor [CNTF], leukemia inhibitory factor [LIF], IL-11). There are two TNF receptors (TNF-R55 and TNF-R75). These receptors

Table 2
Cytokine-Activated Second Messenger Pathways

Cytokine	Phosphatidylcholine-specific phospholipase C (PC-PLC)	Sphingomyelinase (SMase)	Jak-Stat
IL-1α	+	+	–
IL-1β	+	+	–
IL-2	–	–	Jak1/Jak3; Stat 3/Stat 5
IL-6	–	–	Tyk2/Jak1/Jak2; Stat1/Stat3
TNF-α	+	+	–

PC-PLC activation leads to DAG production and subsequent stimulation of PKC. SMase leads to ceramide production and subsequent stimulation of a ceramide-activated serine/threonine kinase. Jak activation by receptor aggregation induces tyrosine-phosphorylation of Stat proteins.

exhibit 30% homology in the extracellular domains, which contain a six-cysteine consensus sequence that is repeated four times. In addition, the TNF receptors exist in the monomeric form, but following binding of ligand are found in a trimeric state. Thus, three receptor molecules are bound to one TNF trimer. Trimerization of TNF-R55 is required for signal transmission. In contrast, TNF-R75 can be activated following dimerization. This receptor also enhances the cytotoxic effects of TNF mediated by TNF-R55. The mechanism of this effect may be owing to an increase of TNF concentration around the target cell caused by the passage of ligand from TNF-R75 to TNF-R55.

3.2. Second Messenger Generation

The cytoplasmic domain of the Type I IL-1 receptor does not possess intrinsic protein kinase activity, and this region is not a substrate for tyrosine kinases. Nevertheless, this portion of the Type I receptor is essential for signal transmission. Thus, a region between 28 and 42 amino acids from the carboxy-terminus is necessary for IL-1 induction of IL-8 expression. After interaction with IL-1, the ligand–receptor complex is internalized and localized to the nucleus; the importance of this translocation to signal transduction is not yet known.

Despite a lack of homology between the cytoplasmic domains of the Type I IL-1 receptor and the TNF receptors, the signaling pathways induced by IL-1 and TNF appear similar (Table 2). In a variety of cells, IL-1 and TNF will induce a number of protein kinases, including protein kinase C (PKC), mitogen-

activated protein (MAP) kinase, and ceramide-activated kinase (a 97-kDa proline-directed serine/threonine kinase). The majority of IL-1 and TNF-induced protein phosphorylations are specific for serine and threonine residues. To account for the activation of this array of protein kinase activity, the breakdown by IL-1 and TNF of two major phospholipid species has been advanced. In Jurkat and U937 cells, diacylglycerol (DAG) production occurs via IL-1 or TNF induction of a phosphatidylcholine-specific phospholipase C. In HL60, EL4, and fibroblast cells, IL-1 and TNF induce a decrease in sphingomyelin and an elevation of ceramide and phosphorylcholine. Regarding IL-1 and TNF, exogenous ceramide or sphingomyelinase activates NFκB and MAP kinase. In addition, IL-1 and TNF increase the activity of the pH-neutral, DAG-independent form of sphingomyelinase in HL60 and EL4 cells. Thus, activation of phospholipase C or sphingomyelinase by IL-1 or TNF can occur depending on the cell type.

The cytokines IL-2 and IL-6 activate protein tyrosine kinase cascades as part of their signal transduction pathways. One of these cascades is termed the Jak-Stat pathway (see Table 2 and Chapter 6 for a complete discussion). The Janus kinase (Jak) family of soluble tyrosine kinases consists of four members (Tyk2, Jak 1–3) that range in molecular wt from 125–135 kDa. These kinases are associated with the cytoplasmic domains of receptor chains (which are devoid of intrinsic tyrosine kinase activity) and are rapidly activated following ligand-induced receptor dimerization or oligomerization.

Table 3
Cytokine Localization in Endocrine Tissues

Cytokine	Hypothalamus	Anterior pituitary	Adrenal	Thyroid	Reproductive Testis	Reproductive Ovary
IL-1α	+	+	?	?	+	?+
IL-1β	+	+	+	?	?+	+
IL-2	?	+	?	?	?	?
IL-6	+	+	+	+	+	+
TNF-α	+	+	+[a]	?	+	+

+[a] = Fetal human and rat adrenal only.
+ = Cytokine present.
? = Presence of cytokine not verified.
?+ = Isoform not verified.

The receptor-associated Jak proteins are activated following crossphosphorylation, and subsequently phosphorylate the receptor itself as well as the signal transducers and activators of transcription (Stat) proteins. Activated Stat proteins may homo- or heterodimerize and translocate to the nucleus for transcriptional activation. Dimerization of the β- and γ-chains of the IL-2 receptor brings Jak1 (associated with the β-chain) and Jak3 (associated with the γ-chain) into close apposition for transphosphorylation and signal transmission. Activated Stat3 and Stat5 proteins subsequently bind specific DNA sequences. Following IL-6 interaction with its receptor α-chain, dimerized gp130 chains associated with activated tyk2, Jak1, and Jak2 tyrosine kinases induce Stat1 and Stat3 activation. Many other cytokines and growth hormones utilize the Jak-Stat pathway of signal transduction.

4. CYTOKINE ENDOCRINE TISSUE EXPRESSION

4.1. Anterior Pituitary

Despite their intial identification within the immune system, several cytokines have now been detected within endocrine tissues (Table 3). As noted below, IL-1 activates the hypothalamic-pituitary–adrenal (HPA) axis. This cytokine is also present within the neuroendocrine system. For instance, IL-1β and its mRNA are present in the cytoplasmic granules of a subpopulation of thyrotropes in the rat anterior pituitary. In addition, both IL-1 receptors (Type I and Type II) are expressed in the anterior lobe of the pituitary as well as in the cor-

ticotrophic cell line AtT20. Importantly, the IL-1ra mRNA is constitutively expressed in the rat anterior pituitary as determined by the polymerase chain reaction (PCR).

Human corticotrophic adenoma cells and the mouse AtT20 cell line contain detectable amounts of the IL-2 mRNA. Human adenoma cells also release IL-2 in vitro. The IL-2 receptor mRNA as well as membrane expression of the cognate protein (p55 α-subunit) is also found on these two cell types. The rat prolactin and growth hormone (GH)-producing cell line GH_3 also displays the IL-2 receptor. In rat anterior pituitary cells, the IL-2 receptor is localized to those cells that release adrenocorticotropin (ACTH), prolactin, and GH. Interestingly, GH_3 cell proliferation is stimulated by IL-2, whereas anterior pituitary cell division is inhibited by this cytokine. Thus, IL-2 may function in the anterior pituitary in a paracrine or autocrine manner to regulate cellular mitosis.

Anterior pituitary cell cultures synthesize and release IL-6. Rat anterior pituitary tissue contains both transcripts for the IL-6 mRNA (1.2 and 2.4 kb). Neurointermediate pituitary lobe cells also synthesize and release IL-6 in vitro. The production of IL-6 by the neurointermediate pituitary lobe is probably owing to the pituicyte, a resident astroglial element of the neural lobe. Because certain hypothalamic projections to the neural lobe contain IL-1 (see Section 4.2.), the neurointermediate pituitary lobe contains at least two cytokines.

Gene expression of IL-6 and the IL-6 receptor is prominant in ACTH- and GH-secreting human pituitary adenomas. Therefore, this cytokine may be cosecreted with ACTH and GH under these conditions. Nontumerous anterior pituitary cell-culture production of IL-6 generally resides within a non-parenchymal element termed the folliculostellate cell, a supportive element for this gland. Almost all IL-6-positive cells in the mouse anterior pituitary will also contain the protein S-100, found only in the folliculostellate cell. A cell line isolated from a rat pituitary thyrotropic tumor (TtT/GF) shares several characteristics with folliculostellate cells, including immunoreactivity for the S-100 protein and the release of IL-6. Because folliculostellate cells extend cytoplasmic processes that are in close apposition to parenchymal elements, a paracrine-mediated role for this cytokine in the anterior pituitary has been hypothesized. In this regard, rat anterior pituitary cells display a single class of specific IL-6-binding sites (170/cell) with a dissociation of constant of 2.7 × 10^{9}M. These cells also contain the IL-6 receptor mRNA, and human gonadotrophs also express an immunoreactive IL-6 receptor.

Adult male rats injected ip with endotoxin have increased accumulation of IL-1α, IL-1β, IL-6, and TNF-α mRNAs in the pituitary 1 h later, as determined by PCR. Thus, several cytokines may be expressed in the anterior pituitary, a component of the neuroendocrine system (*see* Table 3).

4.2. Hypothalamus

The mapping of IL-1β in the brain has been undertaken to determine its possible localization in the central nervous system (CNS). This cytokine is present in hypothalamic and extrahypothalamic brain regions. Immunoreactive IL-1β neuronal processes and terminals are in the hippocampus, specifically in the hilus of the dentate gyrus and extending into the stratum lucidum. In the hypothalamus, IL-1β is present in magnocellular neurons in the paraventricular nucleus. These neurons give rise to projections that terminate in the arcuate and suprachiasmatic nuclei, median eminence, and posterior pituitary. The periventricular and supraoptic nuclei are also positive for IL-1β immunoreactivity. Other IL-1β-immunoreactive cells include blood vessel wall cells and glial-like elements. Binding sites for IL-1α as well as the mRNA for the Type I receptor are found in intrinsic neurons located in the dentate gyrus of the hippocampus. Expression of the Type I receptor is also high in the choroid plexus, but is not detectable in the hypothalamus. Surprisingly, IL-1ra

administration into the hypothalamic median eminence blocks the ability of either IL-1α or IL-1β injected into the same region to enhance ACTH secretion. As noted above, expression of low amounts of the Type I IL-1 receptor may nonetheless allow a biological response.

The IL-6 mRNA can be induced in several brain regions, including hypothalamus, cerebral cortex, thalamus, and hippocampus. Medial basal hypothalamic explants release IL-6 and have increased IL-6 mRNA following endotoxin, but not 56 m*M* K$^+$ treatment in vitro. In addition, bovine hypothalamic membranes have a saturable, specific, and single binding site for this cytokine. The mRNAs for IL-6 and the IL-6 receptor are colocalized in the limbic and hypothalamic brain regions. Thus, *in situ* hybridization using appropriate cDNA probes reveals IL-6 and IL-6 receptor mRNA species in the hippocampal dentate gyrus, habenular nucleus, piriform cortex, and the hypothalamus. The mRNAs for IL-6 and the IL-6 receptor are differentially regulated in the hypothalamus with advancing age. In the rat, hypothalamic IL-6 receptor mRNA increases fourfold from day 2–day 70 of life, whereas the IL-6 mRNA slightly decreases during the same time period. Because the HPA axis undergoes a maturation process that is complete by day 20, the hypothalamic IL-6 system may be involved in the postnatal development of this axis.

In the murine brain, immunoreactive TNF-α is primarily observed in neuronal structures. Neurons positive for TNF-α are present in the hypothalamus, caudal raphe nuclei, bed nucleus of the stria terminalis, and the pons and medullar ventral surface. Fiber pathways both descending and ascending reside in the ventricular system and the medial forebrain bundle. The TNF-α mRNA is inducible in the rat brain in discrete locations (e.g., hypothalamus, hippocampus, striatum, thalamus, and cerebral cortex). In addition, rat astrocytes release TNF-α in response to endotoxin in vitro.

4.3. Adrenal

The human adrenal gland expresses IL-1β. The mRNA for this cytokine is localized to the adrenal cortex, especially the zona fasciculata and the zona reticularis. Steriod-producing cells of the zona reticularis (positive for 17α-hydroxylase cytochrome P450) contain IL-1 and its mRNA. Chromaffin cells of the adrenal medulla contain IL-1 immunoreactivity, but not the mRNA for this cytokine. Because the blood flow within the adrenal is directed from the cortex to the medulla, cortical cell production of IL-1 may regulate medullary cell function and may be the source of intracellular IL-1 in the adrenal medulla. However, the Type I IL-1 receptor mRNA is not detectable in the murine adrenal gland using *in situ* histochemistry. The human adrenal gland also expresses IL-6 mRNA in the inner zone of the cortex, but not in the chromaffin cells of the medulla. In addition, human fetal adrenal, but not the adult adrenal, contains and releases immunoreactive and bioactive TNF (*see* Table 3).

In contrast to the human adrenal gland, cells of the rat zona glomerulosa produce IL-6 in vitro. The zona fasiulata and reticularis have only minor amounts of this cytokine. Similarly, TNF-α is produced mainly by the zona glomerulosa in rat adrenal cell cultures. Therefore, the location of cytokine production within the adrenal gland is species-specific.

4.4. Thyroid

Human thyrocytes express the IL-6 mRNA and release bioactive IL-6. This cytokine is released from thyrocytes obtained from patients with Grave's disease and is also produced by a human thyrocyte cell line (HTori3). The rat thyroid cell line FRTL-5 also constitutively releases IL-6. Thyrocyte production of IL-6 may provide part of an immune response cascade that leads to autoimmune thyroid disease.

4.5. Reproductive

4.5.1. OVARY

Cytokines are expressed in the female reproductive system (*see* Table 3). Immunoreactive IL-1 is present in the follicular fluids of women and pigs. Rat ovarian tissue expresses the IL-1β mRNA exclusively within the theca-interstitial cells of preovulatory follicles. Granulosa cell cultures obtained from diethylstilbestrol-implanted immature rats release IL-6 in vitro. Using Northern blot analysis and PCR, TNF-α mRNA is detectable in rat ovaries. Immunoreactive TNF-α is also present in ovarian follicles, as well as corpora luteal and granulosa cells.

4.5.2. TESTES

The male reproductive system is also a site of cytokine synthesis and release (*see* Table 3). High amounts of IL-1 bioactivity are present in the human and rat testes. Although testicular macrophages express the IL-1 mRNA, Sertoli cells produce IL-1α. In addition, tubular segments from various stages of the seminiferous epithelial cycle release a bioactive IL-1α. Thus, IL-1α concentrations are lowest at stages VIIab and VIIcd and then rise dramatically at stage VIII and remain elevated in stages IX–XIV. The IL-1α mRNA is detectable in rat Leydig cells in vitro, but only after treatment with IL-1β.

Sertoli cells isolated from rats of increasing age have detectable IL-6 bioactivity. The release of IL-6 is age-dependent, with older Sertoli cell donors (day 45) providing maximal production. In contrast to Sertoli cell release of IL-6, pachytene spermatocytes, early spermatids, and peritubular cells do not produce this cytokine. Concerning IL-1α, IL-6 release by the seminiferous epithelium is stage-dependent. Tubular segments from stages VIIab, VIIcd, and VIII release only minimal amounts of IL-6. Only in stage IX (and higher) does IL-6 production increase, a location within the seminiferous epithelium that is already maximal for IL-1α secretion. The synthesis and release of IL-6 occur also in rat Leydig cells. Regarding the IL-1α mRNA, IL-6 transcripts are generally only detectable in Leydig cells following treatment with IL-1β in vitro. Immature and adult rat testes express the IL-6 receptor mRNA. Specifically, Sertoli and Leydig cells contain the 5.1-kb IL-6 receptor mRNA. However, germ cells in the adult testis (pachytene spermatocytes or round spermatids) do not possess IL-6 receptor transcripts. Thus, both IL-6 and its receptor are present only in the functional somatic cells of the testis.

In contrast to IL-1 and IL-6, TNF-α is produced by germ cells in the rat testes. Spermatogenic cells (pachytene spermatocytes and round spermatids) contain the TNF-α mRNA, and round spermatids release this cytokine. Spermatogonia, elongating spermatids, or Leydig cells do not contain the TNF-α mRNA. Interestingly, Sertoli and Leydig cells (but not pachytene spermatocytes or round spermatids) express a TNF-α receptor (TNF-R55).

5. REGULATION OF CYTOKINE SECRETION

5.1. Anterior and Neurointermediate Pituitary Lobe Cells

Circulating cytokine levels are generally low or nondetectable during nonstressed or disease-free conditions. To exert biological effects in endocrine

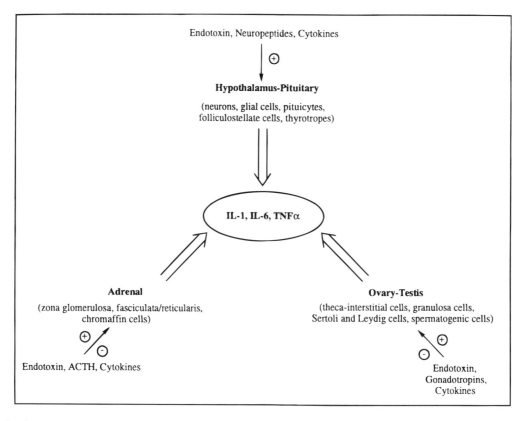

Fig. 1. Endocrine system production of cytokines: cell sources and regulatory agents. Cytokines (IL-1, IL-6, TNF-α) are synthesized and released in the neuroendocrine system as well as the adrenal and reproductive organs. Specific cell types are associated with cytokine production, and endotoxin, hormones, and cytokines may enhance or inhibit this production. *See text* for details.

tissues, one hypothesis holds that localized cytokine production within a tissue results in concentrations sufficient for paracrine- or autocrine-mediated effects. Therefore, the regulation of local cytokine synthesis and release is of paramount importance (Fig. 1).

Endotoxin (or lipopolysaccharide) is a potent inducer of cytokine synthesis and release. Rodents injected with endotoxin have increased anterior pituitary IL-1α, IL-1β, TNF-α, and IL-6 mRNA levels within 2 h. Endotoxin as well as agents that increase intracellular cAMP concentrations (e.g., forskolin, cholera toxin, prostaglandin E_2) enhance IL-6 release in vitro. Certain neuropeptides also increase IL-6 as well as IL-2 production by anterior pituitary cells. Thus, vasoactive intestinal peptide (VIP), pituitary adenylate cyclase-activating peptide (PACAP), and calcitonin gene-related peptide (CGRP) all increase IL-6 release from anterior pituitary cells and the TtT/GF cell line via an increased accumulation of intracellular cAMP. In addition, corticotropin-

releasing hormone (CRH) increases IL-2 mRNA expression in the AtT-20 cell line and human corticotrophic adenoma cells. Cytokines also regulate the production of IL-6 by the anterior pituitary. For example, IL-1α and IL-1β increase IL-6 release from rat anterior pituitary cells and human pituitary adenoma cells. As noted above, neurointermediate lobe cells synthesize and release IL-6. Endotoxin and IL-1β stimulate IL-6 release from these cells, an effect inhibited by oxytocin and vasopressin (the major secretory products of the neural lobe). Concerning the anterior pituitary, neurointermediate pituitary lobe cells express both transcripts for the IL-6 mRNA (1.2 and 2.4 kb).

5.2. Hypothalamus

Intraperitoneal (ip) injection of endotoxin also increases the expression of IL-1α and IL-1β mRNAs in the rat hypothalamus, but not striatum. Endotoxin administration increases immunoreactive IL-1β content 2–4 h later in the rat hypothalamus.

Following central (intracerebroventricular; icv) endotoxin administration, IL-1β mRNA is increased in the hypothalamus, hippocampus, and striatum. Immobilization stress generally increases neuroendocrine activity, including the activity of the HPA axis. This type of stress also increases IL-1β mRNA in the rat hypothalamus (but not other brain regions) 30–60 min after the onset of stress. Thus, this cytokine may be involved in the stimulation of the HPA axis (*see* Section 6.1.1.).

Central injection (icv) of endotoxin induces a robust expression of the IL-6 mRNA in the hypothalamus within 2 h, and increased levels of this cytokine in the cerebrospinal fluid (CSF) as well as the peripheral circulation. In contrast, an ip injection of endotoxin does not substantially change the levels of the IL-6 transcripts in the hypothalamus. As noted above, medial basal hypothalamic explants release IL-6 in response to a 60-min treatment of endotoxin. The 1.2- and 2.4-kb forms of the IL-6 mRNA are also increased by endotoxin in vitro. Although a depolarizing concentration of K^+ (56 mM) increases somatostatin release from these explants, IL-6 release is not affected, indicating a nonneuronal source for this cytokine. Indeed, astrocyte cultures and the rat astrocytoma cell line C6 release IL-6 in response to IL-1α, IL-1β, and endotoxin. Rat astrocytes also produce TNF-α in response to endotoxin, an effect potentiated by the cytokine interferon-γ (IFN-γ).

5.3. Adrenal Cortical Cells

Central (icv) injection of endotoxin leads to a substantial increase in IL-1β and IL-6 mRNAs in the rat adrenal within 1–2 h. Surprisingly, peripheral endotoxin administration induces IL-6 mRNA in the adrenal to a lesser extent than central administration. The mechanism of central endotoxin induction of adrenal cytokine production is speculative, but this response may lead to increased circulating cytokine levels and, thus, has a role during inflammatory CNS diseases.

As noted above, rat adrenal glomerulosa cells release IL-6 in vitro. The anterior pituitary hormone ACTH, endotoxin, as well as IL-1α and IL-1β stimulate glomerulosa cell production of IL-6 (*see* Fig. 1). Similar to the anterior pituitary production of IL-6, agents that enhance intracellular cAMP (e.g., ACTH, forskolin, dibutyryl cAMP) also increase IL-6 release from glomerulosa cells. Interestingly, the

combination of ACTH and IL-1β generates a greater IL-6 release than the sum of their separate effects. This synergistic response may enhance adrenal responses during stress and inflammation. The release of TNF-α is similarly induced by endotoxin, IL-1α, and IL-1β. In contrast, ACTH reduces basal and endotoxin as well as IL-1β- stimulated TNF-α release from zona glomerulosa cells in vitro. Furthermore, agents that increase intracellular cAMP reduce basal and stimulated TNF-α release. Thus, adrenal trophic hormones may either inhibit or stimulate endogenous cytokine production.

5.4. Ovarian Granulosa Cells

Rats injected with the gonadotropins pregnant mare serum gonadotropin (PMSG) and human chorionic gonadotropin (hCG) have increased expression of the IL-1β mRNA in the ovary, especially theca-intersitial cells. Granulosa cells are without IL-1β expression. Dispersed whole ovaries from immature rats treated with IL-1β for 24 h have increased IL-1β mRNA expression. Thus, gonadotropins and cytokines potentially affect IL-1β production in the ovary (*see* Fig. 1).

Follicle-stimulating hormone (FSH) stimulates progesterone, estrogen, and IL-6 release from rat granulosa cells in vitro. The cytokine IFN-γ inhibits FSH-stimulated IL-6 release from these cells. Concerning the anterior pituitary production of IL-6, agents that increase intracellular cAMP also enhance IL-6 release. Dibutyryl cAMP, forskolin, and the phosphodiesterase inhibitor isobutylmethylxanthine (IBMX) each increase IL-6 release from rat granulosa cells in vitro. In addition, endotoxin, IL-1α and IL-1β (but not TNF-α) increase IL-6 release. The bovine thymic preparation thymosin fraction 5 (TF5) decreases FSH-stimulated steroidogenesis. However, this thymic hormonal preparation enhances IL-6 release in the absence or presence of FSH. Therefore, gonadotropins, cytokines, and thymic hormones affect IL-6 production by the ovary.

5.5. Sertoli/Leydig Cells

Mice injected with endotoxin have a 30-fold increase in testicular IL-1β, and a reduction in Type I IL-1 receptor density in the testis and epididymus. The Type I receptor is localized to the interstitial area of the testis and the luminal borders of the epididymus. Endotoxin and IL-1β each increase the expression of the 2.2-kb IL-1α mRNA in purified

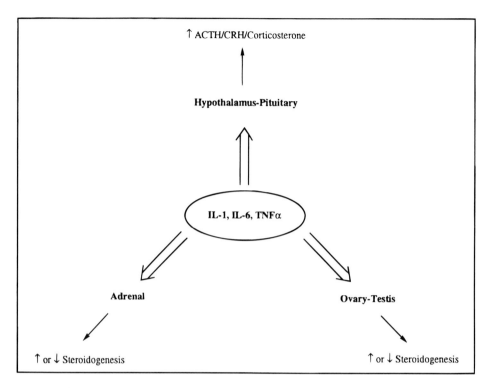

Fig. 2. Endogenous cytokines activate endocrine function. Cytokines (IL-1, IL-6, TNF-α) activate the HPA axis, and either inhibit or stimulate steroidogenesis in adrenal and reproductive tissues. These effects may be exerted by circulating cytokines or local production of these factors acting via paracrine and/or autocrine pathways. *See text* for details.

Leydig cells from rat testes. The cytoplasmic fragments of late spermatids that are shed during the time of sperm release (stage VIII) are termed residual bodies. Within the seminiferous tubule, these bodies remain attached to the Sertoli cells and in vitro also increase IL-1α release from rat Sertoli cells. Stage VIII seminiferous tubules release maximal amounts of IL-1α compared to other stages, presumably because of residual body activation. Endotoxin also induces dramatic increases in Sertoli cell IL-1α production within 6 h of treatment. The release of IL-1α from nongerm cells in the testes is therefore controlled by IL-1β, endotoxin, and residual bodies.

Sertoli cell production of IL-6 is enhanced by FSH, endotoxin, IL-1α, and residual bodies. The induction of Sertoli cell IL-6 by IL-1α is via an eicosanoid cascade involving the 5-lipoxygenase catabolism of arachidonic acid. Because anti-IL-1α antibodies block endotoxin and residual body induction of IL-6, IL-1α may act in an autocrine or paracrine mechanism to increase Sertoli cell IL-6 release. In addition, Sertoli cell expression of the IL-6 receptor mRNA is augmented by FSH, IL-1α, and

IL-6. Leydig cell production of IL-6 is also a regulated event. Thus, hCG and IL-1β increase IL-6 mRNA accumulation within, and IL-6 release from, rat Leydig cells in vitro. Therefore, IL-6 and its receptor are expressed in the interstitial cells and the seminiferous tubular cells of the testis, and this expression is regulated by gonadotropins and cytokines (*see* Fig. 1).

6. CYTOKINE MECHANISM OF ACTION

6.1. Neuroendocrine Function

6.1.1. HPA Axis Activation

Inflammatory responses are often associated with an increase in circulating glucocorticoid levels. Immunosuppressive glucocorticoids are thought to limit the extent of immune activation, preventing nonspecific damage to surrounding tissues. The mechanism of enhanced circulating corticosteroids during disease or inflammation has been extensively studied, resulting in the indentification of the cytokines with a pre-eminent role in the activation of the HPA axis (*see* Fig. 2).

Animals injected with either IL-1α or IL-1β have increased plasma levels of corticosterone, an effect abolished by prior treatment with anti-CRH antibodies. In addition, both cytokines enhance CRH gene expression and peptide release from medial basal hypothalamic explants in vitro. Peripheral injection of IL-1 also increases CRH levels in the hypophysial portal circulation in vivo. A direct effect of IL-1 to increase ACTH release from anterior pituitary cells in vitro is still controversial; however, IL-1 enhancement of CRH secretion is an accepted observation. Increases in circulating IL-1 levels undoubtedly stimulate CRH release from nerve terminals in the median eminence, an area of the hypothalamus outside the blood–brain barrier. The hypothalamic paraventricular nucleus is the primary contributor of CRH to cytokine-enhanced CRH secretion. Because indomethacin partially blocks IL-1-induction of ACTH secretion, prostaglandin (especially prostaglandin E_2) mediation of IL-1 stimulation of CRH secretion from the median eminence is likely.

Central IL-1 administration into the lateral ventricles of the rat increases ACTH secretion and CRH neuronal activity in the paraventricular nucleus. Injection of IL-1β directly into the hippocampus results in increased hippocampal extracellular serotonin concentrations as well as increased plasma ACTH and corticosterone levels. Extrahypothalamic sites may therefore contribute to central IL-1 stimulation of the HPA axis. Thus, both peripherally and centrally administered IL-1 enhances HPA axis activity, with the paraventricular nucleus of the hypothalamus playing an important role.

Although not as effective as IL-1, peripheral injection of IL-6 enhances ACTH secretion within 15 min, and anti-CRH antibodies block this effect. Injection of IL-6 into the third ventricle of the rat also results in increased ACTH secretion for up to 3 h. Concerning IL-1β, circulating IL-6 probably acts at the level of the median eminence to increase CRH and ACTH secretion, with the prostaglandins playing an important role. Peripheral administration of TNF-α, but not central (either third ventricle or upper median eminence), stimulates ACTH secretion, an effect blocked by the cyclooxygenase inhibitor indomethacin. Isolated medial basal hypothalami incubated with IL-2 have an increased release of CRH, but inhibition of cyclooxygenase or lipoxygenase enzymes has no effect on this release.

6.1.2. THE PROBLEM WITH THE BLOOD–BRAIN BARRIER

The blood–brain barrier normally retards entry of circulating proteins to the brain and CSF. This barrier is composed of two parts: the capillary bed of the brain (the endothelial barrier) and the choroid plexus (the ependymal barrier). Because peripheral injection of IL-1β increases CRH mRNA accumulation in the paraventricular nucleus, it is suggested that certain cytokines may cross the blood–brain barrier. Banks and colleagues (1994) have demonstrated that IL-1α and IL-1β cross the blood–brain barrier via a shared, saturable transport system in the mouse. In addition, TNF-α possesses a specific, saturable transport system. In contrast, IL-2 crosses this barrier using a nonsaturable (no self-inhibition) system. These experiments in rodents confirm the ability of these rather large polypeptides to cross the blood–brain barrier and thus exert a central effect.

6.2. Paracrine Effects

6.2.1. ANTERIOR PITUITARY

Because cytokine levels in the blood are usually low or nondetectable, the intrinsic production of these factors in endocrine tissues may allow autocrine- and paracrine-mediated responses to occur. For instance, anterior pituitary thyrotrope production of IL-1β may stimulate GH secretion, since in vitro this cytokine increases GH release from anterior pituitary cells. However, continuous iv infusion of IL-1β actually reduces GH surges in the male rat. Folliculostellate cell production of IL-6 may potentiate pituitary hormone secretion, because this cell type is closely apposed to the parenchymal elements of the pituitary and IL-6 stimulates prolactin, GH, and luteinizing hormone (LH) release in vitro. In contrast to IL-6, IL-2 gene expression in the pituitary is present in the hormone-producing cells (*see* Section 4.1.). Because IL-2 increases proopiomelanocortin gene expression in pituitary cells, this cytokine may stimulate ACTH secretion via an autocrine mechanism. Although the cellular source of anterior pituitary TNF-α has not been identified, this cytokine increases prolactin release in vitro, indicating another probable paracrine network.

6.2.2. ADRENAL

The expression of cytokines in distinct cellular layers of the adrenal provides an opportunity for paracrine actions because these proteins affect glucocorticoid and aldosterone secretion. For instance, IL-1β is present in the zona fasciculata and zona reticularis, and stimulates basal corticosterone (and cortisol) release, but inhibits angiotensin II-induced aldosterone synthesis. The stimulation of corticosterone may involve an intra-adrenal CRH-ACTH pathway, because IL-1β induction of corticosterone release is blocked by competitive inhibitors of these peptides in vitro. Thus, this cytokine may participate in complex paracrine and/or autocrine pathways of steroid regulation. Similarly, IL-6 stimulates corticosterone release in vitro and is expressed predominantly by the zona glomerulosa in the rat, suggesting a paracrine mechanism of action for the regulation of glucocorticoid secretion from the zona fasciculata. Conversely, TNF-α secretion by the rat zona glomerulosa may inhibit aldosterone release via an autocrine mechanism (*see* Fig. 2).

6.2.3. Reproductive

Rat ovarian tissue perifused with IL-1β has a threefold increase in LH-induced ovulation rate and an increase in LH-stimulated progesterone release in vitro. In addition, this cytokine also enhances collagenase biosynthesis, a component of the ovulatory cascade. This effect is noted in whole ovarian as well as in enriched theca-intersitial cell cultures. In contrast, IL-1α inhibits basal and LH-stimulated progesterone production by porcine granulosa cells. Ovarian follicular atresia may result from apoptosis, programmed cell death. Follicular apoptosis is inhibited by IL-1β and hCG, suggesting that IL-1β is a survival factor for ovarian follicles, which is consistent with a facilitating effect of this cytokine on ovulation. IL-6 inhibits FSH-stimulated progesterone production by rat granulosa cells. In contrast to IL-1β, IL-6 stimulates apoptotic DNA-fragmentation in FSH-supported granulosa cells. Progesterone release from rat preovulatory follicles is enhanced by TNF-α. In pig granulosa cell cultures, TNF-α inhibits FSH plus insulin-stimulated progesterone biosynthesis as well as cholesterol side-chain cleavage cytochrome P450 enzyme mRNA accumulation. Thus, cytokines have divergent, species-specific effects on ovarian steroidogenesis and may endogenously regulate ovulation (*see* Fig. 2).

Cytokines also affect testicular steroidogenesis. IL-1α inhibits murine Leydig cell cAMP-induced testosterone release. One mechanism of this inhibi-

tion is the reduction in mRNA levels of 17α-hydroxylase/C17-20 lyase, a cytochrome P450 enzyme required for the production of C19 androgens from C21 steroids. Human chorionic gonadotropin stimulation of testosterone release is inhibited by TNF-α and IL-1β. Leydig cells treated with IL-1β also have decreased expression of the insulin growth factor-1 (IGF-1) mRNA. Although a role for testicular IL-6 is not as well defined, this cytokine enhances Sertoli cell transferrin release. Only those cells obtained from IX–XI and XIII staged segments respond to IL-6. Endogenous cytokine production may therefore affect testicular secretory activity.

6.3. Other Effects

6.3.1. Lipid Metabolism

During inflammation and infection, cytokines may affect the functioning of adipocytes to induce a state of hyperlipidemia. Adipose tissue lipoprotein lipase activity is inhibited by LIF and TNF-α. Other cytokines (e.g., IL-1, IL-6) also decrease lipoprotein lipase activity. In cultured 3T3 adipocytes, TNF-α and LIF decrease lipoprotein lipase mRNA accumulation, suggesting a transcriptional mechanism for the inhibition of lipoprotein lipase activity. Decreased lipoprotein lipase activity inhibits the ability of adipose tissue to accumulate and esterify fatty acids from circulating lipoproteins. Cytokines also increase lipolysis (e.g., TNF-α, IL-1, LIF) and decrease fatty acid synthesis, (e.g., TFN-α, IFN-γ) in cultured adipocytes. These catabolic effects lead to hypertriglyceridemia, a condition that may be protective owing to the ability of lipoproteins to bind endotoxin for a reduction in toxicity.

6.3.2. Bone Metabolism

Cytokines apparently affect both bone resorption (via the osteoclast) and bone formation (via the osteoblast). IL-1 and TNF-α induce local bone resorption in vitro and in vivo. Because neutralizing anti-IL-6 antibodies suppress osteoclast development of mouse bone cells, IL-6 is thought to induce osteoclastogenesis. LIF is also an osteoclast-stimulating factor, inducing bone resorption in murine calvariae via a prostaglandin-dependent mechanism. This cytokine (as well as IL-6 and IL-11) also inhibits osteoprogenitor differentiation and bone formation in fetal rat clavaria cell cultures. Bone resorption stimulated by calcemic hormones (e.g., parathyroid hormone, 1,25-dihyroxyvitamin D_3) or

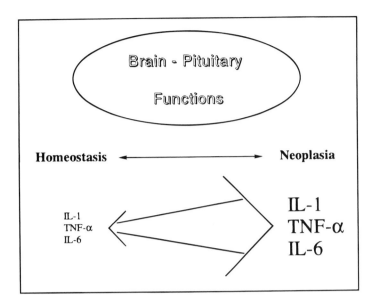

Fig. 3. Dysregulation of cytokine production may be associated with neoplasia in the brain and pituitary. Perturbation of homeostasis leading to neoplasia (e.g., pituitary adenoma, glioma) is associated with enhanced expression of cytokines (IL-1, IL-6, TNF-α), which may affect neoplastic potential. *See text* for details.

cytokines (e.g., IL-1, TNF-α) is inhibited by IFN-γ and IL-4 in vitro. IFN-γ inhibits osteoclast precursor recruitment as well as osteoblast function (e.g., inhibition of collagen and collagenase production). Thus, IFN-γ may cause a net decrease in bone turnover via inhibition of both resorption and bone formation. The B-cell-activating cytokine IL-4 inhibits bone resorption in mice and osteoclast generation in vitro. Bone marrow macrophages committed to the osteoclast pathway are inhibited by IL-4 and IFN-γ, thus preventing osteoclast cell formation. Cytokines may affect bone metabolism during noninflammatory states via paracrine or autocrine pathways, since certain of these proteins are produced within bone tissue (e.g., IL-6 and LIF production by osteoblasts).

7. PATHOPHYSIOLOGY OF HYPERSECRETION

7.1. Pituitary Adenomas

In view of the reported production and activities of cytokines in endocrine tissues, investigators have hypothesized a role for these factors in the progression of endocrine-related pathologic states. Cytokines (e.g., IL-1, IL-2, IL-6) inhibit rat anterior pituitary cell proliferation in vitro, but enhance the proliferation of pituitary adenomas such as the rat mammosoma-

totropic cell line GH$_3$ (e.g., IL-2, IL-6). As noted above, human pituitary adenoma cells contain and release IL-2 and IL-6. In a recent study, approximately one-half of all glioma tumor specimens from human brain tumors coexpressed the IL-1 and IL-6 mRNAs. Thus, the inappropriate expression of cytokine genes may be involved in the growth and development of human pituitary tumors (Fig. 3).

REFERENCES

Banks WA, Kastin AJ, Ehrensing CA. Blood-borne interleukin-1α is transported across the endothelial blood–spinal cord barrier of mice. *J Physiol* 1994; 479:257.

SELECTED READINGS

Akita S, Webster J, Ren SG, Takino H, Said JW, Zand O, Melmed S. Human and murine pituitary expression of leukemia inhibitory factor (LIF): novel intrapituitary regulation of adrenocorticotrophin (ACTH) synthesis and secretion. *J Clin Invest* 1995; 95:1288.

Arai K-I, Lee F, Miyajima A, Miyatake S, Arai N, Yokota T. Cytokines: coordinators of immune and inflammatory responses. *Annu Rev Biochem* 1990; 59:783.

Arzt E, Stelzer, G, Renner U, Lange M, Muller OA, Stalla GK. Interleukin-2 and interleukin-2 receptor expression in human corticotrophic adenoma and murine pituitary cell culture. *J Clin Invest*, 1992; 90:1944.

Boockfor FR, Wang D, Lin T, Nagpal ML, Spangelo BL. Interleukin-6 secretion from rat Leydig cells in culture. *Endocrinology* 1994; 134:2150.

Dinarello CA. The Interleukin-1 family: 10 years of discovery. *FASEB J* 1994; 8:1314.

Green A, Dobias SB, Walters DJA, Brashier AR. Tumor necrosis factor increases the rate of lipolysis in primary cultures of adipocytes without altering levels of hormone-sensitive lipase. *Endocrinology* 1994; 134:2581.

Hughes FM Jr, Fong Y-Y, Gorospe WC. Interleukin-6 stimulates apoptosis in FSH-stimulated rat granulosa cells in vitro: development and utilization of an in vitro model. *Endocrine* 1994; 2:997.

Jones TH. Interleukin-6: an endocrine cytokine. *Clin Endocrinol* 1994; 40:703.

Judd AM, MacLeod RM. Differential release of tumor necrosis factor and IL-6 from adrenal zona glomerulosa cells in vitro. *Am J Physiol* 1995; 268 (*Endocrinol Metab* 31):E114.

Lichtor T, Libermann TA. Coexpression of interleukin-1β and interleukin-6 in human brain tumors. *Neurosurgery* 1994; 34:669

Ray DW, Ren SG, Melmed S. Leukemia inhibitory factor (LIF) stimulates proopiomelanocortin (POMC) expression in a corticotroph cell line: role of stat pathway. *J Clin Invest* 1996; 97:1852.

Rifas L, Kenney JS, Marcelli M, Pacifici R, Cheng SL, Dawson LL, Avioli LV. Production of interleukin-6 in human osteoblasts and human bone marrow stromal cells: evidence that induction by interleukin-1 and tumor necrosis factor-α is not regulated by ovarian steroids. *Endocrinology* 1995; 136:4056.

Rivier C, Rivest S. Mechanisms mediating the effects of cytokines on neuroendocrine functions in the rat. *Ciba Found Symp (Netherlands)* 1993; 172:204.

Schindler C, Darnell JE Jr. Transcriptional responses to polypeptide ligands: the Jak-Stat pathway. *Annu Rev Biochem* 1995; 64:621.

Spangelo BL, Gorospe WC. Role of the cytokines in the neuroendocrine-immune system axis. *Frontiers in Neuroendocrinology* 1995; 16:1.

9   The Neuroendocrine–Immune Interface

Michael S. Harbuz, PhD
and Stafford L. Lightman, PhD

CONTENTS

1. INTRODUCTION

In an era of increased specialization where the trend has been for the individual scientist to delve ever deeper into smaller pools effectively knowing more and more about less and less, one area of research in particular has bucked the trend. The increasing interest in the bidirectional interactions of the immune and the neuroendocrine systems, and the importance of these systems in relation to sickness, inflammation, and immune-mediated diseases has required a sea change to this reductionist approach. Susceptibility to a number of autoimmune diseases, such as rheumatoid arthritis (RA) and multiple sclerosis (MS), have clear genetic components. However, it is also evident that not all individuals with a genetic predisposition go on to develop these

diseases, nor is the disease of equal severity in all individuals. The question of which factors may be responsible in increasing susceptibility to and/or the severity of disease have implicated a whole host of neuroendocrine factors. The anti-inflammatory effects of the glucocorticoids released from the adrenal cortex are well established, and the role of the hypothalamo–pituitary–adrenal (HPA) axis in controlling the release of the glucocorticoids has been of considerable research interest. A proinflammatory role has been proposed for prolactin, which is itself under the positive control of other hormones released from the hypothalamus. Growth hormone has been similarly implicated. The major gender differences associated with many autoimmune diseases have implicated the gonadal steroids. These are under increasing investigation both by neuroendocrinologists (interested in the modulation of neuroendocrine systems by the gonadal steroids) and immunologists (interested in the modulation of other

From: *Endocrinology: Basic and Clinical Principles* (P. M. Conn and S. Melmed, eds.), Humana Press Inc., Totowa, NJ.

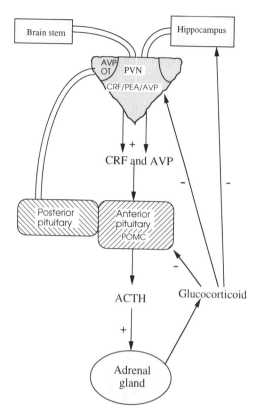

Fig. 1. Representation of the HPA axis (*see* Section 9). Briefly, CRF and AVP are released into the hypophysial portal blood to stimulate the release of ACTH, which stimulates the release of glucocorticoid from the adrenal cortex. The increase in circulating glucocorticoids serves to regulate the system by downregulating the synthesis and release of CRF, AVP, and POMC. Feedback also occurs at the level of the brainstem and the hippocampus. CRF = corticotrophin-releasing factor, AVP = arginine vasopressin, OT = oxytocin, PEA = proenkephalin A, POMC = proopiomelanocortin, and ACTH = adrenocorticotrophin hormone.

immune parameters), in addition to those working at the neuroendocrine–immune interface. Androgens, as we will see later, have a generally favorable effect on a number of diseases, whereas estrogens appear to have variable effects dependent on the disease. This chapter will address the question of susceptibility to disease, and the mechanisms involved particularly at the central and hypothalamic level. We shall begin with the system that has been most extensively investigated, the HPA axis.

2. THE HPA AXIS

The HPA axis, which may also be considered the stress axis, is represented in Fig. 1. Although the

functioning of the axis is covered in greater detail in Chapter 13, a few salient points will be considered here. At the hypothalamic level, corticotrophin-releasing factor$_{1-41}$ (CRF) and arginine vasopressin (AVP) are synthesized in the parvocellular cells of the paraventricular nucleus (PVN). In the normal rat, approx 50% of the CRF-positive neurons also contain AVP. The axons of these neurons terminate in the external zone of the median eminence, where CRF and AVP are released into the hypophysial portal blood and carried to the corticotrophs of the anterior pituitary. CRF is generally considered to be the major corticotrophin-releasing factor. It is able to evoke ACTH release from the anterior pituitary to a greater extent than can AVP alone. However, together these releasing factors act synergistically to evoke the release of ACTH. Importantly, CRF is currently the only factor that has been demonstrated to induce proopiomelanocortin (POMC) mRNA the ACTH precursor. The ACTH released from the anterior pituitary is carried in the general circulation to the adrenal gland, where it stimulates the production and release of glucocorticoid (cortisol in humans; corticosterone in the rat). The glucocorticoid has a negative feedback action at the pituitary and hypothalamic level (and also at other brain sites), to inhibit the synthesis and release of both ACTH and its hypothalamic-releasing factors. To understand the role of the HPA axis in disease, it is first of all necessary to recapitulate the mechanisms activated in response to acute and repeated stress.

2.1. The HPA Response to Acute Stress

In the rat, in response to a variety of acute stressors, there is a general activation of the HPA axis resulting in increased CRF and AVP mRNAs in the PVN, increased release of CRF and AVP into the portal blood, increased POMC mRNA in the anterior pituitary and increased circulating levels of ACTH and corticosterone. The type of stimulus, the duration of the stimulus, and the frequency with which it is applied may all influence the hypothalamic response. Thus, differential activation of the different components of the HPA axis has been demonstrated. Physical stressors, such as footshock, ip hypertonic saline, and naloxone-induced morphine withdrawal, increase CRF mRNA and proenkephalin A (an opiate precursor) mRNA in the PVN. Predominantly psychological stressors, such as restraint or swim stress, only activate CRF mRNA and not proenkephalin A

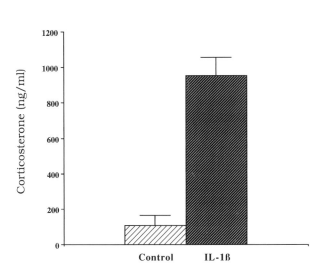

Fig. 2. A single injection of IL-1β directly into the lateral ventricle of the brain of the rat results in a significant increase in plasma corticosterone concentrations 30 min after injection. Values represent means and SEM for *n* = 6 rats/group.

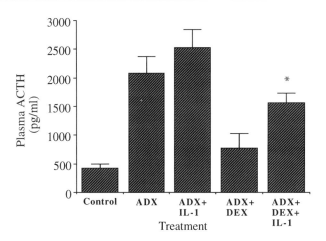

Fig. 3. Plasma ACTH concentrations in control and adrenalectomized rats treated with the synthetic steroid dexamethasone with or without IL-1β. With the removal of steroid-negative feedback following adrenalectomy, there is a significant increase in plasma ACTH levels. Adrenalectomized rats are unable to mount a significant response to ip injection of IL-1β at a concentration previously shown to stimulate release. (Adrenalectomized rats are able to respond to an acute stress). Dexamethasone treatment returns plasma ACTH concentrations to levels similar to those found in intact control animals. These steroid-replaced animals are able to mount a significant increase in response to IL-1β (*see* Section 2.2.).

mRNA. Ether stress, in contrast, results in an increase in proenkephalin A mRNA, while not affecting CRF mRNA. Oxytocin may be important in the response to psychological stress. Studies in anesthetized animals have demonstrated that a conscious appreciation of a physical stress is not necessary for a response to occur. These data suggest a subtle control system operating at the hypothalamus integrating signals from other brain areas to coordinate the release of a cocktail of releasing factors into the portal blood. The prevailing steroid milieu is not of primary importance in the mechanism underlying this response, since a response to stress can be mounted following adrenalectomy, where all endogenous steroid negative feedback has been removed, and also in high-dose glucocorticoid-treated animals, where the activity of the HPA axis is maximally suppressed. Therefore, the stress-responsive trans-synaptic activation of hypothalamic neurons is able to overcome the level of steroid negative feedback. This is in accordance with suggestions that there are mechanisms able to maintain stress responsiveness, despite increased glucocorticoid secretion.

2.2. The HPA Response to Acute Immune Challenge

A major area of research in the last 10 years has concerned the study of the effects of acute challenge with immune activators or mediators, e.g., lipopolysaccharide (LPS), interleukin (1L)-1β, and tumor necrosis factor (TNF)-α, which also stimulate the HPA axis. This aspect is covered in greater detail in Chapter 8. Activation occurs whether the mediator is given peripherally (to mimic the increases seen in infection/disease) or directly into the brain (Fig. 2). A number of studies have demonstrated that IL-1β exerts its stimulatory effect on the HPA axis via CRF and that diminishing the activity of CRF neurons, e.g., by immunoneutralization, ablation of the PVN, and so on, reduces the effectiveness of the stimulus. In the absence of a functioning PVN, and CRF neurons in particular, the ability of immunomodulators to activate the HPA axis is diminished, and hence, the ability to activate corticosteroid-mediated regulation of immunological activity is lost. Although stress-mediated release of corticosteroids normally damps down immunological responses, the presence of corticosteroids is actually necessary to allow rats to respond to IL-1β (Fig. 3). The interrelationship of corticosteroids and immunological responses is clearly a complex one with both permissive and inhibitory effects of corticosteroids.

2.3. The HPA Axis Response to Repeated Stress

The activation of the HPA axis in response to acute stress is relatively well characterized. The response to chronic stress remains less so. In practice, there are few models for chronic stress, and in the literature, the term chronic usually refers to an experimental paradigm where an acute stress is repeated for a number of days. In response to repeated stress, there may be a habituation or adaptation of the HPA axis to this repeated challenge. Therefore, although acute footshock, restraint, or ethanol stress will increase circulating ACTH and corticosterone for up to a week, levels subsequently return to basal levels. At the mRNA level, a number of days of repeated stress may result in elevated CRF mRNA levels (e.g., in response to ip injections of hypertonic saline or immobilization) or levels not different from those seen in controls (e.g., following restraint in a Perspex™ tube), presumably reflecting the nature and severity of the challenge. In the repeated stress situation, although the animals may be refractory to the specific repeated stressor, the system itself has not become refractory to stress; following exposure to a novel stress, a normal or even supranormal response is seen.

2.4. The Effects of Stress on Immune Function

In addition to the effects of immune modulators on neuroendocrine systems, these two systems are also able to interact in the reverse direction (Fig. 4). There is accumulating evidence from both human and animal studies that stress is able to downregulate immune function. Stress can reduce lymphocyte responsiveness to mitogenic stimulation, decrease natural killer cell activity, increase susceptibility to tumors, and decrease thymus growth and differentiation by inducing apoptosis in immature thymocytes.

It is now established that the spleen and thymus are able to synthesize a wide range of neuropeptides (Table 1). Many of these have already been implicated in modulating the response to stress and immune challenge. The role played by these locally produced peptides is unknown, but they may exert a paracrine or autocrine effect on the functioning of these organs. The temporal changes in these neuroimmunopeptides following stress need to be determined.

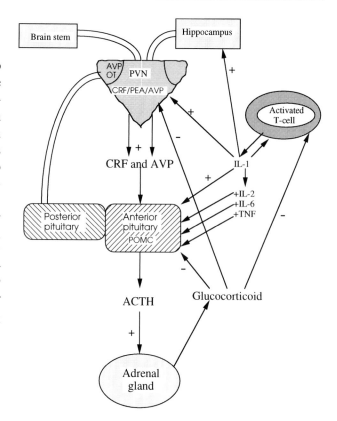

Fig. 4. Representation of the HPA axis demonstrating the interrelationship that exists in the functioning of the neuroendocrine and immune systems. Following immune activation (represented by the activated T-cell), IL-1 is released and sets in motion a series of cascade systems, which result in the increased release of many cytokines and immunomodulators. In addition to exerting effects on the immune system, these immunomodulators are able to stimulate the HPA axis and a number of other brain areas. This communication is bidirectional, since the end point of HPA axis activation is an increase in circulating glucocorticoids, which are able to inhibit synthesis and release cytokines. Other hormones released from the pituitary also have immunomodulatory properties. TNF-α = tumor necrosis factor α.

There is a wealth of evidence supporting the involvement of a variety of cytokines in autoimmune disease, and a discussion of this evidence is beyond the scope of this chapter. It is clear that there is activation of endogenous cytokines at numerous sites from the brain and pituitary through the immune tissues to local production at the affected sites. The balance of pro- and anti-inflammatory effects of these cytokines may be crucial. Targeting of particular cytokines in the cascade may result in novel treatment modalities tailored to meet the needs of each particular disease.

Table 1
An Inexhaustive List of Hormones and
Neurotransmitters Present
in the Spleen and/or Thymus

CRF
AVP
Oxytocin
Luteinizing hormone
   releasing hormone
Luteinizing hormone
ACTH
Proopiomelanocortin
Endorphins
Enkephalins
Thyrotropin-stimulating hormone
Prolactin
Somatostatin
Growth hormone
Noradrenaline
Substance P

3. NEUROENDOCRINE CHANGES ASSOCIATED WITH ADJUVANT-INDUCED ARTHRITIS

Adjuvant-induced arthritis (AA) is a disease model that shares certain characteristics with RA in humans. The model has been used extensively for studies on pain, inflammation, and arthritis. This immune-mediated inflammatory disease, which is T-cell-dependent, can be induced in susceptible strains of rat by a single injection into the base of the tail of heat-killed ground Mycobacterium butyricum (or synthetic adjuvant) in paraffin oil. Twelve to 14 day after the injection of the adjuvant, the animals begin to develop inflammation of the hindpaws. This subsequently spreads to other joints attaining a maximum severity 21 day after injection.

3.1. The Pituitary–Adrenal Response to AA

The hormonal changes in this immune-mediated chronic inflammatory disease model are similar to those seen in the acute and repeated stress situations, and are as one might predict for what is a chronic stress. Associated with the occurrence of hindpaw inflammation, circulating ACTH and corticosterone levels are raised, and POMC mRNA in the anterior pituitary is also increased. The elevation in hormone concentrations occurs in the morning when in the rat the circadian rhythm is at its nadir, and a hormonal

profile reveals a loss of the circadian rhythm with normal high evening levels being present throughout the day. A similar loss of the circadian rhythm has also been reported in humans with RA. A number of immune parameters, for example, variation in total and subset lymphocyte counts, natural killer cell levels together with their cytotoxicity, and the expression of some cytokines also show circadian changes that are correlated with circadian changes in circulating hormone levels. The loss of the normal feedback rhythm may have implications for the disease process.

3.2. Alterations in the Hypothalamic Control Mechanism

In contrast to the activation of the pituitary–adrenal axis in AA, at the hypothalamic level, there is no activation of CRF mRNA. Indeed, in the Piebald-Vital-Glaxo (PVG) strain of rat there is a paradoxical decrease in CRF mRNA, which begins at the time of the first indications of inflammation (day 11) and continues to fall reaching a nadir 21 d after the injection of the adjuvant when disease severity is at its peak (Fig. 5). This decrease occurs irrespective of the adjuvant used to induce the arthritis, which is an important point, since the different adjuvants would have different antigenic determinants. In addition to the decrease in CRF mRNA, CRF peptide release into the hypophysial-portal blood is also significantly reduced, demonstrating a decrease in the activity of CRF neurons associated with the development of the disease. This raises a number of interesting questions.

3.3. With a Reduction in CRF Activity, What Is Driving The Pituitary –Adrenal Axis?

This question is particularly pertinent, since CRF is currently the only factor demonstrated to increase POMC mRNA in the anterior pituitary. Strong evidence suggests that AVP is the factor responsible for driving the HPA axis. AVP in the hypophysial portal blood is increased in a time-dependent fashion associated with the development of AA. AVP mRNA is also increased in the PVN. The anterior pituitaries of AA rats in vitro are more responsive to AVP, and the combination of CRF and AVP, than pituitaries taken from control rats. It would appear therefore that in the presence of permissive levels of CRF, AVP is able to take over as the major CRF in AA. Supporting evidence for the increased role of AVP in chronic stress comes from a number of sources.

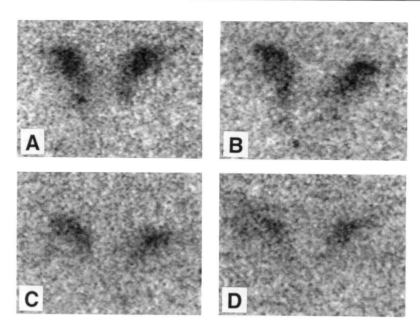

Fig. 5. Representative photomicrographs taken from Hyperfilm-MP (Amersham, Amersham, U. K.) autoradiography film showing hypothalamic paraventricular nucleus hybridized with ^{35}S-labeled probes complementary to CRF mRNA. (**A**) d O: Control. (**B**) d 7: Preclinical. (**C**) d 16: Inflamed. (**D**) d 21: Maximum inflammation. With the onset of adjuvant-induced arthritis, which occurs at around d 14 following injection of adjuvant, there is a significant decrease in CRF mRNA levels in the PVN. As the disease progresses to a maximum severity at d 21, CRF mRNA levels decrease to a nadir at this time. There is good correlation between the decrease in CRF mRNA levels in the PVN and the increase in severity of inflammation. Levels in the d 7 preclinical rats are not significantly different from controls. *See* Section 3.2.

Repeatedly restrained rats are able to mount a response to a novel stress as noted above. However, exogenous injection of CRF is without effect on circulating hormone levels in these animals. In contrast, exogenous AVP elicited a response of both ACTH and corticosterone. This may be explained by the associated loss of CRF receptors in the anterior pituitary. It has been noted in this repeated stress model that there is an increase in AVP stores and increased colocalization of AVP within CRF neurons in the median eminence, leading to the suggestion that in chronic stress situations, endogenous AVP may be essential for sustaining the ability to respond to stress when the axis is refractory to CRF.

3.4. What Is the Inhibitory Mechanism Responsible for the Loss of Hypothalamic CRF Drive?

The identity of the inhibitory factor(s) responsible for the decrease in CRF neuronal activity has yet to be determined. The increase in circulating levels of corticosterone seen in AA is not responsible for the decrease in CRF activity. Following adrenalectomy, although the removal of the negative feedback results

in an increase in CRF mRNA, this is markedly attenuated in arthritic rats, which suggests that the inhibitory influence seen in nonadrenalectomized arthritic rats is also present in the adrenalectomized animals.

Within the PVN of arthritic rats, noradrenaline concentrations are doubled, suggesting a possible role for endogenous noradrenaline in the development of AA. The physiological role of catecholamines in the neuroendocrine response to acute stress is controversial; both inhibitory and excitatory roles have been ascribed. In disease models, it is not too surprising that there have been few studies on the role of catecholamines. In AA, chemical (6-hydroxydopamine) lesions to deplete catecholamines, which resulted in a 75% decrease in hypothalamic noradrenaline, had no effect on CRF mRNA levels, but did lead to an increase in the severity of the hindpaw inflammation. These data suggest a protective role for central catecholamines and also suggest the intriguing possibility of treatments affecting central neurotransmitter systems altering the course of disease. There is also support for a protective role for catecholamines in other disease models. Neonatal treatment of rats with 6-hydroxydopamine to deplete endogenous catecholamines has been shown to increase the severity of experimental autoimmune myasthenia gravis and experimental allergic encephalomyelitis (EAE). Agonists to the β-adrenergic receptor have also been shown to alleviate EAE. In contrast to these studies demonstrating an increase in severity following depletion, other workers have noted that both central and peripheral depletion of catecholamines can reduce the severity of EAE. These latter data are not easily resolved with the above studies and provide an area for future research.

There is both functional and anatomical evidence that the neurokinin substance P can act centrally as an inhibitor of the response to acute stress. Furthermore, there appears to be a direct inhibitory action of substance P on CRF neurons. The role of endogenous substance P in disease models has yet to be investigated fully. There is, however, indirect evidence that substance P may be involved in downregulating CRF activity in AA. However, the precise role of substance P in this model requires further study. Whether substance P synthesized in the arcuate nucleus is responsible or whether this effect is mediated through other inhibitory pathways, e.g., GABA, remains to be determined.

3.5. Is the Defective Stress Response Important to Disease Outcome?

The possibility that a defect in the regulation of the HPA axis may predispose an individual to autoimmune disease has been proposed. The Lewis rat has a hyporesponsive HPA axis, and is unable to mount as effective an increase in plasma corticosterone as the histocompatible Fischer strain to a variety of immune and psychological challenges. The Lewis strain is susceptible to streptoccal cell-wall-induced arthritis, whereas the Fischer strain is resistant. The defect has been localized to the CRF neuron in the PVN. The result of this defect is that in the basal condition, the Lewis rat has low plasma corticosterone levels and exhibits a blunted circadian rhythm. As we have seen previously, the blunted hormonal circadian rhythm has immune consequences. The Lewis strain has smaller adrenal and pituitary glands and larger thymuses, and this correlates with an increased susceptibility to a wide range of T-cell-mediated autoimmune-like diseases, including EAE and streptococcal cell-wall-induced

arthritis. The hyporesponsiveness of the Lewis rat may well be a factor in this susceptibility, although other factors are undoubtedly involved as well. Indeed, although it has been proposed that the resistance of the PVG strain to EAE is based on the hyperresponsiveness to stress, we have found that the PVG is susceptible to AA! It is of interest, however, that when the arthritic PVG rat is subsequently exposed to an acute stress, it is no longer able to produce a significant increase in either CRF mRNA or corticosterone. This may have serious implications for the ability of the organism to cope with additional stressors, such as infections, and this may compromise the individual.

An inability to mount a cortisol response to the stress of surgery has been described in RA, although challenge with CRF resulted in a normal ACTH response in patients with RA, demonstrating no alteration in pituitary function. The adrenal response to CRF was however impaired, suggesting a defect in the responsiveness of the adrenal in RA. This of course does not rule out the possibility of a hypothalamic defect in RA. Although the pituitary ACTH response to CRF is intact in RA, the release of β-endorphin (which is also derived from the POMC gene) is impaired, which suggests a dysfunction in the processing of POMC. The relevance of this is unclear, but β-endorphin has been implicated as a feedback regulator on CRF release.

The crucial role of the HPA axis in the development and severity of disease and in avoiding a fatal outcome has been demonstrated in a number of studies. In the Lewis rat, treatment with corticosterone at physiological doses can reduce the severity of streptococcal cell-wall-induced arthritis. Conversely, Fischer rats can be made susceptible to disease if treated with a corticosteroid receptor antagonist. Adrenalectomy results in an earlier onset and greater severity of AA in PVG rats, and if left unchecked, will prove fatal. This outcome has also been shown in the Lewis rat EAE model. It was proposed by Munck and coworkers (1984) that the increase in endogenous glucocorticoid seen after immune challenge occurs not to protect against the source of the stress itself, but rather to protect against the body's normal reaction to stress. If these responses are allowed to progress unchecked, then they may themselves lead to tissue damage and may even become life-threatening.

4. IS THERE EVIDENCE FOR IMPAIRED HPA AXIS FUNCTION IN OTHER IMMUNE-MEDIATED DISEASES?

Abnormalities in the functioning of the HPA axis have been implicated in a number of autoimmune diseases and also in animal models. African sleeping sickness is a potentially lethal parasitic disease in humans caused by the protozoan *Trypanosoma brucei*. The early acute disease is characterised by fever, rash, weight loss, edema, and chronic fatigue. The parasite may invade the CNS, resulting in a broad spectrum of neurologic and psychiatric symptoms. If left untreated, the disease is fatal. With regard to their HPA axis function, individuals with sleeping sickness are unable to mount an adrenal response to injected ACTH, suggesting adrenal insufficiency. They are also unable to mount a suitable response to injection of CRF, suggesting secondary adrenal insufficiency. However, it does not appear that these individuals have an adrenal insufficiency that predisposes them to the disease, as has been suggested for the Lewis rat. Following antiparasitic treatment and associated with recovery, there is an improvement of the ACTH and cortisol responses to CRF, suggesting the defect is a response to the disease and by inference is not present prior to development.

A similar blunting of the HPA response to challenge has been noted in the obese strain of chicken that develops autoimmune thyroiditis, which is an animal model for Hashimoto disease. These animals show elevated corticosteroid-binding globulin and a decrease in free circulating corticosterone. They exhibit a blunted corticosterone response to IL-1 and other stimulants. The alteration in the response has been localized to the hypothalamo–pituitary part of the axis, although the precise locus remains to be determined. The blunted response to challenge is also evident in a number of inbred strains of mice that develop diseases similar to systemic lupus erythematosus (SLE) and Sjögrens syndrome. Parallel to the development of the diseases in susceptible strains, there is an age-related decline in plasma corticosterone together with a blunted response to challenge with IL-1 and other stimuli.

Determining alterations in the HPA axis in humans is ethically difficult and poses particular problems in attempting to determine the mechanisms likely to be responsible for alterations to the axis.

Some patients with MS have elevated levels of plasma cortisol compared with controls. In one study to ascertain changes in responsiveness, patients were injected with the hypothalamic-releasing factors CRF and AVP. In response to CRF challenge, they responded normally, but the response to AVP was blunted. The cortisol response to insulin-induced hypoglycaemia was also blunted in these patients. These findings support those outlined above, suggesting that in MS AVP may play a more significant role than CRF in maintaining the activity of the HPA axis. These data support the notion that associated with autoimmune disease, there is an alteration in the responsiveness of the HPA axis. However, taken together, it appears that the mechanism involved is not simply a predisposition to autoimmune disease secondary to a defect in the HPA axis, but a more complex interaction between the HPA axis and the disease process.

4.1. Do the Changes in Hypothalamic Control Mechanisms Occur in Other Disease Models?

A question worthy of consideration is whether the alterations in the hypothalamic control mechanisms associated with AA are a feature of this particular disease model or whether a more general mechanism may be inferred. In an adoptive transfer model of EAE (which involves injection of activated spleenocytes, i.e., no adjuvant is directly involved), despite the activation of the pituitary–adrenal axis, there is a similar paradoxical decrease in CRF mRNA in the PVN (Fig. 6). Supporting the contention that the decrease is separate from any question of susceptibility is the observation that when the animals recover from the disease, the decreased CRF mRNA levels return to normal, and the elevated levels of plasma corticosterone and POMC mRNA in the anterior pituitary decline to basal control levels.

Eosinophilia myalgia syndrome (EMS) was originally identified in humans on the West Coast of the US in the summer and fall of 1989, where the cases of the syndrome reached epidemic proportions. EMS is characterized by eosinophilia, muscle pain, and edema in the early stages, followed by inflammation of the muscles and connective tissues, hardening of the skin, and peripheral neuropathy. In a number of cases, the disease proved fatal. The disease was identified as being T-cell-mediated. Painstaking detective work identified the culprit, which turned out to

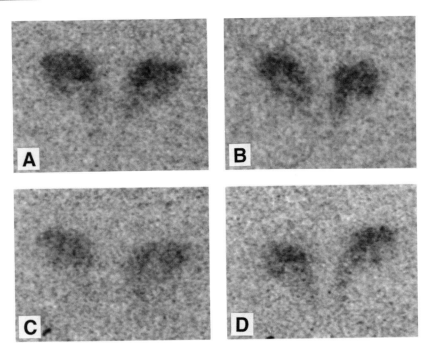

Fig. 6. Representative photomicrographs taken from Hyperfilm-MP (Amersham, Amersham, U. K.) autoradiography film showing hypothalamic paraventricular nucleus hybridized with ^{35}S-labeled probes complementary to CRF mRNA. (**A**) Control. (**B**) Preclinical. (**C**) Clinical. (**D**) Recovery. With the onset of adoptively transferred EAE, there is a decrease in CRF mRNA, which occurs despite the activation of the pituitary–adrenal axis. With recovery, levels return to those seen in controls and at the preclinical stage. *See* Section 4.2.

be a rogue batch of the amino acid L-tryptophan intended for the health food market, where it was sold to treat insomnia, depression, and other disorders. To confirm the cause-and-effect relationship, the suspected compound was fed to Lewis rats who went on to develop histological features consistent with the human disease. Investigation of the HPA axis revealed a tendency to lower plasma corticosterone concentrations in the affected rats. More pertinent for the present discussion, examination of the PVN of the rats with EMS revealed a decrease in CRF mRNA.

Leishmaniasis is a parasitic disease endemic in the Third World that infects the liver. This infection is also T-cell-mediated. Mice infected with *Leischmania donovani* also demonstrate a decrease in CRF mRNA in the PVN. Histocompatible mice show no change in CRF mRNA following inoculation with the parasite. Together these data demonstrate that this adaptive change to these T-cell-mediated diseases results in a paradoxical decrease in CRF mRNA irrespective of the nature of the challenge or of the species investigated.

4.2. What Are the Effects of Stress on the Development and Severity of Disease?

Studies in the rat have shown that a variety of stressful stimuli are able to suppress the development or severity of AA, collagen-induced arthritis, and EAE. In contrast, other studies have demonstrated an increase in severity, and accelerated onset of both collagen-induced arthritis and EAE. These discrepancies may be owing to the stress paradigms employed in the various studies conducted in a number of laboratories around the world. The effect may differ dependent on the type of stress, its duration, and frequency; possibly these and the coping ability of the animals may all be of relevance. What are less well established are the immune consequences of the stressors used. In humans, the indications are that stress, such as death of a loved one, divorce, or separation, can contribute to the onset of or increase the severity of a variety of diseases, e.g., RA, insulin-dependent diabetes, Crohn's disease, uveitis, and Grave's disease. This poses something of a paradox, since stress decreases immunocompetence. It is likely

Table 2
Circulating Hormones and Their Effects on Immune Function

Hormone	Effect on inflammation	Effects on the immune system
ACTH	Anti-inflammatory?	Receptors present on immune tissues
		Stimulatory/inhibitory effects on lymphocyte proliferation
		Suppress antibody production
		Implicated as growth factor
Glucocorticoids	Anti-inflammatory	Receptors present on immune tissues
		Regulates thymocyte maturation and differentiation
		Decreases thymic mass
		Inhibits IL-1 synthesis and secretion
		Inhibits immunoglobulin production
		Stimulates neutrophil egress
Prolactin	Proinflammatory	Receptors present on immune tissues
(also growth hormone)		Stimulates thymocyte maturation and differentiation
		Increases thymic mass
		Immunocompetence compromised by hypophysectomy, but reversed with hormone replacement
Androgens	Anti-inflammatory	Receptors present on immune tissues
		Immunosuppressive on both T- and B-cells
		Decrease thymic mass
		Suppress antibody response
		Increase TGF-β (inhibitor of TH1-mediated functions)
Estrogen	Pro- or anti-inflammatory dependent on the disease	Receptors present on immune tissues
		Decrease thymic mass
		Inhibit suppressive T-cells
		Facilitate T-helper lymphocyte maturation
		Stimulate B-cell-mediated antibody response
DHEA	Anti-inflammatory	DHEA–receptor-binding complex present on tissues
		Inhibits thymic atrophy induced by glucocorticoids
		Suppresses IL-6 production
		Enhances IL-2 production
		Inhibits formation of autoantibodies

that the cytokine profile released in response to stress together with the timing and duration of the anti-inflammatory glucocorticoid release may be crucial.

5. GONADAL STEROIDS

The stress response inhibits the hypothalamo–pituitary–gonadal axis at multiple levels, and glucocorticoids also inhibit the tissue effects of sex steroids. Sex steroids are also able to modulate the activity of the HPA axis, reflecting the bidirectional nature of these systems. The involvement of CRF in the sexually dimorphic response to HPA activation has been proposed because of the estrogen-responsive element in the 5′-regulatory region of the CRF gene. Females (mice, rats, and humans) have a more active HPA axis response than males and are also more prone to

autoimmune diseases, e.g., autoimmune thyroiditis (19:1), SLE (9:1), and RA (4:1). These findings suggest that gonadal steroids have a major role in autoimmune disease (Table 2). Gonadal competence may also be a factor, since young females are many times more susceptible to RA than young males. With increasing age, the ratio is reduced. Under 60 the ratio is about 5:1; with later onset, the female:male ration approaches parity. These changes may reflect the decrease in testosterone associated with increasing age in males, and it has been suggested that androgens may have a role in protecting males from developing autoimmune diseases in both human and in animal models. For example, castration increases the incidence, time of onset, and severity of streptococcal cell-wall-induced arthritis and AA in males. These effects can be reversed by testosterone treatment in AA.

Serum androgen concentrations are reduced in males and females with RA, and also in rats with AA. Female NZB/NZW mice usually die following the development of SLE, but this can be prevented by treatment with the androgen dihydrotestosterone. Intact males have a greater chance of survival, but castration results in increased mortality. In general, it appears that in males, castration increases the severity of the disease, which can be suppressed by androgen replacement.

The role of estrogens in the female is complex and appears to depend on the type of disease. In SLE, estrogen accelerates the progress of the disease, and the influence of estrogen has been suggested to be one of the most important contributors to the female preponderance of the disease. In contrast, estrogen suppresses EAE, collagen-induced arthritis, and AA. One suggestion for this apparent discrepancy concerns the effects of estrogen on B-cell- and T-cell-mediated immune responses. Estrogen enhances the antibody response (B-cell), while suppressing cell-mediated immunity (T-cell). EAE, collagen-induced arthritis, and AA are all considered to be primarily T-cell-mediated disease models. Testosterone acts to suppress both B-cell and T-cell responses, and hence, suppresses disease severity.

The site of action of the gonadal steroids and the mechanism(s) by which these actions are exerted are not fully established. The interactions among the HPA, gonadal, and other neuroendocrine systems are complex. Whether the changes reflect the actions of the gonadal steroids themselves or metabolites is not known. Androgen and estrogen receptors are found on lymphocytes, and androgen receptors are also expressed by synovial cells, suggesting the possibility of direct effects at the site of inflammation.

Further evidence for the important role of the gonadal steroids comes from observations that changes in activity of autoimmune diseases occur at times of change in gonadal axis function, e.g., puberty, pregnancy, postpartum, and menopause. At these times, the hormonal milieu is dramatically altered with not only changes in the gonadal axis, but also with changes in other hormones, such prolactin and growth hormone.

6. DIHYDROEPIANDROSTENEDIONE (DHEAS)

DHEAS is the most abundant adrenal steroid in the circulation in humans. Specific receptors for the free hormone (DHEA) are found in T-cells, and DHEA can prevent the action of dexamethasone on inducing apotosis both on thymocytes and unresponsiveness of peripheral T-cells. DHEA directly enhances Th1 T-cell activity, and indeed, it has been shown that DHEA sulfatase activity regulates the Th1 and Th2 cytokine balance of mouse lymphoid tssue in response to anti-CD3.

DHEA levels fall markedly with aging, and in old mice, DHEA supplements correct many of their immunological deficits. A fall in serum DHEAS has also been reported to herald the progression of HIV to AIDS.

Stress, such as examination time for students, results in a marked fall in the ratio of DHEAS to cortisol together with a loss of delayed hypersensitivity, but sparing of humoral immunity. This infers that stress drives a shift in the Th1/Th2 balance toward Th2, and implicates the fall in DHEA as a likely candidate factor in activating this immunological change.

7. OTHER NEUROENDOCRINE SYSTEMS

Prolactin receptors are found in many neuroendocrine organs and also in immune tissues. Prolactin is required for IL-2 activation of T-cells and also stimulates B-cells. Its release from the pituitary is stimulated by IL-1 and IL-6. Prolactin is therefore ideally suited to play a role in the communication between the neuroendocrine and immune systems. A proinflammatory role for prolactin has been proposed in AA. Removal of the pituitary prevents the development of AA in the rat. Implanting the pituitary under the kidney capsule, which results in hyperprolactinemia, or treatment with either exogenous prolactin or growth hormone (but not any other pituitary hormones) reinstates the susceptibility. Treatment with bromocriptine, which inhibits prolactin release, also prevents AA. These data do not preclude an indirect effect of prolactin, and there are a number of discrepancies in the literature. In RA and AA plasma, prolactin concentrations are not altered from controls. There is evidence in AA that treatments that increase the severity of disease are associated with a decrease in circulating prolactin, thus opposing the proinflammatory view. It may, however, be the balance between circulating levels of the proinflammatory prolactin and anti-inflammatory glucocorticoids that has greater relevance.

8. SUMMARY

The interactions of the neuroendocrine immune systems are complex, and more so in relation to autoimmune/inflammatory disease. These interactions can occur at many levels. Cytokines exert effects on immune tissues, but in addition are able to up-regulate the HPA axis, inhibit the gonadal axis acting both in the brain and on the gonads, suppress thyroid function, suppress appetite, and induce fever. Adrenal and gonadal steroids are important in the regulation of the immune system. Glucocorticoids suppress the host immune response and as such are essential for survival. Other hormones, such as prolactin, growth hormone, and thyroid hormones, are also able to influence the immune system. The recent finding of many neuropeptides and transmitters in the immune tissues has added a further level of complexity. We are only beginning to understand how these systems interact and their implications for disease. The holy grail remains to be the answer to the question, "What are the factors conferring susceptibility and controlling the severity of autoimmune diseases?"

REFERENCES

Munck A, Guyre PM, Holbrook NJ. Physiological functions of glucocorticoids in stress and their relation to pharmacological actions. *Endocr Rev* 1984; 5:25.

SELECTED READINGS

Bateman A, Singh A, Kral T, Solomon S. The immune–hypothalamic–pituitary–adrenal axis. *Endocr Rev* 1989; 10:92.

Chikanza IC, Panayi GS. Hypothalamic-pituitary mediated modulation of immune function: prolactin as a neuroimmune peptide. *Br J Rheumatol* 1991; 30:203.

Grossman CJ, Roselle GA, Mendenhall CL. Sex steroid regulation of autoimmunity. *J Steroid Biochem Molec Biol* 1991; 40:649.

Harbuz MS, Lightman SL. Stress and the hypothalamic–pituitary–adrenal axis: acute, chronic and immunological activation. *J Endocrinol* 1992; 134:327.

Holmdahl R, Carlsten H, Jansson L, Larsson P. Oestrogen is a potent immunomodulator of murine experimental rheumatoid disease. *Br J Rheumatol* 1989; 28:54.

Jorgensen C, Sany J. Modulation of the immune response by the neuro-endocrine axis in rheumatoid arthritis. *Clin Exp Rheumatol* 1994; 12:435.

Rook GAW, Hernandez-Pando R, Lightman SL. Hormones, peripherally acting prohormones and regulation of the Th1/Th2 balance. *Immunol Today* 1994; 15:301.

Sternberg EM, Wilder RL, Chrousos GP, Gold PW. Stress responses and the pathogenesis of arthritis. In: McCubbin JA, Kaufman PG, Nemeroff CB. *Stress, Neuropeptides and Systemic Disease.* Academic, San Diego, CA, 1991:287.

Wick G, Hu Y, Schwarz S. Kroemer G. Immunoendocrine communication via the hypothalamo–pituitary–adrenal axis in autoimmune disease. *Endocr Rev* 1993; 14:539.

Wilder RL. Neuroendocrine-immune system interactions and autoimmunity. *Ann Rev Immunol* 1995; 13:307.

PART III

INSECTS/PLANTS/COMPARATIVE

10 Insect Hormones

Lawrence I. Gilbert, PhD

CONTENTS

1. INTRODUCTION

Recent estimates place the number of insect species at from 2–20 million, more by far than the total of all other animals and plants on earth. Although insects affect the human condition in a variety of ways, primarily as pollinators, competitors for agricultural products, and as vectors of disease, their sheer diversity and numbers make this class of arthropods worthy of study. Indeed, insects have become the model of choice for a variety of research endeavors in genetics, biochemistry, developmental biology, endocrinology, and so forth. Since they are encased in a semirigid exoskeleton (cuticle), insects and other arthropods must shed this cuticle periodically (molt) in order to grow and undergo metamorphosis. Although insect molting and metamorphosis have been scrutinized since the time of Aristotle, the exact control mechanisms have remained elusive. However, research on insect hormones has contributed significantly to the general field of endocrinology.

The now accepted dogma that the nervous system not only controls target organs via action potentials and neurotransmitters, but is also in a sense an

From: *Endocrinology: Basic and Clinical Principles* (P. M. Conn and S. Melmed, eds.), Humana Press Inc., Totowa, NJ.

endocrine system (hence the term neuroendocrinology) was first conceptualized on the basis of data derived from studies on insect development. It was almost eight decades ago that Stefen Kopeć (1922), working on larvae (caterpillars) of the gypsy moth, demonstrated that the insect brain released a substance (hormone) that controls insect molting, i.e., the secretion of a new and larger cuticle to allow growth and the digestion and shedding of the old cuticle (ecdysis). When the brain was extirpated 10 d or more after the final larval–larval molt, pupation ensued, and brainless but otherwise normal moths emerged. If brain extirpation occurred <10 d after the last larval molt, the larvae failed to metamorphose to the pupal stage, although they survived for weeks. These and other studies led Kopeć to conclude that the brain liberated some substance into the hemolymph (blood) that is essential for the larval–pupal molt and that it is released about 10 d after the last larval molt. This was the cornerstone of the field of neuroendocrinology.

Research on this brain factor was extended by the giants of the field in the 1930s and 1940s, and the source of the factor was shown to be specific protocerebral neurosecretory cells. We now know that the brain factor acts on glands in the prothorax of the insect to elicit synthesis and secretion of a steroidal

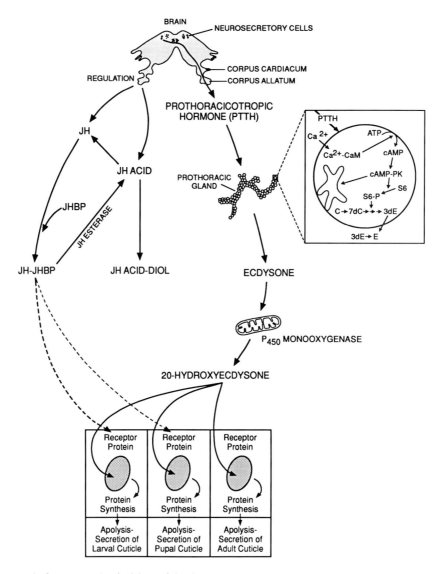

Fig. 1. Endocrine control of metamorphosis. Most of the data contributing to this scheme were derived from studies on *M. sexta* although the scheme applies to all insects in a general sense. Note that in the care of *Manduca*, JH acid rather than JH is released from the corpus allatum toward the end of the last larval stage (Gilbert et al., 1996).

prohormone, an ecdysteroid, which is ultimately responsible for eliciting the molting process. The current name for this neurohormone is prothoracicotropic hormone (PTTH; Fig. 1).

On the basis of subsequent microsurgical studies, it was shown that glands attached to the brain, the corpora allata, were the source of a hormone (juvenile hormone, JH) that controls the quality of the molt, i.e., whether it be larval–larval, larval–pupal, or pupal–adult. Its role is to favor the synthesis of larval (juvenile) structures and inhibit differentiation (metamorphosis) to the pupal and/or adult

stages. Although the action of JH is connected to that of the molting hormone and it therefore does not in a sense act as an independent agent in controlling growth processes, it does act alone in many adult insects as a gonadotropic hormone. Thus, the three major glands controlling insect growth and development are the brain, prothoracic glands, and corpora allata, their respective secretions being a neuropeptide, a steroid, and sesquiterpenoid compounds (Fig. 2).

Figure 1 is a generalized scheme for the Lepidoptera (moths and butterflies) and the details

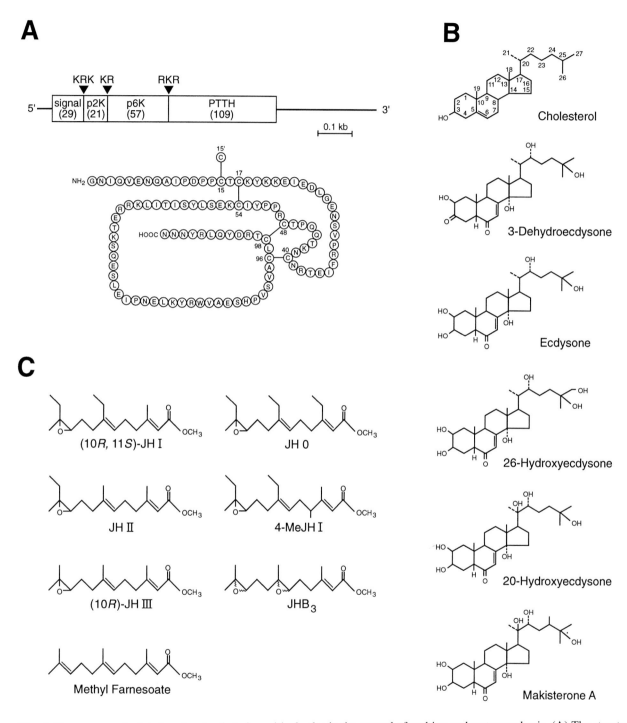

Fig. 2. Hormones and related molecules that play critical roles in the control of molting and metamorphosis. (**A**) The structure of *Bombyx* big PTTH. The upper diagram indicates the predicted organization of the initial translation product. The lower diagram shows the location of inter- and intracellular disulfide bonds. (**B**) The structure of cholesterol and some major ecdysteroids. (**C**) The structure of the various JHs and methyl farnesoate. JH I and JH II are almost entirely restricted to the Lepidoptera, JHB₃ to the cyclorraphan Diptera, whereas JH III is ubiquitous in insects (Gilbert et al., 1996).

may not pertain to all insects. Specific neurosecretory cells (the prothoracicotropes) synthesize PTTH as a prohormone that is cleaved to the true PTTH as it is transported along the axons to the corpora allata, where it is stored in axon endings and ultimately released into the hemolymph. Once released, PTTH acts on the prothoracic glands to stimulate ecdysteroid synthesis. In the Lepidoptera, this stimulation results in the enhanced biosynthesis of 3-dehydroecdysone (3dE), which is converted to ecdysone (E) by a hemolymph ketoreductase and from that to 20-hydroxyecdysone (20E) in target cells, 20E being the principal molting hormone of insects. Additionally, as Fig. 1 notes, the corpora allata synthesize and secrete JH, which is bound to a hemolymph binding protein (JHBP), transported to target tissues, and acts in concert with 20E to determine the quality of the molt. Although the above typifies the endocrine control of molting in most insects, the exact mechanisms are conjectural, although great strides have been made in recent years and are the subject of the remainder of this contribution.

2. PTTH AND PROTHORACIC GLAND ACTIVATION

2.1. Chemistry and Role

Almost all studies on PTTH action have been performed on larvae and pupae of the tobacco hornworm, *Manduca sexta*, but the only PTTH to be purified thus far is that of the commercial silkworm, *Bombyx mori*. After more than 30 years of study using several million *Bombyx* brains, Ishizaki and colleagues (1992) purified and characterized the *Bombyx* PTTH (Fig. 2), and showed that it is synthesized as a prohormone of 224 amino acids and then cleaved to form the mature neurohormone, a homodimer (~26 kDa) containing inter- and intramonomer disulfide bonds, the latter being requisite for hormone activity. The *Bombyx* PTTH antibody reacts with putative prothoracicotropes in a variety of insects, including *Manduca* and *Drosophila*, as judged by *in situ* immunocytochemical and immunogold analyses, but is physiologically inactive in these species.

Correlations have been reported between PTTH levels in the hemolymph and the molting hormone titer for both *Manduca* and *Bombyx*, and in both cases, reflect subsequent increases in the ecdysteroid titer. In *Manduca*, there are two PTTH peaks during

the fifth (final) larval stage as well as two ecdysteroid surges. The first is responsible for an increase in ecdysteroid titer at about day 3.5 of the 9 d fifth instar (stage) when the JH titer is at its nadir, and is responsible for a change in commitment (reprogramming), so that when challenged by a larger ecdysteroid surge 4 d later, target cells respond by synthesizing pupal rather than larval structures. Thus, these two ecdysteroid (and PTTH) peaks are primarily responsible for metamorphosis, and they must be elicited in a very precise manner. Indeed, the precision of the molting process has contributed significantly to the success enjoyed by insects on this planet during the past 600 million years.

The prothoracicotropes apparently receive, directly or indirectly, information from the insect's external (photoperiod, temperature) and internal environment (state of nutrition), and when the appropriate conditions are met, release PTTH from their termini in the corpus allatum. How and where these influences are sensed and then "transmitted" to the neurons that synthesize PTTH is not known.

2.2. Action Via Second Messenger Systems

The only confirmed targets of PTTH are the paired prothoracic glands, which have been well studied in *Manduca*, each gland composed of about 220 monotypic cells surrounded by a basal lamina. Although no candidate PTTH receptor(s) has yet been isolated from the prothoracic glands of any insect, the PTTH–prothoracic gland axis has many similarities to vertebrate steroid hormone-producing pathways, such as the ACTH-adrenal gland system. By analogy, it is probable that PTTH binds to a receptor that spans the plasma membrane multiple times, contains an extracellular ligand-binding domain, and has an intracellular domain that binds G-protein heterotrimers.

PTTH stimulates increased ecdysteroid production in the prothoracic glands via a cascade of events that has yet to be elucidated completely. Early studies on *Manduca* revealed a correlation between circulating ecdysteroid titers and adenylate cyclase activity in the prothoracic gland, suggesting a role for cAMP and also, that at some developmental periods, a cAMP-independent pathway might be involved. In the *Manduca* prothoracic gland, calcium is clearly pivotal in the response to PTTH. Glands incubated in Ca^{2+}-free medium, or medium with a calcium chelator or a calcium channel blocker exhibit a greatly attenuated production of cAMP and ecdysteroids in response to PTTH. More recent studies have implicated the mobilization of internal as well as external Ca^{2+} stores in the PTTH response.

The composite observations suggest that the PTTH-dependent cAMP production by prothoracic glands is generated by a Ca^{2+}-calmodulin-sensitive adenylate cyclase. The interaction between calmodulin and G-protein (presumably $G_{s\alpha}$) is complicated and varies during the final instar. In the first half of this period, calmodulin activates prothoracic gland adenylate cyclase and facilitates G-protein activation of adenylate cyclase. Subsequently, prothoracic gland G-protein activation of adenylate cyclase is refractory to the presence of calmodulin in such assays. Calcium still apparently plays a role in the PTTH transductory cascade after the first half of the fifth instar, since incubation of pupal glands in Ca^{2+}-free medium inhibits PTTH-stimulated ecdysteroidogenesis, and higher levels of Ca^{2+}-calmodulin can still activate adenylate cyclase in prothoracic gland membrane preparations. Regardless of the complicated, developmentally dynamic relationships among calcium, calmodulin, G-proteins, and adenylate cyclase, it is clear that PTTH elicits increased cAMP formation in prothoracic glands leading to activation of a cAMP-dependent protein kinase (PKA) and subsequent protein phosphorylation.

PTTH-stimulated PKA activity appears to be necessary for PTTH-stimulated ecdysteroidogenesis, since such ecdysteroid synthesis by prothoracic glands challenged with a PKA-inhibiting cAMP analog is substantially inhibited. Several PTTH-dependent protein phosphorylations have been described for *Manduca* prothoracic glands, the most striking and consistent of these phosphoproteins being the ribosomal protein S6, the phosphorylation of which has been correlated with increased translation of specific mRNAs in several mammalian cell types. In *Manduca*, rapamycin inhibits both PTTH-stimulated S6 phosphorylation and ecdysteroidogenesis, suggesting that S6 is an integral player in the PTTH transductory cascade. Consistent with this view is the observation that PTTH-stimulated S6 phosphorylation can be readily detected before the PTTH-stimulated increase in ecdysteroid synthesis occurs.

Over the last several years, a number of studies have revealed that PTTH preparations or cAMP analogs stimulate general protein synthesis in the *Manduca* prothoracic gland via a branch of the trans-ductory cascade that is distinct from that leading to the activation of ecdysteroidogenesis. PTTH may, therefore, modulate or control the growth status of the prothoracic gland, perhaps independently of its ability to elicit ecdysteroidogenesis and could play a role in regulating the levels of ecdysteroidogenic enzymes, analogous to peptide regulation of enzymes responsible for vertebrate steroid hormone synthesis. Additional factors, such as JH, could determine whether PTTH stimulates or inhibits gland growth, ecdysteroid synthesis, or both.

Protein synthesis is required for ACTH stimulation of steroidogenesis in the adrenal cortex as well as for the *Manduca* prothoracic gland response to PTTH. It is therefore likely that both in the adrenal cortex and prothoracic glands, the phosphorylation state of ribosomal S6 is critical to the relationship between protein synthesis and steroidogenesis. Presumably, the PKA-promoted multiple phosphorylation of ribosomal S6 imparts information to the translational machinery to synthesize specific proteins, which, in turn, regulate some rate-limiting step in ecdysteroid biosynthesis.

An interesting outcome of this work is the close analogy observed between control of the insect and mammalian steroidogenic systems. It is obviously a "successful" system in an evolutionary sense, since insects appeared on earth several hundred millions of years before mammals, and the ancestors of both groups diverged at least 100 million years before that. Although it is interesting that such divergent groups of animals use the same types of molecules as hormones (peptides, steroids), it is extraordinary that they regulate the synthesis of their steroid hormones in an almost identical manner.

3. ECDYSTEROIDS

3.1. Structure–Activity Relationships

That ecdysteroids, particularly 20E, elicit the molt is no longer in question and has been established as a central dogma of the field. What may not be so obvious is that, in contrast to vertebrate systems, almost the entire insect is the target of ecdysteroids, e.g., regulation of the growth of motor neurons, control of choriogenesis, stimulation of the growth and development of imaginal disks, initiation of the breakdown of larval structures during metamorphosis, induction of the deposition of cuticle by the epidermis, and so on.

It is fitting that recent breakthroughs on the mechanism of action of ecdysteroids (*see* Section 3.3.) were accomplished using *Drosophila melanogaster*, since it was a bioassay developed with another fly that was so well utilized for the initial crystallization of E and then 20E four decades ago. Since that time, a host of ecdysteroids (Fig. 2B), their precursors, and their metabolites have been identified. We know that the *cis*-A-B ring junction is essential for molting hormone activity regardless of whether a hydrogen atom or a hydroxyl group is the 5β substituent, as is the 6-oxo-7-ene system in the B ring. The 3β- and 14 α-hydroxyl groups are required for high activity in vivo, whereas the presence or absence of hydroxyls at C-2, C-5, or C-11 does not appear to affect biological activity. The only essential feature of the side chain appears to be the $22\beta_F$-hydroxyl.

Although E was the first of the ecdysteroids to be crystallized and characterized and thought to be the insect molting hormone 40 years ago, it is actually converted to the principal molting hormone, 20E, by tissues peripheral to the prothoracic glands (Fig. 1), a reaction mediated by an ecdysone 20-monooxygenase. In some insects, particularly the Lepidoptera as exemplified by *Manduca*, the major if not sole ecdysteroid synthesized and secreted by the prothoracic glands is 3dE, which is converted to E by a ketoreductase in the hemolymph, the resulting ecdysone then being hydroxylated to 20E in target tissues.

3.2. Biosynthesis

In most organisms, every carbon atom in cholesterol (Fig. 2A) is derived from either the methyl- or carboxylol-carbon of acetate, but insects (and other arthropods) are incapable of this synthesis owing to one or more metabolic blocks between acetate and cholesterol. Thus, sterols are required in the diet.

The first step in the conversion of cholesterol to E via 3dE is the stereospecific removal of the 7β-hydrogen to form 7-dehydrocholesterol (7dC), a sterol relegated to the prothoracic glands of *Manduca* and other Lepidoptera. This cholesterol 7,8-desaturating activity in the prothoracic glands of *Manduca* is cytochrome P-450-dependent, perhaps via 7β-hydrocholesterol. When [³H]7dC is incubated with prothoracic glands in vitro, there is excellent conversion to both 3dE and E, the kinetics of conversion being highly dependent on developmental stage and experimental paradigm. The desaturation to 7dC

is probably not PTTH-dependent, but the neuropeptide (via S6) may initiate the modulation of enzyme activity responsible for the transformation of 7dC to the next, yet unidentified sterol in the E biosynthetic pathway.

There are a number of postulated intermediates between 7dC and 3dE, e.g. 5α-sterol intermediates, 3-oxo-Δ^4 intermediates, Δ^7-5α-6α-epoxide intermediates, and so on, but their intermediacy remains conjectural. In contrast, more is known about the terminal hydroxylations necessary for the synthesis of the polyhydroxylated ecdysteroids. The enzymes responsible for mediating the hydroxylations at C-2, C-22, and C-25 appear to be classic cytochrome P-450 enzymes, the former two being mitochondrial and the latter microsomal. The sequence of hydroxylation is C-25, C-22, and C-2.

Once formed, 3dE is converted to E through the mediation of a hemolymph ketoreductase, and the E is then transformed to 20E at peripheral (target) tissues. The complete biosynthetic scheme has not been elucidated owing to the difficulty of identifying the extremely short-lived intermediates from minute quantities of tissues and the less than handful of laboratories actively engaged in such investigations. Without the entire sequence of reactions in hand, it is not possible to identify those rate limiting reactions that may be controlled by hormones (PTTH), neuromodulators, or the nervous system.

3.3. Ecdysteroid Receptors

Several cell types in the higher flies and other insects contain polytene chromosomes, the structure and ease of examination of which led to the field of *Drosophila* cytogenetics. At specific developmental stages, discrete regions of these chromosomes undergo puffing, a phenomenon now known to be the morphological manifestation of gene activity, i.e., mRNA synthesis. Thirty-five years ago Clever and Karlson (1960) showed that 20E could elicit a stage-specific puffing pattern in the salivary gland chromosomes of the midge *Chironomus tentans*, the first unequivocal demonstration that steroid hormones act at the level of the gene. This discovery was followed by an exhaustive analysis of salivary gland polytene chromosome puffing during the developmental of *Drosophila* by Ashburner and his colleagues, which involved the testing of E and 20E on the puffing pattern. This led to the "Ashburner Model" of ecdysteroid hormone action, i.e., an intracellular receptor–20E complex elicits elevated transcription of "early puff" genes and, at the same time, represses the transcription of the "late puff" genes. Subsequently, the gene products of the "early puff" genes act on the "late puff" genes to stimulate transcriptional activity while feeding back on the "early puff" genes, resulting in puff regression. This model has withstood the test of time, and several of the "early puff" gene products have been shown to be transcription factors and members of the steroid/thyroid hormone receptor superfamily (nuclear receptor superfamily: *see* Chapters 2 and 4) Indeed, one gene product, E75, was the probe utilized that led to the recent isolation of the *Drosophila* ecdysone receptor gene (*EcR*) by the Hogness Laboratory.

The gene product of *EcR* binds to the proper response elements and to radiolabeled ecdysteroid, but requires a heterodimeric partner to fulfill its function. This critical element is also a member of the nuclear receptor superfamily, ultraspiracle (*Usp*), which is the *Drosophila* homolog of RXR, a receptor for retinoids in mammals that forms heterodimers with a variety of hormones. The *Drosophila* heteromer is stabilized by endogenous 20E, and there are indications that the application of exogenous hormone will increase the amount or affinity of EcR in target cells, although it is not known if this effect is at the level of transcription or translation.

It is of interest that EcR exists in at least three isoforms, which differ from one another in the transactivation domain, and there is some tissue and developmental specificity, although the exact reason for the existence of isoforms remains conjectural. Their presence certainly suggests that there are as yet unidentified *trans*-acting factors with roles in ecdysteroid action. Indirect evidence also suggests that EcR is not monogamous, i.e., can form heterodimeric relationships with gene products other than Usp. Finally, there is a plethora of data indicating that 20E is not the only ecdysteroid with molting hormone activity, and that certain prohormones and "metabolites" of 20E may be hormones in their own right and perhaps interact with specific isoforms of EcR in the EcR–USP complex. As in the field of steroid hormone receptors in general, little is known between the "docking" of the ecdysteroid–receptor complex with the hormone response element and enhanced gene activity in the form of specific mRNA synthesis (puffing).

4. JHs

4.1. Chemistry

The development of structures that distinguish adult forms from larval forms is regulated by a complex interaction between JH and the ecdysteroids. The JHs are a unique group of sesquiterpenoid compounds that have been identified definitively only in insects (Fig. 2) and one plant species, although their structural proximity to retinoids is obvious. To date, six JHs have been identified from various insect orders (Fig. 2). JH III appears to occur in all orders and is the principal product of the corpus allatum in most, with the notable exceptions of the Lepidoptera and the Diptera. In *Drosophila*, the bisepoxide of JH III, JHB_3, is predominant and the sole JH in some species of flies.

The absolute configurations of the epoxide group of only some of the JHs have been resolved (Fig. 2). There are chiral centers at the 10 position of JH III and at the 10 and 11 positions of the other JHs. In addition, JHB_3 from Diptera possesses two chiral centers, at positions 6, 7, and 10. At present, the absolute configurations are known only for JH I, 4-Me-JH I, JHB_3, and JH III. This is important because the unnatural enantiomers appear to be less biologically active or are degraded at different rates by esterolytic enzymes than are the natural enantiomers.

JH acids are also produced by the corpora allata of *Manduca* larvae. The glands lose their ability to methylate JH I and II acid during the final larval stage as a result of the disappearance or inactivation of the methyl transferase enzyme, and thus produce large quantities of these JH acids, which are released into the hemolymph (*see* Section 4.3., on methoprene acid).

4.2. Biosynthesis and Degradation

The JHs are synthesized in the corpora allata from acetate (JH III) and/or propionate (higher JH homologs). The biosynthetic pathway for JH III is identical to that for vertebrate sterol biosynthesis until the production of farnesyl pyrophosphate. As noted previously, insects do not produce cholesterol and related steroids *de novo*; rather, JH is the product of this pathway. It is noteworthy that there is significant sequence similarity between the HMGCoA reductase, the enzyme responsible for the conversion of HMGCoA to mevalonate, of the insect corpus allatum and that of vertebrate liver, a principal site of *de novo* sterol biosynthesis, suggesting that this pathway to farnesyl pyrophosphate is of ancient origin.

The formation of the side chains in the "modified" homologs involves differential utilization of substrates, including propionate and acetate, to give rise to both C5 and C6 pyrophosphate intermediates. Condensation of two C6 units plus one C5 unit results in the formation of JH I, whereas one C6 unit plus two C5 units produce JH II.

The hemolymph JH titer must reflect both the rate of production and the rate of degradation. This estimate is clouded by the presence of JH-specific-binding proteins in the hemolymph, whose function has been hypothesized to be the protection of JH from degradation by both general and specific hemolymph esterases (Fig. 1). JH-specific epoxide hydrolases, capable of hydrating the epoxide function to the diol, also play a role in the catabolism of JH.

4.3. Postulated Action

The JH titer is believed to be the primary endocrine factor influencing the "quality" of developmental events during metamorphosis, (e.g., in Lepidoptera, the nature of the molt—larval–larval, larval–pupal, or pupal–adult) (Fig. 1). It is generally assumed that the absence (or near absence) of JH is required for metamorphosis in holometabolous insects (*see* Fig. 1). Therefore, JH defines the outcome of molts, both metamorphic and nonmetamorphic, and can therefore be regarded as the metamorphic hormone of insects.

Although there are no unequivocal data showing the existence of a JH receptor, there are a multitude of observations that JH can modulate larval and pupal gene activity elicited by the molting hormone, i.e., does not act in the absence of ecdysteroids. There is increasing evidence that JH also acts at the level of the cell membrane via a classical second messenger system (*see* Chapter 3), as it modulates the uptake of vitellogenin from the hemolymph into the developing oocyte. Therefore, JH may have multivalent roles and modes of action, as does, for example, progesterone. In pre-adult stages, JH has an obvious role in preventing precocious development and eliciting larval or pupal synthesis. The prevailing opinion is that JH acts as a "competency determinant", i.e., it affects the target cell's competence to respond to 20E. The mechanism by which JH accomplishes this task is unknown, but it is surely one of the most intriguing problems in endocrinology and developmental biology. Further, very recent work has established that a well-known JH analog, methoprene, as well as its acid metabolite, can activate RXR in vertebrate cells,

but that only the metabolite can bind RXR, indicating that methoprene must be metabolized before it is active in this system. This suggests that perhaps in the case of JH, it is a metabolite (JH acid?) that binds to the receptor, whereas past failures in the search for a receptor utilized the native JH.

5. CONCLUSION

In this abbreviated review, only the essence of the field could be discussed, and there was no opportunity to detail the >50 peptide hormones or hormone-like peptides that have been described in recent years, several of which appear to be identical to vertebrate hormones (e.g., insulin) and others which deal with a variety of homeostatic mechanisms (e.g., hypo-and hyperglycemic, hypolipemic, adipokinetic, and so forth). For the most part, every vertebrate peptide hormone has an immunocytochemically similar (or identical) counterpart in insects, as have estrogens, progesterone, and so on. Therefore, these hormones that play such strategic roles in the life of higher organisms were "discovered" by insects or ancestors of the insects. Thus, the hormones, second messenger systems, receptor mechanisms, neuroendocrine axis, biosynthetic mechanisms, and so forth. are all of very ancient lineage, and their basic essence has been well preserved. With the current use of a genetic organism (*Drosophila*) to study endocrine paradigms, we can look forward to future findings that should allow insights into the myriad of endocrine mechanisms that have survived severe evolutionary pressures.

REFERENCES

Clever U, Karlson P. Induktion von Puff Veranderungen in deu Speicheldrüsenchromosomen von *Chironomus tuitans* deusch ecdgson. *Exp Cell Res;* 20:623.

Gilbert LI, Rybczynski R, Tobe S. Endocrine cascade in insect metamorphosis. In: Gilbert LI, Tata JR, Atkinson BG, eds. *Metamorphosis: Post-Embryonic Reprogramming of Gene Expression in Amphibian and Insect Cells.* San Diego: Academic, 1996:59.

Ishizaki H, Suzuki A. Brain secretory peptides of the silkmoth *Bombyx mori*: prothoracicotropic hormone and bombyxin. In: Joose J, Buijs RM, Tilders FJH, eds. *Progress in Brain Research*, vol 92, Amsterdam: Elsevier, 1992:1.

Kopeć S. Studies on the necessity of the brain for the inception of insect metamorphosis. *Biol Bull* 1922; 42:323.

SELECTED READINGS

Gilbert LI, Combest WL, Smith WA, Meller VH, Rountree DB. Neuropeptides, second messengers and insect molting. *BioEssays* 1988; 8:153.

Grieneisen ML. Recent advances in our knowledge of ecdysteroid biosynthesis in insects and crustaceans. *Insect Biochem Molec Biol* 1994; 24:115.

Harmon MA, Boehm MF, Heyman RA, Mangelsdorf DJ. Activation of mammalian retinoid x receptors by the insect growth regulator methoprene. *Proc Natl Acad Sci USA* 1995; 92:615.

Henrich VC, Brown NE. Insect nuclear receptors: a developmental and comparative perspective. *Insect Biochem Molec Biol* 1995; 25:881.

Koelle MR, Talbot WS, Segraves WA, Bender MT, Cherbas P, Hogness DS. The *Drosophila* EcR gene encodes an ecdysone receptor, a new member of the steroid receptor superfamily. *Cell* 1991; 67:59.

Riddiford LM. Cellular and molecular actions of juvenile hormone. I. General considerations and premetamorphic actions. *Adv Insect Physiol* 1994; 24:213.

Song Q, Gilbert LI. Multiple phosphorylation of ribosomal protein S6 and specific protein synthesis are required for prothoracicotropic hormone-stimulated ecdysteroid biosynthesis in the prothoracic glands of *Manduca sexta. Insect Biochem Molec Biol* 1995; 25:591.

11 Phytohormones and Signal Transduction in Plants

Klaus Palme, PhD Christopher Redhead, PhD and Peter Kristoffersen, PhD

1. INTRODUCTION

We all depend on plant life. Plants produce the oxygen we breathe, the food we eat, and many of the raw materials on which we depend. Plants have developed extraordinary synthetic capacities. They synthesize numerous organic compounds from simple compounds like water, minerals, and carbon dioxide, many of them of medicinal or industrial relevance. Plants use the same principles for their genetics and for the control of their metabolism and molecular physiology as other eukaryotes. They have, however, developed their own growth strategies to accomodate the demands of their sessile and autotrophic life-style. In contrast to animals, which often respond to environmental stimuli by behavioral responses, plants respond by adapting both their development and their metabolism. As a consequence, organogenesis from either active or reactivated meristems is possible throughout the life-span of the plant. The position of a plant cell rather than its lineage is more important during the determination of cell fate. Totipotency, rarely seen in differentiated animal cells, plays a vital role in the growth strategy of plants and provides the capacity for vegetative reproduction. That is, new meristems can be formed within pre-existing organs, allowing the development of new or the replacement of old organs. Frequently, entire plants can be regenerated from single cells of a root, a stem, or a leaf. This enormous plasticity and power of regeneration are tightly regulated by plant signaling molecules, such as the classical phytohormones, and by communication between cells. These signals provide the plant with not only positional information, but also information with regard to its environment.

2. THE NATURE OF PHYTOHORMONES

The idea that plant development is influenced by chemical messengers is not a new one. A hundred

From: *Endocrinology: Basic and Clinical Principles* (P. M. Conn and S. Melmed, eds.), Humana Press Inc., Totowa, NJ.

153

years ago, the German botanist Julius von Sachs suggested the existence of organ-forming substances in plants. His British colleagues, Charles and Francis Darwin concluded from studies of the growing tip of a grass coleoptile that some "influence," probably a chemical substance moving through the coleoptile, existed to regulate the elongation rates on opposite sides of the organ. Because of the low concentration of this substance, its chemical identity was not elucidated until the mid-1930s and even then by purification from human urine. Now we know the substance as auxin (indole-3-acetic acid, Table 1), which was finally identified in plants in 1943. Although the biosynthetic pathways of auxins are not yet completely understood, it has been demonstrated that auxins are produced in meristematic tissues and leaf tips (Normanly et al., 1995). Another group of phytohormones, the cytokinins, was discovered in the 1950s as stimulants of cellular division (for recent overviews, see Kaminek, 1992; Binns, 1994; Brzobohaty et al., 1994). The various cytokinins are now known to differ somewhat in their chemical structure but the majority are adenine-like compounds. They have been found to participate in cell enlargement, the differentiation of tissues, the development of chloroplasts, the stimulation of cotyledon growth, the delay of senescence in leaves, and in many other regulatory events associated with gibberellins and auxins. Auxins and cytokinins interact, often with one compound opposing the activity of the other. The ratio of both compounds seems to be important in determining the responses. In the presence of high concentrations of both auxin and cytokinin, cells grow vigorously to form an undifferentiated callus of parenchyma-like cells. Reducing the concentration of cytokinin under these circumstances causes an immediate formation of roots, whereas lowering the concentration of auxin results in the formation of buds and consequently shoots. Although the molecular basis of these morphogenetic effects is not understood, this phenomenon has nevertheless provided invaluable information for the control of plant transformation, regeneration, and micropropagation.

Gibberellins (Table 1), another group of phytohormones with structural similarity to steroid hormones, were identified from the observation that when rice plants were infected with a fungus (*Gibberella fujikuroi*), they grew twice as long as normal plants. Today more than 80 chemically different gibberellins have been isolated and characterized, many of them differring only in side chains, or the addition of methyl and hydroxyl groups to the molecule's central ring. Gibberellins are involved in many regulatory processes, especially in stimulating cell elongation, a process also known to be affected by auxins. In rossette plants, for example, bolting, the division, and rapid elongation of particular stem cells, and flowering are promoted by high concentrations. Gibberellins induce germination, probably through the induction of several enzymes, such as amylase, and also induce maleness in dioecious flowers.

Abscisic acid was discovered using a bioassay that measured the effects of plant extracts on the abscission of petioles. The compound identified with this simple assay turned out to be a sequiterpenoid that was synthesized from mevalonic acid and composed of three isoprene residues. This structure is similar to the terminal rings of carotenoids (Table 1). This hormone almost always inhibits plant growth. It provides plants with a chemical means of delaying germination until the spring time. Its levels rise in plants when days are getting progressively shorter and, after transport in developing seeds, block in the seeds the metabolic machinery for the initiation of growth. Abscisic acid promotes dormancy, inhibits stem growth, and when water is short, its level quickly rises, thus causing closing of stomata and thus preventing the wilting of the plant.

The fact that volatile compounds have a profound effect on plant development was already noted in 1864, when leaf abscission was reported in response (Table 1) to leaking gas from gas lamps. Ethylene, which is produced from the incomplete combustion of gas, is also naturally produced by various plant tissues (e.g., roots, leaves, seeds, flowers, fruits) and causes fruit ripening, an effect that has been applied industrially to trigger the ripening of fruits that were harvested green to prevent rotting. Now we know that ethylene also plays a fundamental role in germination, sex determination, leaf abscission, flower senescence, adventitious root formation, mechanical stress, and various pathogenic responses. Physiological consequences of ethylene perception by plant tissues include the reorientation of cellulose microfibrils in the secondary cell walls from a transverse to a longitudinal orientation, an effect that probably allows the radial extension of stem tissue. In addition, ethylene affects polar auxin transport,

Table 1
Phytohormones, Chemical Structure, and Properties

Growth factor	Structure	Active concentration	Synthesis	Transport	Biological response
Auxin (IAA)		10^{-11} M – 10^{-5} M	meristems, leaf primordia, developing seeds	phloem, cell to cell	cell division, elongation and differentiation rooting, repression of lateral bud growth, leaf senescence, fruit development, gravitropism, photropism,
Ethylene	$CH_2 = CH_2$	0.1–10 ppm	most tissues	diffusion	fruit ripening, flower and leaf senescence, leaf and fruit abscission, dormancy, "stress" gene activation
Cytokinin (trans-zeatin)		10^{-8} M – 10^{-5} M	root tips, developing seeds	xylem	cell division and differentiation, shooting growth of lateral buds, delay of leaf senescence, fruit development, chloroplast development, morphogenesis.
Abscisic acid		10^{-9} M – 10^{-7} M	mature leaves, roots	phloem, xylem	senescene, water stress, inhibition of shoot growth, defence gene activation upon wounding, induction of storage protein synthesis in seeds
Gibberellin (GA$_1$)		10^{-6} M – 10^{-5} M	young shoot tissue, developing seeds	phloem, xylem	shoot elongation, flower initiation, seed germination
Jasmonic acid		10^{-7} M – 10^{-6} M	leaves	phloem	fruit ripening, senescence, abscission, growth inhibition, wounding, osmotic stress, pathogen defence gene activation
Lipo-chitooligo saccharaide (NodRm-IV (S) from *R. meliloti*)		10^{-15} M – 10^{-13} M	rhizobia	?	cell division and differentiation, morphogenesis

thereby downregulating the cellular auxin concentration and, as a physiological consequence, cell elongation.

Other plant growth regulators (e.g., brassinosteroids, jasmonates, salicylic acid) have attracted much attention over the past few years, but since the scope and size of this chapter is limited, the interested reader should refer to the excellent reviews that summarize the findings on these hormones (Mandava, 1988; Parthier, 1990,1991; Sembdner and Parthier, 1993; Hanke, 1992; Adam, 1994; Vernooji et al., 1994). However, we would like to mention another group of signaling molecules, the lipo-chitooligosaccharides. These molecules are likely to create a good deal of excitement over the next few years. These molecules, used by rhizobial bacteria to trigger nodule growth on infected roots, are composed of a chitinoligosaccharide backbone of three to five sugar units and an unsaturated fatty acid, the structure of which is variable (Table 1). They play an essential role in the formation of root nodule primordia and activate cell-cycle gene expression at pico- or femtomolar concentrations. Several lines of evidence indicate that related molecules will be also produced by animals (Ryan, 1994).

3. SIGNAL TRANSDUCTION PATHWAYS

Signal transduction pathways in plants share many of the essential features of animal signaling pathways. Many of the signaling molecules that were originally identified in animals, such as kinases, G-proteins, and phosphatases, also exist in plants. A comparative study of plant signaling pathways with other pathways reveals how evolution has brought about the fusion of different pathways and genes, which are present in prokaryotes, yeast, and higher animals to meet the special requirements of the plant. The reader interested in more detailed information on plant hormone signaling and signal transduction pathways should refer to a recent volume of *Plant Molecular Biology* (Palme, 1994) and an article by Redhead and Palme (1996). Here we will present only a short and concise overview of general aspects of plant signal transduction pathways.

3.1. Receptor-Like and Other Protein Kinases

In animal cells, a number of peptide growth hormones operate through receptor kinases. These proteins consist of an extracellular receptor domain linked to an intracellular kinase domain via a single transmembrane-spanning segment. Proteins sharing the same topology have also been identified in plants. However, unlike their animal counterparts, in which the target of the kinase is most often a tyrosine residue, the plant receptor kinase is normally a serine/threonine kinase. This is in line with the observation that tyrosine phosphorylation is rare or absent in plants. Since most of the plant receptor kinases have been identified by genetics or molecular biological means, the ligands that bind to them still remain largely a mystery. The first receptor kinases to be identified were from flowers and have been implicated by genetic screens in the mechanism of self-incompatability. This process is the one by which plants prevent self-pollination and thus promote crossfertilization. It is therefore possible that these receptor molecules are involved in the recognition of self-antigens associated with the pollen granules.

Since then, however, other receptor kinase genes have been cloned largely by homology. These are broadly distributed throughout the plant and show a striking variation in their extracellular receptor domains. This indicates that not only do these receptors play a variety of roles throughout the plant, but also that the variety of the ligands that they bind may be extensive. This has led to the suggestion that the classical phytohormones may not be the only extracellular signaling molecules in plants. This idea is supported by the finding that a number of other molecules from plant pathogens, including peptides and lipo-chitooligosaccharides, are able to induce specific responses in plant cells, suggesting perhaps that similar molecules also exist in plants themselves. In general, the signal transduction pathways to which these receptor kinases are connected are unknown.

Recently, however, a phosphatase has been identified that appears to interact directly with one of these receptor molecules, indicating that, like their animal counterparts, these receptor kinases feed into a cascade of interacting kinases and phosphatases. A number of other kinases that are related to animal protein kinases have also been identified in plants. As might be expected, the cell division kinases are highly conserved, as are protein kinases, such as the GSK-3 kinases, and S6 kinases, that are involved in in the global regulation of gene transcription and metabolism. Since many of these genes can complement the relevant yeast mutants, it would appear that these genes perform similar functions. Other protein kinases that do not appear to be present in higher animals, but are present in both yeast and bacteria are also present in plants. One example is the gene *ETR1*. This gene is involved in the perception of the plant hormone ethylene. Sequence analysis suggests that it is related to the two-component systems of bacteria and yeast, and is linked to the initiation of a MAP kinase cascade (refer to Section 5).

A variety of other serine-threonine protein kinases have also been identified in plants, including some that are related to cyclic nucleotide-regulated kinases. A variety of protein phosphatases have been identified. A number of these appear to be involved in cell-cycle regulation, but most are without a known function.

3.2. G-proteins and G-protein-Coupled Receptors

Despite extensive efforts, no G-protein-coupled receptors have been identified in plants. There is, however, a large volume of evidence implicating G-proteins in plant signaling pathways. A large number of GTP-binding proteins have now been cloned in plants, including both large heterotrimeric and small monomeric proteins. Large heterotrimeric proteins have been implicated in a variety of plant signal pathways. One of the clearest examples has come from some elegant microinjection studies (Neuhaus et al., 1993; Bowler et al., 1994). In these experiments, calcium, cyclic nucleotides, and other signaling molecules were microinjected into mutant plant cells with deficiencies in light perception pathways. The influence of these molecules on the light perception pathway was then assayed by measuring the activity of light-regulated gene promoters linked to reporter genes. These experiments showed that the perception of light through the plant red light receptors was followed by a signaling cascade involving G-proteins, calcium, and cGMP. This cascade had echos of the signaling cascade following light transduction by rhodopsin in the eye. However, the two light receptors and phytochromes show no similarity, and phytochromes do not appear to be related to seven-transmembrane domain G-protein-coupled receptors.

Despite the strong evidence for the existence of large heterotrimeric G-proteins from sophisticated biochemical and genetic studies, such as those described above, and from the identification of proteins that both bind GTP and are ADP-ribosylated, only relatively few large heterotrimeric G-protein subunit genes have so far been cloned. These include α and β-subunits, but so far no γ subunits. These genes have been identified from different plants and appear to be homologs. Thus, in fact, only one type of each subunit has so far been identified. Efforts mostly involving homology screening for other members of heterotrimeric G-protein family in plants have been unsuccessful, suggesting that they may be significantly divergent from their animal counterparts.

A large number of plant monomeric G-protein genes have been identified. The majority of these belong to the Rab family of proteins, which are involved in the regulation of vesicular transport. This suggests that, as with yeast, the regulation of membrane transport is highly conserved. Members of other small G-protein families have been identified, including ran, involved in cell-cycle regulation, and rho, involved with the cytoskeleton. One family of monomeric G-proteins that have not so far been identified are those related to ras. The ras G-proteins are involved with the transduction of signals from receptors to intracellular signaling pathways often involving MAP kinases. However, both MAP kinases and raf kinase, a protein that in animals is directly activated by ras, have been identified in plants. This suggests that either ras-like proteins are indeed present in plants, but are sufficiently divergent not to be picked up by standard screens, or that the role of ras in plants is played by another unrelated protein. The answer to these questions will undoubtly be provided by a combination of the implementation of more sophisticated genetic screens involving extensive tagged mutant libraries and the large-scale genomic sequencing efforts that are presently under way in *Arabidopsis thaliana* (mouse ear cress/wall cress) and *Oryza sativa* (rice).

3.3. Calcium and Phosphoinositide Signaling Cascades

There is extensive evidence that, as in animals, calcium is a key second messenger in signal transduction pathways, including responses to temperature movement, or light. A large number of calmodulin genes have been identified and implicated in the transduction of these calcium-mediated pathways. In addition, a number of calcium-dependent protein kinases have been identified. These show a striking resemblence to the calcium-calmodulin-dependent protein kinases of animals. However, in the case of plants, calmodulin and the calmodulin-regulated kinase have evolved into one protein. As with so many of the other plant kinases, the majority of these calcium-regulated kinases genes have been identified by homology and their function is unknown. However, a number have been implicated in salt stress, whereas another appears to be crucial for the growth of the pollen tube.

In addition, two calcium-dependent protein phosphatase genes have been cloned. One of these genes was identified by genetic screening of hormone signal transduction pathways and is necessary for the plant cell response to the phytohormone abscisic acid. This phosphatase gene is of particular interest, since it combines a domain with similarity to the type 2c protein phosphatases with a calcineurin-like calcium-binding site. Thus, it not only represents a totally new type of protein phosphatase, but its existence emphasizes how through evolution, elements that are separate entitities in some organisms exist as one in others. The other calcium-dependent protein phosphatase is also of interest, since it was identified by its ability to bind to a receptor kinase and thus also appears to be involved in the transduction of extracellular signals.

Although the importance of calcium in plant signaling is undisputed, the possible contribution of inositol 1,4,5-triphosphate (IP$_3$) to this calcium signaling has been controversial. A number of studies have suggested that various challenges can give rise to changes in IP$_3$ turnover. More directly, patch-clamp measurements of vacuolar membranes and experiments using caged IP$_3$ have suggested that intracellular IP$_3$-regulated calcium channels may be present, but no IP$_3$ receptors have so far been identified. Recently, however, two inositol lipid-specific phospholipase genes have been cloned, perhaps reinforcing the possiblity for an IP$_3$-mediated second messenger pathway.

3.4. Receptor Proteins

One area where there are significant differences between plants and other organisms is in their receptor proteins. Plants respond both to blue and to red light. Receptors for both responses have been cloned and sequenced. The blue light receptor, CRY1, is structurally related to bacterial photolyases (Ahmad and Cashmore, 1993). These flavoproteins catalyze blue-light-dependent reactions. CRY1 itself does not appear to have photolyase activity, but its similarity to these enzymes might suggest that through similar conformational changes, the protein is able to transduce the light signal to a biochemical pathway. In the case of red light, a small family of proteins, the phytochromes, have been identified. These proteins are cytosolic and contain a tetrapyrrole chromophore. Although some authors have claimed sequence similarities to both serine/threonine and bacterial histidine kinases, they have not yet been shown to possess any protein kinase activity, and the means by which they activate the G-protein-linked, calcium/cGMP pathway to which they are linked remains unknown.

The only other possible receptor proteins that have been identified are those for the phytohormone auxin. These receptors appear to be unlike any other receptors previously identified and are described in detail below.

4. AUXIN

Identification of hormone receptors is one of the "holy grails" of contemporary phytohormone research. Although biochemical and molecular genetic approaches are providing information on components of signal transduction pathways (Redhead and Palme, 1996), identification of the initial receptors in phytohormone–plant cell interactions is just beginning. Because auxins, gibberellins, and abscisic acid are weak acids and diffuse through cell membranes under pH conditions that favor the uncharged form, one of the key questions has been whether to look for receptor proteins extracellularly on the surface of the plasma membrane or for intracellular receptors. Another largely unresolved question is the identity of the intracellular messengers that mediate the responses to phytohormones.

Auxins are widely found throughout the plant kingdom. They have diverse physiological effects on growth and development, and consequently, affect most aspects of plant life (Davies, 1995; Table 1). Cell division, cell elongation, root development, apical dominance, vascular differentiation, and photo- and gravitropisms are all among the responses believed to be controlled by auxins. The mechanism of action is not clear for any of these processes. However, rapid changes in gene expression and a rapid stimulation of proton pumping across the plasma membrane have been shown to be associated with the action of auxin. Thus, both the regulation of proteins at the plasma membrane and the regulation of gene expression are essential for the diverse

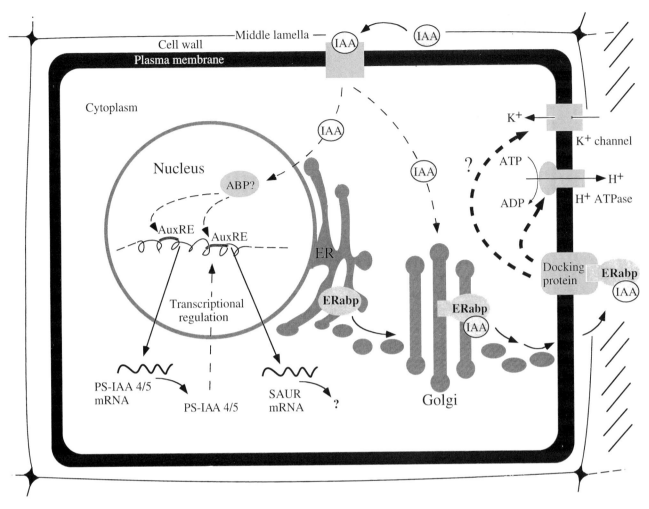

Fig. 1. Scheme illustrating the current view on auxin signaling.

effects described for auxins. These major cellular responses will therefore be described in detail, and the contemporary knowledge on auxin perception and signal transduction discussed. A current scheme on auxin signaling is depicted in Fig. 1.

All compounds with auxin activity stimulate longitudinal elongation of grass coleoptiles, which are the cylindrical sheathing tissue, which surround and protect the primary leaves. Cell division ceases very early in development, and thus cell expansion is the major driving force for the movement of the coleoptile to the surface of the soil. Numerous experiments have established that auxin is the major stimulus for cell elongation in coleoptiles. It has been shown that auxin causes a major change in the cell walls of the coleoptile cells. This wall loosening results in an increase in wall extensibility and allows irreversible expansion of the coleoptile cells. It is probable, but

in most cases still needs experimental confirmation, that active metabolic processes (i.e., synthesis of membrane lipids, membrane proteins, and wall components, such as polysaccharides and cellulosic compounds) and transport of the newly synthesized metabolites to the membranes underly the enormous volume increase during coleoptile cell expansion. It is likely that the control of the secretory pathway plays an important role in the control of cell expansion, and indeed components of the secretory pathway, like small G-proteins, are highly expressed in elongating coleoptiles.

In order to explain the role of auxin in coleoptile expansion, several models have been proposed. The favored hypothesis at the moment suggests that auxin receptors play a crucial role. Several auxin-binding proteins have been identified in maize coleoptiles. One of these proteins binds auxin and has a K_d in the range of 10^{-8} M, which is in the same range as that found for the stimulaion of cell expansion by auxin. This 22-kDa protein is abundantly expressed in maize coleoptiles and was thought to be an auxin receptor. The protein was named ZmERabp1 for Zea mays endoplasmic reticulum-located auxin-binding protein or frequently simply ABP1. Although earlier results suggested a membrane location for this protein, ABP1 was found to contain a C-terminal ER-retention sequence (KDEL) and an N-terminal ER signal peptide, but no membrane-spanning domains. This suggested that ABP1 was a soluble ER protein. This ER location contrasted with the physiological evidence, suggesting a role for ABP1 in mediating auxin induced plasma membrane polarization. Antibodies raised against this protein prevented alterations of auxin-induced transmembrane potential differences of protoplasts when incubated with auxins, suggesting that this protein is involved in the primary perception of auxin. Conversely, incubation of protoplasts with purified ABP1 led to an enhancement of their sensitivity to auxin. These results were further confirmed by the demonstration that antibodies raised against recombinant ABP1 prevented the auxin-induced H^+-ATPase current. The proposition that ABP1 acts at the plasma membrane was further supported by the direct demonstration of ABP1 at the surface of maize coleoptile protoplasts using immunogold-epipolarization microscopy, and the direct demonstration that a peptide comprising the last 14 C-terminal amino acid residues of ABP1 rapidly and reversibly modulated the activity of potassium channels in guard cells. Ion transport processes represent the basis for opening and closing of the stomates, formed by pairs of guard cells surrounding the stomatal pores. Through variation of turgor pressure, guard cells change the aperture of the stomatal pore and thereby act like valves to regulate photosynthetic gas exchange and also to guard plants against excessive water loss. It is well established that auxins stimulate potassium uptake and turgor increase in guard cells in concentration ranges that stimulate elongation growth, which is also a turgor-driven process. Thus, it was of considerable interest to find a reversible modulation of potassium transport in guard cells mediated by a C-terminal ABP1 peptide, again indicating that ABP1 functions at the surface of plant cells to activate both H^+-ATPase and potassium channels through an as yet unknown signal cascade.

Why is ABP1 located inside and outside of plant cells? This intriguing question may have its explanation in the well-known auto- and paracrine hormonal regulation, which takes place between some neighboring animal cells. In plants, a well-functioning circulation system like the blood system is missing. Therefore, novel mechanisms must have been established by plants to allow cell-specific signaling by hormones like auxins. The availability of large physiologically inactive hormone pools may be essential for cell autonomous hormone regulation. Active auxin is found only in relatively small quantities, whereas each cell contains large amounts of auxin conjugates in which auxin is covalently linked to small chemicals (mostly amino acids or sugars). Amidohydrolases or esterases can hydrolyze these inactive conjugates and release physiologically active auxin. Receptor proteins like ABP1 apparently sense auxins both internally and externally, and stimulate different processes, inside and outside of plant cells.

The finding that the auxin stimulation of cell elongation requires the synthesis of proteins, lipids, polysaccharides, and other compounds suggests that part of auxin's action should be to modulate gene expression. This was indeed demonstrated already in very early work where in the presence of auxin, specifically transcribed genes and translated proteins were found in growing plant tissues. Now it is well established that in some plant organs, tissues, or cultured cells, auxin induces the expression, but in others, the repression of specific genes. In most cases, however, the functions of the encoded polypeptides are not known (overview in Takahashi et al., 1995). Of particular interest were genes that in rapidly elongating tissues were rapidly (within 2–3 min) induced after auxin application. These genes, termed *SAUR* for small auxin upregulated RNAs, are apparently involved in some early steps of the auxin response. At present, however, no biochemical function is known for the proteins encoded by the *SAUR* genes. *SAUR* transcripts were found in tissues that are targets for auxin-induced cell elongation and in the elongating cells of tissues responding to gravitropism, a process also thought to involve auxin. These observations indicate that *SAUR*'s are involved in some of the early steps of the auxin response, a view that is further supported by the analysis of the expression of *SAUR* genes in *Arabidopsis* mutants. It was shown, for example, that *Arabidopsis SAUR* gene expression was strongly reduced in an auxin-resistant mutant and in a gravity-response mutant. These observations indicate that these mutant loci encode proteins involved in the auxin signal transduction pathway leading to *SAUR* gene expression. The nature of these mutant loci and the proteins encoded by these genes will be disclosed when positional cloning of these genes will be completed. From studies of these genes, we expect important clues about the molecular mechanisms of auxin signal transduction.

Although the gene products of *SAUR* genes are not known, another interesting group of auxin-induced genes was found belonging to the pea *PS-IAA 4/6* gene family and is present in all plant species studied so far. They encode proteins with very short half-lives (t¹/₂ of 6–8 min). These short-lived proteins contain nuclear localization signals and share structural features of the prokaryotic ARC repressor family. The mechanism of the rapid degradation of these proteins is still unclear (no PEST motifs or ubiquitinylation found). The expression of these unstable proteins precedes the onset of elongation in only a small window of time relative to the elongation response. This has been interpreted to resemble expression patterns of animal growth regulators, such as the *c-fos* oncogene, which seem to establish the conditions for cell proliferation.

Another interesting gene, the *axi*1 gene, was found recently by T-DNA mutagenesis. This mutant search was designed to identify gain of function mutants to allow auxin-independent growth of tobacco protoplasts, which are cells from which walls had been removed by enzymatic digestion, and which depend on the presence of auxin and cytokinin to divide and form undifferentiated callus cells. The *axi*1 gene encodes a protein with nuclear localization signals and seems to be expressed during the onset of proliferation. Its precise function, however, is still unknown.

It is possible that at least part of the signaling chain leading to auxin regulation of gene expression may be transmitted through pathways involving MAP kinases. A number of MAP kinases have been reported in plants (at least nine different MAP kinase genes in *Arabidopsis*) (Nishihama et al., 1995). Most interestingly, auxin seems to affect the expression of some of the kinase genes, suggesting that this pathway could be relevant in plants not only for transducing mechanic stimuli, low temperature, and osmotic stress, but also hormones. The potential importance of the MAP kinase signaling pathway is further illustrated by the findings that the *CTR1* gene, encoding a Raf *homolog* that functions as an activator of MAP kinase kinase (MAPKK), plays a key role in the ethylene signal transduction pathway (*see below*).

5. ETHYLENE

Gaseous signaling molecules, such as NO and CO, have fascinated mammalian biologists over the past few years by their ability to act as second messengers in a wide variety of processes, including long-term memory and blood pressure regulation. The recognition of these effects was, however, relatively recent. In plants, however, it has been recognized for more than 100 years that volatile compounds, such as ethylene are involved in growth coordination and development. The effects of ethylene were first uncovered by the observation that gas from gas lamps, contains up to 5% ethylene-induced plant senescence and leaf abscision. Since then, ethylene has been found to promote both fruit ripening and seed germination while inhibiting flowering (Abeles et al., 1992). Aerial concentrations as low as 0.1 ppm affect seedlings' diageotropic growth, that is, growth upward and downward, and result in the thickening of stems as well as an inhibition of stem elongation. These effects cause an increase in the apical hook curvature (the "triple response"). This phenomenon has allowed the selection of mutants in ethylene's perception and response cascade. The triple response, first described a century ago by Neljubov (1901), results in dark-grown, ethylene-treated *Arabidopsis* seedlings being inhibited in the elongation of the hypocotyl and root, having increased radial swelling of the hypocotyl and increased retention and accentuation of the apical hook. The biological role of these physical changes, which alter hook form, is likely to facilitate soil penetration of the emerging seedling while protecting the delicate shoot apex.

The biosynthetic pathway of ethylene was elucidated in the 1970s, and its genetic elements identified recently (*see* Kende, 1993; Ecker and Theologis, 1994; Fray and Grierson, 1994; Theologis, 1994). Now, however, using the small crucifer *Arabidopsis thaliana*, simple genetic screens of the thousands of small seedlings have allowed the isolation of several mutants with defects in their ethylene responses.

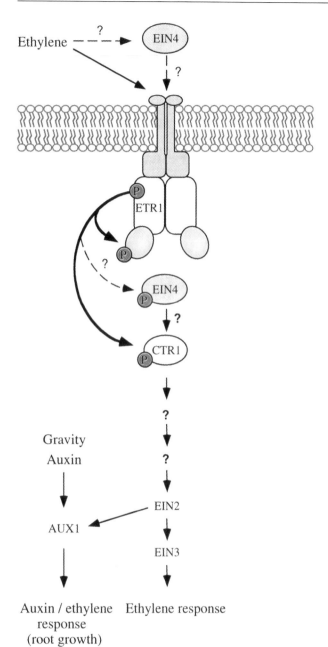

Fig. 2. The ethylene response pathway and its crosstalk to auxin signaling.

These mutants either failed to respond to ethylene, constitutively responded to ethylene, or overproduced ethylene. Thus, using a simple genetic screen, a remarkable dissection of the ethylene response pathway was made possible (Kieber and Ecker, 1993; Fig. 2). The mutants were grouped in classes with respect to their lack of ethylene sensitivity (ethylene insensitive, *ein*), ethylene resistance (*etr*),

ACC (an ethylene precursor) insensitivity (*ain*), constitutive activation of the ethylene response (*ctr*), and ethylene overproduction.

One of the dominant mutants (*etr*) conferred an ethylene-insensitive phenotype (Bleeker et al., 1988) and resulted in the cloning of the *ETR1* gene by chromosome walking (Chang et al., 1993). The amino acid sequence of the protein predicted from the *ETR1* gene shows surprising similarity to a superfamily of proteins well known from prokaryotes as two-component systems and acting as basic signal transduction modules (Chang et al., 1993; Hughes, 1994). These genes encode putative protein kinases related to a histidine kinase, the first component of the so-called two-component systems (Bourett et al., 1991). These signal sensors are composed of an extracellular perception unit and an intracellular histidine kinase domain, which, together with the second intracellularly located receiver component activates gene expression (Fig. 3). A related architecture with a two-component like receptor system and a MAP kinase cascade has been established for the osmosensing pathway of yeast (Maeda et al., 1994). The *CTR1* protein encoded by the *CTR1* locus (constitutive activation of the ethylene response, *ctr*) on the other hand is a member of the Raf family of protein kinases, which in mammals and flies transduce signals from cell-surface receptors to transcriptional factors through activation of the MAP kinase pathway. Thus, the ethylene pathway demonstrates how plants have combined and adapted elements that are present in independent pathways from prokaryotes, yeast, and higher animals. Further detailed understanding of the ethylene signaling pathway will come from cloning of the other mutated loci and the biochemical analysis of the various interacting components.

6. CHALLENGES AND PERSPECTIVES

An understanding of how plants grow is not just of interest to botanists. Challenging questions, such as what molecular events allow plants to overcome injuries, what events activate the meristems, specific centers where cell division starts, and determine how the cells emerging from these centers differentiate into new organs, and what molecular mechanisms allow even fully differentiated cells to embark new developmental programs, are being addressed with the powerful repertoire of molecular and genetic tools. It will be soon (within the next decade) that we obtain a detailed picture of the molecular machinery

Sensor

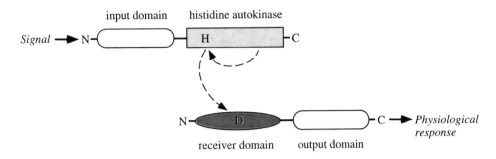

Fig. 3. Schematic illustration of two-component signaling systems.

of plants that transduces hormonal and other signals and of the machinery that regulates metabolism and plant form. Agriculture and environment will benefit from this knowledge.

REFERENCES

Abeles FB, Morgan PW, Saltveit ME. (1992) *Ethylene in Plant Biology.* Academic, New York, 1992.

Adam G. (1994) Brassinosteroide—eine neue Phytohormongruppe? *Naturwissenschaften* 1994; 81:210.

Ahmad M, Cashmore AR. HY4 gene of Arabidopsis encodes a protein with characteristics of a blue-light photoreceptor. *Nature* 1993; 366:162.

Binns AN. Cytokinin accumulation and action: biochemical, genetic, and molecular approaches. *Annu Rev Plant Physiol. Plant Mol Biol* 1994; 45:173.

Bleeker AB, Estelle MA, Somerville C. (1988) Insensitivity to ethylene conferred by a dominant mutation in *Arabidopsis thaliana. Science* 1988; 241:1086.

Bourret RB, Borkovich KA, Simon MI. (1991) Signal transduction pathways involving protein phosphorylation in prokaryotes. *Annu Rev Biochem* 1991; 60:401.

Bowler C, Neuhaus G, Yamagata H, Chua NH. Cyclic GMP and calcium mediate phytochrome phototransdcution. *Cell* 1994; 77:73.

Brzobohaty B, Moore I, Palme K. Cytokinin metabolism: implications for regulation of plant growth and development. *Plant Mol.-Biol.* 1994; 26:1483.

Chang C, Kwok SF, Bleeker AB, Meyerowitz EM. (1993) Arabidopsis ethylene-response gene ETR1: Similarity of product to two-component regulators. *Science* 1993; 266:539.

Davies PJ. (1995) *Plant Hormones, Physiology, Biochemistry and Molecular Biology*, 2nd ed. Dordrecht, The Netherlands, Kluwer Academic Publishers.

Ecker JR, Theologis A. Ethylene: a unique signalling molecule. In:Somerville C, Meyerowitz E, eds. *Arabidopsis* Cold Spring Harbor, NY: Cold Spring Harbor Laboratory Press, 1994:485.

Fray RG, Grierson D. Molecular genetics of tomato fruit ripening. *Trends Genet* 1995; 9:438.

Hanke D. A new signalling role for salicylic acid. *Curr Biolo* 1992; 2:441.

Hughes DA. Histidine kinases hog the lime light. *Nature* 1994; 369:187.

Kaminek M. Progress in cytokinin research. *TibTech* 1992; 10:159.

Kende H. (1993) Ethylene biosynthesis. *Annu Rev Plant Physiol Plant Mol Biol* 1993; 44:283.

Kieber JJ, Ecker JR. Ethylene gas: it's not just for ripening any more. *Trends Genet* 1993; 9:356.

Maeda T, Wurgler-Murphy SM, and Saito H. A two-component system that regulates an osmosensing MAP kinase cascade in yeast. *Nature* 1994; 369:242.

Mandava NB. Plant growth-promoting brassinosteroids. *Annu. Rev. Plant Physiol. Plant Mol. Biol.* 1988; 39:23.

Neljubov DN. Ueber die horizontale Nutation der Stengel von Pisum sativum und einiger anderer Pflanzen. *Ber Bot Zentralblatt* 1901; 10:128.

Neuhaus G, Bowler C, Kern, R, Chua, N-H. Calcium/calmodulin-dependent and -independent phytochrome signal transduction pathways. *Cell* 1993; 73:937.

Nisihihama R, Banno H, Shibata W, Hirano K, Nakashima M, Usami S, Machida J. Plant homologues of components of MAPK (Mitogen-activated protein kinase) signal pathways in yeast and animal cells. *Plant Cell Physiol.* 1995; 36:749–757.

Normanly J, Slovin JP, Cohen JD. Rethinking auxin biosynthesis and metabolism. *Plant Physiol.* 1995; 107:323.

Palme K ed. Signals and signal transduction pathways. Special volume. *Plant Mol. Biol.* 1994; 26:1237.

Parthier B. (1990) Jasmonates: hormonal regulators or stress factors in leaf senescence? *J Plant Growth Regul* 1990; 9,57.

Parthier B. Jasmonates, new regulators of plant growth and development: many facts and few hypotheses on their actions. *Bot Acta* 1991; 104:446.

Redhead CR, Palme K. The genes of plant signal transduction. *Crit Rev Plant Sci* 1996; in press.

Ryan C. (1994) Oligosaccharide signals: from plant defense to parasite offense. *Proc Natl Acad Sci USA* 1994; 91:1.

Sembdner G, Parthier B. The biochemistry and the physiological and molecular actions of jasmonates. *Annu Rev Plant Physiol Plant Mol Biol* 1993; 44:569.

Takahashi Y, Ishida S, Nagata T. Auxin-regulated genes. *Plant Cell Physiol* 1995; 36:383.

Theologis A. Control of ripening. *Curr Opinion Biotechnol.* 1994; 5:152.

Vernooij B, Uknes S, Ward E, Ryals J. Salicylic acid as a signal molecule in plant-pathogenic interaction. *Curr Opinion Cell Biol* 1994; 6:275–279.

SELECTED READINGS

Chang C, Meyerowitz EM. (1995) The ethylene hormone response in Arabidopsis: A eukaryotic two-component signaling system. *Proc Natl Acad Sci USA* 1995; 92:4129.

Kieber JJ, Rothenberg M, Roman G, Feldmann KA, Ecker JR. CTR1, a negtive regulator of the ethylene response pathway in Arabidopsis, encodes a member of the Raf family of protein kinases. *Cell* 1993; 72:427.

12   Comparative Endocrinology

Fredrick Stormshak, PhD

CONTENTS

1. INTRODUCTION

Comparative endocrinology embraces results of research conducted on a plethora of diverse vertebrate and invertebrate animals. Hence, the reader can appreciate the futility of attempting to present an in-depth treatise of this subject within the confines of a single chapter. Rather, an attempt will be made here to present unique and novel aspects of endocrine function that regulate or contribute to behavior, growth, and reproduction in a few select species. Much of what is currently known about general endocrinology evolved from studies in various types of nonprimate animals. This evolution of knowledge continues unabated today. Although much similarity in endocrine organization and function exists among species, there are differences that will be exposed in this chapter.

From: *Endocrinology: Basic and Clinical Principles* (P. M. Conn and S. Melmed, eds.), Humana Press Inc., Totowa, NJ.

2. ENDOCRINE CONTRIBUTIONS TO BEHAVIOR

2.1. Maternal Behavior

Humans, nonhuman primates, and some species as diverse as elephants exhibit spontaneous maternal behavior, but as a general rule, this type of spontaneous behavior is relatively rare among most mammalian species. Perhaps because of confinement and human intervention, more is known about the endocrinological basis of maternal behavior in laboratory and domestic mammals than other animals. Domestic sheep (ewes) are but one example of a species whose maternal behavior is hormonally regulated. Ewes only become maternally responsive toward a lamb after parturition. Nonparturient ewes aggressively reject approaches of lambs by head butting the lamb into retreat. Maternal behavior by the parturient ewe, however, consists of licking of the lamb, low-pitched bleats, and willingness to suckle the lamb. Usually within 2 h of parturition, an exclusive bond is formed between the dam and her offspring. Strange lambs are rejected by the ewe should they attempt to suckle, and this occurs even after loss of her own lamb.

In the pregnant ewe, the placenta near term is the major site of progesterone and estrogen synthesis. In fact, after d 55 of gestation, ovariectomy of ewes does not result in termination of pregnancy. Progesterone and estrogen are essential in facilitating the changes in the chemistry of the central nervous system (CNS) required for normal maternal behavior in this species. As term approaches, the increase in systemic concentrations of estrogen and reduced concentrations of progesterone induce expression of the oxytocin gene in the CNS. Concentrations of oxytocin mRNA are increased in cells in the paraventricular and supraoptic nuclei, posterior portion of the medial preoptic area, and the bed nucleus of the stria terminalis of the hypothalamus immediately after parturition and during subsequent lactation. In the ewe, exogenous estrogen is more effective than exogenous progesterone in increasing oxytocin mRNA in the bed nucleus of the stria terminalis and medial preoptic area, whereas the reverse is true for the supraoptic and paraventricular nuclei. The ability of exogenous progesterone to stimulate significant increases in oxytocin mRNA in several hypothalamic nuclei has not been observed for other species. However, based on immunocytochemical study, estrogen appears to increase storage of oxytocin in the supraoptic and paraventricular nuclei as well as in the olfactory bulb.

The actual process of the young passing through the birth canal resulting in vaginocervical stimulation is what is believed to induce the release of oxytocin. In multiparous ewes, oxytocin is the only peptide, when infused via a intracerebral cannula, that promotes all acceptance behaviors of the ewe toward the lamb.

It must not be assumed, however, that maternal behavior is a phenomenon simply regulated by changing systemic ratios of placental steroids and efferent neural stimuli inducing synthesis and release of oxytocin. There is evidence in the ewe that opiates play a role in promoting maternal behavior. Intracerebral ventricular infusion of naltrexone, an opiate antagonist, reduced the ability of vaginocervical stimulation to induce maternal behavior, and ewes continued to be aggressive to the lamb. Furthermore, intracerebral ventricular infusion of morphine into ewes does not by itself induce significant changes in cerebrospinal or plasma concentrations of oxytocin, but markedly potentiates the ability of vaginocervical stimulation to increase concentrations of this nonapeptide in these biological fluids.

Although there no doubt are other endocrine components that underlie activation of maternal behavior in this species, existing data clearly demonstrate the essentiality of oxytocin in this phenomenon.

The role of oxytocin in promoting maternal behavior in the rat is comparable to its role in sheep. Against rising systemic concentrations of estrogen and decreasing concentrations of progesterone, such as occur as a prelude to parturition, intracerebral ventricular administration of oxytocin to rats rapidly promotes maternal behavior. As in the ewe, the increase in placental secretion of estrogen prior to parturition stimulates synthesis and secretion of oxytocin at parturition. It is not surprising that estrogen can induce increased synthesis of oxytocin in the rat, because in this species the 5′-flanking region of the oxytocin gene has been found to contain estrogen response elements. Administration of oxytocin antiserum to the rat via intracerebral ventricular cannula blocked the onset of maternal behavior, as did lesioning of the paraventricular nucleus in the hypothalamus. Although secretion of oxytocin from the posterior pituitary occurs during parturition and the onset of suckling, it is not this source of the hormone that evokes maternal behavior. This is supported by experimental evidence demonstrating that iv infusion of oxytocin failed to stimulate maternal behavior in rats. It has been demonstrated that oxytocinergic neurons projecting from the medial preoptic area to the ventral tegmental area may be important for initiation of maternal behavior in the rat. Indeed, lesioning of the medial preoptic area in the rat completely prevents the initiation of maternal behavior. Additionally, oxytocinergic neurons have been found to terminate in the amygdala, substantia nigra, olfactory bulb, and ventral hippocampus in rats and sheep. Projections of oxytocinergic neurons to intra- and extrahypothalamic sites are consistent with the detection of oxytocin receptors in the following subsystems of the CNS: the olfactory system, the basal ganglia, the limbic system, the thalamus, hypothalamus, some cortical regions, the brainstem, and the spinal cord. Thus, it is not surprising that intracerebral ventricular rather than in iv infusions of oxytocin are more effective in promoting maternal behavior in rats and sheep.

3. STRESS AND THE AMPLECTIC CLASP

The endocrinology of sexual behavior has been studied in a wide range of vertebrate species, and

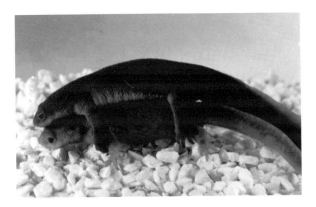

Fig. 1. A rough-skinned male newt (*T. granulosa*) displaying courtship behavior by grasping the female in an amplectic clasp (Courtesy of F. Moore, Oregon State University, Corvallis, OR).

from this research have emerged some common concepts. For example, it is central dogma that estrogen and progesterone in females and testosterone in males are essential for promoting sexual behavior. Similarly, in both females and males, these steroids stimulate secretion of various neuropeptides with which they act in concert to bring about the full complement of physical responses that allow successful reproduction of the particular species.

As in any field of biological study, there occasionally emerges a model that greatly expands our base of knowledge. The rough-skinned newt (*Taricha granulosa*) has proven to be an excellent model for understanding the endocrine basis of sexual behavior. In this amphibian species, reproduction usually extends from late winter through spring. Reproductively active males usually congregate in shallow waters of ponds or lakes awaiting the arrival of gravid females. The male initiates courtship by grasping the female in an amplectic clasp (Fig. 1). Amplexus usually persists for many hours before the male releases the female and deposits a spermatophore on the bottom of the pond or lake. The female then positions herself over the spermatophore and presses the sperm cap of the spermatophore into her cloaca. Females begin to ovulate about 2 wk after being inseminated and clasp underwater objects to which they attach their eggs.

The unique and novel display of reproductive behavior by this amphibian, which can readily be studied in the laboratory, has resulted in new and exciting data about the endocrine regulation of sexual receptivity. In female and male rats, sexual activity is mediated by steroid-induced synthesis of oxytocin and oxytocin receptors in the hypothalamus and extrahypothalamic regions of the CNS. In female rats, oxytocin appears to increase frequency and duration of lordosis, as well as stimulate uterine and oviductal contractions. In male rats, this nonapeptide promotes penile erection, and contractions of the seminiferous tubules and vas deferens. In contrast, in the rough-skinned newt, the reproductive behaviors are mediated by arginine vasotocin, a peptide that like oxytocin, is believed to have evolved from a common ancestral peptide. Like other vertebrate species, reproductive activity in male *T. granulosa* requires secretion of testosterone and dihydrotestosterone, which attain peak concentrations in early spring. In females, estrogen is the primary steroid involved in promoting reproductive activity. As demonstrated by results of gonadectomy/steroid-replacement studies, in both male and female newts, gonadal hormones act to maintain the behavioral actions induced by arginine vasotocin. In both male and female newts, arginine vasotocin administration provokes characteristic changes in sexual behavior of either intact or steroid-treated gonadectomized animals. Administration of arginine vasotocin to males promotes initiation of courtship behavior (amplexus), whereas injection of females with this peptide induces oviposition. In males, several brain regions contain measurable quantities of arginine vasotocin, but during the breeding season, only changes in the optic tectum levels of this peptide and courtship behavior are positively correlated. As might be anticipated, changes in optic tectum concentrations of arginine vasotocin are also highly correlated with seasonal changes in plasma steroid concentrations, further suggesting that gonadal steroids modulate synthesis and (or) secretion of this peptide. Additionally, gonadal steroids have been shown to regulate the number of arginine vasotocin receptors in a site-specific manner in the male and female newt brain. It should be mentioned that newts are not the only species in which reproductive behaviors are modulated by vasotocin. For example, vasotocin administration has been shown to enhance spawning behaviors in fish, sexual receptivity in female frogs, singing in male frogs and birds, and egg-laying behaviors in reptiles and birds.

When males of a given species court and mate, they must be able to recognize conspecific females as potential mates and respond in a species-specific manner to sensory information of various forms telegraphed by the female. Vasotocin in male newts may be responsible for enhancing sensory responsiveness to courtship-related stimuli. Application of cloacal pressure to the male newt causes a contraction of flexor muscles in the hindlegs referred to as "reflexive clasping response," which is particularly enhanced in breeding males. This response is mediated via rostral medullary neurons, which on cloacal pressure, exhibit increased firing. Vasotocin applied to the medulla markedly potentiates the magnitude of neuronal responses to cloacal pressure and increases the spontaneous discharge of rostral medullary neurons. Vasotocin also enhances neuronal responses to light pressure on the jaw, such as occurs during courtship behavior when the male repeatedly contacts the female's snout with his mandible during amplectic clasping. In conclusion, in male newts, the androgen-induced increase in arginine vasotocin enhances sensory responsiveness to courtship-related stimuli.

It should not be inferred from the above discussion that reproductive behaviors, and especially those of newts, are based solely on the integrated functions of a single neuropeptide and gonadal steroids. On the contrary, reproductive behaviors in all classes of animals are controlled by a vast array of hormones and neurotransmitters that exert either stimulatory or inhibitory actions. The above discussion has focused on those chemical messengers that stimulate sexual behavior in the rough-skinned newt. This stimulated sexual behavior is easily visualized because of the amplectic clasp of the male and the somewhat comparable ovipository clasp of the female. Exposure of male newts to a harsh stimulus markedly reduces courtship behavior as reflected by a reduction in amplexus. Such harsh stimuli are stressful and evoke within minutes a marked increase in plasma concentrations of corticosterone. Similarly, it was found through laboratory behavioral testing of sexually active males that administration of corticosterone totally suppressed amplexus. Increased systemic concentrations of corticosterone apparently act to modify brain neuronal activity. In particular, results of neurophysiological studies indicate that exogenous corticosterone rapidly depresses spontaneous activity and sensory responses of the medullary neurons, which normally fire in response to tactile stimuli of the cloaca or

mandible. These observations indicate that the suppressive effects of corticosterone on neuronal processing of sensory stimuli may underlie the ability of this interrenal gland steroid to inhibit reproductive behavior.

Perhaps one of the more important contributions to neuroendocrinology has come from studies of sexual behavior in the rough-skinned newt. Because the effect of exogenous corticosterone in suppressing reproductive behavior was evident within minutes, it was difficult to accept that the action of this steroid was mediated via classical genome transcription pathways. Consequently, studies were undertaken to determine by use of radioligand-binding assays whether neuronal membranes contained specific binding sites for corticoids. Indeed, in highly purified preparations of neuronal membranes, labeled corticosterone specifically bound to sites with high affinity and in a saturable manner. Specific binding of ^{3}H-corticosterone reached equilibrium rapidly and was reversible. Competition studies revealed that the binding sites in neuronal membranes of the newt were highly specific for corticosterone. No other steroid, except cortisol, could compete for the binding sites. The location of the specific high-affinity binding site for corticosterone was subsequently confirmed by autoradiography, which revealed binding of the labeled steroid over synaptic neuropil and not over the cell bodies where intracellular steroid receptors are located. Collectively, results of these studies indicated that the corticosterone receptor in neuronal membranes was distinguishable from the intracellular corticosteroid receptors. Although membrane receptors for progesterone in *Xenopus* oocytes were known to exist, the research with this species was the first to demonstrate that plasma membrane receptors for steroids could exist in the CNS. More recent data suggest that the rapid response of newts to corticosterone is mediated via G-protein-coupled mechanisms. In *T. granulosa*, results of radioligand-binding assays revealed that ^{3}H-corticosterone binding in neuronal membranes is negatively modulated by nonhydrolyzable guanine nucleotide analogs, especially GTPγS. Also, specific binding of ^{3}H-corticosterone to neuronal membranes is enhanced in a concentration-dependent manner by addition of Mg^{2+} to the assay buffer. These results are consistent with known data for G-protein-coupled receptors.

4. ENDOCRINE BASIS OF MALE-ORIENTED BEHAVIOR

Male homosexual behavior is quite widespread among mammals. At least 63 mammalian species have been identified in which male homosexual behavior occurs to some extent. Expression of male homosexual behavior has in general been attributed to social environment to which the individual is exposed either prepubertally or as an adult, and to the influence of hormones on sexual differentiation of the brain. As an example, male–male mounting of prepubertal domestic animals is believed to be important in the development of normal rear orientation in mount interactions. Even adult males of some species that are restricted from contact with females often exhibit homosexual behavior primarily because they have no choice for interaction with the opposite sex.

Sexual differentiation of the female brain of mammals is generally believed to proceed in the absence of hormonal imprinting. Consequently, as adults, most female mammals exhibit a characteristic cyclical pattern of luteinizing hormone (LH) secretion and feminine sexual behavior. However, sexual differentiation of the male brain of mammals is dependent on an interaction of brain cells with testosterone, which can be aromatized to estrogen during a critical prenatal and (or) postnatal period. Male mammals are characterized by an acyclical pattern of LH secretion and a form of sexual behavior characteristic for the species. Sexual differentiation of the brain has received considerable attention from the standpoint of the role of hormones in regulating the development and function of the neuroendocrine system. Comparatively less effort has been devoted to investigate the basis for sexual behavior. Nevertheless, the few studies that have been conducted provide compelling evidence that hormones do function at the level of the brain to establish patterns of sexual behavior. Male rats castrated 24–36 h after birth and treated with testosterone propionate (TP) on d 2 and 4 after birth when tested for sexual preference at 100 d of age preferred females if injected with TP at this time, but males if injected with estradiol benzoate (EB). Similar responses in terms of sexual preference as those observed for male rats have been recorded for male hamsters and pigs castrated shortly after birth, and then as adults treated with TP or EB alone or in combination with proges-

terone. Collectively, these data seem to indicate that postnatal testosterone secretion may be more important than prenatal secretions of gonadal steroids in masculinizing the brain of the male with respect to sexual orientation as an adult. This is also supported by data on sexual preference of male ferrets castrated at various ages after birth. As adults, male ferrets castrated on d 5 after birth chose males in sexual preference tests more often than males castrated on d 20 or 35 after birth. Although the role of testosterone in masculinizing the brain and promoting female-oriented sexual behavior seems fairly well established, it is also quite clear, based on experimental data, that estrogen can induce male homosexual behavior. Perhaps there are other factors produced by the testes of heterosexuals that protect against estrogen-induced homosexual behavior. For example, consider the response of male nonhuman primates to exogenous estrogen. In these males, the hypothalamic–hypophyseal axis responds to exogenous estradiol by releasing surge amounts of LH (ordinarily considered a female response) when the testes are removed, but not if the male is left intact. Treatment of castrated males with testosterone or dihydrotestosterone, or testosterone in combination with physiological levels of estradiol, does not suppress the estradiol-induced LH surge. These observations suggest that the testes of heterosexual males may produce some other substance that interferes with the actions of estradiol in the brain.

Much has been learned about the hormonal induction of homosexual behavior through experimentation, yet in actuality, virtually nothing is known about the endocrinology of male subjects that normally express this behavior. Such a deficiency in our knowledge stems from the inability to identify an adequate number of natural homosexual animals of one species that can be utilized in appropriately planned experiments. From this standpoint, the domestic male sheep, hereafter referred to as rams, may serve as a useful model for studying the endocrine aspects of the homosexual. Homosexual behavior in domestic rams is quite common and even exists in the wild Bighorn and Dall sheep. In these latter populations, rams continue to mature for 5 or 6 yr after puberty, and segregate into groups of their own away from females and juvenile rams. Those rams acting like mature males form all-male societies in which dominant rams act the role of courting males and subordinate rams behave as "estrous" males. Geist (1971), who has studied these populations, generally considers mountain sheep societies to be basically homosexual. Researchers at the US Sheep Experiment Station in Dubois, ID have, through rigorous sexual preference testing, identified an adult population of domestic rams consisting predominantly of heterosexuals, but with a smaller percentage (<10%) of the population consisting of true homosexuals. Those rams exhibiting homosexual behavior were born as singlets or as cotwin with either a male or female, and all were reared prepubertally as a mixed population of males and females. Exposure of homosexual rams to receiver rams for a prolonged period of time (8 h) failed to provoke any change in plasma LH pulse frequency or basal concentration. In contrast, systemic concentrations of LH in heterosexual rams are markedly increased during prolonged exposure of the rams to estrous females. However, plasma concentrations of testosterone in homosexual rams were on the average significantly greater during exposure to receiver males than to receptive estrous females. Homosexual rams compared to contemporary heterosexual rams have been found to be deficient in hypothalamic preoptic area aromatase activity (Resko et al., 1996). This is significant because the preoptic area of the hypothalamus is believed to mediate male reproductive behaviors in most vertebrate species. In rodents, activity of aromatase (which converts androgens to estrogens) in the medial preoptic area is relatively high compared to other parts of the brain. Additional studies have revealed that serum concentrations of testosterone, estrone, and estradiol were significantly lower in homosexual than in heterosexual rams when blood was collected from the rams while not being subjected to sexual preference testing. In support of this, testicular homogenates of homosexual rams incubated with isotopically labeled progesterone produced significantly less labeled testosterone and 17α-hydroxyprogesterone than comparable testes homogenates of heterosexual rams. These data suggest that homosexual rams have a reduced testicular capacity to synthesize androgens. If this deficiency in androgen production is present during the critical period during which brain masculinization occurs, it could be reflected in adulthood by an altered hypothalamic capacity to aromatize androgens to estrogens and hence contribute to or cause the male to become homosexual. Certainly, further study of the homosexual ram may provide additional insight

regarding the endocrine basis for this form of sexual behavior.

5. GROWTH AND DEVELOPMENT

5.1. Characteristics of Prenatal and Postnatal Growth

Body growth in mammals represents a response of the animal to a combination of genetic, nutritional, and endocrine factors. In species, such as rats, cattle, sheep, and pigs, males at birth and maturity are heavier than females. The novice might immediately attribute the weight advantage in males to testicular secretion of androgens. Indeed, if male rats are castrated at birth, they do not attain as great a weight as males castrated at 21 d of age. In contrast, ovariectomized female rats grow to a greater extent than intact females, because estrogens have an inhibitory effect on body growth of rats. In both cattle and sheep, castrated males (steers and wethers, respectively) exhibit superior growth rates characterized by enhanced muscle-to-fat ratios than intact females. Unlike the positive effects of ovariectomy on growth rate of rats, ovariectomy of heifers or ewes has either no effect or a negative effect on growth and body composition. In fact, in these species, exogenous estrogens in appropriate dosages are growth promotants, and the responses they evoke are more consistent in castrated males than in intact females.

The above descriptions of the effects of gonadectomy on body growth of mammals might give one the illusion that gonadal hormones are central in regulating growth. However, it should be recognized that they represent only one of the endocrines involved in this biological process. Endocrine regulation of growth involves interactions among several hormones and growth factors, acting both systemically and locally. In addition to gonadal hormones, pituitary growth hormone (GH) and insulin-like growth factors (IGF) are crucial for normal postnatal growth.

5.2. Patterns of GH Secretion

GH secretion in humans and a wide variety of mammals, such as baboons, monkeys, cattle, sheep, goats, pigs, and rats, is pulsatile in nature. GH hormone secretion in ruminants is asynchronous and episodic. In domestic animals, there is no relationship between sleep phases and GH secretion, as has been reported to be the case for higher primates. As a general rule, systemic concentrations of GH are greatest in prenatal and (or) neonatal mammals and then decrease with age. The rat seems to be an exception to this rule. In fetal lambs, GH secretion is pulsatile as early as day 110 of gestation, and systemic concentrations of this hormone are greater than in the postnatal animal. Within 24 h of birth, GH concentrations decline 10-fold, with a reduction in both pulse amplitude and basal concentration values, to a secretory pattern not different from that of the adult. Similarly, in fetal pigs, serum GH concentrations increase from 40 d of 110-d gestation period to concentrations of nearly 100 ng/mL at parturition. Mean serum concentrations of GH in postnatal pigs decrease with age owing mainly to secretory surges of reduced amplitude. In rats, episodic GH secretion occurs prior to puberty and becomes maximal during early adulthood, after which secretion of the hormone decreases. The pattern of GH secretion is sexually dimorphic in adult male and female rats. Males exhibit a low-frequency, high-amplitude pattern of GH secretion. In contrast, GH secretion in females is characterized by high-frequency, low-amplitude secretory pulses.

It is well established that GH secretion is primarily regulated by two hypothalamic peptides. Somatostatin, which suppresses pituitary secretion and GH-releasing factor (GRF), which stimulates secretion. GRF has been shown to stimulate GH secretion in cattle, goats, sheep, and poultry in a dose-dependent manner. There is convincing evidence that gonadal steroids modulate GH secretion. For example, in rats, steroids appear to modulate basal growth hormone levels as well as the frequency and amplitude of secretory pulses. Administration of testosterone to adult female rats produced male typical secretory patterns of GH, and after withdrawal of treatment, patterns of secretion of growth hormone returned to those typical of female rats. As already alluded to above, gonadal steroids are regulators of growth and development in domestic animals. GH secretion in rams and bulls is characterized by discrete episodic release, which continues even after puberty. Castration increases the frequency of episodic release of GH and reduces amplitude of the pulses. In prepubertal heifers, the pattern of GH secretion is qualitatively similar to that observed in bulls, whereas after puberty, GH secretion in heifers is no longer characterized by discrete episodes of release. A pronounced activational effect of gonadal

steroids on GH secretion has been observed in castrated male sheep (wethers). Administration of diethylstilbestrol or testosterone propionate to wethers increased mean basal plasma concentrations of GH, reduced the frequency of episodic release of the hormone, but did not alter the amplitude of pulses compared to untreated control wethers.

In conclusion, some generalities can be drawn regarding patterns of GH secretion in nonprimate mammals. GH secretion in a wide variety of mammals appears to be greater during fetal development than after birth. Growth hormone secretion is sexually dimorphic in the rat, but apparently not in other species. Patterns of GH secretion are modulated in part by gonadal steroids.

5.3. Regulation of GH Receptors

Two classes of GH receptors defined by affinity (high and low) have been detected in the liver of several species, including the rat, rabbit, cattle, sheep, and pig. In ruminants and pigs, the number of high-affinity sites in the liver correlates with growth rate and plasma IGF-1 levels, whereas there is no such correlation for the low-affinity site. Using ligand-binding assays, little or no binding of GH to liver membranes could be demonstrated until after birth in the calf or lamb. In pig hepatic membranes, binding of GH at birth is very low and gradually increases over 6 mo. Scatchard analysis has revealed a 10-fold increase in the capacity of the high-affinity GH receptor over this period. Chronic treatment of pigs and sheep with GH upregulates the high-affinity receptor found in hepatocytes, but at least in sheep there is no effect of treatment on the low-affinity receptor. Little information is available about effects of GH on its receptor concentrations in other tissues.

5.4. IGF

IGF are important mediators of GH action in mammalian species. Ontogenic development of plasma concentrations of IGF-1 has been studied in rats, sheep, cattle, and pigs. Plasma levels of IGF-1 in rats, sheep, and cattle are low at birth and increase postnatally concomitant with the appearance of GH receptors in the liver, reflecting perhaps the onset of GH-dependent IGF-1 secretion. Similar data exists for systemic concentrations of IGF-1 in pigs, but there are also conflicting data suggesting that serum concentrations of IGF-1 are greater at birth and then decline steadily. In rats and pigs, serum concentrations of IGF-2 are greater at birth and decrease with age. In the bovine, IGF-1 and 2 are not only detectable in serum, but also in colostrum and milk.

Plasma concentrations of IGF-1 in cattle are dependent on nutritional status through both GH-dependent and GH-independent mechanisms. In mature cattle, the ability of GH to maintain plasma IGF-1 is impaired when nutrient intake is markedly reduced. Both basal IGF-1 concentrations and the increment in plasma IGF-1 after GH administration to cattle are most consistently affected by reduced dietary protein intake.

GH acting on the liver stimulates production of IGF-1, which by vascular transport affects distant target cells. Additionally, it is now well established that GH can also act directly on the "distant" target cells to stimulate production of IGF-1, which acts in an autocrine or paracrine fashion. In recent years, bovine somatotropin has received much attention in the popular press because of its commercialization for use in stimulating milk production in dairy cows. Based on the mechanism by which GH promotes production of IGF-1, it is not surprising that when this pituitary hormone is administered daily to cows, systemic concentrations of IGF-1 increase dramatically. Concentrations of IGF-1 in mammary tissue and milk are also increased, but the increase in milk is minor and concentrations remain within the range of values detected in milk from untreated cows. Effects of exogenous bovine GH on plasma concentration of IGF-2 in cattle are equivocal.

5.5. IGF Receptors

Not much is known about receptors for IGF in various species of mammals. Receptors for IGF-1 and 2 are present in bovine mammary gland tissue, bone, capillaries, retina, and adrenals. The receptors for IGF-1 are most abundant in mammary tissue during lactogenesis and decline during lactation. Receptors for IGF-2 predominate in mammary tissue in both the nonlactating and lactating glands, but abundance does not change in response to initiation of lactation.

5.6. IGF Binding Proteins (IGFBP)

Presently, six mammalian IGFBP have been cloned. Within a species, the IGFBP share an overall protein sequence homology of 50%, whereas between species, up to 80% nucleotide sequence homology in corresponding IGFBP is observed. No IGFBP genes have been cloned in nonmammalian vertebrates, yet their likely conservation among vertebrates is attested to by the ability of IGFBP from fish, amphibians, reptiles, birds, and metatherian mammals specifically to bind isotopically labeled mammalian IGF-1. The functional role of IGFBP has not been determined with certainty, but it is obvious that these proteins have become, at least in mammals, complex players in growth and development processes. The IGFBP do prolong the half-life of circulating IGF and separate the activities of these hormones from those of insulin. Additionally, there is now mounting evidence that the IGFBP may play a functional role not only in delivery, but on a local basis, ensure that IGF secreted by a cell are retained in the vicinity, and therefore exert their action on the same (autocrine) or adjacent (paracrine) cell populations.

In mature sheep and cattle, the majority of circulating IGF are bound to IGFBP-3, which is comparable to the situation in humans. There is evidence from studies with domestic animals that treatment with GH significantly increases systemic concentrations of IGFBP-3. In sheep, an increase in systemic IGFBP-3 coincides with the marked increase in hepatic GH receptor that occurs during postnatal development. Reduced nutrient intake causes a reduction in plasma concentrations of IGFBP-3, which are markedly increased after refeeding in the rat and pig. On the other hand, in nutritionally restricted animals, there occurs an increased hepatic expression of genes for IGFBP-1 and 2. The physiological significance of this increased gene expression for these IGFBP is not completely understood.

6. PUBERTY

The phenomenon of puberty has been extensively studied in mammals. Compared to the human, the interval from birth to puberty is of short duration for most mammals. Puberty in the human occurs at a time when growth (weight) is 80–90% complete, whereas in most other mammals, puberty is achieved when the young animal has attained only 30–70% of its adult weight. The Chinese Meishan pig is an example of one mammal that may attain puberty precociously. In this particular breed of pigs, puberty occurs at the age of 3 mo when its body weight is only about 25% of its adult weight.

Puberty represents that stage in life when the hypothalamo–hypophyseal axis and the gonads have achieved a coordinate state of functional maturation sufficient to allow the individual to reproduce. Changes in hypothalamic, pituitary, and gonadal function that characterize this maturational process from before birth to puberty have been well documented for the rat, sheep, and primate. Therefore, this presentation will highlight those similarities and differences in endocrine function and certain environmental factors that contribute to the onset of puberty in these three mammals. When relevant, information on other mammalian species will be included.

6.1. Rats

6.1.1. PRENATAL HYPOTHALAMIC AND HYPOPHYSEAL FUNCTION

In male and female rat fetuses, hypothalamic concentrations of gonadotropin-releasing hormone (GnRH) are low until about days 17 and 18 of gestation, after which concentrations increase to the day of birth. Receptors for GnRH are already detectable in the anterior pituitaries of male rats on day 16 of gestation. Pituitary LH and follicle-stimulating hormone (FSH) have been detected in rat fetuses of both sexes on and after day 17 of gestation. Pituitary LH content in female rats may be greater than in male rats during the late days of gestation.

6.1.2. OVARIAN DEVELOPMENT

In humans, ewes, and cows at birth, the ovary contains antral follicles. This is not the situation for female rats, mice, and pigs in which antral follicles develop only after birth. In the rat, a marked increase in primordial follicles is observed between 24 and 48 h after birth. Apparently the formation of these primordial follicles in the rat is independent of any kind of endogenous gonadotropin stimulation. Neither administration of equine chorionic gonadotropin or FSH is able to stimulate follicular development during the first few days postnatally. Furthermore, receptors of LH and FSH have not been detected in the rat ovary during the first 4 or 5 d after birth.

6.1.3. PREPUBERTAL CHANGES IN HYPOTHALAMIC–HYPOPHYSEAL FUNCTION

In female rats, the first ovulation occurs around 38 d of age. Secretion of FSH in the female increases from birth up to 12 d of age, and thereafter declines so that by about 5–6 d prior to ovulation, plasma concentrations of this gonadotropin are markedly reduced. Secretion of LH also increases up to approx 3 wk of age, but the increase is not as dramatic as for FSH. During the remaining 2–2.5 wk of the prepubertal period, systemic concentrations of LH are low, but quite noticeably pulsatile with the interpulse interval being about 30 min. These changes in FSH and LH secretion during the prepubertal period are believed to reflect the secretion of GnRH. Infrequent release of GnRH is believed to favor a sustained high level of FSH secretion and only generate transient bursts of LH release. However, as frequency of GnRH pulses increases with resultant increased pulsatile secretion of LH, there occurs a decrease in systemic concentrations of FSH. The increased systemic concentrations of gonadotropins evident during the early prepubertal period may also be owing in part to reduced sensitivity of the anterior pituitary to estradiol negative feedback and to greater responsiveness of the pituitary to GnRH. The anterior pituitary during the early prepubertal period contains a greater percentage of gonadotropins. Additionally, the systemic concentrations of α-fetoprotein that bind endogenous estrogens with relatively high affinity remain elevated until at least day 16 of age. Rat milk contains a GnRH-like substance that is chromatographically indistinguishable from hypothalamic GnRH. During the first 2 wk after birth, this milk GnRH is believed to cross the gastrointestinal epithelium of the pup in sufficient quantities to bind to GnRH receptors in the ovary with a consequent inhibition of gonadotropin-induced estrogen and progesterone production. Such a phenomenon would theoretically suppress ovarian function and hence preclude any type of hormonal feedback on the hypothalamo–hypophyseal system of the young female.

During the latter half of the prepubertal period, the ovary grows in response to the low systemic levels of FSH and LH. Waves of follicles begin to develop and undergo atresia, but it should be emphasized that none attain the ovulatory stage. Concomitantly, there is an increase in the number of gonadotropin receptors, especially the receptors for LH, and a decrease in GnRH receptors that continues until the first proestrus. Two additional pituitary hormones play a role in regulating prepubertal ovarian function in the rat. Both prolactin and GH have been shown to contribute to ovarian maturation by facilitating the effects of gonadotropins. Prolactin enhances ovarian steroidogenesis in response to exogenous human chorionic gonadotropin (hCG) and FSH. Although GH may act directly on the ovary, there is considerable evidence that the actions of GH are mediated by IGF-1. IGF-1 is produced by granulosa cells and facilitates FSH induction of aromatase activity, progesterone secretion, and formation of LH receptors. Approximately 8–9 d prior to first proestrus, the diurnal pattern of LH release changes in the female rat. Both basal LH levels and LH pulse amplitude become greater in the afternoon than in the morning. Some peripubertal females also exhibit a more sustained midafternoon episode of LH secretion, which has been termed a "minisurge." These "minisurges" of LH may promote increased synthesis of estrogen by the ovary. However, the afternoon increase in LH pulse amplitude is not estradiol-induced, whereas the "minisurges" of LH do appear to be caused by increases in systemic concentrations of estradiol.

The ovary of the rat during the transition to proestrus produces increasing quantities of estradiol, progesterone, and testosterone, and reduced quantities of 3α-androstanediol. Reduction in the synthesis and secretion of the latter steroid may be elicited in part by the rising levels of prolactin. It has been proposed that 3α-androstanediol may be involved in delaying onset of puberty, but this has not been substantiated experimentally. Secretion of estradiol is the key event that ultimately triggers the onset of puberty in the rat. Estradiol acts on both the anterior pituitary and the hypothalamus to promote the proestrus surge of LH that causes ovulation. In the hypothalamus, estradiol evokes a release of GnRH, and in the pituitary, it sensitizes the gonadotropes to the stimulatory effect of GnRH. The increase in ovarian progesterone production prior to proestrus may have a role in facilitating the stimulatory effect of estradiol on GnRH release. Perhaps this effect of progesterone on GnRH release may be owing in part to the ability of this steroid to increase GnRH gene expression.

Hypothalamic concentrations of GnRH in the male rat increase throughout postnatal development and even into adulthood. Pituitary concentrations of GnRH receptors and LH are maximal at about 30 d of age, and then receptor levels decline to adult levels detected around 60–70 d of age. This reduction in GnRH receptors is inversely related to testicular testosterone feedback action on the hypothalamo–hypophyseal axis.

During neonatal development serum concentrations of gonadotropins in males are increased, but are significantly lower than levels detected in females. Subsequently the systemic levels of these gonadotropins decrease. The nature of LH secretion during the peripubertal period in the male rat is equivocal. Some reports suggest that LH secretion increases, whereas other reports indicate a decrease or no change. Onset of puberty in the male is, however, associated with an increase in FSH secretion. Serum FSH levels rise postnatally and attain maximal levels usually between 30 and 40 d of age. Thereafter, serum concentrations of FSH decline as serum levels of testosterone increase.

During the interval between 1 and 4 wk of age, testosterone is not the primary androgen produced by the rat testes. During this time, the activity of 5α-reductase in the testes is markedly increased. Consequently, the primary androgens produced by the immature rat testes are androstenedione, 5α-androstanediol, and 5α-dihydrotestosterone. After day 40 of age, 5α-reductase activity decreases, and because of enhanced activity of 17α-hydroxylase, C_{17-20} lyase and 17β-hydroxysteroid dehydrogenase, testosterone becomes the major androgen synthesized and secreted. As in males of other species, actual testosterone secretion is highly correlated, but phase-delayed, with pulses of LH release.

6.2. Sheep

6.2.1. Puberty in Females

In most North American breeds of sheep, the females born in late winter and early spring usually attain puberty at about 7 mo of age. The ovaries of ewe lambs, although possessing antral follicles at birth, do not respond to exogenous gonadotropins until after 2–4 wk of age. After 5–6 wk, exogenous gonadotropins can induce ovulation and formation of corpora lutea. In the prepubertal ewe lamb, pulsatile secretion of LH has been detected as early as the second week after birth. The amplitude of the LH pulses is similar to that detected in the adult ewe, but the frequency is lower being on the order of 90–120 min apart. From time of birth to puberty, systemic concentrations of FSH are greater than basal or pulsatile concentrations of LH. Changes in systemic concentrations of FSH are, however, positively correlated with pulsatile release of LH in the intact and ovariectomized ewe lamb. A functional ovarian negative feedback system is apparently not operational in the ewe lamb during the first few weeks after birth. This is supported by data demonstrating that ovariectomy of ewe lambs is followed by a lag period of 2–3 wk or more before pulsatile secretion of LH occurs, with a frequency and amplitude resembling that found in ovariectomized mature ewes. This is similar to the situation in the neonatal female rat in which ovariectomy during the first few postnatal days of life fails to activate gonadotropin release. The fact that ovariectomy of ewe lambs results in high-frequency LH pulses during prepuberty may also be interpreted as indirect evidence that the pituitary is able to respond accordingly to GnRH. Indeed, it has been demonstrated that each LH pulse in ovariectomized prepubertal lambs is preceded by a GnRH pulse. In the ewe lamb, onset of puberty appears to be dictated by sensitivity of the hypothalamo–hypophyseal axis to the negative feedback of ovarian estradiol. Sensitivity of the hypothalamo–hypophyseal axis to the negative feedback of estradiol decreases with the age of the ewe lamb, thus allowing increased gonadotropin secretion, which in turn stimulates the ovary to produce sufficient estrogen to provoke the preovulatory surge of LH. This role of estradiol in regulating gonadotropin secretion in the ewe lamb has been demonstrated experimentally. Chronic treatment of ovariectomized ewe lambs with estradiol beginning at an early age suppressed high-frequency pulsatile secretion of LH up until the time that intact controls began exhibiting pubertal estrus. At this time, pulsatile secretion of LH began occurring in the ovariectomized ewe lambs.

In ewe lambs approaching puberty, frequency of pulsatile LH secretion increases, and amplitude of the pulses decreases. This is similar to the pattern of LH secretion during the follicular phase of the cycle of mature ewes. Ultimately, this pattern of LH secretion promotes increased synthesis of estradiol by ovarian follicles, which then feeds back positively to trigger the first ovulatory surge of LH. However, this ovulatory surge of LH is rarely accompanied by expression of behavioral estrus. In most cases, the corpus luteum or luteinized follicle developing from the first ovulatory surge is short-lived, resulting in a so-called short luteal phase of about 6–7 d duration, and characterized by a transient increase in systemic concentrations of progesterone. This short luteal phase may be followed by an ovulatory surge of LH accompanied by expression of behavioral estrus, which results in a cycle of normal duration (15–17 d) in ewes, or the ovulatory surge may result in another

short luteal phase before ovulation with estrus occurs. In mature ewes that are seasonal breeders, short luteal phases also precede the expression of estrus with ovulation during the transition from anestrus to cyclic activity. A short luteal phase, or at least a transient increase in systemic concentration of progesterone, has been found to precede first ovulation with estrus in prepubertal heifers. In female pigs, pubertal estrus and ovulation are not preceded by a transient increase in progesterone secretion. It appears that prepubertal short luteal phases may be a characteristic common to ruminants.

6.2.2. Photoperiod Can Affect Puberty in Female Sheep

In seasonal breeding sheep, changes in sensitivity of the hypothalamo–hypophyseal axis to estradiol that characterize onset of puberty are modulated by photoperiod signals to which the animal is exposed. In sheep, changes in photoperiod (hours of light and hours of darkness) are perceived by the retina and the information telegraphed via a neuronal pathway ultimately to affect synthesis of melatonin by the pineal gland. During darkness, the pineal gland of sheep secretes rather copious quantities of melatonin in a pulsatile fashion. The pattern of melatonin secretion constitutes a form of neuroendocrine record of changes in photoperiod that modulates the frequency of GnRH secretion and, hence, pulsatile LH secretion required for onset of puberty. In order for puberty to be attained in the correct season for mating (autumn in the Northern Hemisphere), the lamb must be born in late winter or spring. In other words, these lambs must be exposed to long days (long hours of daylight) followed by short days. Lambs born out of season, i.e., born in autumn or winter, are exposed to short days followed by long days. Although these lambs attain a state of maturity and somatic development commensurate with attainment of puberty during the following spring, puberty is delayed until autumn. The reason for the delay in puberty arises from continued hypersensitivity of the hypothalamo–hypophyseal axis to estradiol-negative feedback. Consequently, tonic LH secretion is low in autumn-born lambs during the spring and summer, thus preventing preovulatory follicular development. In conclusion, photoperiod regulates onset of puberty in some breeds of sheep through changes in hypothalamo–hypophyseal sensitivity to estradiol inhibition of LH secretion.

6.2.3. Onset of Puberty in Males

Spring-born male lambs begin reproductive development at about 10 wk of age as evidenced by onset of the spermatogenic cycle. In ram lambs, the first pulsatile release of LH occurs on the average at about 3 wk of age, but can occur as early as 1 wk of age. Frequency of pulsatile LH release increases with age reaching a maximum near 8 wk and decreasing thereafter. Serum concentrations of LH increase concomitant with frequency of pulses attaining maximal levels at 8 wk and then decreasing. Pulsatile release of LH in ram lambs stimulates a rise in systemic concentrations of testosterone that are maximal by 1 h after the pulse of LH. The testes of the neonatal lamb are responsive to stimulation by gonadotropins. Administration of hCG to a 2-d-old ram lamb provoked an increase in testosterone secretion. It has been proposed that during prenatal development, androgens from the testes both masculinize (male traits) and defeminize (female traits) mechanisms controlling LH secretion in the male sheep. Presumably, the androgens would act to alter the neural components that process and relay information about photoperiod to the neural network governing GnRH secretion. Consequently, tonic secretion of LH would be masculinized, and defeminization of the LH surge mechanism would occur, thus preventing activation of the GnRH surge in response to estradiol. In essence, this would prevent the preovulatory gonadotropin surge from becoming operative in the male. The pattern of melatonin secretion in the ram and ewe in response to changing photoperiod is similar. However, unlike the ewe, the ram's GnRH pulse generator appears to be rather insensitive to changes in the photoperiod. Precisely why males do not respond to photoperiod but females do is unknown.

6.3. Primate

6.3.1. Ovary and Testis Development

In primates, growth and atresia of ovarian follicles occur throughout infancy and the juvenile period of development, but follicles never attain preovulatory size. In juvenile rhesus monkeys, ovarian vein concentrations of estradiol increase, suggesting that follicles in prepubertal primates synthesize and secrete steroids. Growth and steroidogenic potential of follicles continues in the human female with approaching onset of puberty. This is manifested by development of secondary sex characteristics and by menarche, which usually occurs between 12 and 13 yr of age. Menarche is frequently used as a marker of puberty in humans and other primates. However, in most young women, ovulation does not occur until several months later.

Testes of prepubertal rhesus monkeys and humans contain few, if any, Leydig cells, and testosterone secretion during this phase of development is minimal. Studies of humans and rhesus monkeys suggest that initial activation of testicular testosterone secretion during early puberty occurs nocturnally. In humans, daytime levels of plasma testosterone begin to rise above prepubertal concentrations during the 10th yr of life and continue to increase steadily to attain maximal concentrations at 15–16 yr of age.

6.3.2. Pre- and Postnatal Gonadotropin Secretion

Secretion of gonadotropins by the human and rhesus monkey fetus increases during mid- to late gestation with peak plasma concentrations occurring between 100 and 150 d of pregnancy. Concentrations of gonadotropins in females are greater than in males. The lower levels of LH and FSH in males are believed to be owing to the inhibitory feedback of testicular hormones. During the latter half of gestation in humans and rhesus monkeys, FSH and LH concentrations in fetal blood decrease with lowest levels present at birth. After parturition, systemic concentrations of LH and FSH in the male neonate markedly increase. In males of some primate species, the increased secretion of gonadotropins at this stage of development promote increased testosterone secretion comparable to that of adult males. Bilateral orchidectomy after 1 wk of age causes an increase in LH and FSH secretion similar in magnitude to that observed after castration of sexually mature males. This response indicates the existence of a negative feedback system during infantile development. Furthermore, in such neonate castrates, LH secretion is episodic, having an interpulse interval of 60 min. Collectively, these observations suggest that in male primates, the hypothalamo–hypophyseal unit that governs testicular function differentiates to full maturity during fetal development.

Secretion of FSH and LH in female primate neonates is increased as in males, and depending on the species, the levels of these gonadotropins are maintained for a variable period of time. Subsequently the levels of FSH and LH decrease to levels characteristic of the prepubertal state. However, in contrast to the levels of FSH and LH in infantile human males, the ratio of FSH to LH in systemic circulation of infantile girls is markedly increased. This sex difference in secretion of gonadotropins may be attributed to the fact that the GnRH pulse generator in the infantile female primate does not operate at the adult circhoral frequency as in the male.

Following the infantile period of development, gonadotropin secretion in male and female primates declines to low levels characteristic of the prepubertal primate, and these levels are sustained throughout the juvenile period. In human and rhesus monkey males, the reactivation or reawakening of the hypothalamo–hypophyseal–gonadal axis is characterized by nocturnal increases in both LH and testosterone secretion. In rhesus monkey males, these nighttime increases in LH and testosterone are not unique, but rather similar to increases in these hormones observed during infancy and adulthood. The pubertal activation of the hypothalamo–hypophyseal system in the female is also characterized by nocturnal elevations in LH secretion, which in the human are sleep-related. During the pubertal phase of development, spontaneous preovulatory gonadotropin surges are first observed in females. These surges are owing to the positive feedback of estradiol acting to elicit the release of LH and FSH. However, absence of preovulatory-type surges of LH during the early pubertal period cannot be attributed entirely to failure of the ovaries to generate an adequate estrogen stimulus sufficient to provoke a release of gonadotropin. Thus, in the primate, changing sensitivity of the hypothalamo–hypophyseal system to the feedback action of estradiol may not be the explanation for onset of puberty.

6.4. The Gonadostat Hypothesis

No treatise on puberty would be complete without mentioning the gonadostat hypothesis. According to this hypothesis, at least in the case of the female, the hypothalamo–hypophyseal axis is initially supersensitive to the inhibitory feedback action of estradiol. During the peripubertal period, sensitivity to estradiol decreases, thereby allowing gonadotropin secretion to increase, and consequently, the ovary is stimulated to become functional. This hypothesis is best exemplified by the changing pattern of gonadotropin secretion from birth to puberty in the ewe lamb. However,

puberty in the rat and primate is not as easily explained by this hypothesis. For example, ovariectomy of the rhesus monkey during any phase of prepubertal development when gonadotropin secretion is diminished should result in immediate hypersecretion of LH and FSH, yet, this does not happen. Similarly, in female rats ovariectomized at different stages of prepubertal development and implanted with Silastic capsules containing estradiol, a very low concentration of estradiol was just as effective in suppressing serum gonadotropin levels regardless of stage of development even on the day of first proestrus. These data suggest no changes in sensitivity of the hypothalamo–pituitary system as the female rat matures to puberty. Hence, in the primate and rat, other factors must be involved other than simple gonadal hormone feedback to regulate neuroendocrine function for attainment of puberty.

6.5. Somatic Development

In virtually all species, the interval from birth to puberty is negatively correlated with body weight. Animals that grow at a faster rate to achieve a critical body weight will become pubertal at an earlier age. Obviously then, any condition that impairs the normal growth process for a particular species of animal, such as malnutrition, weight loss owing to physical exertion, or diseases will delay the onset of puberty. In ewe lambs whose growth is somewhat retarded, fasting can cause an almost immediate suppression of LH secretion, whereas caloric intake can have the opposite effect. Although various constituents of foodstuffs, such as amino acids and fatty acids, have been shown to alter gonadotropin secretion, no conclusive data have emerged implicating these biochemicals as being magic in promoting onset of puberty. Thus, the connection between somatic development and puberty remains a mystery still to be solved.

7. ENDOCRINOLOGY OF THE ESTROUS CYCLE

7.1. Patterns of Hormone Secretion

The sequences of neuroendocrine and gonadal hormones secreted during the course of the estrous or menstrual cycles of mammals are coordinated to promote successful reproduction of the species. Characteristics of the estrous cycle of a number of mammalian species are presented in Table 1. As can

Table 1
Characteristics of the Estrous Cycles of Some Mammals

Species	Duration of cycle, d	Duration of estrus, h	Time of ovulation relative to onset or end of estrus
Cow	19–23	13–18	10–12 h after end
Elephant	120	96	Not defined
Goat	21	30–40	30–36 h after beginning
Guinea pig	16–19	12	8–10 h after beginning
Hamster	4	24	8–12 h after beginning
Mare	19–25	96–192	24–48 h before end
Mouse	4	10	2–3 h after beginning
Pig	18–22	48–72	36–46 h after beginning
Rat	4–5	13–15	8–10 h after beginning
Sheep	15–17	24–48	24–30 h after beginning

be appreciated from these data, time of spontaneous ovulation occurs coincident with expression of behavioral estrus, thus ensuring that mating will occur when a viable ovum is available to be fertilized. In the primate, ovulation occurs midway in the menstrual cycle (duration of 28 d) and is not overtly associated with expression of mating behavior as occurs in other mammals. In contrast to the protracted follicular phase of the menstrual cycle, the follicular phase during the estrous cycle is of relatively short duration (1–3 d) and occurs during proestrus. The granulosa and theca cells of the ovulated follicle luteinize to form one or more corpora lutea, depending on whether the animal is monovular or polyovular. The formation and growth of the corpus luteum that occur during metestrus and diestrus, respectively, and the progesterone produced by this gland dictate, in part, the duration of the cycle. For most domestic and laboratory animals, duration of the estrous cycle is long compared to that of rats, mice, and hamsters, whose cycles are 4–5 d in duration. Hence, during the estrous cycles of rats and mice, in which no mating occurs, corpora lutea develop rapidly after ovulation, but produce little progesterone, and within 2–3 d the corpora lutea undergo functional regression. A typical pattern of hormone secretion that occurs during the estrous cycle of domestic animals is presented in Fig. 2.

7.1.1. FOLLICULOGENESIS

Ovulatory size follicles do not develop during the luteal phase of the primate menstrual cycle, but a cohort of growing follicles emerges during the early follicular phase. Towards the end of the follicular phase, only one follicle usually continues to become the ovulatory follicle, and the others undergo atresia. Although follicular development occurs during the luteal phase of the estrous cycle of pigs, no follicles attain ovulatory size. Similarly, during the luteal phase of the cycle of sheep, follicular development in polyovular ewes apparently occurs as a continuum, with no clear evidence for follicular dominance until corpora lutea regress. In contrast, in cows, waves of follicular development occur during the luteal phase of the cycle. Usually there are three waves of follicles that develop beginning on days 2, 9, and 16 of the cycle. Some animals have only two waves that begin developing on days 2 and 11. Each wave consists of three to six follicles. Duration of the luteal phase of the cycle appears to determine, at least in part, the number of follicular waves during the cycle. After several days, one follicle grows to near ovulatory size to become a dominant follicle, whereas the subordinate follicles regress. Eventually, the dominant follicle in each wave, except the last one, also regresses. In the last wave, the dominant follicle becomes the ovulatory follicle. Mares usually have one wave of follicular development that occurs during the midluteal phase of the cycle, but about one-third of the mares have two waves, one beginning shortly after ovulation and the other during the mid- to late luteal phase.

Recruitment of follicles is owing to secretion of FSH. For example, in rats, a secondary surge of FSH occurs on the day of estrus, just before the next cohort of ovulatory follicles is recruited. In the cow, there is

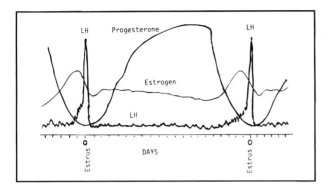

Fig. 2. Temporal patterns of pituitary and ovarian hormones secreted during the estrous cycle of domestic animals. Although variable among species, serum concentrations of progesterone and LH are in nanograms/mL, whereas those of estrogen are in picograms/mL.

not only a secondary surge of FSH on the day of ovulation (day 1) that precedes the first follicular wave of the cycle, but also slight increases in systemic FSH that precede the second and third follicular waves.

In most mammalian species, follicular estradiol synthesis requires the coordinated function of both follicular endocrine cell types and both LH and FSH: theca cells producing androgens in response to LH and granulosa cells aromatizing the androgens to estradiol in response to FSH and later in follicular development in response to both FSH and LH. Theca cells from dominant follicles secrete significantly more androgen, and granulosa cells possess a greater capacity to convert androgens to estradiol than follicular cells from subordinate follicles. Subordinate follicles destined for atresia usually are characterized by presence of follicular fluid containing high concentrations of androgens. The increased production of estradiol by the dominant preovulatory follicle(s) feeds back to the hypothalamo–pituitary axis to stimulate the pulsatile secretion of LH, which ultimately constitutes the ovulatory surge of this gonadotropin.

7.1.2. Corpus Luteum Characteristics

The mature corpus luteum varies in size depending on the species of mammal. In the rat, the corpus luteum weighs a few milligrams, whereas in the cow, one corpus luteum may weigh in excess of 5 g. Corpora lutea of the rat, cow, ewe, sow, monkey, and rabbit have been found to consist of two steroidogenic cell types referred to most commonly as small and large cells. This designation is based primarily on cell diameter along with distinguishing morphological

characteristics. Large luteal cells possess both rough and smooth endoplasmic reticulum, whereas small luteal cells possess only the smooth endoplasmic reticulum characteristic of steroidogenic cells. The major secretory product of the corpus luteum is progesterone, but in addition, this endocrine gland produces other steroids, the nature and quantity of which vary among the mammalian species. This variation in steroid secretory products indicates that differences do exist in the complexity of luteal steroidogenic pathways. Extremes in steroidogenesis are exemplified on the one hand by the bovine corpus luteum, which secretes progesterone, 20β-hydroxy-4-pregnen-3-one, and pregnenolone, and on the other hand, by the human corpus luteum, which secretes progesterone, 20α-hydroxy-4-pregnen-3-one, pregnenolone, 17β-hydroxyprogesterone, 4-androstenedione, estrone, and estradiol. In bovine and ovine corpora lutea, although large cells are fewer in number than small cells, they account for the majority of progesterone synthesized and secreted.

7.1.3. Luteotropins

Large and small luteal cells are endowed with LH receptors. Therefore, it is not surprising that LH is luteotropic during the estrous cycle of such species as the cow, ewe, mare, and primate. Tonic secretion of LH, which occurs during the cycle of these animals, is apparently able to sustain the maintenance and function of the corpus luteum until response to the gonadotropin is overridden by the endogenous luteolysin. Designation of this gonadotropin as a luteotropin is based on research demonstrating that exogenous LH prolongs luteal life-span, and by its ability to stimulate luteal progesterone synthesis in vivo and in vitro. Interestingly, stimulation of progesterone production in response to LH is based on its effect on small luteal cells. Large luteal cells, at least in the cow and ewe, are unresponsive to stimulation by LH, although, as mentioned above, these cells do possess LH receptors as well as adenylyl cyclase capable of being activated by forskolin and cholera toxin. Steroidogenesis in the large luteal cell appears to be "free running" until induced to undergo apoptosis.

Whether LH is luteotropic in the sow is debatable, because hypophysectomy shortly after onset of estrus allows ovulation and development of corpora lutea that are slightly smaller in size by days 13–14 of the cycle, but otherwise fully functional. However, an injection of hCG given to the sow near the midluteal

Table 2
Duration of Pseudopregnancy and Pregnancy in Select Mammals

Species	Type of ovulation	Duration of pseudopregnancy, d	Duration of pregnancy, d
Cat	Induced	30–40	65
Dog	Spontaneous	60[a]	58–63
Fox	Spontaneous	40–50[a]	52
Hamster	Spontaneous	7–13	16–19
Mink	Induced	Variable	Variable[b]
Mouse	Spontaneous	10–12	19
Rabbit	Induced	16–17	30–32
Rat	Spontaneous	12–14	22

[a]Pseudopregnancy follows even without copulation.
[b]Variable owing to delayed implantation; the duration, depending on time of mating during the breeding season.

phase of the cycle prolongs the functional life-span of the corpora lutea.

Some species of mammals that ovulate spontaneously and have relatively short estrous cycles will, on cervical stimulation at estrus resulting from an infertile mating or experimental manipulation, become pseudopregnant. Similarly, some mammals become pseudopregnant if ovulation is induced as a result of an infertile mating or if injected with LH or hCG. Characteristics of pseudopregnancy in a select group of spontaneous and induced ovulators are presented in Table 2. Corpora lutea of pseudopregnancy have unique requirements for luteotropic support. The rabbit is one species in which corpora lutea maintenance and function during pseudopregnancy, as well as during pregnancy are dependent on estrogen. In the Northern Hemisphere, mink, an induced ovulator, mate only in late February to March. The corpora lutea that form remain nonfunctional until after the vernal equinox when the lengthening hours of daylight to which the animal is exposed promote increased secretion of prolactin. This pituitary hormone serves as a luteotropin in mink, and activates the corpora lutea to begin producing large quantities of progesterone in the pseudopregnant or pregnant animal. In the pseudopregnant or pregnant rat, the stimulus of mating results in prolactin being secreted as two daily surges for the first 8 d and as a single nocturnal surge on day 9. Prolactin is luteotropic in the rat and also functions to suppress the activity of 20α-hydroxysteroid dehydrogenase, activation of which is associated with luteal regression in this

species. Pituitary LH is also luteotropic in the pseudopregnant and pregnant rat, and is required from days 8–12 for the synthesis of ovarian estrogen, the third luteotropic hormone. If the rat is pregnant, additional luteotropic support in the form of decidual and placental lactogens is provided throughout gestation. After day 12, hormones of the pituitary gland are no longer required. The placenta of the rat also synthesizes androgens, which are aromatized to estrogens by the corpora lutea.

7.1.4. LUTEAL PEPTIDE HORMONES

Oxytocin and the related peptide, vasopressin, are synthesized in the large luteal cells and granulosa cells in ovaries of humans, nonhuman primates, cattle, sheep, goats, and pigs. In cattle and sheep, the ovulatory surge of LH initiates oxytocin gene transcription and oxytocin synthesis and secretion by granulosa cells. After ovulation and luteinization of granulosa cells, mRNA for this nonapeptide continues to increase dramatically, attaining maximal luteal concentrations by about day 3 of the cycle. Thereafter, luteal concentrations of oxytocin mRNA decrease, whereas luteal concentrations of the hormone actually increase, reaching maximal levels by the midluteal phase of the estrous cycle and then gradually decreasing. Why oxytocin levels in the corpora lutea of domestic animals increase early in the cycle is not known. It has been suggested that oxytocin may serve as an autocrine or paracrine modulator of luteal cell function in the developing corpus luteum.

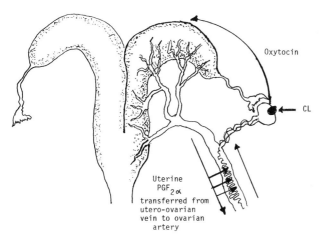

Fig. 3. PGF$_{2\alpha}$ secreted by the uterus is transferred from the utero-ovarian vein by a countercurrent mechanism to the ovarian artery. The action of this eicosanoid on the corpus luteum stimulates luteal secretion of oxytocin, which acts back on the uterus to stimulate additional pulsatile release of PGF$_{2\alpha}$. Successive pulsatile releases of PGF$_{2\alpha}$ cause luteal regression.

7.1.5. LUTEOLYSIS

It is well established that regression of the corpus luteum in most mammals is initiated by exposure of the gland to endogenous prostaglandin F$_{2\alpha}$ (PGF$_{2\alpha}$) synthesized and secreted by the uterus or the corpus luteum itself. In the cow and ewe, with two distinct uterine horns, the uterine vein draining each horn lies in close apposition to the ovarian artery. Regression of the corpus luteum in these species during the estrous cycle is the consequence of a functional inter-relationship between the ovary and adjacent uterine horn. At the end of the estrous cycle, uterine concentrations of oxytocin receptors are increased in the cow and ewe. Oxytocin, most probably of pituitary origin, binds to uterine oxytocin receptors to stimulate endometrial synthesis and secretion of PGF$_{2\alpha}$, which is transferred via a countercurrent mechanism from the uterine vein to the ovarian artery. This pulsatile release of PGF$_{2\alpha}$ acts on the corpus luteum to stimulate secretion of oxytocin, which acts back on the uterus to provoke another pulse of PGF$_{2\alpha}$ release. This double positive feedback system between the adjacent ovary and uterine horn (Fig. 3) ensures the generation of several pulsatile releases of PGF$_{2\alpha}$ that ultimately cause luteal regression. In species in which the anatomical arrangement of the vascular system precludes a local effect of the uterus on ovarian function, such as in the mare, the PGF$_{2\alpha}$ generated by the uterus must travel via the general systemic route to reach the ovary. In primates, it is believed that the corpus luteum brings about its own demise through synthesis of PGF$_{2\alpha}$.

SELECTED READINGS

Adkins-Regan E. Sex hormones and sexual orientation in animals. *Psychobiology* 1988; 16:335.

Brier BH, Gluckman PD. The regulation of postnatal growth: nutritional influences on endocrine pathways and function of the somatotrophic axis. *Livestock Prod Sci* 1991; 27:77.

Ford JJ, Klindt J. Sexual differentiation and the growth process. In: Campion DR, Hausman GJ, Martin RJ, eds. *Animal Growth Regulation*. New York: Plenum, 1989:317.

Fortune JE. Ovarian follicular growth and development in mammals. *Biol Reprod* 1994; 50:225.

Foster DL, Ebling FJP, Claypool LE, Wood RI. Photoperiodic timing of puberty in sheep. In: Reppert SM, ed. *Development of Circadian Rhythmicity and Photoperiodism in Mammals. Research in Perinatal Medicine (IX)*. Ithaca, NY: Perinatology, 1989:103

Geist V. *Mountain Sheep. A Study in Behavior and Evolution*. Chicago: University of Chicago Press, 1971.

Herbosa CG, Wood RI, Foster DL. Prenatal androgens modify the reproductive response to photoperiod in the developing sheep. *Biol Reprod* 1995; 52:163.

Keverne EB, Kendrick KM. Oxytocin facilitation of maternal behavior in sheep. In: Pederson CA, Caldwell JD, Jirikowski GF, Insel TR, eds. *Oxytocin in Maternal, Sexual, and Social Behaviors. Ann NY Acad Sci* 1992; 262:83.

Millard WJ. Central regulation of growth hormone secretion. In: Campion DR, Hausman GJ, Martin RJ, eds. *Animal Growth Regulation*. New York: Plenum, 1989:237.

Moore FL, Lowry CA, Rose JD. Steroid-neuropeptide interactions that control reproductive behaviors in an amphibian. *Psychoneuroendocrinology* 1994; 19:581.

Moore FL, Orchinik M, Lowry C. Functional studies of corticosterone receptors in neuronal membranes. *Receptor* 1994; 5:21.

Ojeda SR, Urbanski HF. Puberty in the rat. In: Knobil E, Neill JD, eds. *The Physiology of Reproduction*, 2nd ed., vol 2. New York: Raven, 1994:363.

Perkins A, Fitzgerald JA. Luteinizing hormone, testosterone, and behavioral response of male-oriented rams to estrous ewes and rams. *J Anim Sci* 1992; 70:1787.

Plant TM. Puberty in primates. In: Knobil E, Neill JD, eds. *The Physiology of Reproduction*, 2nd ed., vol 2. New York: Raven, 1994:453.

Resko JA, Perkins A, Roselli CE, Fitzgerald JA, Choate JVA, Stormshak F. Endocrine correlates of partner preference behavior in rams. *Biol Reprod* 1996; 55:120.

Stormshak F. Zelinski-Wooten MB, Abdelgadir SE. Comparative aspects of the regulation of corpus luteum function in various species. In: Mahesh VB, Dhindsa DS, Anderson E, Kalra SP, eds. *Regulation of Ovarian and Testicular Function. Advances in Experimental Medicine and Biology*. New York: Plenum, 1987:327.

Straus DS. Nutritional regulation of hormones and growth factors that control mammalian growth. *FASEB J* 1994; 8:6.

PART IV

HYPOTHALAMIC–PITUITARY

13 Hypothalamic Hormones
GnRH, TRH, GHRH, SRIF, CRH, and Dopamine

Constantine A. Stratakis, MD, DSc
and George P. Chrousos, MD

CONTENTS

INTRODUCTION
GNRH
TRH
GHRH
SRIF
CRH
DOPAMINE

1. INTRODUCTION

Alkmeon, a 6th century B.C. physiologist and philosopher, introduced the brain as the center of human thinking, organizer of the senses, and coordinator for survival. However, the need for a visible connection between the brain and the rest of the body to explain a rapid and effective way of communication that would maintain homeostasis led Aristotle to the erroneous conclusion that the heart was the central coordinating organ and blood the means of information transmission. In contemporary medicine, the two ancient concepts are integrated in the exciting field of neuroendocrinology. The traditional distinctions between neural (brain) and hormonal (blood) control have become blurred. Endocrine secretions are influenced directly or indirectly by the central nervous system (CNS), and many hormones influence brain function. The hypothalamic–pituitary unit is the mainstay of this nonstop, interactive, and highly efficient

connection between the two systems. Its function is mediated by hypothalamic-releasing or hypothalamic-inhibiting hormones, including gonadotropin-releasing hormone (GnRH), thyrotropin-releasing hormone (TRH), growth hormone-releasing hormone (GHRH), somatostatin (SRIF), corticotropin-releasing hormone (CRH), and the neurotransmitter dopamine.

2. GnRH

2.1. GnRH Protein and Its Structure

The existence of GnRH as a hypothalamic factor was demonstrated in 1960. Systemic injection of acid hypothalamic extracts released LH from rat anterior pituitaries. The structure of GnRH was elucidated in 1971. The decapeptide pyroGlu-His-Trp-Ser-Tyr-Gly-Leu-Arg-Pro-Gly-amide was named luteinizing hormone-releasing hormone (LHRH). This term has been supplanted by GnRH, since this peptide not only releases LH from the gonadotrophs, but also follicle-stimulating hormone (FSH). An FSH-specific hypothalamic-releasing hormone,

From: *Endocrinology: Basic and Clinical Principles* (P. M. Conn and S. Melmed, eds.), Humana Press Inc., Totowa, NJ.

however, may also exist and be similar to the LHRH/GnRH protein, explaining the difficulty researchers have met with its purification.

GnRH plays a pivotal role in reproduction. Phylogenetically, this protein has been a releasing factor for pituitary gonadotropins, since the appearance of vertebrates. The structures of its gene and encoded protein have been highly preserved. Only one form of GnRH has been identified in most placental mammals, but six additional highly homologous GnRH forms have been found in other more primitive vertebrates. Only three amino acids vary in these six molecules, which together with the mammalian protein (mGnRH) form a family of molecules with diversity of function, including stimulation of gonadotropin release, regulation of sexual behavior and placental secretion, immunostimulation, and possibly, mediation of olfactory stimuli. In the human brain, placenta, and other tissues, where the gene is expressed, GnRH protein is the same. In other species, however, several GnRH forms are expressed in the various tissues and have different functions. In amphibians, mGnRH releases gonadotropins from the pituitary, but another, nonmammalian GnRH is responsible for slow neurotransmission in sympathetic ganglia.

Marked diversification of function exists within the relatively small GnRH peptide. The residues at the amino (N) and carboxy (C)-termini appear to be primarily responsible for binding to the GnRH receptor, whereas release of LH and FSH depends on the presence of residues 1–4. These critical residues are conserved in evolution. In addition, residues 5, 7, and 8 form a structural unit, which is important for the biological activity of GnRH receptors. Thus, the functional unit formed by the side chains of His^2, Tyr^5, and Arg^8 is necessary for full biological activity of mGnRH. Substitution of the Arg residue reduces potency in releasing both LH and FSH, whereas replacement of the Leu^7 increases the potency for LH release, but does not alter that for FSH. Similar structure–function specificity is present in the remaining GnRH family members. The secondary structure of all GnRH peptides is highly conserved, too. A β-turn, formed by residues 5–8, creates a hairpin loop, which aligns the N- and C-termini of the GnRH molecule, and provides the active domain of the hormone.

2.2. GnRH Gene and Its Expression

GnRH is synthesized as part of a larger peptide, the prepro-GnRH precursor. The latter contains a signal sequence, immediately followed by the GnRH decapeptide, a processing sequence (Gly-Lys-Arg) necessary for amidation, and a 56 amino acid-long fragment, called GnRH-associated peptide, or GAP. Thus, the structure of prepro-GnRH is similar to that of many secreted proteins, in which the active sequence is coded along with a signal and processing sequences, and an "associated" peptide that is cleaved prior to secretion. GAP appears to coexist with GnRH in hypothalamic neurons, but its function remains elusive. Its sequence is considerably less preserved among species, and it does not appear to bind to specific receptors. GAP was initially thought to inhibit the secretion of prolactin (PRL), but this was not confirmed in vivo.

The human GnRH gene is located on the short arm of chromosome 8 (Table 1) and in all mammals, consists of four exons. The first exon encodes the 5′-untranslated region. The second exon encodes prepro-GnRH up to the first 11 amino acids of GAP. The third and fourth exons encode the remaining sequence of the GAP and the 3′-untranslated region. Interestingly, the opposite strand of DNA is also transcribed in the hypothalamus and the heart. The function of this transcript, named SH, is unknown, and may be involved in GnRH gene regulation. Despite the presence of many sequence changes between the GnRH genes of different species, the intron/exon boundaries have been preserved through evolution. The presence of highly homologous other GnRH forms in nonmammalian vertebrates suggests a common evolutionary process, that of the duplication of one common ancestor gene.

The expresion of the GnRH gene is subject to significant species- and tissue-specific regulation. One example is the alternative splicing of the first GnRH gene exon in the mammalian brain and placenta. The promoter region of the rat GnRH gene has been sequenced and studied extensively. Sequences that can bind transcription factors, such as Pit-1, Oct-1, and Tst-1, as well as estrogen and other steroid hormone response elements exist in the 5′-flanking region of the rat GnRH gene, suggesting a quite complex and extensive hormonal regulation of its expression.

2.3. GnRH Receptor

The first step in GnRH action is recognition of the hormone by a specific cell membrane receptor (GnRH-R). The latter was recently cloned from several species, including human. It is a member of the seven-transmembrane segment (TMS) class, charac-

Table 1
Hypothalamic Hormones: Genes, Pathophysiology, and Clinical Use

Hormone	Chromosome	Receptor	Associated disorders	Clinical use
GnRH	8p	GnRH-R	Kallman syndrome, precocious puberty, *hpg* mouse.	GnRH-test, GnRH superagonists and antagonists
TRH	3	TRH-R	"Hypothalamic" hypothyroidism	TRH test
GHRH	20p	GHRH-R	*lit*-mouse, *dw*-and *dwj*-mice, "hypo– thalamic" GH deficiency	GHRH test, GHRH– analogs and antagonists
SRIF	3q	SSTR-1–5	—	SRIF analogs
CRH	8q	CRH-R 1Δ, 1β CRH-R2	"Hypothalamic" adrenal insuf., chronic fatigue, fibromyalgia, atypical and melancholic depression, stress, autoimmune states	CRH test, CRH– analogs and antagonists
Dopamine		D-1R–D-5R (pituitary: D2-R)	Nonadenomatous hyperprolactinemia	D-2R agonists

teristic of G-protein-linked receptors. Several differences exist, however, between the GnRH-R and the other members of this superfamily of membrane proteins. The highly conserved Asp-Glu, which is essential for function and is found in the second TMS of many receptors, is replaced in the GnRH-R by Asp. In addition, the GnRH-R lacks a polar cytoplasmic C-terminal region, and has a novel phosphorylation site adjacent to the third TMS.

The concentration of GnRH-Rs in the pituitary gland is tightly regulated and changes with the physiologic state of the organism. During the estrous cycle of rats, hamsters, ewes, and cows, the maximum number of receptors is observed just prior to the preovulatory surge of LH; thereafter, the number decreases and may require several days to achieve proestrous levels. Ovariectomy increases the number of pituitary GnRH-Rs, whereas this number decreases significantly after exposure to androgens and during pregnancy and lactation. Several in vitro models employing pituitary cell cultures have indicated a biphasic response of GnRH-R to physiological concentrations of GnRH. An initial desensitization of gonadotropes to GnRH is associated with downregulation of the receptor. This phase is fol-

lowed by an upregulation of the receptor number, which, however, is not associated with increased sensitivity to GnRH, since gonadotropes respond with near-maximal LH release, when only 20% of available GnRH-Rs are occupied.

The regulation of GnRH-R gene expression and protein function by GnRH provides the basis for the effects of constant GnRH infusion or GnRH-superagonists on LH and FSH secretion. Whereas low or physiological concentrations of GnRH stimulate the synthesis of GnRH-R, constantly high concentrations of this hormone downregulate the receptor in a process that involves physical internalization of agonist-occupied receptors. This is accompanied by loss of a functional calcium channel and other mechanisms. Indeed, GnRH regulates pituitary LH and FSH synthesis and release by a Ca^{2+}-dependent mechanism involving GnRH-R-mediated phosphoinositide hydrolysis and protein kinase C (PKC) activation. A G-protein or multiple G-proteins coupled to GnRH-R also play(s) an intermediatary role. This protein appears to be different from G_s or G_i, and similar to that hypothesized to be involved in TRH mediation of action. Following GnRH stimulation, an increase in phospholipid metabolism and intracellular Ca^{2+} and accumulation of inositol phosphates occur in pituitary gonadotropes. Calmodulin and its dependent protein system are important intracellular mediators of the Ca^{2+} signal in the gonadotropes.

In addition to its action on the gonadotropes, GnRH exerts a variety of effects in the CNS. Lordosis and mounting behaviors are facilitated by intraventricular and subarachnoid administration of GnRH, or local infusion of this peptide in the rat hypothalamic ventromedial nucleus (VMN) and central gray. GnRH can change the firing patterns of many neurons and is present in presynaptic nerve terminals. These actions are mediated through the GnRH-R. The latter has been found to be widely distributed in the rat brain, in areas such as the hypothalamic VMN and arcuate nucleus (but not the preoptic region), the olfactory bulb and the nucleus olfactorius, the septum, and the amygdala and hippocampus. With few exceptions, the CNS GnRH-R binds to GnRH analogs with the same affinity that the pituitary GnRH-R does. However, the former may not share the same second messenger system(s) with the latter, since it is unclear whether Ca^{2+} is needed for hippocampal GnRH action. Aside from the CNS, the GnRH-R is present in the gonads (rat and human ovary, rat testis) and rat immune system. GnRH has also been demonstrated to stimulate the production of ovarian steroidogenesis from isolated rat ovaries. The physiologic significance of these actions, however, remains unclear.

2.4. GnRH-Secreting Neurons: Embryology and Expression

Almost all the GnRH in mammalian brains is present in the hypothalamus and regions of the limbic system, the hippocampus, cingulate cortex, and olfactory bulb. GnRH-expressing neurons migrate during development from their original place on the medial side of the olfactory placode into the forebrain. The GnRH neurons, which are generated by cells of the medial olfactory pit, do not have a GnRH secretory function before they attain their target sites in the basal forebrain. They do, however, express the GnRH gene, a feature that allowed their detection by *in situ* hybridization. In mice, these cells are first noted in the olfactory epithelium by day 11 of embryonic life. By days 12 and 13, they are seen migrating across the nasal septum toward the forebrain, arriving at the preoptic area of the developing hypothalamus by days 16–20. GnRH neuron migra-

tion is dependent on a neural cell adhesion molecule (NCAM), a cell-surface protein that mediates cell-to-cell adhesion, is expressed by cells surrounding the GnRH neurons, and appears to be a "guide" for their migration.

By immunocytochemistry, GnRH cell bodies are found scattered in their final destination, the preoptic area, among the fibers of the diagonal band of Broca and in the septum, with fibers projecting not only to to the median eminence, but also through the hypothalamus and midbrain. In primates, more anterior-placed cell bodies in the preoptic area and septum are connected with dorsally projecting fibers that enter extrahypothalamic pathways presumably involved in reproductive behavior, whereas more posteriorly placed cell bodies in the medial hypothalamus itself give rise to axons that terminate in the median eminence. The two types of GnRH neurons are also morphologically different, since the former have a smooth cytoplasmic contour, whereas the latter has "spiny" protrusions. Similar anatomical and functional plasticity has been documented at the level of the GnRH neuronal terminal.

GnRH may be present in other areas of the nervous system. In frogs, a GnRH-like peptide in sympathetic ganglia is thought to be an important neurotransmitter. GnRH can enhance or suppress the electrical activity of certain neurons in vitro. GnRH is also present in the placenta, where its mRNA was first isolated from. Interestingly, GnRH, like TRH, is secreted into milk.

2.5. GnRH Secretion and Action

Secretion of hypothalamic GnRH is required for reproductive function in all species of mammals studied. Its secretion is subject to regulation by many hormones and neurotransmitters that act on the endogenous GnRH secretory rhythm, the "GnRH pulse generator." The latter provides a GnRH pulse into the hypophyseal-portal vessels at approx 90 intervals, which can be slowed down or accelerated by gonadal hormones. Testosterone and progesterone in physiologic concentrations and hyperprolactinemia slow the discharge rate of the generator, whereas estrogens have no effect on the frequency of the GnRH pulses. Females of all species respond to estrogens with an acute increase of LH, and to a lesser degree, FSH, a phenomenon that explains the "ovulatory LH surge" via positive estrogen feedback on the pituitary.

The mechanism of the estrogen-induced LH release has yet to be elucidated. The presence of testicular tissue prevents the estrogen-stimulatory effect on GnRH and LH secretion, but testosterone, although it slows down the GnRH pacemaker, does not completely abolish the estrogen effect. Since estrogen releases LH in castrated male monkeys, a nontestosterone testicular hormone, other than inhibin, may be responsible for this blocking effect in males.

GnRH secretion responds to emotional stress, changes in light–dark cycle, and sexual stimuli through the inputs that GnRH neurons receive from the rest of the CNS. Norepinephrine stimulates LH release through the activation of α-adrenergic receptors, and administration of α-antagonists blocks ovulation. A population of β-adrenergic neurons, which are inhibitory to GnRH secretion, has also been identified. Dopamine has inhibitory effects, but the role of epinephrine, GABA, and serotonin is less clear. Acetylcholine may increase GnRH secretion, since it can induce estrous in the rat that is blocked by atropine. Glutamate stimulates GnRH secretion via the NMDA receptor. Naloxone can stimulate LH secretion in humans, but this effect is modulated by the hormonal milieu. Thus, administration of naloxone increases LH levels in the late follicular and luteal phases, but not in the early follicular phase or in postmenopausal women. It has been postulated that endogenous opioids may mediate the effects of gonadal steroids on GnRH secretion, since β-endorphin levels are markedly increased by estrogen and progesterone administration.

Disruption of reproductive function in mammals is a well-known consequence of stress. This effect is thought to be mediated through activation of both the central and peripheral stress system. CRH directly inhibits hypothalamic GnRH secretion via synaptic contacts between CRH axon terminals and dendrites of GnRH neurons in the medial preoptic area. The role of CRH regulation of GnRH secretion may be species-specific with important differences noted between rodents and primates. Endogenous opioids mediate some of these effects of CRH, but their importance varies with species, as well as with the period of the cycle and the gender of the animals. CNS cytokines also regulate GnRH secretion and function. Central injection of interleukin-1 (IL-1) inhibits GnRH neuronal activity and reduces GnRH synthesis and release. These effects are in part mediated through endogenous opioids and CNS prostaglandins. IL-1 and possibly other central cytokines may act as endogenous mediators of the inflammatory stress-induced inhibition of reproductive function.

2.6. Gonadotropin Deficiency— Kallmann Syndrome

A clinical syndrome of hypogonadism and anosmia affecting both men and women was described in 1943 by Kallman and associates. The pathologic documentation of the characteristic neuroanatomical defects of the syndrome led to the term "olfactory-genital dysplasia" for what is now known as "Kallman syndrome." With the discovery of GnRH in 1971, the defect was determined to be hypothalamic in all patients with the syndrome, who subsequently were shown to resume normal gonadotropin secretion after repeated and/or pulsatile administration of GnRH.

The genetic basis of Kallman syndrome, which has in most cases an X-linked inheritance, was recently elucidated at the molecular level. The earlier evidence that GnRH-secreting neurons migrate to the hypothalamus from the olfactory placode during development, combined with the observation that many patients with the X-linked form of ichthyosis that is caused by steroid sulfatase deficiency also had deafness and hypogonadotropic hypogonadism, led to identification of the *KAL* gene. The latter maps at chromosome Xp22.3, is contiguous to the steroid sulfatase gene, and codes for a protein that is homologous to the fibronectins, with an important role in neural chemotaxis and cell adhesion.

Since the identification of the *KAL* gene, several defects have been described in patients with Kallman syndrome. Contiguous gene deletions have been found in patients with other genetic defects, such as ichthyosis, blindness, and/or deafness, whereas smaller deletions of the *KAL* gene are found in patients with anosmia and GnRH deficiency. These patients also demonstrate cerebellar dysfunction, oculomotor abnormalities, and mirror movements. Mutations of the gene that cause only anosmia in some affected patients have been described, and recently, *KAL* gene defects were reported in a few patients with isolated gonadotropin deficiency.

Selective, idiopathic GnRH deficiency (IGD) is thought to be caused by various genetic defects that may include the GnRH gene itself. Patients with IGD and hereditary spherocytosis were recently described and are believed to have contiguous gene deletions involving the 8p11-p21.1 locus. In a murine model of hypogonadotropic hypogonadism (the *hpg* mouse), the defect was found to be caused by a deletion of the GnRH gene and was recently repaired by gene replacement therapy.

2.7. Clinical Uses of GnRH

GnRH and its long-acting agonist analogs are, respectively, used in the treatment of GnRH deficiency, including menstrual and fertility disorders in women and hypothalamic hypogonadism in both sexes, and the treatment of central precocious puberty (CPP) in both boys and girls. Soon after the pulsatile nature of gonadotropin secretion was characterized, the requirement for intermittent stimulation by GnRH to elicit physiologic pituitary responses was determined. This led to the development of long-acting GnRH analogs, which provide the means of medical castration not only in CPP, but in a variety of disorders, ranging from endometriosis to uterine leiomyomas and prostate cancer. GnRH antagonists are currently being developed for the treatment of hormone-dependent cancers, such as prostate cancer, and for potential use as a male contraceptive in combination with testosterone.

GnRH is also used in clinical testing for the identification of CPP in children and the diagnosis of GnRH deficiency in all age groups. The gonadotropin response to 100 μcg GnRH (intravenously [iv]) changes from an FSH-predominant response during the prepubertal years to an LH-predominant response during puberty. Significant gender differences exist in the peak hormonal values attained following GnRH stimulation, and the test is used in combination with other criteria for the establishment of the diagnosis of precocious puberty. The same test is used in adults with suspected central hypogonadism. The lack of LH and FSH response to 100 μcg GnRH iv is compatible with GnRH deficiency or pituitary hypogonadism, and repeated stimulation with GnRH may be needed to distinguish patients with Kallman syndrome or selective IGD. The GnRH stimulation test is particularly useful in testing the efficacy of medical castration by GnRH agonists.

3. TRH

3.1. Prepro-TRH and Its Structure

TRH was the first hypothalamic-releasing factor to be isolated in 1969. Its discovery was followed by

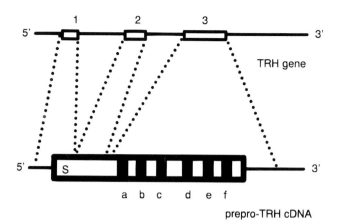

Fig. 1. Schematic representation of the human TRH gene and its encoded cDNA. Three exons (1, 2, and 3) code for a transcript that contains a signal peptide (S) and six potential copies (a–f) of the TRH tripeptide. This structure is highly preserved in evolution and is considered a model mechanism by which multiple copies of small peptides are produced from a single transcript.

the description of the GnRH, somatostatin, CRH, and GHRH, all in the early 1970s. TRH is a tripeptideamide (pGlu-His-Pro-NH$_2$), synthesized as part of a large prohormone termed prepro-TRH. The latter contains repeating sequences (Gln-His-Pro-Gly), the number of which varies from species to species. There are five of these repeats in the rat and six in the human preprohormone, and each can give rise to a TRH molecule after extensive posttranslational processing, which includes enzymatic cleavage of the prepro-TRH transcript, cyclization of the amino-terminal glutamic acid, and exchange of an amide for the carboxy-terminal glycine (Fig. 1). This structure, highly conserved in the mammalian genome, is considered a model of large production of small molecules from a single gene copy.

The human prepro-TRH gene is on chromosome 3, has three exons, and encodes a cDNA that extends 3.7 kb. Exon 1 encodes the 5′-untranslated region of the mRNA, exon 2 encodes the signal sequence and part of the amino-terminal peptide, and exon 3 codes for the six potential copies of TRH and the C-terminal peptide (Fig. 1). The rat prepro-TRH gene has a similar structure and size, but the exon 3 codes for only five potential copies of TRH. The human prepro-TRH protein is smaller than the rat (242 amino acids long compared to 255 in the rat) and has a 60% homology to the latter.

Analysis of the rat 5′-flanking sequences has revealed the presence of many regulatory sequences that underline the complex regulation and determine the tissue-specific expression of the gene. A glucocorticoid-responsive element and an SP-1 transcription factor-binding sequence are located 100–200 bp upstream, whereas closer to the start site are sequences that are imperfect copies of the cAMP regulatory element (CRE), and those that bind the triidothyronine receptor (c-*erb* A) and the AP-1 trancription factor. As is the case in other pluripotential prohormone proteins, the connecting sequences between the repeat TRH units in the prepro-TRH transcript have the potential to modulate the biologic activity of TRH and are involved in long-term storage of the uncleaved molecule.

3.2. TRH-Receptor

The pituitary TRH receptor (TRH-R) is a member of the seven-TMS–G-protein-coupled receptor family. The gene that codes for the human TRH-R is located on chromosome 8q23. It consists of two exons, and its coded peptide has 398 amino acids. Although highly homologous to the rat and mouse TRH-Rs, the human transcript has a distinct C-terminal. Arg-283 and Arg-306, in transmembrane helices 6 and 7, respectively, appear to be important for binding and activation. A binding pocket formed by the third TMS domain is also important for binding with TRH. Recently, two TRH-R cDNAs encoding for a long and a short isoform have been identified in the rat. Their regulation of expression and second messenger systems appears to be cell-specific. The exact pattern of their distribution in the brain and elsewhere has not been determined.

The evidence supports a central role for the phosphoinositol/Ca^{2+} system mediating TRH actions. Following binding to TRH, the TRH-R stimulates hydrolysis of the membrane lipid phosphatidylinositol 4,5-biphosphate to yield inositol 1,4,5-triphosphate and diacylglycerol. Both function as second messengers of the TRH-R and stimulate pKC. The response is Ca^{2+}-dependent and involves a G-protein as an intermediary. TRH stimulates a rapid, biphasic elevation of intracellular Ca^{2+}. The early phase is believed to come from intracellular Ca^{2+} stores and the sustained second phase from the influx of extracellular Ca^{2+} through voltage-dependent Ca^{2+} channels. A rapid translocation of pKC to the membrane has also been reported in response to TRH. As a result of TRH-R activation, a series of proteins are phosphorylated.

TRH does not appear to have a primary action on adenylate cyclase activity, despite the unequivocal evidence that cAMP stimulates thyroid-stimulating hormone (TSH) secretion from pituitary thyrotrophs. However, cAMP-induced TSH secretion may not be TRH-dependent. TRH action is exerted on the membrane and does not depend on internalization of the TRH-R, although the latter does take place. The TRH-R C-terminus is important for receptor-mediated endocytosis, a process that is clathrin-mediated and acidic pH-dependent.

The receptor is specific for TRH and does not bind to any other known peptides. Several TRH-analogs have been designed that bind to the TRH-R with high affinity and mimic TRH action. The receptor is widely distributed in the CNS and many nonneuronal tissues, but its second messenger systems in tissues other than the pituitary have not been elucidated. Rat TRH-R mRNA, indistinguishable from that of the pituitary thyrotrophs, is found in the hypothalamus, cerebrum, cerebellum, brainstem, spinal cord, and the retina. Extraneuronal sites include the immune system and the gonads.

3.3. TRH-Secreting Cells

In addition to anticipated regions of immunostaining for pro-TRH in the hypothalamus, immunoreactivity for this prohormone is detected in many other regions of the rat brain. The latter include the reticular nucleus of the thalamus, pyramidal cells of the hippocampus, cerebral cortex, the external plexiform layers of the olfactory bulb, sexually bimorphic nucleus of the preoptic area, anterior commissural nucleus, caudate-putamen nucleus, supraoptic nucleus, substantia nigra, pontine nuclei, the external cuneate nucleus, and dorsal motor nucleus of the vagus. TRH is also present in the pineal gland and the spinal cord. The extensive extrahypothalamic distribution of TRH, its localization in nerve endings, and the presence of TRH receptors in brain tissue suggest that TRH serves as a neurotransmitter or neuromodulator in many areas of the brain. There is also evidence that posttranslational processing of the prepro-TRH transcript is not identical throughout the CNS. In many areas of the rat brain, C- but not N-terminal extensions of TRH are found, indicating that the dibasic residues of the latter are subject to enhanced cleavage as compared to the former.

Differential processing of the prepro-TRH transcript amplifies the biological significance of its gene product, and is similar to that of other potent propeptides with wide distribution and array of action in the mammalian brain, such as the preproenkephalins (-A and -B) and propiomelanocortin (POMC).

In extraneuronal tissues, prepro-TRH mRNA that is identical to that of the hypothalamus is found in mammalian pancreas, normal thyroid tissue, and medullary thyroid carcinoma cell lines. In the rabbit prostate, a TRH-related peptide was found that is believed to be derived from a precursor distinct from the hypothalamic TRH prohormone. In nonmammals and as the phylogenetic scale is descended, TRH concentration in nonhypothalamic areas of the brain and extraneural tissues increases. TRH is present and functions solely as a neurotransmitter in primitive vertebrates that do not synthesize TSH. The peptide is also found in the skin of some species of frogs, which provides testimony to the common embryological origin of the brain and skin from the neuroectoderm.

3.4. Regulation of TRH Synthesis and Secretion

TSH secretion by the anterior pituitary thyrotrophs is characterized by a circadian rhythm with a maximum around midnight and a minimum in the late afternoon hours. Superimposed to the basic rhythm are smaller, ultradian TSH peaks occurring every 2–4 h. TRH appears to be responsible for the ultradian TSH release that is also regulated by somatostatin. Input from the suprachiasmatic nucleus and potentially other circadian pacemakers is required for this part of hypothalamic TRH secretion. Several other brain regions have been implicated in the regulation of TRH secretion, including the limbic system, the pineal gland, and CNS areas involved in the stress response.

Hypothyroidism, induced either pharmacologically or by thyroidectomy, increases the concentration of prepro-TRH mRNA at least twofold in the medial and periventricular parvocellular neurons of experimental animals. This response occurrs shortly after thyroxine (T4) falls to undetectable levels, and parallels the gradual rise in serum TSH. This response is not TSH-mediated, since hypophysectomy has no effect, whereas the administration of T4 completely prevents it and supraphysiologic doses of T4 cause an even further decline. Interestingly, the

increase of prepro-TRH mRNA levels in hypothyroid animals occurs over several weeks, whereas its decline following T4 administration is faster, occurring within 24 h. Because of the absence of Type II deiodinase in the paraventricular nucleus (PVN), the feedback regulation of prepro-TRH gene expression is mediated by circulating levels of free T3 rather than by intracellular conversion of T4 to T3. This serves to increase the sensitivity of TRH neurons to declining levels of thyroid hormone. The hypothalamic TRH neuron thus determines the set point of thyroid hormone feedback control.

The dramatic feedback effects of thyroid hormone on TRH synthesis appear to be limited to the TRH-synthesizing neurons of the hypothalamic PVN. In contrast to the medial and periventricular parvocellular PVN neurons, no increase in prepro-TRH mRNA was observed in the anterior parvocellular subdivision cells of hypothyroid animals, a hypothalamic region that is functionally diverse. Similarly, no change was detectable in any other TRH neuronal population in the hypothalamus or the thalamus. Thus, the nonhypophysiotropic TRH neurons of the CNS may not be subject to thyroid hormone control. Their function is regulated via a variety of neurotrasmitters, including catecholamines, other neuropeptides, and perhaps excitatory amino acids.

Catecholamines have an important regulatory role in the secretion of hyphothalamic TRH. The stimulation of ascending α_1-adrenergic neurons from the brainstem causes activation of hypothalamic TRH neurons, and norepinephrine induces TRH secretion in vitro. Dopamine inhibits TSH release and the administration of α-methyl-*p*-tyrosine, a tyrosine hydroxylase inhibitor, diminishes the cold-induced TSH release. The action of serotonin is unclear, since both stimulatory and inhibitory responses have been found.

Endogenous opioids inhibit TRH release and so does somatostatin, which inhibits TSH secretion as well. Glucocorticoids decrease hypothalamic prepro-TRH mRNA synthesis both directly and indirectly via somatostatin. However, in vitro studies have shown upregulation of the prepro-TRH transcript by dexamethasone in several cell lines. This discrepancy may be explained by the in vivo complexity of prepro-TRH gene regulation vs the deafferentiated in vitro system. Thus, even though the direct effect of glucocorticoids on hypothalamic TRH synthesis is stimulatory, the in vivo effect is normally overridden by inhibitory neuronal influences, such as those emanating from the hippocampus via the fornix.

3.5. Endocrine and Nonendocrine Actions of TRH

The iv administration of TRH in humans is followed by a robust increase in serum TSH and prolactin (PRL) levels. TRH is the primary determinant of TSH secretion by the pituitary thyrotrophs, but its physiologic role in prolactin secretion is unclear. PRL, but not TSH, is elevated in nursing women. The administration of anti-TRH antibody does not block the physiologic prolactin rise during pregnancy or suckling. On the other hand, the prolactin response to TRH is dose-dependent and suppressible by thyroid hormone pretreatment. Hyperprolactinemia and galactorrhea have been observed in primary hypothyroidism.

Normally, TRH does not stimulate secretion of other pituitary hormones. However, growth hormone release is stimulated by TRH administration in many subjects with acromegaly, occasionally in midpuberty, and in patients with renal failure, anorexia nervosa, and depression. TRH can also stimulate ACTH release by corticotropinomas in Cushing's disease and Nelson syndrome, and FSH and α subunit by pituitary gonadotropinomas and clinically nonfunctioning adenomas.

As a neurotransmitter, TRH has a general stimulant activity, with its most significant roles being thermoregulation and potentiation of noradrenergic and dopaminergic actions. Directly, TRH regulates temperature homeostasis, by stimulating the hypothalamic preoptic region, which is responsible for raising body temperarure in response to signals received from the skin and elsewhere in the brain. Indirectly, TRH elevates body temperature by activating thyroid gland function and regulating sympathetic nerve activity in the brainstem and spinal cord. TRH participates in the regulation of the animal stress response by increasing blood pressure and spontaneous motor activity. Other TRH actions include potentiation of NMDA receptor activation, by changing the electrical properties of NMDA neurons and alteration of human sleep patterns.

TRH appears to function as a neurotrophic factor in addition to being a neurotransmitter. Its administration in animals decreases the severity of spinal shock, and increases muscle tone and the intensity of spinal reflexes. Recently, TRH was found to play an important role in fetal extrathymic immune cell differentiation and, thus, appears to be involved in the neuroendocrine regulation of the immune system.

In the CNS, a TRH-degrading ectoenzyme (TRH-DE) degrades TRH to acid TRH and a cyclic dipeptide (cyclic His-Pro). The former has some of the TRH actions, but the latter may function as a separate neurotransmitter with its own distinct actions, such as increase of stereotypical and inhibition of eating behaviors. TRH-DE is regulated in a manner that is the mirror image of that of the TRH-R; thus, its mRNA levels are increased by thyroid hormone and decreased by antithyroid agents.

3.6. Clinical Uses of TRH

The oral, im, or iv administration of TRH stimulates the immediate secretion of TSH and PRL from the anterior pituitary. The maximal response is obtained after a 400-µcg TRH iv injection, but the most frequently administered dose is 200–250 µcg. The peak serum TSH concentration is achieved 20–30 min after the iv bolus of TRH, but in individuals with central (hypothalamic) hypothyroidism, this response is delayed and prolonged. In primary hypothyroidism, the TSH response to TRH stimulation is accentuated, and in patients with isolated TSH deficiency, TRH fails to elicit an increase in serum TSH, whereas the PRL response is normal. In thyrotoxicosis, because even minute amounts of supraphysiologic thyroid hormone suppress the hypothalamic–pituitary–thyroid axis, TSH responses to TRH are blunted. However, owing to the wide variation in TRH-induced increases in serum TSH levels in normal individuals, interpretation of the test is difficult, and the latter is seldomly necessary in clinical practice.

The most frequent use of TRH testing, prior to the advent of third-generation TSH assays, was in patients with mild or borderline thyrotoxicosis and equivocal levels of thyroid hormone. Another application of the TRH test was in the diagnosis of central hypothyroidism, caused by lesions of the hypothalamic–pituitary area. However, the loss of circadian TSH variation is a far more sensitive test than TRH stimulation for the diagnosis of secondary (central) hypothyroidism, and has replaced the latter in clinical practice. Currently, the TRH stimulation test is most useful in the differential diagnosis of TSH-secreting adenomas and thyroid resistance with determination of the plasma α subunit vs intact TSH concentration ratio. A ratio >1 suggests the presence of a TSH-secreting adenoma. The test is also useful in the identification of gonadotropinomas and clinically nonfunctioning pituitary adenomas, which respond to TRH with a FSH and/or glycoprotein α subunit predominant gonadotropin response, whereas normal individuals do not have a gonadotropin or α subunit response to TRH. The observation that acromegalic patients respond to TRH with an increase in their GH levels has been in clinical use as a diagnostic provocative test and as a way to monitor the therapeutic response of acromegalic patients to transsphenoidal surgery, pituitary radiation, or somatostatin analog treatment.

4. GHRH

4.1. The Prepro-GHRH Gene and Its Product

In contrast to GnRH and TRH, a deca- and tripeptide, respectively, GHRH is larger and exists in more than one isoforms in the human hypothalamus. The first evidence for an hypothalamic substance with growth hormone-releasing action became available in 1960, when it was shown that rat hypothalamic extracts could release GH from pituitary cells in vitro. It was not until 1980 that part of the peptide was purified from an nonhypothalamic tumor in a patient with acromegaly. Subsequently, three isoforms of the peptide were identified and sequenced from pancreatic islet cell adenomas with ectopic GHRH production. Two of the three isoforms were also present in human hypothalamus (GHRH-[1–44]NH$_2$ and GHRH[1–40]OH) and differ only by four amino acids at the C-terminus. GHRH-(1–44)NH$_2$ is the most abundant form and homologous to the GHRH of other species, but the shorter, 40 amino acid isoform has equipotent bioactivity and is physiologically important. The third form, GHRH(1–37)OH, has only been found in neuroendocrine tumors from acromegalic patients and is less potent in releasing GH. The shortest prepro-GHRH sequence with GH-releasing activity consists of the first 29 amino acids of the intact GHRH, whereas the GHRH(1–27) form has no biologic activity.

The human GHRH gene is on chromosome 20p12 (Table 1). It is 10-kb long and consists of five exons. The mRNA transcript is 750-bp long and generates one GHRH molecule, but exhibits heterogeneity owing to an alternative splice site present in the fifth exon. Like the other hypothalamic peptides, GHRH

is coded in a larger prohormone molecule. Prepro-GHRH contains a 30-residue signal peptide and the GHRH(1–44) sequence, followed by an amidation signal and a 30- or 31-residue C-terminus peptide (GCTP). The prepro-GHRH peptide undergoes extensive posttranslational processing during which the signal peptide is removed and the rest of the molecule is cleaved by endopeptidases to GHRH(1–45)-glycine and GCTP. GHR(1–45) is then converted to GHRH(1–44)NH$_2$ by peptidylglycine α-amidating monooxygenase. In the human hypothalamus, pituitary, extrahypothalamic brain, and several other normal and tumor tissues, endopeptidases convert GHRH(1–44)NH$_2$ to GHRH(1–40)OH, a form that is absent in other species studied to date.

The human prepro-GHRH transcript has been identified in hypothalamus, nonhypothalamic areas of the brain, testicular germ cells, and a variety of neuroendocrine tissues and tumors. The hypothalamic expression of the gene is primarily under the control of GH. Deficiency of the latter, caused by hypophysectomy or defects of the GH gene, is associated with increased GHRH mRNA steady-state levels. Conversely, GH treatment decreases the synthesis of GHRH. These effects are exerted directly on the GHRH-secreting neurons, since GH receptor mRNA has been colocalized with prepro-GHRH mRNA in many areas of the brain, including the hypothalamus and thalamus, septal region, hippocampus, dentate gyrus, and amygdala. Preliminary results also indicate an inhibitory effect of insulin-like growth factor-I (IGF-1) on prepro-GHRH mRNA.

Baseline GHRH mRNA levels are greater in hypothalami of male rats compared to hypothalami of female rats. This sexually bimorphic expression of the prepro-GHRH gene in the rat is significantly regulated by gonadal steroids. Administration of dihydrotestosterone to ovariectomized rats masculinizes their GH-secretion pattern and increases hypothalamic prepro-GHRH mRNA content. Conversely, administration of estrogens to male rats decreases GHRH synthesis, althought the latter is not a consistent finding. GH-feedback inhibition of GHRH synthesis appears to be sex-specific, also. In addition, after caloric deprivation of genetically obese and/or diabetic animal models, GHRH synthesis is decreased in a GH-independent fashion.

Tissue-specific regulation is exhibited by the prepro-GHRH gene in the mouse placenta. The transcript in this tissue contains a first exon which is approximately 8 to 12 kb upstream from the mouse hypothalamic first exon, indicating a different trascription start site. The human placenta does not contain the prepro-GHRH transcript. A GHRH-like mRNA and peptide have been detected in rat and human testes.

4.2. The GHRH Receptor

The GHRH receptor (GHRH-R) is a single 26-kDa protein that resembles the other members of the seven-TMS-domain G-protein-linked receptor family, although little information is currently available about its stucture and its tissue distribution. Recently, three transcriptional variants of the GHRH-R mRNA were identified in normal pituitary and in somatotropic adenomas. Form a is identical to the previously reported GHRH-R, whereas forms b and c are predicted to form truncated proteins and are the products of alternative splicing of the human GHRH-R gene.

The main action of the activated GHRH-R is GH release from the pituitary somatotrophs. Only partial occupancy of the hypothalamic GHRH-R is needed for maximal GH response. At least four intracellular second messenger systems are mediating the actions of the activated GHRH-R. The evidence that cAMP was involved in GHRH function preceded the isolation of this hormone by 15 years and was based on the GH-releasing effects of theophylline, a phosphodiesterase inhibitor, and of cAMP analogs. The activation of the receptor is followed by a marked and dose-dependent increase of adenylate cyclase activity and cAMP production in pituitary somatotropes. The occupied GHRH-R activates a stimulatory G-protein by catalyzing the binding of GTP to the G_s-α subunit. The latter, then, dissociates from the β-γ complex and activates the catalytic subunit of adenylate cyclase. Agents that increase intracellular cAMP levels, like cholera toxin and forskolin, stimulate GH release, mimicking activated GHRH action.

The activation of GHRH-R is followed by a rapid increase of intracellular Ca^{2+} levels. In the absence of extracellular Ca^{2+} or in the presence of Ca^{2+}-channel blockers or antagonists, GH secretion is greatly diminished or abolished. In the initial phase of the Ca^{2+} response, inositol triphosphate, produced after the activation of GHRH-R, stimulates the release of Ca^{2+} from the endoplasmic reticulum stores. During the second phase of Ca^{2+} increase, which is regulated primarily by cAMP- or Ca^{2+}-dependent protein kinases and/or inositol phosphate, net extracellular Ca^{2+} influx and efflux occur through Ca^{2+} channels

in the plasma membrane. Ca^{2+}-binding proteins, such as calmodulin, modulate many of the intracellular events that follow the activation of the GHRH-R.

Activation of the GHRH-R initiates the hydrolysis of phosphatidylinositol 4,5-biphosphate by phospholipase C through an intermediary G-binding protein (Gp). The products, 1,2-diacylglycerol and 1,4,5-inositol phosphate, serve as endogenous substrates for mobilization of intracellular Ca^{2+} stores and activation of pKC. Phorbol esters that activate pKC stimulate GH secretion in a dose-dependent manner. To the contrary, the addition of a pKC inhibitor or the depletion of pKC by prolonged exposure to phorbol ester did not affect GHR -stimulated GH release.

Additional factors that play a role in GHRH-R action are arachidonic acid and its metabolites. Prostaglandins E_1 and E_2 and prostacyclin markedly enhance GH secretion from rat somatotrophs in vitro. Lipoxygenase and epoxygenase metabolites of arachidonic acid inhibit and stimulate, respectively, GH secretion. These effects are specific, since they can be abolished by the respective antagonists, and appear to be mediated in part by cAMP. A novel peptide, the pituitary adenylate cyclase-activating polypeptide (PACAP), participates in GHRH-stimulated GH release. PACAP has its own receptor (PACAP-R), which in the rat has significant homology with the GHRH-R as well as with the secretin and glucagon receptors.

Regulation of the GHRH-R and/or its second messenger systems influences the sensitivity of the somatotrophs to GHRH. Prolonged exposure of pituitary cells to GHRH causes a time-dependent, reversible desensitization to this peptide and downregulation of the GHRH-R. Glucocorticoids increase the number and sensitivity of GHRH-binding sites in pituitary cells in vitro. The effect of gonadal steroids on GHRH-R synthesis and function is unclear. Starvation does not affect GHRH-R number or sensitivity, whereas aging decreases adenylate cyclase activity, despite the presence of increased levels of the enzyme.

4.3. GHRH Secretion

GHRH-containing nerve fibers arise from neurons of the ventromedial and arcuate nuclei of the hypothalamus. These neurons receive a variety of inputs from diverse areas of the CNS. Signals from sleep centers are excitatory and linked to the sleep cycle, whereas signals from the amygdala and ascending noradrenergic neurons from the brainstem are linked to activation

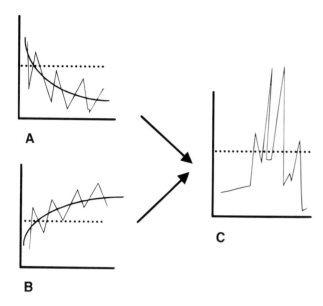

Fig. 2. Regulation of GH secretion: The theory proposed by Tannenbaum and Ling suggests that every secretory pulse of GH (panel **C**) is the product of a GHRH pulse (panel **B**) and a SRIF trough (panel **A**).

of the stress system and responsible for stress-induced GH release. The ventromedial nucleus integrates the secretion of glucoregulatory hormones and also influences GHRH release in response to hypoglycemia.

The secretion of GH is regulated by the excitatory GHRH and the inhibitory somatostatin (SRIF) (Fig. 2). Functional and anatomical reciprocal interactions exist between GHRH and SRIF neurons, in the ventromedial/arcuate and periventricular nuclei, respectively. Endogenous SRIF blocks GHRH release from the median eminence, whereas intracerebral administration of SRIF stimulates GHRH secretion from the specific neurons. The importance of SRIF in the regulation of GHRH secretion is demonstrated by the presence of high-affinity SRIF receptors in the GHRH neurons of the ventrolateral portion of the arcuate nucleus. Regulation by SRIF and the endogenous zeitgeber in the suprachiasmatic nucleus and elsewhere are responsible for the ultradian GHRH secretion. The latter, along with the tonic pulses of SRIF, define the GH-circadian release, which is synchronized with the sleep cycle.

Neuronal inputs to the GHRH-secreting neurons are transmitted via a variety of neurotransmitters. Sleep-induced GH release is mediated mainly by seretoninergic and cholinergic fibers. The spontaneous ultradian pulses of GH, caused by GHRH or transient inhibition of SRIF, can be blocked by α-antagonists or drugs that inhibit catecholamine biosynthesis. β_2-agonists stimulate GH secretion, presumably by inhibiting SRIF release. Anticholinergic substances block all GH-stimulatory responses, with the exception of that of hypoglycemia. L-Dopa and dopamine stimulate GH release in humans, though in vitro dopamine inhibits GH secretion by normal pituitary or somatotropinomas. It has been postulated that the in vivo stimulatory effect of L-Dopa and dopamine is owing to their local conversion to norepinephrine.

In addition to SRIF, many other CNS peptides interact with GHRH and affect GH secretion. Endogenous opiates, particularly β-endorphin, stimulate the GHRH neuron and induce GH release. Vasoactive intestinal peptide (VIP) and peptide histidine isoleucine (PHI) stimulate rat GH and PRL secretion. Since VIP and PHI do not bind to the GHRH-R, it is not clear whether these effects on GH secretion are mediated at the hypothalamic or the pituitary level, or both. In humans, VIP-induced GH secretion has been observed only in acromegaly. PACAP has been shown to stimulate GH release in rats in vitro; however, this action may not be specific, since it also enhances the secretion of PRL, ACTH, and LH. Central administration of TRH induces GH release by a Ca^{2+}-dependent, cAMP-independent mechanism that is modified by the presence of GHRH and is species-specific. In humans, TRH-induced GH secretion is observed only in acromegaly. Galanin, motilin, and NPY enhance GHRH-induced GH release from rat pituitary cells. NPY and a structurally similar hormone, the pancreatic polypeptide, have opposite effects on GH secretion, depending on the dose and the route of administration. A subset of GHRH neurons contain NPY, which appears to enhance GH secretion in vitro. After intracerebroventricular administration, however, NPY inhibits GH release, demonstrating additional function at the level of the GHRH or SRIF neuron. This may be via inhbition of ascending noradrenergic neurons from the brainstem, which normally stimulates GH secretion via GHRH.

4.4. Pathophysiology of GHRH Action

GHRH secretion and GHRH-R binding to its ligand in rodents are decreased with aging. The GH reponse to GHRH stimulation is similarly decreased in elderly humans. Studies in children with short stature have failed to demonstrate deficiency in either

GHRH synthesis or action, although GHRH-induced GH secretion may be augmented in young adults with idiopathic tall stature. The human prepro-GHRH gene was recently excluded as a cause for short stature in familial GH deficiency by linkage and single-strand conformation analysis. Nevertheless, mutations in this gene and those of the GHRH-R and its second messengers are still candidates for familial disorders of human growth. In support of the latter is a well-studied rodent model of GHRH deficiency. The GHRH-R of the *lit* mouse contains a missense mutation in the extracellular domain that disrupts receptor function. Another animal model, the *dw* rat, demonstrates a defect in the ability of GHRH-activated $G_S\alpha$ to stimulate adenylate cyclase, which results in low or undetectable GH levels. In contrast to the *dw* (Snell) and *dwJ* (Jackson) dwarf mice with similarly low GH levels, in which mutations are present in the Pit-1 pituitary transcription factor, the dw rat defect has not been elucidated. Recent studies have shown normal Pit-1 and GHRH mRNA levels, and a normal $G_S\alpha$ sequence, indicating that another or other proteins are responsible for this phenotype.

Hypersecretion of GHRH causes sustained GH secretion, somatotroph hyperplasia, and adenoma formation. A transgenic mouse expressing the human GHRH gene exhibits GH hypersecretion associated with somatotroph and lactotroph hyperplasia that eventually leads to adenoma formation. Indeed, approximately half of human GH-secreting tumors contain point mutations of the $G_S\alpha$ gene that interfere with the intrinsic GTPase activity of G_S and lead to constitutive activation. A similar pathophysiologic mechanism explains the presence of somatotropinomas in patients with McCune-Albright syndrome.

4.5. Clinical Uses of GHRH and Its Analogs

The GHRH stimulation test is rarely used in clinical practice because of the wide variability of GH responses in normal individuals. In the diagnosis of GH deficiency, pharmacologic agents, such as clonidine, arginine, and L-dopa, provide more sensitive and specific GH stimulation tests.

GH-releasing peptides (GHRPs) are oligopeptides with GH-releasing effects that bind to receptors different from the GHRH-R in the hypothalamus and elsewhere in the CNS. The original GHRP was a synthetic, met-enkephalin-derived hexapeptide (His-D-Trp-Ala-Trp-D-Phe-Lys-NH$_2$), which was a much more potent GH-secretagog than GHRH both in vivo

and in vitro. When administered in big doses, GHRPs enhance ACTH and PRL release from the pituitary, whereas in smaller doses and/or after prolonged oral administration, only GH is secreted. Recently, a peptide analog (hexarelin) has been shown to be a relatively specific and potent GH secretagog after oral administration in GH-deficient adults and children. Nonpeptide, equipotent analogs were subsequently synthesized that could be administered orally. Their use is still investigational.

5. SRIF

5.1. Somatostatin Gene and Protein

The first evidence for the existence of SRIF was provided in 1968, when hypothalamic extracts were shown to inhibit GH secretion from pituitary cells in vitro. A tetradecapeptide was isolated a few years later in parallel to the discovery of a factor in pancreatic islet extracts that inhibited insulin secretion. The term somatostatin was applied to the originally described cyclic peptide (S-14), but today it is used for other members of this family of proteins, which in mammals include the 28 amino acid form (S-28) and a fragment corresponding to the first 12 amino acids of S-28 (S-28[1–12]). S-14 contains two cysteine residues connected by a disulfide bond that is essential for biologic activity, as are residues 6–9, which are contained within its ring structure.

The mammalian SRIF gene is located on chromosome 3q28 (Table 1), spans a region of 1.2 kb, and contains two exons. The SRIF mRNA is 600 nucleotides in length, and codes for a 116 amino acid precursor, preprosomatostatin. Unlike GHRH, the sequence of the SRIF gene is highly conserved in evolution. Single-cell protozoan organisms have a somatostatin-like peptide, whereas the mammalian and one of the two anglerfish somatostatins are identical. A total of seven genes coding for the somatostatin family of peptides have been described in the animal kingdom. Posttranslational processing of preprosomatostatin by a number of peptidases/convertases is also conserved, and results in various molecular forms with some degree of functional specificity. S-14 is the predominant form in the brain, whereas S-28 predominates in the gastrointestinal tract, especially the colon. Somatostatin form specificity appears to be determined by the presence of different convertases in the various tissues and cell lines examined.

The 5′-untranslated region of the SRIF gene contains several cAMP and other nuclear transcription factor-responsive elements. GH administration increases SRIF mRNA levels in the hypothalamus, whereas GH deficiency doses not always cause a decrease in the level of SRIF gene expression. Glucocorticoids enhance hypothalamic somatostatin expression, but the effect may be indirect through the activation of β- adrenergic neurons. T3 also regulates brain somatostatin mRNA levels in vitro. Extensive SRIF gene tissue-specific regulation has been described, a necessary phenomenon for a gene that is so widely expressed and has so many functions.

5.2. Somatostatin Receptors

In 1992, five different somatostatin receptor genes (SSTR-1–5) were identified, which belong to the seven-TMS-domain receptor family. The tissue expression of these receptors matches with the distribution of the classic binding sites of somatostatin in the brain, pituitary, islet cells, and adrenals. The pituitary SRIF receptor appears to be SSTR-2, but other actions of the different forms of somatostatin have not yet been attributed to a single receptor subtype. The clinically useful somatostatin agonists (octreotide, lancreotide, and vapreotide) bind specifically to SSTR-2 and less to SSTR-3, and are inactive for SSTR-1 and SSTR-4.

All five SRIF receptors are expressed in rat brain and pituitary, whereas the exact distribution of the receptor subtypes is not known for the periphery. In the fetal pituitary, SSTR-4 is not expressed. SSTR-4 is coexpressed with SSTR-3 in cells of the rat brain, in the hippocampus, the subiculum, and layer IV of the cortex. SSTR-3 alone is expressed in the olfactory bulb, dentate gyrus, several metencephalic nuclei, and the cerebellum, whereas SSTR-4 is primarily in the amygdala, pyramidal hippocampus, and anterior olfactory nuclei. Human pituitary adenomas express multiple SSTR transcripts from all five genes, although SSTR-2 predominates. SSTR-5 mRNA, which has not been reported in other human tumors, is expressed in neoplastic pituitary tissues, including GH-secreting adenomas.

The main pituitary SRIF receptor, SSTR-2, demonstrates heterogeneity by alternative splicing. Two isoforms (SSTR-2A and SSTR-SB) have been identified, and their expression is subject to tissue-specific regulation. In human tumors, the predominant form is SSTR-2A. In the mouse brain, SSTR-2A was mainly present in the cortex, but both mRNAs were found in hippocampus, hypothalamus, striatum, mesencephalon, cerebellum, pituitary, and testis. The promoter region of the human SSTR-2 gene shares many characteristics with the promoters of other G-protein-coupled receptor-encoding genes, including a number of GC-rich regions, binding sites for several transcription factors, and the absence of coupled TATAA and CAAT sequences.

SRIF inhibits adenylate cyclase activity on binding to the SSTRs. The latter are coupled to the adenylate cyclase-inhibitory G-protein, G_i, which is activated in a manner similar to that for G_S. Additionally, SRIF induces a dose-dependent reduction in the basal intracellular Ca^{2+} levels. Ca^{2+} channel agonists abolish this effect, indicating that SRIF acts by reducing Ca^{2+} influx through voltage-sensitive channels. Voltage on either side of the cell membrane is altered via K^+ channels that are stimulated by SRIF, resulting in hyperpolarization of the cell and a decrease of the open Ca^{2+} channels. The role of the inositol phosphate-diacylglycerol-pKC and arachidonic acid-eicosanoid pathways in mediating SRIF action is uncertain.

Recently, evidence was presented that the widespread inhibitory actions of somatostatin may be mediated by its ability to inhibit the expression of the c-fos and c-jun genes. Interference with AP-1 effects results in inhibition of cellular proliferation, but this could be important for the control of tumor growth. It is not clear how the SSTRs mediate this action of somatostatin, but one way may be the stimulation of several protein phosphatases that inhibit AP-1 binding and transcriptional activity.

5.3. SRIF Secretion

Somatostatin-secreting cells, in contrast to GHRH-secreting cells, are widely dispersed throughout the CNS, the peripheral nervous system, tissues of neuroectodermal origin, the placenta, gastrointestinal tract, and immune system. Those neurons secreting SRIF and involved in GH regulation are present in the periventricular nuclei of the anterior hypothalamus. The axonal fibers sweep laterally and inferiorly to terminate in the outer layer of the median eminence. SRIF neurons are also present in the ventromedial and arcuate nuclei, where they contact GHRH-containing perikarya providing the anatomical basis for the concerted action of the two hormones on the pituitary somatotropes.

The secretory pattern of GH is dependent on the interaction between GHRH and SRIF at the level of the somatotroph (Fig. 2). Both hormones are required for pulsatile secretion of GH, since GHRH and/or SRIF antibodies can abolish spontaneous GH pulses in vivo. The manner by which the two proteins maintain GH secretion has been the subject of intense investigation for over two decades. The prevailing theory is that proposed by Tannenbaum and Ling, who suggested that GH pulses are the consequence of GHRH pulses together with troughs of SRIF release (Fig. 2). Additional factors, however, appear to contribute to this basic model of GH secretion, such as the regulation of the SSTRs, the IGFs (particularly IGF-1), other hypothalamic hormones (CRH and perhaps TRH), the glucocorticoids, and gonadal steroids.

GH stimulates SRIF secretion, and SRIF mRNA levels are increased by GH and/or IGF-1. Hypothalamic SRIF mRNA levels are decreased by gonadectomy in both male and female rats, whereas E_2 and testosterone reverse these changes in female and male rats, respectively. In humans GH-pulse frequency does not appear to be different in the two genders, but GH-trough levels are higher and peaks lower in women than men. Pulsatile GH secretion in the rat is diminished in states of altered nutrition (diabetes, obesity, deprivation). In vivo administration of SRIF antiserum restores GH secretion in food-deprived rats. During stress, CRH-mediated SRIF secretion provides the basis for inhibition of GH secretion observed in this state. TRH appears to stimulate SRIF release, whereas galanin increases hypothalamic SRIF secretion. Acetylcholine inhibits SRIF release and induces GHRH secretion. Similarly, the other neurotransmitter-mediated regulation of hypothalamic SRIF secretion mirrors that of the GHRH, although studying SRIF neurons has been proven to be a task of considerable difficulty, because of their multiple connections and widespread presence.

In the pituitary, SRIF inhibits GH and TSH secretion and occasionally that of ACTH and PRL. In the gastrointestinal tract, pancreas, and genitourinary tract, somatostatin inhibits gastrin, secretin, GIP, VIP, motilin, insulin, glucagon, and renin. These actions are the result of a combined endocrine, autocrine, and paracrine function of somatostatin, which is supported by its widespread gene expression and receptor distribution.

5.4. SRIF Analogs

In view of its ability to affect so many physiologic regulations, SRIF was expected to be of therapeutic value in clinical conditions associated with hyperactivity of endocrine and other systems. The finding that many tumors from neuroendocrine and other tissues expressed the SSTR subtypes raised these expectations, which, however, were hampered by the short half-life need for iv administration and nonspecific activity of the native peptide. These problems were recently overcome with the introduction of a number of SRIF analogs, which are more potent, have longer action and different activities than somatostatin, and do not require iv administration. The best-studied among these analogs is octreotide (D-Phe-Cys-Phe-D-Trp-Lys-Thr-Cys-Thr[ol]), which is currently used extensively in neuroendocrine tumor chemotherapy, the treatment of acromegaly, and for radioisotopic detection of these and other neoplasms.

6. CRH

6.1. CRH Gene and PreproCRH

The idea that the hypothalamus controlled pituitary corticotropin (ACTH) secretion was first suggested in the late 1940s, whereas experimental support for the existence of a hypothalamic CRH that regulates the hypothalamic–pituitary–adrenal (HPA) axis was obtained in 1955. In 1981, the sequence of a 41 amino acid peptide from ovine hypothalami, designated CRH, was reported. This peptide showed greater ACTH releasing potency in vitro and in vivo than any other previously identified endogenous or synthetic peptide.

CRH is synthesized as part of a prohormone. It is processed enzymatically and undergoes enzymatic modification to the amidated form ($CRH[1–41]NH_2$). Mammalian CRH has homologies with nonmammalian vertebrate peptides xCRH and sauvagine in amphibia (from frog brain/spleen and skin, respectively, and urotensin-I in teleost fish. It also has homologies with the two diuretic peptides Mas-DPI and Mas-DPII from the tobacco hornworm *Manduca sexta*. The vertebrate homologs have been tested and found to possess potent mammalian and fish pituitary ACTH-releasing activity. In addition, they decrease peripheral vascular resistance and cause hypotension when injected into mammals.

The N-terminal of CRH is not essential for binding to the receptor, whereas absence of the C-terminal amide abolishes specific CRH binding to its target cells. Oxidation of a methionine residue abolishes the biological activity of CRH, and this may be a mechanism for neutralization of the peptide in vivo. CRH bioavailability is also regulated by binding to CRH-binding protein (CRHBP), with which it partially colocalizes in the rat CNS and other tissues. CHBP is present in the circulation, where it determines the bioavailability of CRH. In the CNS, CRHBP plays a role analogous to that of enzymes and transporters that decrease the synaptic concentration of neurotransmitters by either breaking it down (acetylcholinesterase) or by taking it up at the presynaptic site (dopamine, serotonine).

The CRH gene is expressed widely in mammalian tissues, including the hypothalamus, brain and peripheral nervous system, lung, liver, gastrointestinal tract, immune cells and organs, gonads, and placenta. The biological roles of extraneural CRH have not yet been fully elucidated, although it is likely that it might participate in the auto/paracrine regulation of opioid production and analgesia, and that it may modulate immune/inflammatory responses and gonadal function.

The human CRH gene has been mapped to chromosome 8 (8q13) (Table 1). It consists of two exons. The 3′-untranslated region of the hCRH gene contains several polyadenylation sites, which may be utilized differentially in a potentially tissue-specific manner. CRH mRNA polyA-tail length is regulated by phorbol esters in the human hepatoma CRH-expressing cell line NPLC, and this may have potential relevance for differential stability of CRH mRNA in various tissues in vivo. Alignment of the human, rat, and ovine CRH gene sequences has allowed the comparison of the relative degree of evolutionary conservation of their various segments. These comparisons revealed that the 330-bp-long proximal segment of the 5′-flanking region of the hCRH gene had the highest degree of homology (94%), suggesting that it may play a very important role in CRH gene regulation throughout phylogeny. A conserved polypurine sequence feature of unknown biological significance is present at –829 of hCRH (–801 of the ovine CRH gene) as well as in the –400 bp 5′-flanking region of POMC, rat GH, and other hormone genes. A segment at position 2213–2580 of the 5′-flanking region of the hCRH gene has > 80% homology to members of the type-O family of repetitive elements, and another at –2835

to –2972 has homology to the 3′-terminal half of the Alu I family of repetitive elements.

CRH regulation by the protein kinase A (pKA) pathway is well documented. Administration of cAMP increases CRH secretion from perfused rat hypothalami, and forskolin, an activator of adenylate cyclase, increases CRH secretion and CRH mRNA levels in primary cultures of rat hypothalamic cells. Regulation of the hCRH gene by cAMP has also been demonstrated in the mouse tumorous anterior pituitary cell line AtT-20, stably or transiently transfected with the hCRH gene. The hCRH 5′-flanking sequence contains a perfect consensus CRE element that is conserved in the rat and sheep.

TPA, an activator of pKC and ligand of the TPA-response element (TPE) that mediates epidermal growth factor (EGF) function and binds AP-1, stimulates CRH mRNA levels and peptide secretion in vitro. TPA also increases CRH mRNA levels by almost 16-fold and CRH mRNA poly-A tail length by about 100 nucleotides in the human hepatoma cell line NPLC. The proximal 0.9 kb 5′-flanking the hCRH gene confers, TPA inducibility to a CAT reporter in transient expression assays. In the absence of a clearly discernible perfect TRE in this region, it has been suggested that the CRE of the CRH promoter may, under certain conditions, elicit TRE-like responses, thus conferring TPA responsivity to the CRE site. Further upstream into the 5′-flanking region of the hCRH gene, eight perfect consensus AP-1-binding sites have been detected. Their ability to mediate TPA-directed enhancement of hCRH gene expression has not yet been tested by conventional reporter gene assays. EGF, however, has been shown to stimulate ACTH secretion in the primate and to stimulate directly CRH secretion by rat hypothalami in vitro.

Glucocorticoids play a key regulatory role in the biosynthesis and release of CRH. They downregulate rat and ovine hypothalamic CRH content. However, adrenalectomy and dexamethasone administration in the rat elicits differential CRH mRNA responses in the PVN and the cerebral cortex, respectively, stimulating and suppressing it in the former, but not influencing it in the latter. Glucocorticoids can also stimulate hCRH gene expression in other tissues, such as the human placenta and the central nucleus of the amygdala. A construct containing the proximal 900 bp of the 5′-flanking region of the hCRH gene was found to confer negative and positive glucocorticoid effects, depending on the coexpression of a glucocorticoid receptor-containing plasmid. The molecular mechanism by which glucocorticoids regulate hCRH gene expression is somewhat obscure. Suppression might be mediated by the inhibitory interaction of the activated GR with the *c-jun* component of the AP-1 complex. On the other hand, glucocorticoid enhancement of hCRH gene expression might be mediated by the potentially active half-perfect glucocorticoid-responsive elements (GREs) present in the 5'-flanking region of the gene, since half-GREs have been shown to confer delayed secondary glucocorticoid responses in other genes.

Gonadal steroids may modulate hGRH gene expression. Human female hypothalami have higher CRH content than the male ones. E_2 stimulates rat PVN CRH mRNA levels. A bidirectional interaction between the HPA and gonadal axes has been suggested on the basis of hCRH gene responsiveness to gonadal hormones. A direct E_2 enhancement of the CAT reporter was found by using two overlapping hCRH 5'-flanking region-driven constructs. Furthermore, the two perfect half-palindromic estrogen-responsive elements (EREs) present in the common area of both CRH constructs bound specifically to a synthetic peptide spanning the DNA-binding domain of the human estrogen receptor, suggesting that hCRH gene is under direct E_2 regulation.

Tissue-specific regulation of hCRH gene expression has been suggested for the human decidua and placenta. In rodents, such regulation was absent, which probably accounts for the differences in placental CRH expression between these species and primates. Differential distribution of short and long hCRH mRNA transcripts has been detected in several tissues and under varying physiological conditions. Tissue-specific and/or stress-dependent differential utilization of the two hCRH promoters may explain these observations. Differential mRNA stability would then be a particularly important feature in CRH homeostasis, primarily in conditions of chronic stress, since in the latter case, sustained production of CRH would be required, and the long stable mRNAs produced by activation of the distal promoter would be beneficial to the organism.

6.2. CRH Receptors

In the pituitary, CRH acts by binding to membrane receptors (CRH-R) on corticotrophs, which couple to guanine nucleotide-binding proteins and stimulate the release of ACTH in the presence of Ca^{2+} by a cAMP-dependent mechanism. CRH stimulation of cAMP production increases in parallel with the secretion of ACTH in rat pituitary corticotrophs and human corticotroph cells. In addition to enhancing the secretion of ACTH, CRH also stimulates the *de novo* biosynthesis of POMC. CRH regulation of POMC gene expression in mouse AtT-20 cells involves the induction of *c-fos* expression by cAMP and Ca^{2+}-dependent mechanisms.

Sequence analysis of hCRH-R cDNAs isolated from cDNA libraries prepared from human corticotropinoma or total human brain mRNA revealed homology to the G-protein-coupled receptor superfamily. The hCRH-R cDNA sequences of the tumor and normal brain were aligned and found to be identical. The hCRH-R gene has been assigned to 17q12-qter. Human/rodent CRH-R protein sequences differ primarily in their extracellular domains. In particular, positively charged arginine amino acids are present in the third and fourth positions of the extracellular amino-terminal domain sequences of the rodent, but not the hCRH-R peptide. This might be responsible for the differential activity of the α-helical 9–41 CRH antagonist between rodents and primates.

Central sites of CRH-R expression include the hypothalamus, the cerebral cortex, the limbic system, the cerebellum, and the spinal cord, consistent with the broad range of neural effects of icv-administered CRH, including arousal, increase of sympathetic system activity, elevations in systemic blood pressure, tachycardia, suppression of the hypothalamic component of gonadotropin regulation (GnRH), suppression of growth, and inhibition of feeding and sexual behaviors characteristic of emotional and physical stress.

A splice variant of the hypothalamic hCRH-R, referred to as hCRH-R1A$_2$, was identified in a human Cushing's disease (CD) tumor cDNA library, in which 29 amino acids were inserted into the first intracellular loop. This protein has a pattern of distribution similar to the hypothalamic hCRH-R (hCRH-R1A). A different CRH-R, designated CRH-R2, was recently cloned from a mouse heart cDNA library. It is expressed in the heart, epididymis, brain, and gastrointestinal tract, and has its own splice variant expressed in the hypothalamus. The pattern of expression of the CRH-R2 protein differs from that of CRH-R1A, but its functional significance is currently unknown. Apparently, both rodents and humans express the CRH-R2 type.

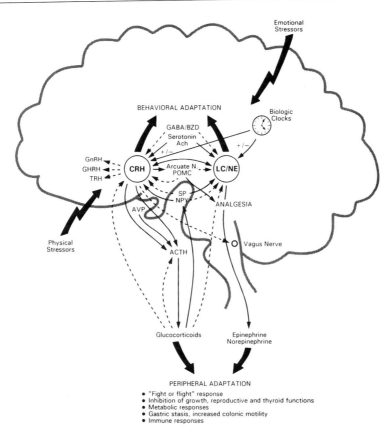

Fig. 3. A simplified representation of the central and peripheral components of the stress system, their functional interrelations, and their relations to other CNS systems involved in the stress response. Solid lines represent direct or indirect activation, and dashed lines represent direct or indirect inhibition. (Abbreviations: Ach = acetylcholine, ACTH = corticotropin, AVP = vasopressin, Arcuate N = arcuate nucleus, RH = corticotropin-releasing hormone, GABA/BZD = γ-aminobutyric acid/benzodiazepine receptor system, GHRH = growth hormone-releasing hormone, GnRH = gonadotropin-releasing hormone, LC = locus cerulus, NE = norepinephrine, NPY = neuropeptide Y, PAF = platelet-activating factor, POMC = propiomelanocortin, SP = substance P, TRH = thyrotropin-releasing hormone).

6.3. CRH Neurons: Regulation and the Central Stress System

CRH is the primary hormonal regulator of the body's stress response. Exciting information collected from anatomic, pharmacologic, and behavioral studies in the past 14 years has suggested a broader role for CRH in coordinating the stress response than had been suspected previously (Fig. 3). The presence of CRH and CRH-R in many extrahypothalamic sites of the brain, including parts of the limbic system and the central arousal-sympathetic systems in the brainstem and spinal cord provide the basis for this role. Central administration of CRH was shown to set into motion the coordinated series of physiologic and behavioral responses, which included activation of the pituitary–adrenal axis and the sympathetic nervous system, enhanced arousal, suppression of feeding and sexual behaviors, hypothalamic hypogonadism, and changes in motor activity, all characteristics of stress behaviors. Factors other than CRH also exert major regulatory influences on the corticotrophs.

It appears that there is a reciprocal positive interaction between CRH and vasopressin (AVP) at the level of the hypothalamic–pituitary unit. Thus, AVP stimulates CRH secretion, whereas CRH causes AVP secretion in vitro. In nonstressful situations, both CRH and AVP are secreted in the portal system in a pulsatile fashion, with approx 80% concordancy of the pulses. During stress, the amplitude of the pulsation increases, whereas if the magnocellular AVP-secreting neurons are involved, continuous elevations of plasma AVP concentrations are seen.

Both CRH and AVP are released following stimulation with catecholamines. Indeed, the two components of the stress system in the brain, the CRH/AVP and the locus cerulus/noradrenergic (LC/NE) neurons, are tightly connected, and regulated in parallel by mostly the same factors. Reciprocal neural connections exist between the CRH and noradrenergic neurons, and there are autoregulatory ultrashort negative-feedback loops on the CRH neurons exerted by CRH and on the catecholaminergic neurons exerted by NE via collateral fibers and presynaptic receptors. Both CRH and noradrenergic neurons are stimulated by serotonin and acetylcholine, and inhibited by glucocorticoids, by the γ-aminobutyric acid (GABA)/benzodiazepine (BZD) receptor system and by POMC-derived peptides (ACTH, α-MSH, β-endorphin) or other opioid peptides, such as dynorphin. Administration (icv) of NE acutely increases CRH, AVP, and ACTH concentrations, whereas NE does not affect pituitary ACTH secretion. Thus, catecholamines act mainly on suprahypophyseal brain sites and increase CRH and AVP release.

Activation of the stress system stimulates hypothalamic POMC-peptide secretion, which reciprocally inhibits the activity of the stress system and, in addition, through projections to the hindbrain and spinal cord, produces analgesia. CRH and AVP neurons cosecrete dynorphin, a potent endogenous opioid derived from the cleavage of prodynorphin, which acts oppositely at the target cells. NPY- and substance P (SP)-secreting neurons also participate in the regulation of the central stress system by resetting the activity of the CRH and AVP neurons. Activation of the central NPY system overrides the glucocorticoid negative feedback exercised at hypothalamic and other suprahypophyseal areas, since icv administration of NPY causes sustained hypersecretion of CRH and AVP, despite high plasma cortisol levels. NPY on the other hand suppresses the LC/NE sympathetic system through central actions on these neurons. The importance of NPY lies into the fact that it is the most potent appetite stimulant known in the organism and may be involved in the regulation of the HPA axis in malnutrition, anorexia nervosa, and obesity. SP is an 11 amino acid peptide that belongs to the tachykinin family, together with neurokinins-A and B. SP is present in the median eminence and elsewhere in the central and peripheral nervous systems. In the hypothalamus, it exerts negative effects on the CRH neurons, whereas it regulates positively

the LC/NE neurons of the brainstem. SP plays a major role in the neurotransmission of pain and may be involved in the regulation of the HPA axis in chronic inflammatory or infectious states. NPY, somatostatin, and galanin are colocalized in noradrenergic vasoconstrictive neurons, whereas VIP and SP are colocalized in cholinergic neurons.

CRH neurons may be affected during stress by other factors, such as angiotensin-II, the inflammatory cytokines, and lipid mediators of inflammation. The latter two are particularly important, since they may account for the activation of the HPA axis observed during the stress of inflammation. In the human, interleukin-6 (IL-6) is an extremely potent stimulus of the HPA axis. The elevations of ACTH and cortisol attained by IL-6 are well above those observed with maximal stimulatory doses of CRH, suggesting that parvocellular AVP and other ACTH secretagogs are also stimulated by this cytokine. In a dose–response, maximal levels of ACTH are seen at doses at which no peripheral AVP levels are increased. At higher doses, however, IL-6 stimulates peripheral elevations of AVP, indicating that this cytokine is also able to activate magnocellular AVP-secreting neurons. The route of access of the inflammatory cytokines to the central CRH and AVP-secreting neurons is not clear, given that the cellular bodies of both are protected by the blood–brain barrier. It has been suggested that they may act on nerve terminals of these neurons at the median eminence through the fenestrated endothelia of this circumventricular organ. Other possibilities include stimulation of intermediate neurons located in the organum vasculosum of the lamina terminalis, another circumventricular organ. In addition, crossing the blood–brain barrier with the help of a specific transport system has not been excluded. Also, and quite likely, each of these cytokines might initiate a cascade of paracrine and autocrine events with sequential secretion of local mediators of inflammation by nonfenestrated endothelial cells, glial cells, and/or cytokinergic neurons, finally causing activation of CRH and AVP-secreting neurons.

In addition to setting the level of arousal and influencing the vital signs, the stress system also interacts with two other major CNS elements, the mesocorticolimbic dopaminergic system and the amygdala/hippocampus. Both of these are activated during stress and, in turn, influence the activity of the stress system. Both the mesocortical and mesolimbic components of the dopaminergic system are innervated by the LC/NE sympathetic system and are activated during stress. The mesocortical system contains neurons whose bodies are in the ventral tegmentum, and whose projections terminate in the prefrontal cortex and are thought to be involved in anticipatory phenomena and cognitive functions. The mesolimbic system, which also consists of neurons of the ventral tegmentum that innervate the nucleus accumbens, is believed to play a principal role in motivational/reinforcement/reward phenomena.

The amygdala/hippocampus complex is activated during stress primarily by ascending catecholaminergic neurons originating in the brainstem or by inner emotional stressors, such as conditioned fear, possibly from cortical association areas. Activation of the amygdala is important for retrieval and emotional analysis of relevant information for any given stressor. In response to emotional stressors, the amygdala can directly stimulate both central components of the stress system as well as the mesocorticolimbic dopaminergic system. Interestingly, there are CRH peptidergic neurons in the central nucleus of the amygdala that respond positively to glucocorticoids and whose activation leads to anxiety. The hippocampus exerts important, primarily inhibitory influences on the activity of the amygdala, as well as on the PVN/CRH and LC/NE sympathetic systems.

6.4. CRH Secretion and Pathophysiology

ACTH, a 39 amino acid peptide-proteolytic product of POMC, is the key effector of CRH action, as a regulator of glucocorticoid secretion by the adrenal cortex. The regulatory influence of CRH on pituitary ACTH secretion varies diurnally and changes during stress. The highest plasma ACTH concentrations are found at 6 AM to 8 AM, and the lowest concentrations are seen around midnight with episodic bursts of secretion appearing throughout the day. The mechanisms responsible for the circadian release of CRH, AVP, and ACTH are not completely understood, but appear to be controlled by one or more pacemakers, including the suprachiasmatic nucleus. The diurnal variation of ACTH secretion is disrupted if a stressor is imposed and/or changes occur in zeitgebers, e.g., lighting and activity. These changes affect CRH secretion, which in turn regulates ACTH responses.

Glucocorticoids are the final effectors of the HPA axis and participate in the control of whole-body homeostasis and the organism's response to stress. They play a key regulatory role in CRH secretion and

the basal activity of the HPA axis, and in the termination of the stress response by exerting negative feedback at the CNS components of the stress system. The other component of the peripheral stress system is the systemic sympathetic and adrenomedullary divisions of the ANS. It widely innervates vascular smooth muscle cells, as well as the adipose tissue and the kidney, gut, and many other organs. In addition to acetylcholine, norepinephrine, and epinephrine, both the sympathetic and the parasympathetic divisions of the ANS secrete a variety of neuropeptides, including CRH itself.

Several states seem to represent dysregulation of the generalized stress response, normally regulated by the CRH neurons and the stress system. In melancholic depression, the cardinal symptoms are the hyperarousal (anxiety) and suppression of feeding and sexual behaviors (anorexia, loss of libido), and excessive and prolonged redirection of energy (tachycardia, hypertension), all of which are extremes of the classic manifestations of the stress reaction. Both the HPA axis and the sympathetic system are chronically activated in melancholic depression. In a postmortem study, depressed individuals were found to have a three- to four-fold increase in the number of their hypothalamic PVN CRH neurons, when compared to normal age-matched controls. This could be an inherent feature of melancholic depression or a result of the chronic, although intermittent hyperactivity of the HPA axis that is known to occur in these patients.

Chronic activation of the HPA axis has been shown also in a host of other conditions, such as anorexia nervosa, panic anxiety, obsessive-compulsive disorder, chronic active alcoholism, alcohol and narcotic withdrawal, excessive exercising, malnutrition, and more recently, in sexually abused girls. Animal data are rather confirmatory of the association of chronic activation of the HPA axis and affective disorders. Traumatic separation of infant rhesus monkeys and laboratory rats from their mothers causes behavioral agitation and elevated plasma ACTH and cortisol responses to stress that are sustained later in life. Such activation of the CRH system was originally thought to be an epiphenomenon, as a result of stress. Administration of CRH to experimental animals, however, with its profound effect on totally reproducing the stress response suggested that CRH is a major participant in the initiation and/or propagation of a vicious cycle.

Interaction of CRH with the other hormone regulatory systems provides the basis for the various

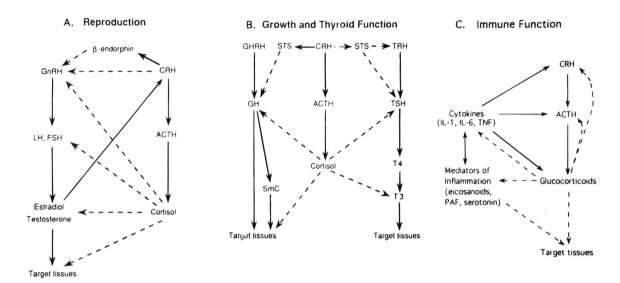

Fig. 4. Interactions of the HPA axis and the systems that subserve reproduction, growth, and metabolism. **(A)** Interactions between the HPA and reproductive axes. **(B)** Interactions between the HPA and and growth and thyroid axes. **(C)** Interaction between the HPA axis and the immune system. (Solid lines represent direct or indirect activation, and dashed lines, direct or indirect inhibition [abbreviations are the same as the ones used in Fig. 3, and STS = somatostatin {SRIF}, IL-1 and IL-6 = interleukin-1 and 6, TNF-α = tumor necrosis factor-α, PAF = platelet-activating factor) (Modified with permission from Chrousos and Gold, 1992.)

endocrine manifestations of CRH hypersecretion/ chronic hyperactivity of the stress system. CRH suppresses the secretion of GnRH by the arcuate neurons of the hypothalamus either directly or via the stimulation of arcuate POMC peptide-secreting neurons, whereas glucocorticoids exert inhibitory effects at all levels of the reproductive axis, including the gonads and the target tissues of sex steroids (Fig. 4A). Suppression of gonadal function caused by chronic HPA activation has been demonstrated in highly trained runners of both sexes and ballet dancers. These subjects have increased evening plasma cortisol and ACTH levels, increased urinary free cortisol excretion, and blunted ACTH responses to exogenous CRH; males have low LH and testosterone levels, and females have amenorrhea. Obligate athletes go through withdrawal symptoms and signs if, for any reason, they have to discontinue their exercise routine. This syndrome is possibly the result of withdrawal from the daily exercise-induced elevation of opioid peptides and from similarly induced stimulation of the mesocorticolimbic system. The interaction between CRH and the gonadal axis appears to be bidirectional. The presence of estrogen responsive elements in the promoter area of the human CRH gene and direct stimulatory estrogen

effects on CRH gene expression implicate CRH, and therefore, the HPA axis, as a potentially important target of ovarian steroids and a potential mediator of gender-related differences in the stress response.

In parallel to its effects on the gonadal axis, the stress system suppresses thyroid axis function via a number of known pathways, including SRIF-induced suppression of TRH and TSH secretion and glucocorticoid-mediated suppression of TSH secretion and the 5′-deiodinase enzyme (Fig. 4B). Thus, during stress, there is suppressed secretion of TRH and TSH and decreased conversion of T4 to T3 in peripheral tissues. This situation is similar to what is observed in the "euthyroid sick" syndrome, a phenomenon that serves to conserve energy during stress. The mediators of these changes in thyroid function include the CRH neurons, glucocorticoids, somatostatin, and cytokines. Accordingly, patients with melancholic depression, anorectics, highly trained athletes, and patients with chronic, inflammatory diseases have significantly lower thyroid hormone concentrations than normal controls.

Prolonged activation of the HPA axis leads to suppression of GH and inhibition of IGF-1 effects on target tissues (Fig. 4B). CRH-induced increases of somatostatinergic tone have been implicated as a potential mechanism of stress-induced suppression of GH secretion. In several stress system-related mood disorders, GH and/or IGF-1 levels are significantly decreased in animals and humans. Nervous pointer dogs, an animal model of anxiety with mixed panic and phobic features, were found to have low IGF-1 levels and lower body growth than nonaffected animals. Patients with panic disorder, compared to normal control subjects, had blunted GH responses to iv administered clonidine, and children with anxiety disorders can be short in stature.

The association between chronic, experimentally induced psychosocial stress and a hypercortisolism/metabolic syndrome-X (MS-X)-like state, with increased incidence of atherosclerosis, was recently reported in cynomolgus monkeys. In these animals, chronic psychosocial stress-induced activation of the HPA axis led to hypercortisolism, dexamethasone nonsuppression, visceral obesity, insulin resistance, hypertension, suppression of GH secretion, and osteoporosis.

Gastrointestinal (GI) function is also affected by chronic CRH hypersecretion. During stress, gastric emptying is delayed, whereas colonic motor activity increases in animals and humans. Innervations by the vagus nerve and the LC/NE sympathetic system provide the network for the rapid responses of the GI system to stress. CRH microinjected into the PVN was shown to reproduce the stress responses of the GI system in an animal model, including inhibition of gastric emptying and stimulation of colonic transit and fecal excretion. This effect was abolished by the intrathecal administration of a CRH-antagonist. CRH may be implicated in mediating the gastric stasis observed during the stress of surgery and/or anesthesia. IL-1β, a potent cytokine that is found increased during surgery and in the immediate postoperative period, also inhibits gastric motility. Intrathecal administration of a CRH antagonist prevented surgery-induced rises of IL-1β in rats, thus suggesting that CRH may be an important mediator of IL-1β-induced gastric stasis. CRH hypersecretion could be the hidden link between the symptoms of chronic GI pain and history of abuse, since young victims of abuse demonstrate CRH hypersecretion.

A large infrastructure of anatomical, chemical, and molecular connections allows communication within and between the neuroendocrine and immune systems (Fig. 4C). In addition to the HPA axis, which via glucocorticoids exerts major immunosup-

pressive and anti-inflammatory effects, the efferent sympathetic/adrenomedullary system participates in the restraint immune/inflammatory reaction by transmitting neural signals to the immune system. This is mediated through a dense innervation of both primary and secondary lymphoid organs, and by reaching all sites of inflammation via postganglionic sympathetic neurons. The sympathetic system, when activated, causes systemic secretion of IL-6, which by inhibiting the other two inflammatory cytokines, tumor necrosis factor-α (TNF-α) and IL-1, and by activating the HPA axis, participates in the stress-induced suppression of the immune inflammatory reactions. Stress-associated CRH hypersecretion, and the resultant glucocor-ticoid- , catecholamine-, and IL6-mediated immunosuppression correlate well with such clinical observations as the suppression of the immune and inflammatory reaction during chronic psychological and physical stress, the reactivation of autoimmune diseases during the postpartum period or following cure of Cushing's syndrome (CS), and the decreased ability of the stressed organism to fight viral infections and neoplasms.

In contrast to states with a hyperactive stress system, there is a host of different conditions, such as atypical or seasonal depression in the dark months of the year, the postpartum period, the period following the cessation of smoking, rheumatoid arthritis, and the chronic fatigue and fibromyalgia syndromes, which represent hypoarousal states. In these conditions, CRH secretion is decreased and symptoms, such as increase in appetite and weight gain, somnolence, and fatigue, are seen.

6.5. Clinical Uses of CRH

The CRH stimulation test (ovine CRH [oCRH]) 1 μcg/kg iv) is used clinically in the differential diagnosis of CS alone or in combination with inferior petrosal sinus sampling (IPSS). Over 80% of patients with CD respond to iv oCRH with an increase of ACTH and cortisol in the first 30–45 min of the test. Most patients with ACTH-independent CS do not respond to this test, whereas ectopic ACTH-producing tumors occasionally respond. IPSS is the best available test for the diagnosis of CD, since over 95% of the patients with CD respond to iv-administered oCRH with a twofold increase in their petrosal sinus over peripheral ACTH levels in the first 3–10 min of the test, and 100% of the patients with CS from other causes do not respond. The administration of dexamethasone prior to oCRH test has been suggested for the differential diagnosis of CS vs pseudo-Cushing states. In primary adrenal insufficiency, patients respond to oCRH with markedly elevated ACTH levels, whereas two patterns have been described in patients with secondary arterial insufficiency: a pituitary pattern with absence of an ACTH response, and an hypothalamic pattern with a delayed and prolonged ACTH response to oCRH.

In the clinical investigation of depression and other disorders of the HPA axis, including anorexia nervosa, panic anxiety, abuse, malnutrition, addiction, and withdrawal syndromes and autoimmune diseases, the oCRH-stimulation test, as a sensitive indicator of corticotroph function, has been proven to be an invaluable tool. A variety of CRH analogs have recently been synthesized, but not used in clinical trials. They bind specifically to the CRH-Rs, and in vitro studies have suggested that they might find therapeutic use in the treatment of disorders of the HPA axis.

Recently, two groups of substances were discovered that might be therapeutically useful. Nonpeptide CRH antagonists might prove useful in the treatment of melancholic depression, anorexia nervosa, panic anxiety, withdrawal from addiction agents, and in other conditions associated with hyperactivation of the HPA axis. Conversely, CRH-BP antagonists might provide a means of increasing levels of CRH in states characterized by low CRH, such as atypical depression, chronic fatigue/fibromyalgia syndromes, and autoimmune disorders.

7. DOPAMINE

7.1. Dopamine Synthesis and Dopaminergic Neurons

Dopamine is a catecholamine neurotransmitter and a hormone with a wide distribution and array of functions in the animal kingdom. It differs from the other catecholamines in that it is present in many nonneuronal tissues, but in relatively limited areas of the brain. It is a hypothalamic hormone directly involved in the regulation of PRL secretion from pituitary lactotropes, where, unlike other neurotrasmitters, it forms its own short-feedback loop and is released in great quantities.

Dopamine is endogenously synthesized by hydroxylation of L-tyrosine (by tyrosine hydroxylase [TH]) and subsequent decarboxylation of the product (L-Dopa) by the aromatic-L-amino acid decarboxylase.

The TH step is the rate-limiting step in the synthesis of dopamine. An increase in hydroxylation of tyrosine can be demonstrated rapidly after the stimulation of catecholaminergic neurons. Tetrahydrobiopterin is an important cofactor in the TH reaction, and its availability plays a regulatory role in the in vivo stimulation of TH activity. TH exhibits product inhibition by catecholamines, and is stimulated by acetylcholine and by phosphorylation from a cAMP-dependent kinase. The TH gene is located on chromosome 11p and codes for a cDNA that is approxi 1900 bp long, Multiple mRNA species have been identified, indicating that tissue-specific regulation of TH gene expression is extensive. Unlike TH, which is only located in catecholamine-producing neurons and neuroendocrine cells, the L-dopa decarboxylase is expressed in many neuronal and nonneuronal tissues. It is not substrate-specific and decarboxylates a variety of amino acids.

There are four major dopamine pathways in the mammalian forebrain. Nerve cell bodies of origin are clustered in nuclei in the rostral midbrain of three of these pathways, with the borders between the nuclei not always well defined. These nuclei have been shown to contain dopamine neurons. Anatomically, the most distinctive nuclei are the paired substantia nigra neurons, whose axons ascend rostrally in the nigrostriatal pathway to provide dopaminergic innervation of the corpus striatum (caudate and putamen). The substantia nigra neurons selectively degenerate in Parkinson's disease. A closely paired nucleus, the ventral tegmental area lies medially and dorsally to the substantia nigra, and its dopamine neurons provide two ascending pathways: (1) the mesolimbic, which provides dopamine innervation to forebrain limbic structures, especially the nucleus accumbens in the ventral striatum, and (2) the mesocortical, which provides dopamine innervation to the frontal and cingulate cortex. The fourth dopamine nucleus, the arcuate, is in the hypothalamus, projects to the median eminence through the tuberoinfundibular pathway and the intermediate lobe (in species that have this structure) through the tuberohypophyseal pathway, and releases dopamine directly into the hypophyseal portal circulation.

Although all of these groups of neurons synthesize dopamine by identical mechanisms, they are not identical functionally. Alterations in pituitary function related to changes in dopamine secretion by tuberoinfundibular neurons do not necessarily reflect alterations in other central dopaminergic systems. Tuberoinfundibular neurons are components of the short-loop feedback control of PRL secretion by the pituitary lactotrophs, and they possess PRL receptors but not dopamine receptors. Thus, dopaminergic drugs and their antagonists act directly on the mesolimbic and nigrostriatal systems and on the pituitary, but not on the tuberoinfondibular system.

7.2. Dopamine Regulation of PRL Secretion

The synthesis and release of PRL from lactotrophs have been extensively studied over the past two decades. Unlike other anterior pituitary cells, lactotrophs release their hormone at a high rate in the absence of hypothalamic regulation. Lesioning the median eminence, transecting the pituitary stalk, and grafting the pituitary beneath the kidney capsule, all result in hyperprolactinemia. The incubation of pituitary fragments or dispersed cells in vitro is also associated with a sustained release of PRL.

Dopamine is the long-sought hypothalamic PRL-release inhibiting factor (PIF) and the main modulator of the pleiotropic regulation of PRL secretion. Concentrations of dopamine in portal blood are maintained at physiologically active levels, and lactotropes contain dopamine receptors. PRL levels increase after treatment with dopamine antagonists and when dopamine is removed from the perfusion medium of cultured pituitary cells. Neither dopamine nor hypothalamic function is necessary for the pulsatile release of PRL from the pituitary, but tonic inhibition by the former synchronizes PRL secretion.

Both TRH and VIP stimulate PRL release, although only the former appears to be affected by dopamine. Part of the suckling-induced release of PRL appears to be mediated by TRH, and this effect can be prevented by the administration of a dopamine agonist. A trough in vivo or removal of dopamine secretion in vitro appears to enhance PRL release by TRH. In contrast, the transient removal of dopamine has no effects on VIP-induced PRL release, and blockade of dopamine receptors does not potentiate VIP or oxytocin-stimulated PRL release. Significant reduction of the rat portal concentrations of dopamine is observed immediately before large releases of PRL, such as during the last day of pregnancy and in response to suckling and estradiol, the latter on the afternoon of proestrus.

7.3. Dopamine Receptors

Pituitary lactotrope regulation by dopamine is primarily through dopamine type-2 receptors (D2-R). Five DRs exist (D-1R–5R) and all their genes were cloned before 1991. They belong to the seven-TMS-domain G-protein-coupled receptor family, and have common structural organization and some homology with serotoninergic and adrenergic receptors. D-1R and D-5R activate, whereas D-2R, D-3R, and D-4R inhibit adenylate cyclase. The third cytoplasmic loop is short in the former, and long in the latter. It is generally believed that receptors with a short third cytoplasmic loop couple to stimulatory G-proteins (G_s) and, thus, activate adenylate cyclase, whereas those with long third cytoplasmic loop react with G_i and G_o, which inhibit adenylate cyclase, and G_q, which couples with phospholipase C. Although the structures of the extra- and intracellular loops of the DRs vary with each receptor, the transmembrane domains are highly homologous. The genes for these receptors are located on different chromosomes in humans (5q34, 11q22, 3q13, 4p16, and 4p16 for the D-1R, D-2R, D-3R, D-4R, and D-5R, respectively) and are intronless for the activating D-1R and D-5R, but contain 6, 5, and 4 introns for the inhibitory D-2R, D-3R, and D-4R, respectively. Posttranslational processing is extensive for the latter three receptors, resulting in a greater number of receptor isoforms.

The action of dopamine on pituitary PRL release is mediated through D-2R, the first DR to be cloned, and a receptor that is abundant in the pituitary, striatum, nucleus accumbens, olfactory tubercle, and substantia nigra. There are two isoforms of the D-2R that differ in length by 29 amino acids owing to an insertion in the third cytoplasmic loop. Both forms are expressed in all the tissues in which D-2Rs are present, including the pituitary and are equipotent in inhibiting adenylate cyclase and activating K^+ channels, the latter an action unique to D-2Rs among the dopamine receptors.

Dopamine administration decreases cAMP concentration in pituitary cells in vitro. It also inhibits the Ca^{2+} second messenger system and decreases intracellular Ca^{2+} concentration. PRL release is inhibited in Ca^{2+}-deficient medium and by Ca^{2+} channel blockers. Dopamine effects on Ca^{2+} are mediated by a G-protein-dependent mechanism or by direct coupling to Ca^{2+} channels. The effects of dopamine on phospholipase C are less clear, and although PKC is involved in regulating PRL secretion, the evidence that dopamine regulates PKC activity is scant. Basal activity of phospholipase C in the lactotropes is low, but dopamine dissociation from its receptor is associated with its activation. The latter is not dependent on adenylate cyclase activity, which is also significantly activated on dissociation of dopamine from the pituitary D-2R.

7.4. Hyperprolactinemia and the Use of D-2R-Agonists

The anatomical (by surgery, or mass effects of a large pituitary or hypothalamic tumor) or functional (by the use of dopamine antagonists) uncoupling of the pituitary lactotrophs from hypothalamic dopaminergic control results in hyperprolactinemia. The latter is a manifestation of a number of disorders of the hypothalamic–pituitary unit, and leads to hypogonadism, decreased libido, and/or galactorrhea. It can also develop from the administration of neuroleptic drugs, like reserpine (a catecholamine depletor), and phenothiazines, such as chlorpromazine and haloperidol. The PRL response to the latter is an excellent predictor of their antipsychotic effects.

Dopamine agonists have been developed and have been in clinical use for the management of hyperprolactinemia. Bromocriptine and, recently, pergolide, are D-2R agonists that restore effectively PRL inhibition and are used in the medical management of pituitary prolactinomas. Only 10% of the latter are resistant to the action of bromocriptine; the rest respond with significant reduction of their size and resolution of hyperprolactinemia. Although dopamine agonists are useful for the reduction of PRL levels induced by disruption of hypothalamic function by other pituitary tumors, they are not effective in decreasing the size of non-PRL-secreting tumors.

The response to dopamine receptor stimulation and blockade is not specific for the central, pituitary, or peripheral actions of dopamine. Indeed, bromocriptine can induce schizophrenic psychosis in a small proportion of individuals with no prior history of mental disorders. In general, however, dopamine agonists have few side effects, and bromocriptine can be safely used during pregnancy, if needed.

REFERENCE

Chrousos GP, Gold PW. The concepts of stress and stress system disorders. An overview of physical and behavioral homeostasis. *JAMA* 1992;21:833.

Frohman LA, Downs TR, Chomzynski P. Regulation of growth hormone secretion. *Frontiers in Neuroendocrinol* 1992;13:344.

Reichlin S. Neuroendocrinology. In: Wilson JD, Foster DW, eds. *Williams Textbook of Endocrinology*, 8th ed. Philadelphia: W.B. Saunders 1992:135.

Sherwood NM, Lovejoy DA, Coe IR. Origin of mammalian gonadotropin-releasing hormones. *Endocr Rev* 1993;14:241.

SELECTED READING

Chrousos GP. The hypothalamic–pituitary–adrenal axis and immune-mediated inflammation. *N Engl J Med* 1995;332:1351.

Conn PM, Janovick JA, Stanislaus D, Kuphal D, Jennes L. Molecular and cellular bases of GnRH action in the pituitary and central nervous system. *Vitam Horm* 1995;50:151.

De La Escalera GM, Weiner RI. Dissociation of dopamine from its receptor as a signal in the pleitropic hypothalamic regulation of prolactin secretion. *Endocr Rev* 1992;13:241.

Jackson IMD, Lechan RM, Lee SL. TRH-prohormone:biosynthesis, anatomic distribution and processing. *Frontiers in Neuroendocrinol* 1990;11:267.

King JC, Rubin BS. Dynamic changes in LHRH neurovascular terminals with various endocrine conditions in adults. *Horm Behav* 1994;28:349.

Korbonits M, Grossman AB. Growth hormone-releasing peptide and its analogues. Novel stimuli to growth hormone release. *Trends Endocrinol Metab* 1995;6:43.

Ogawa N. Molecular and chemical neuropharmacology of dopamine receptor subtypes. *Acta Med Okayama* 1995;49:1.

Rivest S, Rivier C. The role of corticotropin-releasing factor and interleukin-1 in the regulations of neurons controlling reproductive functions. *Endocr Rev* 1995;16:177.

Schwanzel-Fukuda M, Jorgenson KL, Bergen HT, Weesner GD, Pfaff DW. Biology of normal LHRH neurons during and after their migration from olfactory placode. *Endocr Rev* 1992;13:623.

Spada A, Faglia G. G-proteins and hormonal signalling in human pituitary tumors: genetic mutations and functional alterations. *Front Neuroendocrinol* 1993;14:214.

Stratakis CA, Chrousos GP. Neuroendocrinology of stress: implications for growth and development. *Horm Res* 1995;43:162.

Vamvakopoulos NC, Chrousos GP. Hormonal regulation of human corticotropin-releasing hormone gene expression: implications for the stress response and immune/inflammatory reaction. *Endocr Rev* 1994;15:409.

Viollet C, Prevost G, Maubert E, et al. Molecular pharmacology of somatostatin receptors. *Fundam Clin Pharmacol* 1995;9:107.

Wehrenberg WB, Giustina A. Basic counterpoint: mechanisms and pathways of gonadal steroid stimulation of growth hormone secretion. *Endocr Rev* 1992;13:299.

14 Anterior Pituitary Hormones

Ilan Shimon, MD, and Shlomo Melmed, MD

CONTENTS

1. INTRODUCTION

The human anterior pituitary gland contains at least five distinct hormone-producing cell populations, expressing six different hormones: proopiomelanocortin (POMC), growth hormone (GH), prolactin (PRL), thyroid-stimulating hormone (TSH), follicle-stimulating hormone (FSH) and luteinizing hormone (LH).

2. POMC

2.1. Corticotrope Embryology and Cytogenesis

The corticotrope is the first cell type to develop in the human fetal pituitary, as early as 6 wk of gestation (Table 1) and 2 wk later ACTH is detectable by radioimmunoassay (RIA) of both fetal pituitary tissue and fetal blood. The corticotropes constitute between 15 and 20% of the adenohypophyseal cell population, are initially identified by their basophilic staining, and express strong granular cytoplasmic immunopositivity for adrenocorticotropic hormone (ACTH) and for other fragments of the POMC molecule. By electron microscopy (EM), the cells are oval with spheri-

From: *Endocrinology: Basic and Clinical Principles* (P. M. Conn and S. Melmed, eds.), Humana Press Inc., Totowa, NJ.

cal eccentric nuclei and a large membrane-bound lysosomal structure, the "enigmatic body".

2.2. POMC Gene

The human POMC gene (Fig. 1) is an 8-kb single-copy gene located on chromosome 2p25. It consists of a 400–700 bp promoter, three exons, and two introns. The majority of the 266 amino acid POMC precursor protein is encoded by exon 3, which contains all the known peptide products of the gene, including the 39 amino acid ACTH, α-melanocyte-stimulating hormone (α-MSH), β-MSH, β-lipotropin (β-LPH), β-endorphin, and corticotropin-like intermediate lobe peptide (CLIP). Human POMC is digested at either Lys-Arg or Arg-Arg residues by two endopeptidases, prohormone convertase 1 (PC1), abundant in anterior pituitary corticotropes, and prohormone convertase 2 (PC2), expressed in the brain as well as in pancreatic islet cells, but absent from the anterior pituitary. This tissue-specific enzyme distribution correlates well with the different enzymatic cleavage of the prohormone to its products. Thus, in the pituitary corticotrope, POMC is cleaved into ACTH, β-LPH, and other peptides including N-terminal glycopeptide and joining peptide, whereas in brain, ACTH is further cleaved to

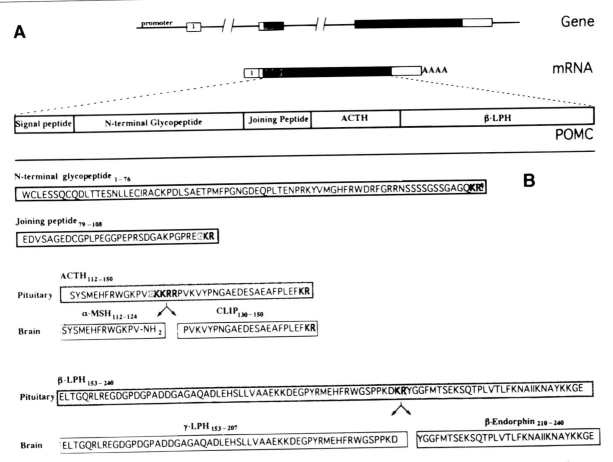

Fig. 1. Schematic structure of POMC gene, mRNA, and protein products. **(A)** The gene (top) contains the promoter, three exons (thick bars, translated regions are stippled), separated by two introns (thin broken lines). The mRNA transcript (middle) consists of the three exons and the polyadenylation site. The POMC precursor protein (bottom) consists of the signal peptide, N-terminal glycopeptide, joining peptide, ACTH, and β-LPH. **(B)** Tissue-specific enzymatic cleavage of POMC to its products. POMC is cleaved into N-terminal glycopeptide and joining peptide in the pituitary coticotropes and the brain. In brain, ACTH is further cleaved to α-MSH and CLIP, and β-LPH is digested into γ-LPH and β-endorphin. KR = dibasic amino acids at proteolytic cleavage sites. From Holm and Majzoub (Adrenocorticotropin) in Melmed (1995).

α-MSH and CLIP (Fig. 1). Exon 1 is not translated and there is only a 45% nucleotide sequence homology in exon 1 and the promoter region of the human, bovine, and other mammals. In contrast, exons 2 and 3 bear 80–95% homology among human, other mammals, and mice. The main regulators of POMC transcription are corticotropin-releasing hormone (CRH) and glucocorticoids, which exert opposite effects on POMC transcription rates. CRH increases POMC mRNA and protein content via cAMP, whereas the glucocorticoid negative-feedback effect is probably mediated through binding of the glucocorticoid receptor complex to cis-acting POMC promoter sequences. POMC transcription is also stimulated by β-adrenergic catecholamines and insulin-induced hypoglycemia.

2.3. Regulation of ACTH Secretion

The endogenous circadian rhythm of ACTH pulsatile secretion leads to a parallel diurnal pattern of glucocorticoid release. Both ACTH and cortisol are higher in the early morning, and decline through the day to the lower levels during the night. This rhythmicity of ACTH pulse amplitude may be controlled by the concomitant diurnal variation of CRH secretion. CRH and AVP are the main secretagogs of ACTH, and glucocorticoids inhibit its secretion. CRH, by binding to CRH receptors on the corticotrope, stimulates ACTH synthesis as well as release. In addition, physical stress, exercise, acute illness, and hypoglycemia increase ACTH levels. Inflammatory cytokines—tumor necrosis factor-α,

Table 1
Human Anterior Pituitary Hormone Gene Expression and Protein Action

	POMC	GH	PRL	TSH	FSH	LH
Cell	Corticotrope	Somatotrope	Lactotrope	Thyrotrope	Gonadotrope	
Fetal appearance	6 wk	8 wk	12 wk	12 wk	12 wk	
Chromosomal gene locus	2p	17q	6	α—6q; β—1p	β—11p;	β—19q
Protein	Polypeptide	Polypeptide	Polypeptide	Glycoprotein α, β subunits	glycoprotein α, β subunits	
Protein length, kDa	ACTH- 4.5	22	23	28	34	28.5
Amino acid no.	266 (ACTH-39)	191	199	211	210	204
Normal range	ACTH, 4–22 pmol/L	<0.5^a µg/L	M < 15; F < 20 µg/L	0.1–5 mU/L	M, 5–20 IU/L; F, (basal), 5–20 IU/L	
Secretion regulators*						
Stimulators	CRH, AVP	GHRH	Estrogen, TRH	TRH	GnRH, estrogen	
Inhibitors	Glucocorticoids	Somatostatin, IGF-1	Dopamine, T_3	T_3, T_4, Dopamine Somatostatin, Glucocorticoids	Estrogen, inhibin	
Receptor	GSTD	Singletransmembrane	Single transmembrane	GSTD	GSTD	
Location	Adrenal	Liver, other tissues	Breast, other tissues	Thyroid	Ovary	Testis
Trophic effects	Steroid production	IGF-1 production, growth induction	Milk production	T_3, T_4 Synthesis and secretion	Testosterone synthesis Follicle growth	

^{a} Integrated over 24 h.
*Only stimulators and inhibitors are under "secretion regulators".
GSTD = G_s protein coupled with seven-transmembrane domains.

interleukin-1, interleukin-6, and leukemia-inhibitory factor—stimulate pituitary corticotropin secretion, whereas oxytocin, opiates, and somatostatin inhibit ACTH release.

2.4. ACTH Receptor Gene

ACTH receptors have been detected in human adrenal glands, adrenal tumors, and on human mononuclear leukocytes and rat lymphocytes. The ACTH receptor gene encodes a 297 amino acid protein that belongs to the G_s-protein-coupled superfamily of receptors containing seven-transmembrane domains. The ACTH effect is mediated by adenylate cyclase activation, cAMP production, and protein kinase A induction in the adrenal.

2.5. ACTH Action

ACTH stimulates steroidogenesis in the adrenocortical cells. Lipoprotein uptake from the plasma is enhanced, and steroid hormone enzyme gene transcription is increased. The prolonged effects of ACTH may promote growth of adrenal size and act with β-LPH on melanocytes to increase skin pigmentation.

2.6. Hypersecretion

2.6.1. PITUITARY ADENOMA

ACTH-producing tumors are usually monoclonal, well-differentiated microadenomas. About 10–15% of all pituitary adenomas are clinically active ACTH-producing tumors, and 5% are silent corticotrope adenomas. In addition to POMC glycoprotein, secretory granules in tumor cells stain for ACTH, β-endorphin, β-LPH, and N-terminal peptide. Some corticotrope adenomas contain altered forms of gastrin, cholecystokinin, and also vasoactive intestinal peptide (VIP), neurophysin, α subunit, and chromogranin-A. Cell cultures of corticotrope adenomas secrete ACTH in response to CRH and AVP, and ACTH is suppressible by glucocorticoids, but to a lesser extent as compared with normal corticotropes.

2.6.2. ECTOPIC ACTH SECRETION

Small-cell carcinomas of the lung, and bronchial and thymic carcinoids can produce ACTH, leading to Cushing's syndrome. These tumors express other neuroendocrine markers, including chromogranins, synaptophysin, and neurotensin. POMC mRNA from nonpituitary tumors may be longer than normal or pituitary tumor POMC mRNA. In addition, CLIP and β-MSH are detected in ectopic tumors, indicat-

ing an alternative POMC processing. POMC mRNA and ACTH are not suppressed in small-cell lung carcinoma cell lines by glucocorticoids.

2.7. Hyposecretion

Pituitary failure owing to irradiation, hypophysectomy, large macroadenomas, pituitary apoplexy, trauma, postpartum necrosis, hypophysitis, glucocorticoids withdrawal, or CRH deficiency results in ACTH hyposecretion and hypocortisolism. This is usually a late manifestation of pituitary failure and indicates severely compromised pituitary function.

2.8. ACTH Receptor Defects

Familial glucocorticoid deficiency is a rare autosomal recessive disorder of adrenal unresponsiveness to ACTH, characterized by glucocorticoid deficiency in the presence of elevated circulating ACTH and normal mineralocorticoid production. Affected children usually have hypoglycemic episodes, hyperpigmentation, failure to thrive, and chronic asthenia. They have no cortisol or aldosterone responses to exogenous ACTH. Recently, homozygous and compound heterozygous point mutations have been reported in the ACTH receptor gene.

2.9. Clinical Testing

The low-dose (1-mg) overnight dexamethasone suppression test and the measurement of 24-h urinary-free cortisol are the standard screening tests for Cushing's syndrome. The 48-hour low-dose dexamethasone suppression test (2 mg/d) is usually performed to diagnose Cushing's syndrome, and the high-dose (8 mg/d) suppression test will usually differentiate pituitary from nonpituitary tumor source of ACTH. Once the diagnosis of Cushing's syndrome is made, measuring ACTH concentration in plasma is important for etiologic evaluation. The normal levels of ACTH are 4–22 pmol/L. In Cushing's disease, ACTH is moderately increased to 10–50 pmol/L, and ectopic ACTH syndrome usually results in highly elevated levels. Patients with adrenal adenoma have low or undetectable ACTH. The CRH stimulation test may serve to differentiate patients with Cushing's disease who have exaggerated ACTH and cortisol response to CRH, from patients with ectopic ACTH-producing tumors that, in general, do not respond further to CRH. To screen the functional adrenal reserve for cortisol production, the rapid cortrosyn (ACTH 1–24, 1–250 μg) stimulation test is used. Patients with ACTH hyposecretion have a blunted cortisol response to cortrosyn administration.

2.10. Clinical Syndromes

2.10.1. CUSHING'S SYNDROME

In 1932, Harvey Cushing described a syndrome resulting from long-term exposure to glucocorticoids. Most patients (70%) have pituitary corticotrope adenomas (Cushing's disease). Other etiologies include ectopic ACTH (12%), cortisol-producing adrenal adenoma, carcinoma and hyperplasia (18%), and the rare ectopic CRH syndrome. Prolonged administration of glucocorticoids produces a similar syndrome. Patients have a typical habitus, including "moon facies," "buffalo hump," truncal obesity, cutaneous striae, as well as muscle weakness, osteoporosis, impaired glucose tolerance, hirsutism, acne, hypertension, depression, and ovarian dysfunction. Usually the clinical presentation is insidious, but the ectopic syndrome associated with small-cell lung carcinoma may be acute with rapid onset of hypertension, edema, hypokalemia, glucose intolerance, and hyperpigmentation. When a probable diagnosis of Cushing's disease is made, the most direct way to demonstrate pituitary ACTH hypersecretion is by catheterization of the inferior petrosal venous sinuses, which drain the pituitary. ACTH measurements in petrosal and peripheral venous plasma before and after CRH stimulation can document a central-to-peripheral gradient of ACTH in blood draining an adenoma.

High-resolution MRI of the sella turcica, enhanced by gadolinium, is useful in determining the location of corticotrope adenomas with a sensitivity of 2 mm. The treatment of choice is transsphenoidal adenomectomy, and the cure rate is 70–80%.

2.10.2. HYPOCORTISOLISM

Hypocortisolism can be either primary (Addison's disease), secondary to pituitary ACTH deficiency, or tertiary resulting from CRH deficiency. Primary adrenal insufficiency can result from autoimmune adrenocortical destruction, AIDS, tuberculosis, bilateral hemorrhage, and metastatic disease. Clinically, patients present with fatigue, weakness, nausea and vomiting, weight loss, hypotension, hypoglycemia, and hyperpigmentation (only in primary hypocortisolism). Treatment of Addison's patients includes glucocorticoids and mineralocorticoids, whereas patients with secondary adrenal insufficiency do not usually require mineralocorticoid replacement.

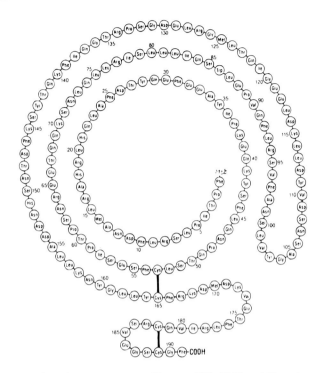

Fig. 2. Primary structure of human GH. GH is a 191-amino acid single-chain 22-kDa polypeptide with two intramolecular disulfide bonds. From Fryklund et al., 1986.

3. GH

3.1. Somatotrope Embryology and Cytogenesis

Somatotropes that contain GH immunoreactivity are identified at 8 wk of gestation, and circulating GH is measurable in fetal serum at the end of the first trimester. Somatotropes comprise 40–50% of pituitary cells and are located in the lateral wings of the gland. These acidophilic cells reveal intense cytoplasmic immunopositivity for GH.

3.2. GH Gene

The human GH genomic locus contains a cluster of five highly conserved genes, and spans approx 66 kb on the long arm of chromosome 17 (q22–24). All these genes have the same basic structure consisting of five exons separated by four introns. The hGH gene codes for a 22-kDa protein (Fig. 2), containing 191 amino acids, and is exclusively expressed in somatotropes, whereas the others are expressed in placental tissue. The GH promoter, 300 bp of 5′-flanking DNA, contains cis-elements, which mediate both pituitary-specific and hormone-specific signaling.

Pit-1, a 33-kDa tissue-specific transcription factor, binds to specific sites on the promoter. This factor is expressed in lactotropes, somatotropes, and thyrotropes, and is critical for GH, PRL, and TSH-β gene transcription. GH releasing hormone (GHRH) stimulates GH transcription, and insulin-like growth factor 1 (IGF-1) inhibits GH mRNA expression.

3.3. GH Secretion

GH is secreted as a 22-kDa single-chain polypeptide hormone, or a less abundant 20-kDa monomer, formed by alternative mRNA splicing. The secretion is pulsatile, with low or undetectable basal levels between peaks. In children, maximum GH secretory peaks are detected within 1 h of deep sleep onset. Somatostatin (SRIF) and GHRH interact to generate pulsatile GH release, whereas SRIF appears to be the primary regulator of GH pulses in response to physiologic stimuli. GHRH stimulates GH synthesis and secretion, whereas SRIF, as well as IGF-1, inhibit GH secretion. Thyroid-releasing hormone (TRH) does not stimulate GH secretion in normal subjects, but induces GH release in patients with acromegaly.

3.4. GH Receptor and Binding Proteins

In addition to the liver, which contains the highest concentration of GH receptors, many other tissues also express these receptors. The human GH receptor is a 620 amino acid protein (130 kDa) with an extracellular hormone-binding domain of 246 amino acids, a single transmembrane region, and a cytoplasmic domain of 350 residues. The human GH receptor gene has been assigned to chromosome 5p13. The GH-binding proteins (GHBPs), soluble short forms (60 kDa) of the hepatic GH receptor, and identical to the extracellular domain, bind half of circulating GH. They prolong GH plasma half-life by decreasing the GH metabolic clearance rate and also inhibit GH binding to surface receptors by ligand competition.

3.5. GH Action

GH acts both directly, via its own receptor, and indirectly, via IGF-1, on peripheral target tissues. Longitudinal bone growth-promoting actions on the chondrocytes in the epiphyseal growth plate are probably stimulated indirectly by GH, through local as well as hepatic-derived circulating IGF-1. GH itself has chronic anti-insulin effects, resulting in glucose intolerance, and the hormone increases muscle volume and lean body mass, and significantly decreases body fat when administered to GH-deficient adults.

3.6. Clinical Testing

GH immunoradiometric assays (IRMA), employing a double-monoclonal antibody (MAb) sandwich system, are now widely used because of their sensitivity and accuracy, compared with RIAs. Random GH measurements are not helpful in the diagnosis of GH hypersecretory or deficiency states because of the pulsatile nature of pituitary GH secretion, and integrated measurements over time are required. Serum IGF-1 levels are invariably high in acromegaly, and correlate better with the clinical manifestations of hypersomatotrophism than single GH measurements. Therefore, high IGF-1 levels are highly specific for diagnosing acromegaly. IGF-1 is less helpful in evaluation of GH deficiency (GHD), since its levels are low in infancy and the normal range overlaps with values measured in GH-deficient children.

3.6.1. PROVOCATIVE TESTS

These dynamic tests assess GH reserve in the evaluation of GHD, by pharmacologic stimulation of the somatotropes. The diagnosis is determined by an inadequate GH response to at least two separate provocative tests.

3.6.2. GHRH

This test (1 μg/kg, iv) may help in the diagnosis of GH insufficiency, when GH does not increase within 60 min subsequent to injection. If the somatotropes are first primed with intermittent GHRH pulses, the acute GHRH test may sometimes distinguish between hypothalamic and pituitary GHD.

3.6.3. INSULIN-INDUCED HYPOGLYCEMIA

This is the most reliable provocative stimulus for the diagnosis of GHD. Clonidine, arginine, L-Dopa, and propranolol are other stimulants used in GH reserve evaluation. The diagnosis of GHD in adults is currently being re-evaluated, since the sensitive new IRMAs indicate "normal" integrated GH levels of <0.5 μg/L.

3.6.4. SUPPRESSION TESTS

In acromegalic patients, the elevated GH levels fail to suppress (<2 μg/L) after an oral glucose load.

3.7. GH Hypersecretion

3.7.1. ACROMEGALY

Over 95% of patients with acromegaly harbor a pituitary adenoma, two-thirds have pure GH-cell tumors, and the others have plurihormonal tumors, usually expressing PRL in addition to GH. These patients have elevated GH and IGF-1 levels, and normal GHRH concentrations. Ectopic acromegaly may be central owing to excess GHRH production by functional hypothalamic tumors or peripheral rare extrapituitary GH-secreting tumors (pancreas), and the more common tumors secreting GHRH (carcinoid, pancreas, small-cell lung cancer). Patients with ectopic acromegaly manifest normal (central) or elevated (peripheral) GHRH levels. The clinical manifestations of acromegaly include generalized visceromegaly with enlargement of the tongue, bones, salivary glands, thyroid, heart, and soft organs; characteristic facial features with wide spacing of the teeth, large fleshy nose, and frontal bossing; and skeletal overgrowth leading to mandibular overgrowth with proganthism, increased hand, foot, and hat size. Patients present with voice deepening, headaches, arthropathy and carpal tunnel syndrome, muscle weekness and fatigue, oily skin and hyperhydrosis, hypertension and left ventricular hypertrophy, sleep apnea, menstrual abnormalities, depression, and glucose intolerance. Acromegalic patients have a significant increase in overall mortality because of cardiovascular disorders, malignancy, and respiratory disease. Selective transsphenoidal resection is the indicated treatment for GH-secreting pituitary adenoma. Octreotide (an octapeptide somatostatin analog) significantly attenuates GH and IGF-1 levels in most patients, and chronic administration is accompanied by marked clinical improvement.

3.8. GH Hyposecretion

GHD in children may be isolated or combined with deficiencies of other pituitary hormones. Its incidence approaches 1:5,000 to 1:10,000, and only between 25 and 30% of affected children exhibit identifiable underlying disorders. Several types of hereditary GHD with different modes of inheritance have been described. Molecular defects include GH gene deletion or lack of synthesis or secretion of GHRH. Excess somatostatin secretion has also been postulated. A group of children with growth failure may secrete immunoreactive, but a bioinactive GH molecule. Point mutations or major deletion of the *PIT-1* gene result in strains of transgenic dwarf mice that fail to develop pituitary somatotrope, lactotrope, and thyrotrope cells. This may be a potential mechanism for human GHD. Children with GHD are short and fail to grow at a normal rate, and are usually diagnosed by 12–18 mo of age. Patients tend to be overweight for their height, but are normally proportioned. These children have low stimulated GH levels, and low IGFBP-3. IGF-1 levels are normally very low before 3 yr of age, and do not correlate with stimulated GH levels. GH replacement with recombinant hGH (rhGH) should be started as early as possible, as total height gain is inversely proportional to pretreatment chronologic and bone age. Adult GHD may be isolated or the result of panhypopituitarism from several causes. These include pituitary apoplexy, large pituitary tumors, surgical trauma, hemochromatosis, hypophysitis, and other sellar lesions. GH-deficient adults have altered body composition with increased fat and decreased muscle volume and strength, lower psychosocial achievement, and altered glucose and lipid metabolism. These patients have low stimulated GH, low or normal IGF-1, and low IGFBP-3. The clinical effects of rhGH replacement in pituitary-deficient adults are currently being evaluated.

3.9. GH Receptor Defects (Laron Dwarfism)

Growth retardation may occur owing to failure of the liver and peripheral tissues to generate IGF-1 in response to GH. The genetic defect appears to be in the GH receptor itself, but the clinical characteristics of Laron dwarfism are identical to those in GH-deficient children. Basal and stimulated GH levels are high, but IGF-1 values are low and do not respond to GH therapy. Recently, successful response of Laron dwarfs to recombinant IGF-1 therapy was reported.

4. PRL

4.1. Lactotrope Embryology and Cytogenesis

Lactotropes are the last cells to differentiate in the human fetal pituitary. PRL is found only at 12 wk of gestation, and until 24 wk is localized in mammosomatotropes. These cells produce both GH and PRL, and appear to be the source of differentiated lactotropes, which are found only after that time. The lactotropes are acidophilic cells, contain

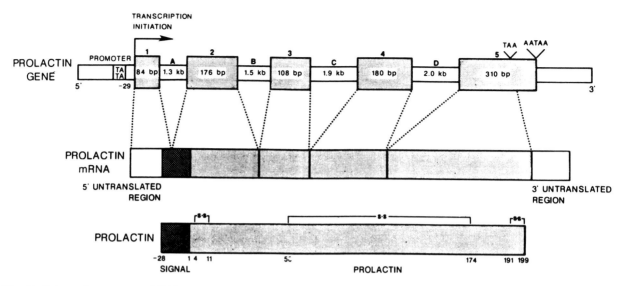

Fig. 3. Schematic structure of PRL gene, mRNA, and protein. The PRL gene (top) consits of the promoter, and five exons (1–5), separated by four introns (A–D). The PRL protein is a 199 amino acid 23-kDa polypeptide with three intraprotein disulfide bonds. From Melmed, 1995.

PRL-immunostained secretory granules, and constitute 15% of adenohypophysial cells. However, in multiparous women they represent up to a third of the cells, and during pregnancy and lactation, they may constitute 70% of the pituitary cells.

4.2. PRL Gene

The human PRL gene is approx 10 kb long, consists of five exons separated by four large introns, and encodes the 199 amino acid PRL peptide (23 kDa) (Fig. 3). The gene, located on chromosome 6, has two regions responsible for lactotrope-specific trnscription activation—a proximal promoter (–422 to +33) and a distal enhancer element (–1831 to –1530 bp)—both containing specific binding sites for Pit-1. PRL is homologous to GH and placental lactogen (PL), and they are thought to have arisen from a common original ancestral gene. Sequence homology among human PRL, bovine, and other mammals is in the range of 70–80%. Dopamine, the major PRL inhibitory factor, acts through the D_2 dopamine receptor to decrease intracellular cAMP, PRL gene transcription, synthesis, and release, mediated by the phosphoinositide/calcium pathway. VIP induces PRL synthesis and secretion, whereas glucocorticoids and thyroid hormones exert an inhibitory effect on PRL transcription and secretion. Estrogens, by binding of the estrogen receptor to the PRL-enhancer element, and TRH through the phospho-

inositide–protein kinase C pathway, induce PRL transcription and secretion.

4.3. PRL Secretion

PRL is under tonic inhibitory hypothalamic control and is secreted in pulses with an increase in amplitude during sleep. Basal levels increase throughout the course of pregnancy, up to 10-fold by term. In the postpartum period, basal PRL levels remain elevated in lactating women, and suckling triggers a rapid release of PRL. TRH is a pharmacologic stimulator of PRL release, and dopamine is the predominant physiologic inhibitor factor.

4.4. PRL Receptor

The human PRL receptor is a 598 amino acid protein, encoded by a gene on chromosome 5 (p13-p14). The receptor contains a long extracellular region, a single transmembrane region, and a short cytoplasmic domain. There is a high sequence homology among the human, rat, and rabbit PRL receptors, and between the human PRL and GH receptors, which are colocalized to the same area on chromosome 5. PRL receptors are widely distributed, and their hormonal regulation is tissue-specific. In the mammary gland, high progesterone levels during pregnancy limit PRL receptor numbers, and early in lactation, the numbers increase markedly. Testosterone increases and estrogens decrease PRL receptor levels in the prostate. In most organs studied, PRL is able to up- and downregulate the level of its own receptor.

4.5. PRL Action

PRL contibutes to breast development during pregnancy, with estrogen, progesterone, and placental lactogen. After delivery, PRL stimulates milk production. Hyperprolactinemia suppresses gonadotropin-releasing hormone (GnRH) pulses at the hypothalamus, pituitary gonadotropin pulsatile secretion, and ovarian progesterone and estrogen release. In men, testosterone levels are low. PRL may induce mild glucose intolerance and has a role as an immune modulator.

4.6. RIA

Most assays for human PRL are based on the double-antibody method. Normal concentrations are slightly higher (<20 µg/L) in women than in men (<15 µg/L).

4.7. Hyperprolactinemia

The differential diagnosis of hyperprolactinemia includes PRL-secreting pituitary adenomas, pituitary stalk compression blocking dopamine access (because of large nonfunctioning adenomas), acromegaly, chronic breast stimulation, pregnancy, hypothyroidism, chronic renal failure, hypothalamic disorders, and medications (estrogens, phenothiazines, methyldopa, metoclopramide, and verapamil). PRL serum levels over 200 µg/L are usually associated with prolactinoma. Hyperprolactinemia presents as amenorrhea and galactorrhea in women, and impotence and infertility in men.

4.8. PRL-Secreting Pituitary Adenomas

Prolactinomas are the most common hormone-secreting pituitary adenomas. These monoclonal tumors are classified as microprolactinomas (<10 mm, 90% are women) or macroprolactinomas (>10 mm, 60% are men). In macroadenomas, the clinical presentation of hyperprolactinemia may be associated with mass effect signs of headaches and visual field disturbances. Some tumors secrete both GH and PRL. Most patients (70%) are successfully treated with dopamine agonists (usually bromocriptine). Transsphenoidal surgery is reserved for drug-resistant tumors.

4.9. Immune System Interaction

Lymphocytes express PRL receptors. In the rat hypoprolactinemic states are associated with impaired lymphocyte proliferation, decreased macrophage activation, and other manifestations of immunosuppression, which can be restored with PRL treatment.

5. TSH

5.1. Thyrotrope Embryology and Cytogenesis

Differentiated thyrotropes are found in the fetal pituitary at 12 wk of gestation, when TSH β subunits are immunolocalized and also found in the circulation. However, TSH levels remain low until week 18, when fetal levels increase significantly. Thyrotropes comprise only 5% of the anterior pituitary cell population.

5.2. TSH Gene

Human TSH is a 211 amino acid glycoprotein with a molecular mass of 28 kDa, structurally related to LH, FSH, and human chorionic gonadotropin (hCG). They are composed of a heterodimer of two noncovalently linked subunits, α and β. The α subunits of all four glycoproteins are identical and are encoded by a 13.5-kb gene (Fig. 4), located on chromosome 6q21–23 containing four exons and three introns. The α subunit is expressed in thyrotropes, gonadotropes, and placental cells, but cell-specific expression is dependent on different regions of the promoter. The β subunits of the glycoproteins define tissue specifity despite a 75% similarity in their primary structure and cysteine residues. The TSH β subunit gene is 4.9 kb in size, located on chromosome 1p22, and consists of three exons and two introns. The pituitary transcription factor Pit-1 binds to the β subunit promoter, but is not required for α-subunit gene expression. Both α and β subunit transcription are induced by TRH and inhibited by triiodothyronine (T_3) and dopamine.

5.3. TSH Secretion

TSH pulsatile secretion occurs every 2–3 h and is superimposed on basal hormone release from the pituitary. TSH has a circadian pattern of secretion, with nocturnal levels measuring up to twice daytime levels. TSH secretion is enhanced by TRH, whereas T_3, thyroxine (T_4), dopamine, SRIF, and glucocorticoids suppress TSH secretion.

5.4. TSH Receptor

The TSH receptor is located on the plasma membrane of thyroid follicular cells. It consists of a

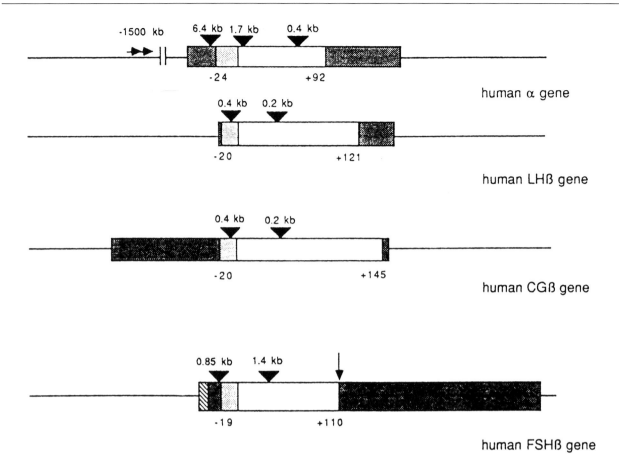

Fig. 4. Schematic structures of the human α, hLH-β, hCG-β, and hFSH-β genes. Untranslated regions are represented by dark regions, signal peptides are depicted by stippled regions, and mature proteins are represented by unshaded areas; hatched region—extended 5′-untranslated sequence; solid triangles represent the introns; the pair of horizontal arrows in the α-gene diagram—cAMP regulatory element; the solid arrow—polyadenylation site used by some of the FSH-β transcripts. From Gharib et al., 1990.

polypeptide chain of 764 amino acids, containing a 398 amino acid extracellular domain, seven-transmembrane segments, and a short intracellular domain of 82 amino acids. Receptor-ligand-binding activates G_s protein and adenylate cyclase cascade. The TSH receptor gene is located on chromosome 14 (q31), consisting of 10 exons. The extracellular domain and parts of the transmembrane domain contribute to TSH binding, and binding specifity is conferred by the TSH β subunit, although LH and hCG can activate the human TSH receptor to a certain degree. Recently, germ-line mutations in the transmembrane domain of the TSH receptor gene, resulting in constitutive cAMP activation, were reported in congenital hyperthyroidism, and somatic mutations in this domain were also found in patients with hyperfunctioning thyroid adenomas. Moreover, resistance to thyrotropin, caused by mutations in the

extracellular domain of the TSH receptor gene, has been described.

5.5. TSH Action

TSH induces morphological changes of the follicular cells, causes thyroid gland enlargement owing to hyperplasia and hypertrophy, stimulates iodide uptake and organification, thyroglobulin gene transcription, and thyroid hormone secretion.

5.6. Clinical Testing

RIA for TSH, the "first-generation assay," uses labeled antigen and is useful in distinguishing elevated TSH levels in primary hypothyroidism from normal euthyroid values, but is unable to differentiate euthyroid and hyperthyroid subjects. The new sensitive immunometric assays employ labeled antibody and a "capture antibody" in sandwich formation, and clearly discriminate euthyroid from hyperthyroid patients. TRH (200–500 µg, iv. or im) stimulates TSH release in euthyroid subjects. Hyperthyroid patients have no response, and primary hypothyroid patients demonstrate augmented TSH response to TRH stimulation. However, elevated basal TSH levels in TSH-secreting pituitary tumors fail to respond to TRH, whereas patients with hypothyroidism secondary to pituitary or hypothalamic disease have attenuated TSH response.

5.7. TSH Hypersecretion

Most cases of elevated serum TSH levels are a result of primary thyroid failure. Thyroid hormone resistance is a rare syndrome that includes clinical euthyroidism, elevated levels of thyroid hormones, and inappropriately normal to slightly increased TSH levels. TSH-producing pituitary adenomas comprises < 1% of all pituitary tumors, and secrete the TSH α and β subunits characteristic of the normal thyrotropes. However, the α subunit is synthesized in excess of the β subunit, a useful characteristic in the diagnosis of these tumors. TSH secretion by these tumors fails to respond to TRH stimulation or to normal thyroid hormone negative feedback. However, somatostatin suppresses TSH release from the tumors. Most patients present with hyperthyroidism and diffuse goiter. TSH is elevated or inappropriately normal in the presence of elevated thyroid hormones. Cosecretion of other pituitary hormones, GH, PRL, and FSH, is common, resulting in acromegaly, amenorrhea, galactorrhea, and impotence. Since tumors are usually large macroadenomas, local intracranial mass effects are common. Transsphenoidal pituitary surgery is the preferred initial approach, but most patients are not cured and require adjuvant medical or radiation therapy. The somatostatin analog, octreotide, is a promising treatment modality for these tumors. Thyroid ablation or surgery is not recommended because of the potential risk of pituitary tumor expansion owing to release of the thyrotrope cells from negative feedback inhibition.

6. FSH AND LH

6.1. Gonadotrope Embryology and Cytogenesis

Gonadotropes are found in the fetal pituitary at 12 wk of gestation, when β subunits are immunolocalized and first detected in blood. Gonadotropes represent up to 10% of the pituitary cell population. These basophilic cells reveal cytoplasmic positivity for FSH and LH, usually both in the same cell. However, some cells contain only one of the two hormones.

6.2. FSH and LH Genes

The gonadotropins, FSH and LH, are members of the glycoprotein hormone family, and share many structural similarities with TSH and hCG. The α subunits of all four members of this hormone family are identical, and the β subunits share considerable amino acid homology with one another, indicating evolution from a common precursor. The FSH and LH β subunits are both expressed in the gonadotropes, and possess three exons and two introns (Fig. 4). FSH β subunit, located on the short arm of human chromosome 11p13, is highly conserved between different species. LH β-gene, approx 1.5 kb in length, is one of the hCG β-like gene clusters, arranged on human chromosome 19q, and encodes a 121 amino acid mature protein. Human FSH is a 34-kDa protein with 210 amino acids, and LH is a 28.5-kDa protein consisting of 204 amino acid residues. GnRH pulses increase transcription rates of all three gonadotropin subunits, namely α, LH β, and FSH β. Testosterone increases FSH β mRNA levels in pituitary cell cultures, but has no effect on LH β mRNA. Estrogen negatively regulates transcription of all three subunits. However, estrogen exerts a positive-feedback effect at the pituitary level under several physiologic conditions and increases LH-β mRNA.

6.3. Regulation of Secretion

GnRH is the major regulator of gonadotropin secretion from pituitary cells. The frequency and amplitude of GnRH pulses are critical for stimulating LH and FSH output. Estrogens can exert both stimulatory and inhibitory effects on gonadotropin secretion, depending on the dose, duration, and other physiologic factors. Testosterone inhibits in vivo serum FSH levels, but its direct effects on FSH release at the pituitary level are stimulatory. Another regulator of FSH secretion is inhibin, a gonadal peptide produced by Sertoli cells, that inhibits FSH release and, under some conditions, may also regulate LH output.

6.4. Gonadotropin Receptor

FSH, LH, and TSH receptors have similar structure and belong to the subfamily of G$_s$-protein-coupled receptors having seven hydrophobic transmembrane segments. The specific, high-affinity interaction between hormone and receptor is owing to the large extracellular N-terminal domain of the receptor (LH—340 amino acids). The LH receptor is a single 75 kDa polypeptide of 700 amino acids. FSH receptor is also a single polypeptide, consisting of four subunits of similar mass (60 kDa).

6.5. Gonadotropin Action

In the male, LH binds to receptors on the Leydig cells and stimulates testosterone synthesis. High intratesticular testosterone levels are important for spermatogenesis. FSH is probably essential for the maturation process of the spermatids. In the female, LH and FSH are major regulators of ovarian steroid production. FSH plays a critical role in follicle growth and cytodifferentiation of granulosa cells.

6.6. Clinical Testing

RIAs of FSH and LH suffer from limited sensitivity and specificity owing to crossreactivity of free α subunits and other pituitary glycoprotein hormones. Recently, new two site-directed IRMA and nonisotopic assays have been introduced. These more sensitive measurements with no α-crossreactivity, are extremely useful in studying physiologic events characterized by low gonadotropin levels. The GnRH (25–100 µg, iv) stimulation test has limited usefulness in the diagnosis of hypothalamic–pituitary disorders. Patients with primary testicular failure exhibit an exaggerated increase in serum FSH and LH response within 30 min after injection. However, patients with hypothalamic and pituitary disorders cannot be distinguished. Repetitive administration of GnRH pulses may normalize gonadotropin responses in patients with hypothalamic disease, indicating pituitary integrity.

6.7. Gonadotrope-Cell Tumors

Gonadotrope adenomas are the most common pituitary adenomas. In the past, they were termed "nonsecreting" adenomas, because the gonadotropins and their subunits produced by them are either not released or inefficiently secreted, and usually do not produce a distinct clinical syndrome. These tumors produce supranormal (up to 10 times normal) serum levels of α and FSH β subunits, but rarely of LH β. Usually, the subunits are not secreted in the same proportions. Some gonadotrope adenomas produce α subunits, but not intact FSH or LH. TRH administration to patients with gonadotrope adenomas usually results in secretion of gonadotropins or their subunits, compared with no stimulation in normal subjects. Most of the "nonsecreting adenomas" immunostain either for intact FSH and LH, or α, FSH β, and LH β subunits. Mass effects, including optic chiasm pressure and other neurologic symptoms, may be the first symptoms of large gonadotrope tumors. Excessive secretion of FSH or LH may actually downregulate the reproductive axis.

REFERENCES

Fryklund LM, Bierich JR, Ranke MB. Recombinant human growth hormone. *Clin Endocrinol Metab* 1986; 15:511.

Gharib SD, Wierman ME, Shupnik MA, Chin WW. Molecular biology of the pituitary gonadotropins. *Endocr Rev* 1990; 11:177.

Melmed, S. (ed.) *The Pituitary*. Cambridge, MA. Blackwell Science, 1995.

SELECTED READINGS

Asa SL, Kovacs K. Functional morphology of the human fetal pituitary. In: Sommers SC, Rosen PP, (eds). Pathology Annual, part 1, vol. 19 Appleton-Century-Crofts. Norwalk, CT: pp 275–315.

Baumann G. Growth hormone heterogeneity: Genes, isohormones, variants, and binding proteins. *Endocr Rev* 1991; 12:424.

Combarnous Y. Molecular basis of the specificity of binding of glycoprotein hormones to their receptors. *Endocr Rev* 1992; 13:670.

Eyde Theill L, Karin M. Transcriptional control of GH expression and anterior pituitary development. *Endocr Rev* 1993; 14:670.

Kelly PA, Djiane J, Postel-Vinay MC, Edery M. The prolactin/growth hormone receptor family. *Endocr Rev* 1991; 12:235.

Magner JA. Thyroid-stimulating hormone: Biosynthesis, cell biology, and bioactivity. *Endocr Rev* 1990; 11:354.

Mountjoy KG, Robbins LS, Mortrud MT, Cone RD. The cloning of a family of genes that encode the melanocortin receptors. *Science* 1992; 257:1248.

Tsigos C, Arai K, Hung W, Chrousos GP. Hereditary isolated glucocorticoid deficiency is associated with abnormalities of the adrenocorticotropin receptor gene. *J Clin Invest* 1993; 92:2458.

Vassart G, Dumont JE. The thyrotropin receptor and the regulation of thyrocyte function and growth. *Endocr Rev* 1992; 13:596.

15 Posterior Pituitary Hormones

Daniel G. Bichet, MD

CONTENTS

1. STRUCTURE OF NEUROHYPOPHYSIS: ANATOMY OF VASOPRESSIN-PRODUCING CELLS

The hypothalamus (Fig. 1) embodies a group of nuclei that form the floor and ventrolateral walls of the triangular-shaped third ventricle. A thin membrane called the lamina terminalis forms the anterior wall of this compartment and is believed to contain osmoreceptor cells in a structure known as the organum vasculosum. The subfornical organ (SFO) is also believed to contain these cells. The organum vasculosum of the lamina terminalis (OVLT), the SFO, and the pituitary gland lack a blood–brain barrier. The supraoptic nucleus (SON) lies just dorsal to the optic chiasm and approx 2 mm from the third ventricle. The paraventricular nucleus (PVN) lies closer to the thalamus in the suprachiasmatic portion of the hypothalamus, but it borders on the third ventricular space. These well-defined nuclei contain the majority of the large neuroendocrine cell bodies, known as the magnocellular or neurosecretory cells, that manufacture arginine-vasopressin and oxytocin.

The neurohypophysis consists of:

1. A set of hypothalamic nuclei: the supraoptic and paraventricular nuclei, which house the pericarya of the magnocellular neurons;

2. The axonal processes of the magnocellular neurons form the supraoptical hypophyseal tract; and,

3. The neurosecretory material of these neurons, which is carried on to the posterior pituitary gland (Fig. 1).

Oxytocin and vasopressin are synthesized in separate populations of the supraoptic nuclei and the paraventricular nuclei neurons. The axonal

From: *Endocrinology: Basic and Clinical Principles* (P. M. Conn and S. Melmed, eds.), Humana Press Inc., Totowa, NJ.

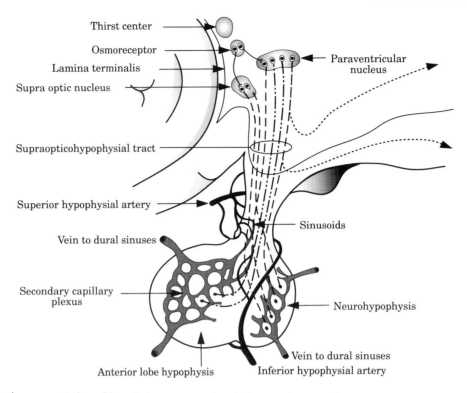

Fig. 1.   Schematic representation of hypothalamus, posterior pituitary and surrounding structures. Four major neuronal tracts originate from the supraoptic and paraventricular nuclei: (1) to the posterior lobe of the pituitary (– –); (2) to the hypophysial portal system (— - - —) (3) to the brainstem and the spinal cord; (4) to the forebrain. Afferent fibers to these nuclei originate from the osmoreceptors and baroreceptors (not represented).

projections of vasopressin and oxytocin-producing neurons from these nuclei reflect the dual function of vasopressin and oxytocin as hormones and as neuropeptides, since they project their axons to several brain areas or to the neurohypophysis. A second vasopressin neurosecretory pathway to the hypophysial portal system transports high concentrations of the hormone to the anterior pituitary gland. Vasopressin produced by this pathway seems to play a role in the secretion of adrenocorticotropic hormone (ACTH) from the anterior pituitary gland.

2. THE VASOPRESSIN AND OXYTOCIN GENES

2.1. A Gene Structure

Vasopressin and its corresponding carrier protein are synthesized as a composite precursor (Fig. 2) by the magnocellular neurons described above. The pre-

cursor is packaged into neurosecretory granules and transported axonally in the stalk of the posterior pituitary. On route to the neurohypophysis, the precursor is processed into the active hormone. The vasopressin prohormone includes the neurophysin II and a glycopeptide. The oxytocin prohormone only includes the neurophysin I, and the glycopeptide part is not represented. This prohormone is targeted from the trans-Golgi network into secretory granules of the regulated secretory pathway. Once the prohormone has entered the granule, the biosynthesis of vasopressin as a hormone is completed: vasopressin is excised from the prohormone, and the C-terminal is amidated. Preprovasopressin (prepro-VP) is encoded by the 2.5-kb arginine-vasopressin (AVP)-neurophysin II gene on chromosome 20 (20p13). Exon 1 of the AVP-neurophysin II gene encodes the putative signal peptide, vasopressin, and the NH_2-terminal region of neurophysin II. Exon 2 gives rise to the central region of neurophysin II and exon 3

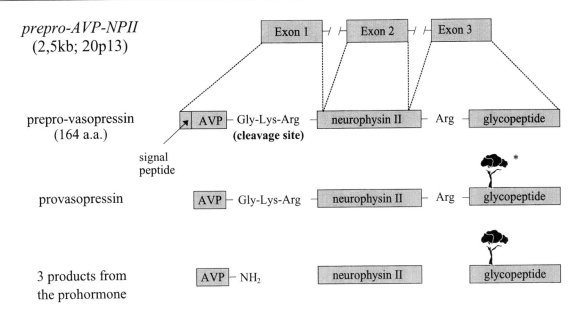

prepro-AVP-NPII
(2,5kb; 20p13)

prepro-vasopressin
(164 a.a.)

signal
peptide

provasopressin

3 products from
the prohormone

* addition of a carbohydrate chain

Fig. 2. Structure of the human vasopressin gene and prohormone.

accounts for the COOH-terminal region of neurophysin and glycoprotein. Provasopressin is generated by the removal of the signal peptide from prepro-VP and the addition of carbohydrate to its glycoprotein domain in magnocellular neurons in the hypothalamus. Additional posttranslational processing occurs within neurosecretory vesicles during transport of the precursor protein to axon terminals in the posterior pituitary, yielding vasopressin, neurophysin, and glycoprotein. Mammalian vasopressin and oxytocin hormones are encoded by distinct, but structurally related genes. These genes are transcribed on opposite DNA strands (tail to tail) in humans and rats on chromosome 20, where they are separated by approx 8–10 kb of intergenic sequences. A similarity in the nucleotide sequence encoding the neuropeptides, vasopressin and oxytocin, suggests that they may have arisen from a common ancestor by gene duplication. However, gene inversion would also be required. A considerable homology is observed in exon B of both genes (specifically the region encoding amino acids residues 10–76 of neurophysins I and II). There is a head-to-tail arrangement in other evolutionarily

duplicated gene systems, such as the β subunits of human chorionic gonadotrophin or the C4/steroid 21-hydroxylase/gene X locus.

2.2. Gene Regulation

The regulation of mammalian vasopressin gene expression is closely correlated with the expression of its structural counterpart oxytocin. Both genes are similar in their protein-encoding sequences, yet their translational products control different functions and hence their expression should depend on quite distinct physiological stimuli. This is consistent with the finding that these two genes show very little homology in their promoter regions, suggesting independent transcriptional control mechanisms. However, osmotic stimulation has been shown to upregulate both vasopressin and oxytocin gene transcription. Late gestation and lactation also trigger the transcription of both vasopressin and oxytocin genes. Cyclic 3', 5'-adenosine monophosphate has been shown to regulate bovine vasopressin expression in vitro via cis-acting element within the vasopressin promoter.

In rats, the vasopressin- and oxytocin-encoding genes are expressed in distinct sets of hypothalamic magnocellular neurons, which are specific for either vasopressin (vasopressinergic neurons) or oxytocin (oxytocinergic neurons). *In situ* hybridization experiments have demonstrated that, during osmotic stimulation, vasopressin and oxytocin genes are expressed exclusively in vasopressinergic and oxytocinergic neurons, respectively. No coexpression of the neuropeptides in the same neurons has been observed.

2.3. Expression of the Vasopressin Gene in Diabetes Insipidus (Brattleboro Rats)

The animal model of diabetes insipidus that has been most extensively studied is the Brattleboro rat. Discovered in 1961, the rat lacks vasopressin and its neurophysin, whereas the synthesis of the structurally related hormone oxytocin is not affected by the mutation. Its inability to synthesize vasopressin is inherited as an autosomal semirecessive trait. Schmale and Richter (Czernichow et al., 1985) isolated and sequenced the vasopressin gene from homozygous Brattleboro rats and found that the defect is owing to a single nucleotide deletion of a G-residue within the second exon encoding the carrier protein neurophysin. The shift in the reading frame caused by this deletion predicts a precursor with an entirely different C-terminus. The messenger RNA produced by the mutated gene encodes a normal AVP, but an abnormal neurophysin II moiety, which impairs transport and processing of the AVP-NP II precursor and its retention in the endoplasmic reticulum of the magnocellular neurons where it is produced.

3. CHEMISTRY, PROCESSING, AND METABOLISM OF AVP

Arginine-vasopressin is a nonapeptide with a mol wt of 1084 Dalton. The chemical structure of AVP and related peptides is given in Table 1. It is a strongly basic molecule (isoelectric point pH 10.9) because of the amidation of three carboxyl groups. Lysine-vasopressin, the antidiuretic hormone of the pig family, has the less basic amino acid lysine at position 8, resulting in a lower isoelectric point (pH 10.0). Biological activity of these hormones is destroyed by oxidation or reduction of the disulfide bond.

Members of the vasopressin hormone family have been detected throughout the animal kingdom comprising more than half a dozen variants, including peptides such as vasotocin of nonmammalian vertebrates, the diuretic hormone of insects, and the conopressins of molluscs. In vertebrates, their endocrine hormonal activity—controlling mainly water retention—is well documented, whereas in invertebrates, they may function primarily as neurotransmitters, although a hormonal diuretic activity has been demonstrated in the locust. Acher and Chauvet postulated the existence of a single ancestral peptide that developed along two evolutionary lines, one vasotocin-vasopressin and the other isotocin-mesotocin-oxytocin (Saito et al., 1995). However, recent evidence suggests that multiple genes, which code for numerous vasopressin-like hormones, are present in Australian macropods.

Neurophysins were first thought to be carrier proteins for vasopressin and oxytocin. It is now recognized that neurophysin I (for oxytocin) and neurophysin II (for vasopressin) belong to the precursor of the respective hormone. Neurophysins exist in monomer-dimer equilibrium in aqueous solution. Hormone binding increases the dimerization constant with a factor variably estimated as 10–100. A three-dimensional structure of a bovine peptide–neurophysin monomer complex has been proposed by Chen and coworkers (Rittig et al., 1996). The structure of each monomer is 12% helix and 40% β-sheet. The chain is folded into two domains as predicted by disulfide-pairing studies. The time from synthesis to release of the hormone into the systemic circulation is about 1.5 h. Pulse-chase experiments indicate that cleavage occurs continuously during axonal transport, but both cleaved and uncleaved precursors are present in the neurosecretory granules of the posterior pituitary. Only a small percentage of the synthetic peptide is released; some of the vasopressin-containing neurosecretory granules move away from the nerve endings and are unavailable for release. Once secreted into the circulation, vasopressin is accompanied, but not bound, by its specific neurophysin. Neurophysins themselves do not appear to have any biological activity, but since they are synthesized and released with vasopressin and oxytocin, their concentrations in the plasma reflect any changes in the release of the active hormones (*vide infra*). The plasma half-life of vasopressin is short,

Table 1
Amino Acid Sequence of AVP and Related Neurohypophyseal Nonapeptides

	1 2 3 4	5	6 7 8 9	Distribution
AVP	Cys-Tyr-Phe-Glu(NH$_2$)-Asp(NH$_2$)-Cys-Pro-Arg-Gly(NH$_2$)			Most mammals
Lysine vasopressin	Phe Glu(NH$_2$)		Lys	Pig family
Arginine vasotocin	Ile Glu(NH$_2$)		Arg	Nonmammalian vertebrates
Oxytocin	Ile Glu(NH$_2$)		Leu	Mammals, birds
Mesotocin	Ile Glu(NH$_2$)		Ile	Reptiles
Isotocin	Ile Ser		Ile	Fish
Glumitocin	Ile Ser		Glu(NH$_2$)	Fish
Valitocin	Ile Glu(NH$_2$)		Val	Fish
Aspartocin	Ile Asp(NH$_2$)		Leu	Fish

From Baylis, 1989.

being about 5–15 min. Platelet-rich plasma AVP concentrations are approximately five- to sixfold higher than those of platelet-depleted plasma. Furthermore, irreversible platelet aggregation could bring about intraplatelet arginine-vasopressin release. However, osmotic stimulation of AVP release does not influence platelet-associated AVP concentrations.

4. CONTROL OF AVP SECRETION

4.1. Osmotic Stimulation

Osmotic stimulation is the principal determinant of vasopressin release and has been the subject of a recent review by Bourque and coworkers (1995). Cerebral osmoreceptors respond to changes in blood osmolality of 1% or less, and all of the available evidence leads to the conclusion that they are located in the anterior part of the brain, presumably in the anterior hypothalamus.

4.1.1. ESSENTIAL CRITERIA FOR OSMORECEPTORS

Three criteria must be met for cells to be identified as osmoreceptive. First, increasing the osmolality of the perfusing fluid should result in an increase in firing frequency, but no response should be obtained if the osmolality is increased with solutes, such as urea or glycerol, since these solutes are able to diffuse across the cell membrane. Furthermore, the osmoreceptor cells should display a sensitivity to changes in osmolality, which approaches that observed in vivo. Second, the putative osmoreceptors must, if they are not the

magnocellular neurons themselves, have neuroanatomical connections with the magnocellular neurons. Third, if the osmoreceptors are separated from the magnocellular neurons, alterations in vasopressin secretion secondary to changes in plasma osmolality should occur. The following candidates fulfill these criteria for osmoreceptors: magnocellular cells, which synthesize vasopressin in the SON and PVN; the perinuclear zone around the SON; cells in the SFO and OVLT; cells in the lateral preoptic area.

4.1.2. THE BLOOD–BRAIN BARRIER AND OSMORECEPTORS

The blood–brain barrier is impermeable to all solutes, except for lipid-soluble compounds. The hypothesis that the circumventricular organ (CVO), with its fenestrated perfusing capillaries, contains osmoreceptors is supported by the fact that all the aforementioned criteria for osmoreceptors are fulfilled. The CVO then seems to provide essential osmoreceptive input to the vasopressin-secreting cells in the SON and PVN. Functional deficits observed after lesions of the SFO and OVLT and extensive electrophysiological evidence also suggest that cells in both the OVLT and SFO are osmosensitive.

4.1.3. OSMOTIC CONTROL OF ELECTRICAL ACTIVITY IN SUPRAOPTIC NUCLEUS NEURONS

Patch-clamp analysis revealed that the supraoptic nucleus neurons are, respectively, depolarized and hyperpolarized by increases and decreases in external osmolality, and that these intrinsic responses resulted from changes in the activity of mechanosensitive cationic channels. Moreover, intracellular recordings in hypothalamic explants have shown that changes in electrical activity are associated with proportional changes in the frequency of glutamatergic excitatory postsynaptic potentials derived from osmosensitive OVLT neurons.

4.1.4. Osmotic Threshold: Sensitivity or Gain of the Osmoreceptor/Arginine-Vasopressin/Releasing Unit

The level of plasma osmolality at which hydrated subjects first responded to an IV infusion of 5% saline with a statistically significant fall in free water clearance (without a fall in osmolal clearance or creatinine excretion) was termed the osmotic threshold for vasopressin release. This osmotic threshold (288.5 mosM/kg), was raised by the administration of hydrocortisone, and plasma volume expansion, and lowered by plasma volume contraction.

With the development of sensitive radioimmunoassays, it was later demonstrated that, in healthy adults, the infusion of concentrated saline (850 mmol/L) caused a progressive rise in plasma osmolality and in plasma arginine-vasopressin concentrations. A direct correlation between the two variables was established, defined by the function: pAVP = 0.30 (PosM – 280) (Fig. 3). The abscissal intercept, 280 mmol/kg, is the osmotic threshold. Because this intercept falls below the limit of detection of the assay methods, this "set" of the osmoreceptor mechanisms should be referred to as the theoretical for vasopressin release. Whether AVP secretion can be completely suppressed or whether a linear vs an exponential model should be used remains unclear. A very close relationship has also been demonstrated between urine osmolality and AVP concentrations, except in patients with nephrogenic diabetes insipidus (Fig. 3). The exquisite sensitivity and gain of the osmoreceptor—AVP—renal reflex is given by the following example (Fig. 4). A normally hydrated human may have a plasma osmolality of 287 mmol/kg, a plasma vasopressin concentration of 2 pg/mL, and a urinary osmolality of 500 mmol/kg. With an increase of 1% in total body water, plasma osmolality will fall by 1% (2.8 mmol/kg), plasma AVP will decrease to 1 pg/mL, and urinary osmolality will diminish to 250 mmol/kg. Similarly, it is only necessary to increase total body water by 2% to suppress the plasma AVP maximally (<0.25 pg/mL) and to dilute the urine maximally (<100 mmol/kg). In the opposite direction, a 2% decrease in total body water will increase plasma osmolality by 2% (5.6 mmol/kg), plasma AVP will rise from 2–4 pg/mL, and urine will be maximally concentrated (>1000 mmol/kg). Thus, in the context of these sensitivity changes, a 1-mmol rise in plasma osmolality would be expected to increase plasma AVP by 0.38 pg/mL and urinary osmolality by 100 mmol/kg. Such a small change in plasma osmolality (measured by freezing point depression) or plasma AVP (by radioimmunoassay) may be undetectable, yet of extreme physiological importance. For example, a patient with a 24-h urinary solute load of 600 mmol must excrete 6 L of urine with an osmolality of 100 mmol/kg to eliminate the solute; however, if the urine osmolality increases from 100–200 mmol/kg (owing to an undetectable rise of 1 mmol in plasma osmolality and 0.38 pg/mL in plasma AVP), the obligatory 24-h urine volume to excrete the 600-mmol solute load decreases substantially from 6–3 L. Examination of Fig. 4 demonstrates that a maximal antidiuresis is obtained when the plasma AVP concentrations reaches 5 pg/mL. Greater hyperosmolality, although releasing more AVP, fails to conserve any more renal water, thus exposing the body to the potential of severe dehydration. This can be avoided by the stimulation of the thirst osmoreceptor at a plasma osmolality of 298 mmol/kg. However, recent studies, using a visual analog scale, have demonstrated that the onset of thirst occurs at a considerably lower plasma osmolality than was previously recognized; the values were similar to those of the threshold for vasopressin release. It has been shown in both animals and humans that the act of drinking ameliorates thirst and inhibits the secretion of vasopressin before changes occur in the extracellular fluid volume or osmolality. In humans, it has been shown that AVP secretion is inhibited independently of osmotic or gastric factors by the activation of the cold-sensitive oropharyngeal receptors. The presence of such cold-sensitive oropharyngeal receptors may explain the desire of severely dehydrated patients,

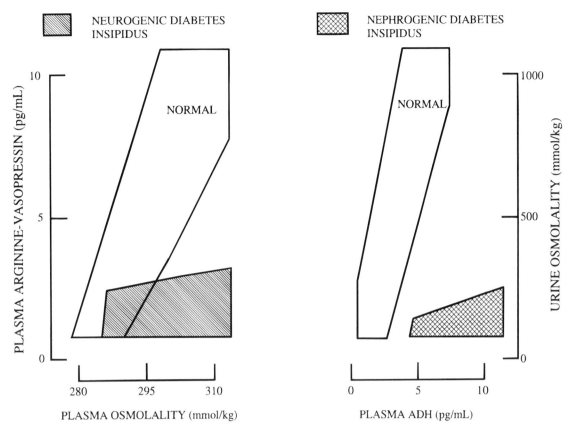

Fig. 3. The relationship between plasma AVP and plasma osmolality during the infusion of hypertonic saline solution (left part of the figure). Patients with primary polydipsia and nephrogenic diabetes insipidus have values within the normal range (open area) in contrast to patients with neurogenic diabetes insipidus, who show subnormal plasma ADH responses (hatched area).

Relationship between urine osmolality and plasma ADH during dehydration and water loading (right part of the figure). Patients with neurogenic diabetes insipidus and primary polydipsia have values within the normal range (open area) in contrast to patients with nephrogenic diabetes insipidus, who have hypotonic urine despite high plasma ADH (crosshatched area). (From Zerbe and Robertson, 1984, with permission.)

i.e., patients with diabetes insipidus (neurogenic or nephrogenic), for cold liquids.

4.2. Baroregulation

It is now well established that afferent neural impulses arising from stretch receptors in the left atrium, carotid sinus, and aortic arch inhibit the secretion of vasopressin. Conversely, when the discharge rate of these receptors is reduced, vasopressin secretion is enhanced. Moreover, the relative potency of the cardiac and sino-aortic reflexes in the release of vasopressin appears to vary among species. For example, the increase in plasma vaso-

pressin that occurs during moderate hemorrhage in the dog is attributable primarily to reflex effects from cardiac receptors; sino-aortic receptors appear to exert only minor influences on vasopressin release in this situation. In contrast, sino-aortic receptors appear to play the dominant role in eliciting vasopressin secretion during blood loss in nonhuman primates and humans. In humans, blood pressure reductions of as little as 5%, induced by the ganglion blocking agent trimetaphan, significantly altered plasma AVP concentration. Furthermore, an exponential relationship between plasma vasopressin and the percentage decline in mean arterial blood

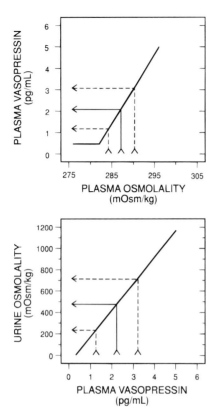

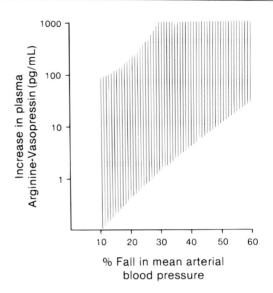

Fig. 5.   Increase in plasma AVP during hypotension (vertical lines). Note that a large diminution in blood pressure in normal humans induces large increments in AVP (From Vokes and Robertson, 1985, with permission.)

Fig. 4.   Schematic representation of the effect of small alterations in the basal plasma osmolality on plasma vasopressin and urinary osmolality in healthy adults. (From Robertson et al., 1976, with permission.)

pressure has been observed with large decreases in blood pressure (Fig. 5). Since an interdependence exists between osmoregulated and baroregulated AVP secretion (Fig. 6), under conditions of moderate hypovolemia, renal water excretion can be maintained around a lower set point of plasma osmolality, thus preserving osmoregulation. As hypovolemia becomes more severe, plasma AVP concentrations attain extremely high values, and baroregulation overrides the osmoregulatory system.

4.3. Hormonal Influences on the Secretion of Vasopressin

Studies on the direct effects of various peptides and other biological substances on the release of vasopressin may be confounded by the hemodynamic effects of these substances, which indirectly modulate vasopressin release via the cardiovascular reflexes. For example, the infusion of pressor doses

of norepinephrine increases both arterial blood pressure and left atrial pressure. Each of these changes is capable of eliciting a reflex inhibition of vasopressin release that should reduce plasma vasopressin. However, the inhibitory effects of the sino-aortic and cardiac reflexes on vasopressin release seem to be offset by the direct stimulatory effect of circulating norepinephrine. A similar situation may exist with the possible stimulation of vasopressin release by angiotensin. The direct stimulatory effect of angiotensin may be offset by inhibitory influences elicited from the cardiovascular reflexes. Angiotensin is a well-known dipsogen and has been shown to cause drinking in all the species tested.

Physiological concentrations of angiotensin II do not cause an increase in plasma vasopressin concentration in normal subjects. However, the complex interaction between the direct stimulatory and cardiovascular inhibitory influences has not been studied.

5. CELLULAR ACTIONS OF VASOPRESSIN: VASOPRESSIN ISORECEPTORS POSTRECEPTOR EVENTS, VASOPRESSIN AGONISTS, AND ANTAGONISTS

There is evidence that vasopressin:

1. Participates in the short-term regulation of arterial blood pressure by its direct vascular action and

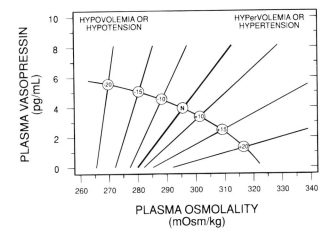

Fig. 6. Schematic representation of the relationship between plasma vasopressin and plasma osmolality in the presence of differing states of blood volume and/or pressure. The line labeled N represents normovolemic normotensive conditions. Minus numbers to the left indicate percent fall, and positive numbers to the right, percent rise in blood volume or pressure (From Robertson, 1985a, with permission).

that it interacts with the central nervous system baroreceptor pathways;

2. Is one component of the multifactorial regulation of adrenocorticotropin release by the adenohypophysis;

3. Acts specifically on anterior pituitary cells to enhance the release of the thyroid-stimulating hormone (TSH);

4. Induces contraction of glomerular mesangial cells;

5. Increases prostaglandin synthesis by medullary interstitial cells;

6. Causes platelet aggregation and the release of at least three coagulation factors: factor VIIIc, von Willebrand factor, and tissue plasminogen activator;

7. Has a mitogenic effect on several cell types; and

8. Increases the firing rate of the hippocampal neurons and affects several brain functions, such as memory consolidation.

The signal molecule arginine-vasopressin is thus involved in endocrine, paracrine, neurotransmitters, and neuromodulator functions.

These multiple actions of AVP could be explained by the interaction of AVP with at least three types of G-protein-coupled receptors; the V_{1a} (vascular

hepatic) and V_{1b} (anterior pituitary) receptors act through phosphatidylinositol hydrolysis to mobilize calcium, and the V_2 (kidney) receptor is coupled to adenylate cyclase. Molecular cloning and the expression of vasopressin and oxytocin receptors have confirmed that these receptors belong to the G-protein-coupled receptor family characterized by seven putative transmembrane helices. To date, more than 10 related complementary DNAs have been cloned and sequenced: they encode the rat and human vasopressin V_{1a} receptors, the human vasopressin V_{1b} (or V_3) receptor, the rat and human vasopressin V_2 receptors, the rat and human oxytocin receptors, the [Lys^8]VP V_2 receptor and the oxytocin receptor from a pig kidney cell line, and the [Arg^8] vasotocin receptors from teleost fish and toad. These receptors are strikingly similar in both size and amino acid sequences. The rat V_{1a} and the human oxytocin receptors have 48% similarity with the human V_2 receptor. The V_2[Lys^8]VP receptor from the pig kidney cell line and the human V_2 receptor (V_2[Arg^8]VP receptor) demonstrate more than 90% identity within their putative transmembrane domains, 80% identity for their C-terminal regions, and a relatively low identity of 62% for their N-terminal regions. These differences could be responsible for different ligand affinities. As expected, the messenger RNA (mRNA) encoding the V_{1a} receptor is abundant in rat liver and kidney and present in brain. V_2 receptor transcripts are heavily expressed in cells of the renal collecting ducts and thick ascending limbs of the loops of Henle. RT-PCR and Northern blot analysis showed that the human V_3 receptor was expressed in normal pituitary.

The first step in the action of AVP on water excretion is its binding to arginine-vasopressin type 2 receptors (V_2 receptors) on the basolateral membrane of the collecting duct cells (Fig. 7). The human V_2 receptor gene, AVPR2, is located in chromosome region Xq28, and has three exons and two small introns. The sequence of the cDNA predicts a polypeptide of 371 amino acids with a structure typical of guanine-nucleotide (G) protein-coupled receptors with seven-transmembrane, four-extracellular, and four-cytoplasmic domains (*see also* Fig. 8). A three-dimensional model of the V_{1a} vasopressin receptor subtyped has been constructed by Mouillac and coworkers (1995) to dock its endogenous ligand AVP. It is likely that this model will be applicable to the binding characteristics of AVP to its V_2 receptor.

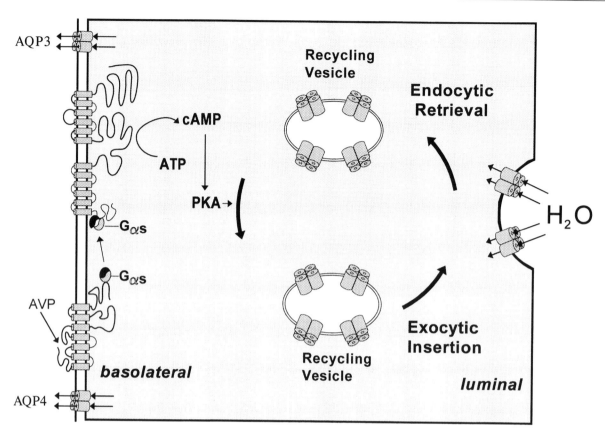

Fig. 7.   Schematic view of the intracellular action of the antidiuretic hormone, AVP. The hormone is bound to the vasopressin V_2 receptor (a G-protein-linked receptor) on the basolateral membrane. AVP activates adenylate cyclase increasing the intracellular concentration of cyclic AMP (cAMP). The topology of adenylyl cyclase is characterized by two tandem repeats of six hydrophobic putative transmembrane domains separated by a large cytoplasmic loop and terminating in a large intracellular tail. cAMP generation follows receptor-linked activation of the heterometric G-protein (G_s) and interaction of the free $G_{\alpha s}$-chain with the adenylyl cyclase catalyst. A cAMP-dependent protein kinase (pKA) is the target of the generated cAMP. Cytoplasmic vesicles carrying the water channel proteins (represented as homotetrameric complexes) are fused to the luminal membrane in response to vasopressin, thereby increasing the water permeability of this membrane. When vasopressin is not available, water channels are retrieved by an endocytic process, and water permeability returns to its original low rate. AQP3 and AQP4 are expressed on the basolateral membrane.

AVP was found to be completely buried into a 15–20 Å deep cleft defined by the transmembrane helices of the receptor (Fig. 9) and to interact with amino acids located within this region (Fig. 10). The activation of the V_2 receptor on renal-collecting tubules stimulates adenylyl cyclase via the stimulatory G-protein (G_s) and promotes the cyclic adenosine monophosphate (cAMP)-mediated incorporation of water channels (aquaporins) into the luminal surface of these cells. This process is the molecular basis of the vasopressin-induced increase in the osmotic water permeability of the apical membrane of the collecting tubule. Aquaporin-1 (AQP1, also

knowns as CHIP, channel-forming integral membrane protein of 28 kDa) was the first protein shown to function as a molecular water channel and is constitutively expressed in mammalian red cells, renal proximal tubules, thin descending limbs, and other water-permeable epithelia. At the subcellular level, AQP1 is localized in both apical and basolateral plasma membranes, which may represent entrance and exit routes for transepithelial water transport. In contrast to aquaporin-2 (AQP2) (*vide infra*), limited amounts of AQP1 are localized in membranes of vesicles or vacuoles. In the basolateral membranes, AQP1 is localized to both basal

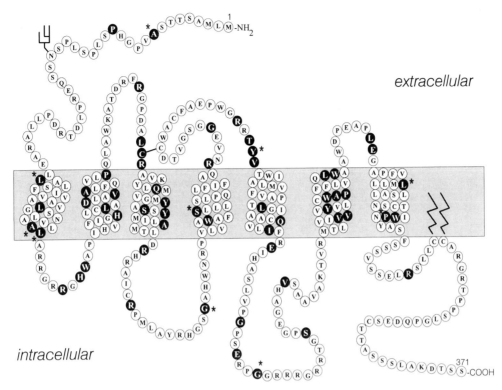

Fig. 8. Schematic representation of the V$_2$ receptor and identification of 72 *AVPR2* mutations, which include 37 missense, 10 nonsense, 18 frameshift, 2 inframe deletion, 1 splice-site, and 4 large deletion mutations. The four large deletions are incompletely characterized and are not included in the figure. Predicted amino acids are given as the one-letter code. Solid symbols indicate the predicted location of the mutations; an asterisk indicates two different mutations in the same codon. The names of the mutations were assigned according to the conventional nomenclature. The extracellular (E$_I$–N$_{IV}$), cytoplasmic (C$_I$–C$_V$), and transmembrane domains (TM$_I$–TM$_{VII}$) are labeled according to Sharif and Hanley (Saito et al., 1995). E$_I$: 98del28, 98ins28, 113delCT. TM$_I$: L44F, L44P, L53R, A61V, L62P. TM$_I$ and C$_I$: 253del35, 255del9. C$_I$: 274insG, W71X. TM$_{II}$: H80R, L83P, D85N, V88M, 337delCT, P95L. E$_{II}$: R106C, 402delCT, C112R, R113W. TM$_{III}$: Q119X, Y124X, S126F, Y128S, A132D. C$_{II}$: R137H, R143P, 528del7, 528delG. TM$_{IV}$: W164S, S167L, S167T. E$_{III}$: R181C, G185C, R202C, T204N, 684delTA, Y205C, V206D. TM$_V$: L219R, Q225X, 753insC. C$_{III}$: E231X, 763delA, 786delG, E242X, 804insG, 804delG, 834delA, 855delG. TM$_{VI}$: V277A, ΔV278, Y280C, W284X, A285P, P286L, P286R, L292P, W293X. E$_{IV}$: 977delG, 980A → G. TM$_{VII}$: L312X, P322H, P322S, W323R. C$_{IV}$: R337X.

and lateral. AQP2 is the vasopressin-regulated water channel in renal collecting ducts. It is exclusively present in principal cells of inner medullary collecting duct cells and is diffusely distributed in the cytoplasm in the euhydrated condition, whereas apical staining of AQP2 is intensified in the dehydrated condition or after vasopressin administration. These observations are thought to represent the exocytic insertion of preformed water channels from intracellular vesicles into the apical plasma membrane (the shuttle hypothesis) (Fig. 7). AQP3 is the water channel in basolateral membranes of renal medullary collecting ducts. AQP4

is abundantly expressed in brain, and could be the osmoreceptor that regulates body water balance and mediates water flow within the central nervous system.

The gene that codes for the water channel of the apical membrane of the kidney-collecting tubule has been designated AQP2 and was cloned by homology to the rat aquaporin of collecting duct. The human AQP2 gene is located in chromosome region 12q13, and has four exons and three introns. It is predicted to code for a polypeptide of 271 amino acids that is organized into two repeats oriented at 180° to each other and has six membrane-spanning

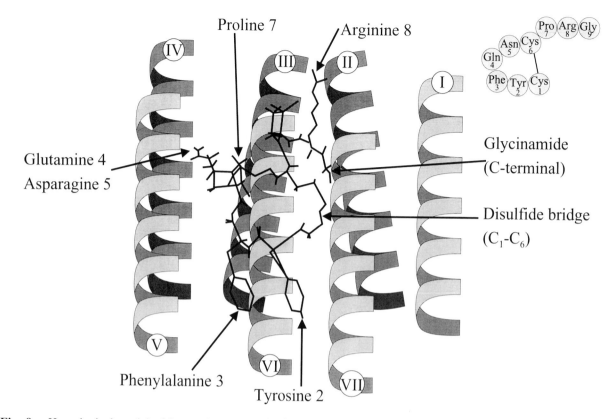

Fig. 9. Hypothetical model of interaction between AVP and its V_{1a} receptor. A schematic lateral view of the seven-transmembrane α-helices (I–VII) of the receptor and of the vasopressin docked in the rat V_{1a} receptor is represented. Each individual amino acid of the vasopressin molecule is represented. Redrawn from data published by Mouillac et al., 1995.

domains, both terminal ends located intracellularly, and conserved Asn-Pro-Ala boxes (Fig. 11). These features are characteristic of the major intrinsic protein family. AQP2 is detectable in urine and changes in urinary excretion of this protein can be used as an index of the action of vasopressin on the kidney.

6. HYPOTHALAMIC DIABETES INSIPIDUS

Diabetes insipidus is a disorder characterized by the excretion of abnormally large volumes (30 mL/kg of body wt/pd for an adult patient) of dilute urine (<250 mmol/kg). Four basic defects can be involved. The most common, a deficient secretion of the antidiuretic hormone (ADH) AVP, is referred to as neurogenic (or central, neurohypophysial, cranial, or hypothalamic) diabetes insipidus. Diabetes insipidus can also result from renal insensitivity to the antidiuretic effect of AVP, which is referred to

as nephrogenic diabetes insipidus. Excessive water intake can result in polyuria, which is referred to as primary polydipsia: it can be the result of an abnormality in the thirst mechanism and referred to as dipsogenic diabetes insipidus; it can also be associated with a severe emotional cognitive dysfunction and is referred to as psychogenic polydipsia. Finally, increased metabolism of vasopressin during pregnancy is referred to as gestational diabetes insipidus.

6.1. Common Forms

Failure to synthesize or secrete vasopressin normally limits maximal urinary concentration and, depending on the severity of the disease, causes varying degrees of polyuria and polydipsia. Experimental destruction of the vasopressin-synthesizing areas of the hypothalamus (supraoptic

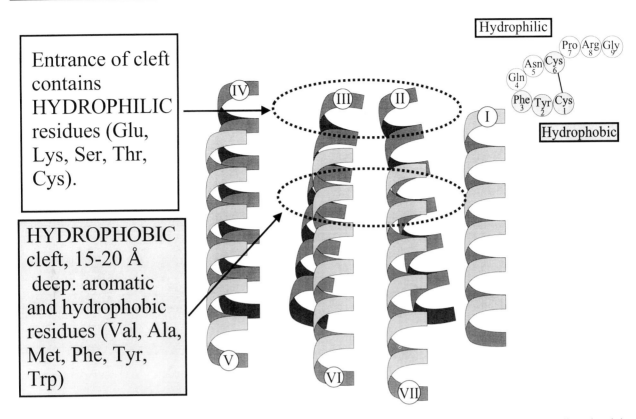

Fig. 10. Docking of arginine-vasopressin in the V_{1a} receptor cavity taking into account the polarity of both the ligand and the receptor. The schematic lateral view of the preceding figure is used. Redrawn from data published by Mouillac et al., 1995.

and paraventricular nuclei) causes a permanent form of the disease. Similar results are obtained by sectioning the hypophyseal hypothalamic tract above the median eminence. Sections below the median eminence, however, produce only transient diabetes insipidus. Lesions to the hypothalamic—pituitary tract are frequently associated with a three-stage response both in experimental animals and in humans:

1. An initial diuretic phase lasting from a few hours to 5–6 d;
2. A period of antidiuresis unresponsive to fluid administration. This antidiuresis is probably owing to vasopressin release from injured axons and may last from a few hours to several days. Since urinary dilution is impaired during this phase, continued water administration can cause severe hyponatremia; and
3. A final period of diabetes insipidus.

The extent of the injury determines the completeness of the diabetes insipidus, and as already discussed, the site of the lesion determines whether the disease will or will not be permanent. The etiologies of central diabetes insipidus in adults and in children are listed in Table 2. No underlying pathologic condition (idiopathic form) could be recognized in 12–29% of the child and adult cases.

6.2. Rare Forms: Autosomal Dominant Central Diabetes Insipidus and the DIDMOAD Syndrome

In familial central diabetes insipidus, the polyuria-polydipsia symptoms usually occur after the first year of life, and some limited capacity to release vasopressin can be demonstrated. As a consequence, no severe episodes of dehydration have been described in the affected individuals during their first year of life. The physical and mental development of

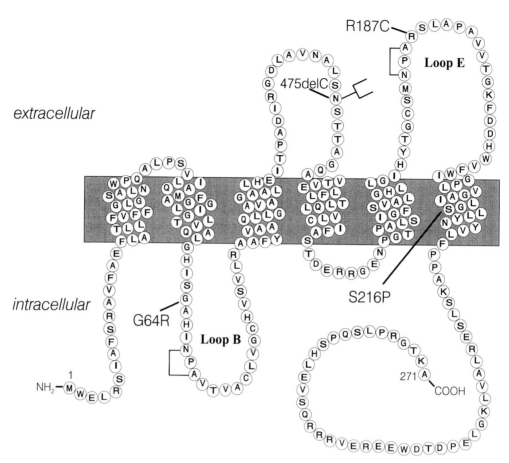

Fig. 11. Schematic representation of AQP2 protein and identification of four AQP2 mutations. (Deen et al., 1994; van Lieburg et al., 1994).

Table 2
Etiology of Hypothalamic Diabetes
Insipidus in Children and Adults

	Children %	Adults %
Primary brain tumor	49.5	30
Before surgery	33.5	13
After surgery	16.0	17
Idiopathic (isolated or familial)	29	25
Histiocytosis	16	
Metastatic cancer	—	8
Trauma	2.2	17
Postinfectious disease	2.2	—

Data from Czernichow et al., 1985; Greger et al., 1986; Moses et al., 1985.

the affected children are normal. These characteristics are in sharp contrast to X-linked and autosomal recessive nephrogenic diabetes insipidus, where the polyuro-polydipsic symptoms are present during the first week of life. The early severe polyuria can lead to repeated episodes of severe dehydration and eventual mental retardation if left untreated. Familial cases of diabetes insipidus can thus be clearly diagnosed through their mode of inheritance, their clinical characteristics, and their molecular alterations (Table 3).

Autosomal dominant neurogenic diabetes insipidus is secondary to mutations in the *prepro-AVP-NPII* gene. The classical animal model for studying diabetes insipidus has been the Brattleboro rat with autosomal recessive diabetes insipidus, *di/di*, a

Table 3
Inherited Diabetes Insipidus

	Neurohypophyseal		Nephrogenic
Inheritance	Autosomal dominant	Autosomal recessive: DIDMOAD	X-linked and non-X-linked
First clinical manifestations:	Variable, usually >1 yr	Variable: infancy	First week of life
Mental retardation	Absent	Absent	Severe if repeated unrecognized episodes of dehydration occur during infancy

form of hereditary diabetes insipidus not described in humans. *di/di* Rats are homozygous for a 1-bp deletion in the second exon that results in a frameshift mutation in the coding sequence of the carrier NPII. The mutant allele encodes a normal AVP, but an abnormal NPII moiety, which impairs transport and processing of the AVP-NPII precursor and results in retention of the abnormal polypeptide in the endoplasmic reticulum of the magnocellular cells.

Twenty *prepro-AVP-NPII* mutations segregating with autosomal dominant neurogenic diabetes insipidus have been described (Table 4). The mechanism(s) by which a mutant allele causes neurogenic diabetes insipidus could be by a gain of function of the mutant protein; a loss of function owing to insufficient normal product; or by an interaction of the mutant and normal product by degradation, functional inactivation of an oligomer, or interference with processing. If defective protein slowly accumulates and leads to the death of magnocellular neurons, this could explain the absence of symptoms in the first years of life of a heterozygote, when expression of the normal allele is sufficient to mount an appropriate antidiuretic response.

The acronym DIDMOAD describes the following clinical features of a syndrome: diabetes insipidus, diabetes mellitus, optic atrophy, sensorineural deafness. The syndrome (also known as Wolfram syndrome [MIM222300]) is an autosomal recessive disorder and has been linked to markers on the short arm of chromosome 4. The diabetes insipidus is usually partial and of gradual onset, and the polyuria can be wrongly attributed to poor glycemic control. A severe hyperosmolar state can occur if untreated diabetes mellitus is associated with an unrecognized pituitary deficiency. In Wolfram syndrome, an autosomal locus seems responsible for the occurrence of mitochondrial deletions (Barrientos et al., 1996a, b).

7. NEPHROGENIC DIABETES INSIPIDUS

7.1. Congenital

In congenital nephrogenic diabetes insipidus, the renal-collecting ducts are resistant to the antidiuretic action of AVP, or to its antidiuretic analog, dDAVP). This is a rare, but now well-described entity secondary to either mutations in the gene (*AVPR2*) coding for the vasopressin antidiuretic (V2) receptor or to mutations in the gene (*AQP2*) coding for the vasopressin-dependent water channel (see Section 5). Of 75 families with congenital nephrogenic diabetes insipidus referred to our laboratory in Montreal, 71 families bear *AVPR2* mutations and four have *AQP2* mutations. The *AVPR2* gene is localized on the distal (*Xq28*) part of the X chromosome, and as a consequence, *AVPR2* mutations are X-linked: males have a full phenotype characterized by early (first week of life) dehydration episodes, hypernatremia, and hyperthermia. The dehydration episodes are so severe that they lower arterial blood perfusion pressure to a degree that will not be sufficient to sustain adequate oxygenation to the brain, the kidneys, and other organs. As a consequence, mental and physical retardations and renal failure are the classical "historical" consequences of a late diagnosis and treatment. The *AQP2* gene is localized on chromosome 12. Male or female homozygous or compound heterozygous mutants have been described.

There are now many other hereditary endocrine and non-endocrine diseases that have been found to

Table 4
***prepro-AVP-NPII* Mutations Causing Autosomal-Dominant Neurogenic Diabetes Insipidus**

Name[a]	Type of mutation	Nucleotide change	Predicted amino acid change	Restriction enzyme analysis	Comments and putative functional consequence	References
S17F	Missense	C → T at nucleotide 274	Ser → Phe at codon 17	*Mbo*II site created		Rittig et al. (1996)
A19T	Missense	G → A at nucleotide 279	Ala → Thr at codon 19	*Bst*UI site abolished, *Pml*I site created the leader peptide	CG → CA: alteration of the cleavage of	Ito et al. (1993), Krishnamani et al. (1993), McLeod et al. (1993), Rittig et al. (1996) (total of five families)
A19V	Missense	C → T at 280	Ala → Val at codon 19	*Bst*UI site abolished		Rittig et al. (1996)
G45R	Missense	G → C at 1730	Gly → Arg at codon 45 (NP$_{14}$)	*Bsl*I site created		Rittig et al. (1996)
G48V	Missense	G → T at nucleotide 1740	Gly → Val at codon 48 (NP$_{17}$)	*Bgl*I site abolished	Disruption of a β-turn in AVP-NPII precursor	Bahnsen et al. (1992)
R51C	Missense	C → T at 1748	Arg → Cys at codon 51 (NP$_{20}$)			Rittig et al (1996)
P55L	Missense	C → T at nucleotide 1761	Pro → Leu at codon 55 (NP$_{24}$)	*Dde*I site created	*De novo* mutation, amino acid substitution in NPII	Repaske and Browning (1994)
ΔE77	Inframe deletion	Deletion of three nucltides in region 1824–1829	Deletion of Glu (glutamic acid) at codon 77 (NP$_{46}$)	*Mnl*I site abolished tandem repeats; unable to form a salt bridge between AVP and NPII	Two sets of staggered 3-bp	Yuasa et al. (1993), Rittig et al. (1996)
E78G	Missense	A → G at 1830	Glu → Gly at codon 78 (NP$_{47}$)			Rittig et al. (1996)
L81P	Missense	T → C at 1839 (NP$_{50}$)	Leu → Pro at codon 81			Rittig et al. (1996)

Continued

Table 4 *(continued)*

Name[a]	Type of mutation	Nucleotide change	Predicted amino acid change	Restriction enzyme analysis	Comments and putative functional consequence	References
G88R	Missense	G→C at 1859	Gly→Arg at codon 88 (NP$_{57}$)	MspI and BglI sites abolished		Rittig et al. (1996)
G88S	Missense nucleotide 1859	G→A at (NP$_{57}$)	Gly→Ser at codon 88 abolished	MspI and BglI sites of NPII, alteration of axonal transport, or posttranslational processing	Failure of dimerization Rittig et al. (1996)	Ito et al. (1991), (two families)
C92S	Missense	G→C at 1872 (NP$_{61}$)	Cys→Ser at codon 92	HgaI site created		Rittig et al. (1996)
C92X	Nonsense	C→A at 1873 (NP$_{61}$)	Cys→stop at codon 92	MnlI site created		Rittig et al. (1996)
G93W	Missense	G→T a nucleotide 1874	Gly→Trp at codon 93 (NP$_{62}$)	BpmI site created		Nagasaki et al. (1995)
G96C	Missense	G→T at 1883	Gly→Cys at codon 96 (NP$_{65}$)			Rittig et al. (1996)
C98X	Nonsense	C→A at nucleotide 1891	Cys→Stop at codon 99 (NP$_{68}$)	DdeI site created		Nagasaki et al. (1995)
C110X	Nonsense	C→A at 2094	Cys→Stop at codon 110 (NP$_{79}$)	BbvI site abolished		Rittig et al. (1996)
2106 CG→GT	Nonsense	C→G at 2106	Pro→Pro at 114 (NP$_{83}$)			Rittig et al. (1996)
E118X	Nonsense	G→T at 2107; G→T at 2116	Glu→Stop at 115 (NP$_{84}$); Glu→Stop at 118 (NP$_{87}$)	MaeI site created		Rittig et al. (1996)

[a]The names were assigned following the suggested nomenclature for mutations (Beaudet and Tsui, 1993). The nucleotides and amino acids are numbered according to the *prepro-AVP-NPII* gene sequence published by Sausville et al. (1985). The human vasopressin gene is linked to the oxytocin gene and is selectively expressed in a cultured lung cancer cell ligne. *J Biol Chem* 1985; 260(18):10,236 and GenBank accession number M11166; The codons corresponding to the moieties are 1–19—signal peptide, 20–28—AVP, 29–31—cleavage site, 32–124—NPII, and 126–164—glycopeptide. NP$_{14}$ means the 14th amino acid of the protein neurophysin. References are found in Rittig et al. (1996).

be secondary to mutations inducing a loss of function of G-protein-linked receptors. However, naturally occurring *AVPR2* mutations are of interest for many aspects:

1. They are diverse, numerous, and described in many ethnic groups;
2. They encompass missense, nonsense, frameshift mutations, and large deletion mutations, and thus recapitulate the genomic alterations seen in many other genes; and
3. These mutations are distributed almost evenly in the four-extracellular, five-cytoplasmic, and seven-transmembrane domains of the 371 amino acids receptor molecule (Fig. 8); as a consequence, the *in vitro* expression of these mutations help us to understand the processing, sorting, and function of seven-transmembrane proteins involved in signal transduction. Seventy-two different putative disease-causing mutations in *AVPR2* have now been reported in 97, presumably unrelated families with X-linked nephrogenic diabetes insipidus (Fig. 8).

The cause of loss of function of mutant V2 receptors have ben studied in in vitro expression systems. Truncated proteins generated by nonsense mutations or frameshift mutations are expected to be nonfunctional. For missense mutations, Tsukaguchi and coworkers (1995) suggested three phenotypes: Type 1 mutants will reach the cell surface, but will not bind; Type 2 are intracellularly trapped; and Type 3 are not produced. More recently, Schöneberg et al. (1996) (Fig. 12) pharmacologically rescued truncated vasopressin receptors by supplying by coexpression individual lacking domains. Of potential "futuristic" therapeutic importance, several of the nine mutant receptors tested (E242X, E242-frameshift, G254-frameshift, W284X, L312X) regained considerable functional activity as demonstrated by stimulation of adenylate cyclase. Diagnosis of X-linked NDI was accomplished by mutation testing of a sample of cord blood in three of our patients. The more common causes of acquired nephrogenic diabetes insipidus are listed in Table 5.

8. PRIMARY POLYDIPSIA

Primary polydipsia is a state of hypotonic polyuria secondary to excessive fluid intake. Polyuric female

subjects might be heterozygous for a *de novo* or previously unrecognized *AVPR2* mutations, and may be classified as compulsive water drinkers. Therefore, the diagnosis of compulsive water drinking must be made with care and may represent our ignorance of yet undescribed pathophysiological mechanisms.

9. DIFFERENTIAL DIAGNOSIS AND TREATMENT OF POLYURIC STATES

9.1. Carrier Detection and Postnatal Diagnosis

As described earlier in this chapter, the identification, characterization, and mutational analysis of three different genes, namely, the prepro-arginine-vasopressin-neurophysin II gene (*prepro-AVP-NPII*), the arginine-vasopressin receptor 2 gene (*AVPR2*), and the vasopressin-sensitive water channel gene (aquaporin-2, *AQP2*) provide the basis for the understanding of three different hereditary forms of diabetes insipidus, autosomal dominant neurogenic diabetes insipidus, X-linked nephrogenic diabetes insipidus, and autosomal recessive nephrogenic diabetes insipidus, respectively. The identification of mutations in these three genes that cause diabetes insipidus enables the early diagnosis and management of at-risk members of families with identified mutations.

9.2. Treatment

In most patients with complete hypothalamic diabetes insipidus, the thirst mechanism remains intact. Thus, these patients do not develop hypernatremia, and suffer only from the inconvenience associated with marked polyuria and polydipsia. If hypodipsia develops or access to water is limited, then severe hypernatremia can supervene. The treatment of choice for patients with severe hypothalamic diabetes insipidus is dDAVP, a synthetic, long-acting vasopressin analog, with minimal vasopressor activity, but a large antidiuretic potency. The usual intranasal daily dose is between 5 and 20 µg.

10. SYNDROME OF INAPPROPRIATE SECRETION OF THE ANTIDIURETIC HORMONE (SIADH)

Hyponatremia (defined as a plasma sodium below 130 meq/L) is the most common disorder of

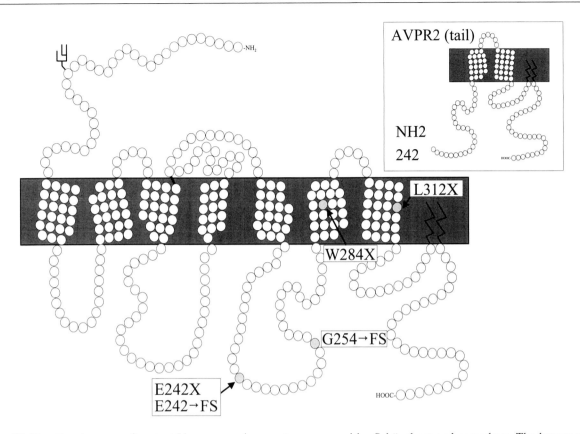

Fig. 12. Functional rescue of mutant V₂ vasopressin receptors proposed by Schöneberg and coworkers. The human vasopressin V₂ receptor amino acid sequence is represented and naturally occurring mutations responsible for nephrogenic diabetes insipidus are indicated (E242X, E242 frameshift, G254 frameshift, W284X, L312X). The insert in the upper part of the figure is representing the V₂ (tail) polypeptide (Glu 242 to Ser 371) used by Schöneberg and coworkers to complement the various truncated receptor mutants and restore, in vitro, cAMP stimulation. Redrawn from the data of Schöneberg et al., 1996.

body fluid and electrolyte balance encountered in clinical practice of medicine, with incidences ranging from 1–2% in both acutely and chronically hospitalized patients. Because a defect in renal water excretion, as reflected by hypoosmolality, may occur in the presence of an excess or deficit of total body sodium or nearly normal total body sodium, it is useful to classify the hyponatremic states accordingly (Fig. 13). Moreover, since total-body sodium is the primary determinant of the extracellular fluid (ECF) volume, bedside evaluation of the ECF volume allows for a convenient means of classifying hyponatremic patients.

Since 1957 when Schwartz and coworkers (Berl and Schrier, 1992) first described SIADH in two patients with bronchogenic carcinoma who were hyponatremic, clinically euvolemic with normal renal and adrenal function, and who had less than maximally dilute urine with appreciable urinary sodium concentrations (>20 meq/L), SIADH has been recognized in a variety of pathological processes. Various diseases that may be accompanied by SIADH are listed in Table 6. These diseases generally fall into three categories: malignancies, pulmonary disorders, and central nervous system disorders.

In spite of the hyponatremia, patients with SIADH have a concentrated urine in which the urinary sodium concentration closely parallels the sodium intake, i.e., it is usually above 20 meq/L. However, in the presence of sodium restriction or volume depletion, these patients can conserve sodium normally and decrease their urinary

Table 5 Acquired Causes of Nephrogenic Diabetes Insipidus	Table 6 Disorders Associated with SIADH

Chronic renal disease
  Polycystic disease
  Medullary cystic disease
  Pyelonephritis
  Ureteral obstruction
  Far-advanced renal failure
Electrolyte disorders
  Hypokalemia
  Hypercalcemia
Drugs
  Alcohol
  Phenytoin
  Lithium
  Demeclocycline
  Acetohexamide
  Tolazamide
  Glyburide
  Propoxyphene
  Amphotericin
  Methoxyflurane
  Norepinephrine
  Vinblastine
  Colchicine
  Gentamicin
  Methicillin
  Isophosphamide
  Angiographic dyes
  Osmotic diuretics
  Furosemide and ethacrynic acid
Sickle cell disease
Dietary abnormalities
  Excessive water intake
  Decreased sodium chloride intake
  Decreased protein intake
Miscellaneous
  Multiple myeloma
  Amyloidosis
  Sjögren's disease
  Sarcoidosis
	Carcinomas
	  CNS disorders
	  Small-cell carcinoma of the lung
	  Carcinoma of the duodenum
	  Carcinoma of pancreas
	  Thymoma
	  Carcinoma of the ureter
	  Lymphoma
	  Ewing's sarcoma
	  Mesothelioma
	  Carcinoma of the bladder
	  Prostatic carcinoma
	  Olfactory neuroblastoma
	  Encephalitis (viral or bacterial)
	  Meningitis (viral, bacterial, tuberculous, fungal)
	  Head trauma
	  Brain abscess
	  Brain tumors
	  Guillain-Barré syndrome
	  Acute intermittent porphyria
	  Subarachnoid hemorrhage or subdural hematoma
	  Cerebellar and cerebral atrophy
	Cavernous sinus thrombosis
	  Neonatal hypoxia
	  Hydrocephalus
	Pulmonary disorders
	  Viral pneumonia
	  Bacterial pneumonia
	  Pulmonary abscess
	  Tuberculosis
	  Aspergilosis
	  Positive-pressure breathing
	  Asthma
	  Pneumothorax
	  Cystic fibrosis
	Shy-Drager syndrome
	  Rocky Mountain spotter fever
	  Delirium tremens
	  Cerebrovascular accident (cerebral thrombosis or
	    hemorrhage)
	  Acute psychosis
	  Peripheral neuropathy
	  Multiple sclerosis

sodium concentration to <10 meq/L. Serum uric acid has been found to be reduced in SIADH patients, whereas patients with other causes of hyponatremia have normal concentrations of serum uric acid. Uric acid and phosphate clearances were found to be increased in patients with SIADH as the consequence of volume expansion and decreased tubular reabsorption. Similarly, low-serum BUN concentrations have been found in SIADH. This is probably owing to an increase in total body water, where urea is normally distributed, but a decrease in protein intake could also

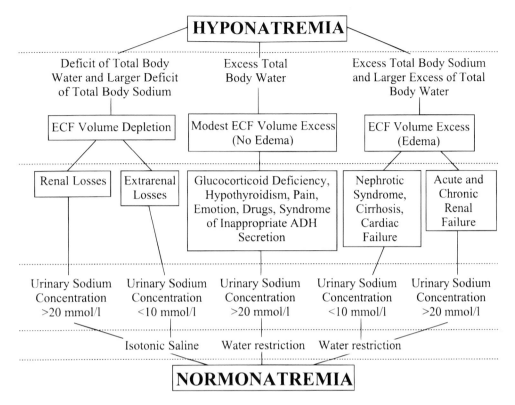

Fig. 13. Diagnostic and therapeutic approach to the hyponatremic patient. (Modified from Berl and Schrier, 1992.)

contribute. Plasma atrial natriuretic factor concentration has been found to be increased in patients with SIADH and to correlate with urinary sodium excretion.

11. SIGNS, SYMPTOMS, AND TREATMENT OF HYPONATREMIA

The majority of the manifestations of hyponatremia are of a neuropsychiatric nature, and include lethargy, psychosis, seizures, and coma. The elderly and young children with hyponatremia are most likely to become symptomatic. The degree of the clinical impairment is not strictly related to the absolute value of the lowered serum sodium concentration, but, rather, it relates to both the rate and the extent of the fall of ECF osmolality. Arieff quotes a mortality rate of approx 50%. On the other hand, none of the 10 acutely hyponatremic patients reported by Sterns had permanent neurologic seque-

lae. Most patients who have seizures and coma have plasma sodium concentrations <120 meq/L. The signs and symptoms are most likely related to the cellular swelling and cerebral edema that are associated with hyponatremia.

The treatment of symptomatic hyponatremic patients has recently been the subject of a large-scale debate in the literature. This debate has been prompted by the description of both pontine (central pontine myelinolysis ([CPM]) and extrapontine demyelinating lesions in patients whose hyponatremia has been treated. Numerous experiments (reviewed by Berl [1990]) have demonstrated that hyponatremia *per se* is not the underlying cause of CPM, but that the corrections of hyponatremia of greater than 24-h duration may play a central role in the development of CPM. The critical rate and the magnitude of the correction have been addressed, and a "prudent" approach to the treatment has been published (Table 7).

Table 7
A Prudent Approach to the Treatment of Hyponatremia

Guiding principles in the treatment of hyponatremia

Neurologic disease can follow both the failure to treat promptly and the injudicious rapid treatment of hyponatremia

The presence or absence of significant neurologicsigns and symptoms must guide the treatment

The acuteness or chronicity of the electrolyte disturbance influences the rate at which the correction should be undertaken.

Acute symptomatic hyponatremia:

The risk of the complications of cerebral edema are greater than the risk of the complications of the treatment

Treat with furosemide and hypertonic NaCl until convulsions subside

Asymptomatic hyponatremia

Almost always chronic

Treat with water restriction regardless of how low the serum sodium concentration is

Symptomatic hyponatremia (chronic or unknown duration)

Increase serum sodium promptly by 10%, that is, approx 10 meq/L, and then restrict water intake

Do not exceed a correction rate of 2 meq/L/h at any given time

Do not increase serum sodium by more than 20 meq/d

From Berl (1990).

REFERENCES

Barrientos a: Barrientos A, Volpini V, Casademont J, Genis D, Manzanares J-M, Ferrer I, Corral J, Cardellach F, Urbano-Márquez, Estivill X, Nunes V. A nuclear defect in the 4p16 region predisposes to multiple mitochondial DNA deletions in families with Wolfram syndrome. *J. Clin. Invest.* 97: 1570–1576, 1996.

Barrientos b: Barrientos A, Casademont J, Saiz A, Cardellach F, Volpini V, Solans A, Tolosa E, Urbano-Márquez, Estivill X, Nunes V. Autosomal recessive Wolfram syndrome associated with an 8.5-kb mtDNA single deletion. *Am. J. Hum. Genet.* 59:963–970, 1996.

Berl T. Treating hyponatremia: damned if we do and damned if we don't. *Kidney Int* 1990; 37:1006.

Berl T, Schrier RW. In: Schrier RW, ed. *Disorders of Water Metabolism in Renal and Electrolyte Disorders*, 4th ed., 1992.

Baylis PH. Vasopressin and its neurophysin. In: DeGroot LJ, Besser JM, Cahill GF Jr, et al., eds. *Endocrinology*, 2nd ed. Philadelphia: W.B. Saunders Company, 1989:213.

Beaudet AL, Tsui LC. A suggested nomenclature for designating mutations. *Hum Mutat* 1993;2:245.

Bourque CW, Oliet SHR, Richard D. Osmoreceptors, osmoreception, and Osmoregulation. In: *Frontiers in Neuroendocrinology*, 1995: 231.

Czernichow P, Pomarede R, Braumer R, Rappaport R. Neurogenic diabetes insipidus. In: Czernichow P, Robinson AG, eds. Frontiers of Hormone Research. Diabetes Insipidus in Man, vol. 13. Basel: S. Karger, 1985:190.

Deen PMT, Verdijk MAJ, Knoers NVAM, et al. Requirement of human renal water channel aquaporin-2 for vaso-pressin-dependent concentration of urine. *Science* 1994; 264:92.

Greger NG, Kirkland RT, Clayton GW, Kirkland JL. Central diabetes insipidus: 22 years' experience. *Am J Dis Child* 1986 140(6):551.

Ito M, Mori Y, Oiso Y, Saito H. A single base substitution in the coding region for neurophysin-II associated with familial central diabetes insipidus. *J. Clin. Invest.* 87:725–738, 1991.

Miller M, Dalakos T, Moses A, et al. Recognition of partial defects in antidiuretic hormone secretion. *Ann Intern Med* 1970;73:721.

Moses AM, Blumenthal SA, Streeten DHP. Acid-base and electrolyte disorders associated with endocrine disease: pituitary and thyroid. In: Arieff AI, de Fronzo RA, eds. *Fluid, Electrolyte and Acid-Base Disorders*. New York: Churchill Livingstone, 1985:851.

Mouillac B, Chini B, Balestre M-N, Elands J, Trumpp-Kallmeyer S, Hoflack J, Hibert M, Jard S, Barberis C. The binding site of neuropeptide vasopressin V_{1a} receptor. Evidence for a major localization within transmembrane regions. *J Biol Chem* 1995;43:25,771–2.

Nagasaki H, Ito M, Yuasa H, Saito H, Fukase M, Hamada K, Ishikawa E, Katakami H, Oiso Y. Two novel mutations in the coding region for neurophysin-II associated with familial central diabetes insipidus. *J. Clin. Endocrinol. Metab.* 80:1352–1356, 1995.

Repaske DR, Browning JE. A *de novo* mutation in the coding sequence for neurophysin-II (Pro[24]-Leu) is associated with onset and transmission of autosomal dominant neurohypophyseal diabetes insipidus. *J. Clin. Endocrinol. Metab* 79:42–427, 1994.

Rittig R, Robertson GL, Siggaard C, Kovacs L, Gregersen N, Nyborg J, Pedersen EB. Identification of 13 new mutations in the vasopressin-neurophysin II gene in 17 kindreds with familial autosomal-dominant neurohypophyseal diabetes insipidus. *Am J Hum Genet* 1996;107.

Robertson GL. The pathology of ADH secretion. In: Tolis G et al., eds. *Clinical Neuroendocrinology: A Pathophysiological Approach*. New York: Raven, 1979: 247.

Robertson GL. Diseases of the posterior pituitary. In: Felig P, Baxter JD, Broadus AE, Frohman LA, eds. *Endocrinology and Metabolism*. New York: McGraw-Hill, 1981:251.

Robertson GL. Regulation of vasopressin secretion. In: Seldin DW, Giebisch G, eds. *The Kidney: Physiology and Pathophysiology*, New York: Raven, 1985a: 869.

Robertson GL. Diagnosis of diabetes insipidus. In Czernichow P, Robinson AG, eds. *Front Horm Res.* Basel: S. Karger, 1985b: 176.

Robertson GL, Shelton RL, Athar S. The osmoregulation of vasopressin. *Kidney Int* 1976;10(1):25.

Sausville E, Carney D, Battey J. The human vasopressin gene is linked to the oxytocin gene and is selectively expressed in a cultured lung cancer cell ligne. *J Biol Chem* 1985; 260(18):10,236.

Schöneberg T, Yun J, Wenkert D, Wess J. Functional rescue of mutant V_2 vasopressin receptors causing nephrogenic diabetes insipidus by a coexpressed receptor polypeptide. *EMBO* 1996: 15:1283–91.

Tsukaguchi H, Matsubara H, Taketani S, Mori Y, Seido T, Inada M. Binding-, intracellular transport-, and biosynthesis-defective mutants of vasopressin type 2 receptor in aptients with X-linked nephrogenic diabetes insipidus. *J Clin Invest* 1995;97:2043.

van Lieburg AF, Verdijk MAJ, Knoers NVAM, et al. Patients with autosomal nephrogenic diabetes insipidus: homozygous for mutations in the aquaporin 2 water-channel gene. *Am J Hum Genet* 1994;55:648.

Vokes T, Robertson GL. Physiology of secretion of vasopressin. In: Czernichow P, Robinson AG, eds. *Frontiers of Hormone Research*, Basel: S. Karger, 1985:127.

Yuasa H, Ito M, Nagasaki H, Oiso Y, Miyamoto S, Sasaki N, Saito H. Glu-47, which forms a salt bridge between neurophysin-II and arginine vasopressin, is deleted in patients with familial central diabetes insipidus. *J. Clin. Endocrinol. Metab.* 77:600–604, 1993.

Zerbe RL, Robertson GL. Disorders of ADH. *Med North Am* 1984;13:1570.

SELECTED READINGS

Bichet DG, Kluge R, Howard RL, Schrier RW. Hyponatremic states. In Seldin DW, Giebish G, eds. *The Kidney: Physiology and Pathophysiology*, 2nd ed., New York: Raven, 1992:1727.

Czernichow P, Robinson AG, eds. Diabetes insipidus in man. In: *Frontiers of Hormone Research*, vol. 13. Basel: S. Karger, 1985:1.

Fujiwara TM, Morgan K, Bichet DG. Molecular biology of diabetes insipidus. In CH Coggins, ed. *Annual Review of Medicine*, vol. 46. Palo Alto, CA: Annual Reviews Inc., 1995: 331.

Gross P, Richter D, Robertson GL, eds. Vasopressin. IVth International Vasopressin Conference. Berlin: John Libbey Eurotex, 1993:1.

Howard RL, Bichet DG, Schrier RW. Hypernatremic and polyuric states. In: Seldin DW, Giebish G, eds. *The Kidney: Physiology and Pathophysiology*, 2nd ed. New York: Raven, 1992:1753.

Kanno K, Sasaki S, Hirata Y, Ishikawa S-E, Fushimi K, Nakanishi S, Bichet DG, Marumo F. Urinary excretion of aquaporin-2 in patients with diabetes insipidus. *N Engl J Med* 1995;332:1540.

Knoers N, Monnens LAH. Invited review: Nephrogenic diabetes insipidus: clinical symptoms, pathogenesis, genetics and treatment. *Pediatr Nephrol* 1992;6:476.

Kovács L, Lichardus B, eds. *Vasopressin: Disturbed Secretion and Its Effects.* Dordrecht, The Netherlands: Kluwer Academic Publisher, 1989:1.

Nielsen S, Agre P. The aquaporin family of water channel in kidney. *Kidney Int* 1995;48:1057.

Saito T, Kurokawa K, Yoshida S, eds. Neurohypophysis: Recent Progress of Vasopressin and Oxytocin Research. Proceedings of the 1st Joint World Congress of Neurohypophysis and Vasopressin. Tochigi, Japan: Elsevier, 1995:1.

DISEASES AND SYSTEMS

16 Endocrine Disease

Value for Understanding Hormonal Actions

Glenn D. Braunstein, MD

CONTENTS

INTRODUCTION
PATHOPHYSIOLOGY OF ENDOCRINE DISEASES
EXAMPLES OF CLINICAL SYNDROMES WITH MULTIPLE PATHOPHYSIOLOGIC
    MECHANISMS
CONCLUSIONS

1. INTRODUCTION

Disorders involving the endocrine glands, their hormones, and the targets of the hormones may cover the full spectrum ranging from an incidentally found, insignificant abnormality that is clinically silent to a flagrant, life-threatening metabolic derangement. Some endocrine diseases, such as well-differentiated thyroid carcinoma, present as neoplastic growths that rarely are associated with evidence of endocrine dysfunction. However, most clinically relevant endocrine disorders are associated with overexpression or underexpression of hormone action. There is a great deal of phenotypic variability in the clinical manifestations of each of the endocrine disorders reflecting in part the severity of the derangement and the underlying pathophysiologic mechanisms. Although most of the individual clinical endocrine syndromes have multiple pathophysiologic mechanisms, the qualitative manifestations of the disease states are similar owing to the relatively limited

From: *Endocrinology: Basic and Clinical Principles* (P. M. Conn and S. Melmed, eds.), Humana Press Inc., Totowa, NJ.

ways in which the body responds to too much or too little hormone action.

This chapter will emphasize the diversity of pathophysiologic mechanisms responsible for endocrine diseases, and will illustrate the concept that despite the underlying pathophysiology, the clinical manifestations of diseases leading to overexpression or underexpression of hormone action are quite similar.

2. PATHOPHYSIOLOGY OF ENDOCRINE DISEASES

Endocrine diseases can occur on a congenital, often genetic, basis or can be acquired. Many of the congenital abnormalities are owing to mutations that result in structural abnormalities, defects in hormone biosynthesis, or abnormalities in hormone receptor structure or postreceptor signaling mechanisms. Tables 1 and 2 provide examples of identified mutations that result in over- and underexpression of hormone action. Most endocrine diseases are acquired and fit broadly into the categories of neoplasia, destruction or impairment of function of the endocrine gland through infection,

Table 1
Examples of Mutations That Cause Endocrine Hyperfunction

Type of mutation	Disorder
Membrane receptor	
TSH receptor constitutive activation	Thyroid adenoma; hyperthyroidism
LH/hCG receptor constitutive activation	Familial male precocious puberty (testotoxicosis)
Calcium-sensing receptor defect	Familial hypocalciuric hypocalcemia; neonatal hyperparathyroidism
Signal pathway	
Pituitary $G_s\alpha$ activation	Acromegaly
Thyroid $G_s\alpha$ activation	Thyroid adenoma; hyperthyroidism
Generalized $G_s\alpha$ activation	McCune-Albright syndrome
Temperature-sensitive $G_s\alpha$ activation	Testotoxicosis and pseudohypoparathyroidism
Thyroid p53	Neoplasia
Ret proto-oncogene	Multiple Endocrine Neoplasia IIa
Cyclin D1 fusion to PTH promoter (PRAD-1) activation	Parathyroid adenoma
$G_i\alpha$ (gip oncogene in adrenal and ovaries)	Adrenocortical and ovarian tumors
Enzyme	
Aldosterone synthase-11β-hydroxylase chimera	Glucocorticoid-remediable hypertension

Modified from Jameson (1995).

infiltrative processes, vascular disorders, trauma, or immune-mediated injury, as well as functional aberrations owing to multiorgan dysfunction, metabolic abnormalities, or drugs.

The above processes may disrupt the biosynthesis of protein hormones through interference with transcription, mRNA processing, translation, posttranslational protein modifications, protein storage, or secretion. Abnormalities in steroid hormone, thyroid hormone, and calcitriol production may result from loss of the orderly enzymatic conversion of precursor molecules to active hormones. Many disease states as well as medications may alter the transport and metabolism of hormones. Finally, there are a multitude of lesions that can affect hormone–receptor interaction, as well as postreceptor signal pathways.

From a functional standpoint, clinical endocrine disease can be broadly classified into diseases of the endocrine glands that are not associated with hormonal dysfunction, diseases from overexpression of hormone action, and diseases characterized by underexpression of hormone action (Table 3).

Endocrine diseases without hormonal aberrations are generally nonfunctional neoplasms, such as thyroid carcinoma or the frequently found incidental pituitary and adrenal adenomas. These neoplasms generally cause symptoms through their anatomical effects on the surrounding structures or, in the case of some malignant neoplasms, through their metastases.

Most endocrine disorders that result in overexpression of hormone action do so through excessive production of hormones. Such production may be eutopic in which the normal physiologic source of the hormone secretes excessive quantities of that hormone, or ectopic in which a neoplasm or other pathology involving a tissue that is not the known physiologic source of the hormone produces excessive quantities of the hormone. Eutopic hypersecretion may be the result of autonomous production of the hormone with loss of normal target organ product feedback regulation. This is found in many hormone-secreting benign and malignant neoplasms. An example would be a cortisol-secreting adrenal cortical adenoma that continues to secrete cortisol despite the suppression of endogenous ACTH levels. Dysfunction of endocrine glands leading to hyperplasia may be found in situations when there is excessive physiologic stimulation, such as occurs in secondary hyperaldosteronism owing to cirrhosis or congestive heart failure, in which there is decreased effective vascular volume, resulting in stimulation of aldosterone secretion through the renin-angiotensin system. Alterations in the normal feedback set point also cause dysfunction of the endocrine gland, as is

Table 2
Examples of Mutations That Cause Endocrine Hypofunction

Type of mutation	Disorder
Hormone/hormone precursor	
GH gene deletion	Growth retardation
TSH β subunit gene	Hypothyroidism
LH β subunit gene	Hypogonadism
Neurophysin/ADH processing	Central diabetes insipidus
Parathyroid hormone processing	Hypoparathyroidism
Proinsulin processing	Diabetes mellitus
Insulin gene	Diabetes mellitus
Thyroglobulin	Hypothyroidism with goiter
Membrane receptor	
GH	Laron dwarfism
TSH	Hypothyroidism
LH/hCG	Resistant testes syndrome
FSH	Resistant ovary syndrome
ACTH	Familial glucocorticoid deficiency
Vasopressin V2	Nephrogenic diabetes insipidus
Parathyroid hormone	Pseudohypoparathyroidism
Insulin	Insulin resistance
β_3-adrenergic	Obesity
Nuclear receptor	
Thyroid hormone	Thyroid hormone resistance syndrome (generalized or pituitary)
Glucocorticoid	Glucocorticoid resistance syndrome
Androgen	Androgen insensitivity syndromes
Estrogen	Delayed epiphyseal closure, osteoporosis
Mineralocorticoid	Generalized pseudohypoaldosteronism
Progesterone	Progesterone resistance
Vitamin D	Vitamin D-resistant rickets
DAX-1	X-linked congenital adrenal hypoplasia
Signal pathway	
$G_s\alpha$ inactivation	Albright hereditary osteodystrophy (pseudohypoparathyroidism with resistance to PTH, TSH, gonadotropins)
Transcription factors	
SRY translocation	XX Male
SRY mutation	XY Female
Pit-1 mutation	Growth retardation and hypothyroidism (GH, TSH, and PRL deficiencies)
Enzymes	
Thyroid	
Peroxidase	Hypothyroidism with goiter
Iodotyrosine deiodinase	Goiter $\pm$ hypothyroidism
Adrenal and testes	
Cholesterol side-chain cleavage (20,22-desmolase)	CAH with hypogonadism
3β-hydroxysteroid dehydrogenase	CAH with ambiguous genitalia
17α-hydroxylase	CAH with androgen deficiency and hypertension
Adrenal	
11β-hydroxylase	CAH, androgen excess, hypertension
21-hydroxylase	CAH with androgen excess $\pm$ salt wasting

(continued)

Table 2 (*continued*)

Type of mutation	*Disorder*
Testes	
17,20-desmolase	Hypogonadism
17-ketosteroid reductase	Hypogonadism
Pancreas and Liver	
Glucokinase gene	Maturity-onset diabetes of the young
Multiple tissues	
Aromatase	Estrogen deficiency with virilization, delayed epiphyseal closure, tall stature
5α-reductase	Male pseudohermaphroditism
Other	
KAL protein deficiency	Kallmann's syndrome
Aquaporin-water channel	Nephrogenic diabetes insipidus

Modified from Jameson (1995).
Abbreviation: CAH, congenital adrenal hyperplasia.

seen in the hypercalcemia found in patients with familial hypocalciuric hypercalcemia or in hypercalcemic patients receiving lithium. In both situations, there are alterations in the calcium-sensing mechanism in parathyroid cells that require higher serum calcium concentrations than normal to suppress parathormone production. The concept of an altered set point for feedback regulation also forms the basis for the low and high-dose dexamethasone suppression tests in patients with pituitary-dependent Cushing's disease. Such patients do not suppress their ACTH and cortisol production normally following low-dose dexamethasone, but generally do suppress following a high dose of dexamethasone.

A wide variety of hormones have been found to be secreted ectopically by tumors, especially solid tumors of the lung, kidney, liver, and head and neck region. These tumors may directly secrete excessive quantities of a prohormone or active hormone, or in some instances, may secrete releasing factors that, in turn stimulates the release of hormone from the normal endocrine glands. Thus, the ectopic ACTH syndrome may be found in patients with oat cell carcinoma of the lung resulting from ectopic production of ACTH by the tumor, and may also be found in patients with bronchial carcinoid tumors that secrete corticotropin-releasing factor, which in turn, stimulates the pituitary to secrete ACTH. Another form of ectopic hormone production is found with some benign and malignant diseases in which there is dysregulation of metabolic pathways. Patients with sarcoidosis or other granulomatous processes,

as well as patients with some forms of lymphoma may develop hypercalcemia owing to excessive quantities of 1,25(OH)$_2$-vitamin D produced from normal circulating quantities of 25 (OH)-vitamin D because of dysregulation of macrophage 1α-hydroxylase in the lesions.

A second broad mechanism responsible for overexpression of hormone action is through excessive activation of hormone receptors. Constitutive activation of thyroid-stimulating hormones (TSH) receptors owing to point mutations are found in some patients with toxic thyroid adenomas, and several families with constitutive activation of the luteinizing hormone (LH) receptor in the testes have been described who present with familial male precocious puberty (testotoxicosis). Hormone receptors may also be activated by hormones that share close homology with the hormone for which the receptor is the primary target. Thus, human chorionic gonadotropin (hCG) when present in high concentrations, as occurs in some women with large hydatidiform moles, may stimulate the thyroid TSH receptor resulting in hyperthyroidism. Other examples of receptor crossreaction include insulin binding to the insulin-like growth factor-1 (IGF-1) receptor in the ovary-stimulating androgen production, and growth hormone interaction with the prolactin receptor resulting in galactorrhea in some patients with acromegaly. Some nonhormonal substances can mimic hormone action through interreaction with the hormone receptor. The thyroid-stimulating immunoglobulins present in the sera of patients with Graves'

Table 3
Pathophysiology of Endocrine Diseases

Neoplastic growth of endocrine glands without hyper- or hypofunction
Overexpression of hormone action
  Excessive Production of Hormones
    Eutopic
      Autonomous
      Excessive physiologic stimulation
      Altered regulatory feedback set point
    Ectopic
      Direct secretion by tumor
      Indirect
      Dysregulation
  Excessive activation of hormone receptors
    Constitutively activated receptors
    Hormone mimicry
    Receptor crossreactivity
  Postreceptor activation of hormone action
  Altered metabolism of hormones
Underexpression of hormone action
  Aplasia or hypoplasia of hormone source
  Acquired destruction of source of hormone
  Congenital absence of hormone
  Production of inactive forms of hormone
  Substrate insufficiency
  Destruction of target organ
  Enzyme defects in hormone production
  Antihormone antibodies
  Hormone resistance
    Absent or altered receptor
    Receptor occupancy
    Down regulation of normal receptors
    Postreceptor defects
  Altered metabolism of hormones

disease and the hypoglycemia found in some patients with Type B insulin resistance with insulin receptor autoantibodies are examples of this phenomenon.

There are several intracellular signalling pathways that regulate hormone function. Among these are the adenylyl cyclase-cAMP system, tyrosine kinase, guanylyl cyclase and activation of phospholipase-C. Many of these regulatory processes involve the guanylyl nucleotide-binding proteins (G-proteins). Some activating mutations of the G-protein subunits "turn on" these signaling pathways, which results in the hyperfunction of an endocrine cell. This occurs in some somatotrophs associated with acromegaly or thyroid follicular cells-associated neonatal hyperthyroidism. This also occurs in the endocrine target cells, which when activated through a G-protein mutation function as if they were exposed to excessive quantities of the hormone. This mechanism is responsible for the precocious puberty and other clinical manifestations of the McCune-Albright syndrome (Table 1).

Hormone metabolism may be altered by disease states and medications. Hyperthyroidism, obesity, liver disease, and spironolactone increase the aromatization of testosterone and androstenedione, leading to enhanced production of estradiol and estrone, respectively, which can cause gynecomastia in affected individuals. Clinicians caring for patients with Type I diabetes mellitus have long known that the unexpected onset of frequent hypoglycemic reactions necessitating the reduction in insulin dosages may herald the onset of renal insufficiency with loss of the ability of the kidneys to metabolize the exogenous insulin.

Multiple mechanisms also exist resulting in the underexpression of hormone action. Certainly, congenital aplasia or hypoplasia of endocrine tissue will prevent the normal synthesis or secretion of hormones by that tissue. Anencephaly, which is associated with an absence or maldevelopment of the hypothalamus, leads to a loss of hypothalamic-releasing hormones that, in turn, leads to profound panhypopituitarism. Another example of an abnormal development of at least a portion of the hypothalamus is X-chromosome-linked Kallmann's syndrome. Mutations in the KAL gene result in a loss of KAL protein, which is an adhesion molecule that is reasonable for the coordinated migration of the GnRH-secreting neurons from the olfactory placode into the hypothalamus. Loss of this normal migration results in inadequate production and secretion of GnRH, leading to a hypogonadotropic hypogonadism. In addition to congenital structural defects, destruction of endocrine organs can occur from replacement by tumor or involvement with one of the many processes listed earlier.

Congenital absence of a hormone owing to a gene deletion is rare and has been described for growth hormone. More commonly, point mutations in the genes encoding a hormone or a hormone subunit may result in a biologically inactive form of the hormone that may or may not retain its immunologic activity. Since many hormones are produced in a prohormone form, some point mutations may result in a defect that prevents the normal processing of the biologically inactive prohormone to the biologically active hormone (Table 2).

Substrate required for hormone production may be limited as occurs in individuals with vitamin D deficiency resulting from inadequate intake, lack of sun exposure, or the presence of malabsorption. Without an appropriate amount of native vitamin D, insufficient quantities of 25(OH)-vitamin D and 1,25(OH)$_2$-vitamin D may be produced. The target organ may not appropriately respond to hormonal stimulation because of structural defects, acquired disease, or in the case of thyroid hormones, steroid hormones and vitamin D, congenital or acquired defects in the enzymes responsible for active hormone production (Table 2). Antibodies that bind circulating hormone usually do not cause a major interference in hormone action. However, some antibodies may sufficiently interfere with hormone action to result in a hormone insufficiency state. Examples include the high-titer, high-affinity antibodies against insulin that occasionally cause insulin resistance, gonadotropin antibodies that occasionally form in individuals with hypogonadotropic hypogonadism receiving exogenous gonadotropins, and the extremely rare growth hormone-inactivating antibody found in some growth hormone-deficient children receiving exogenous growth hormone. Spontaneous antihormone antibodies are occasionally seen in patients with autoimmune diseases, but rarely cause clinical manifestations.

Another mechanism for the underexpression of hormone action is hormone resistance at the target organ level owing to receptor or postreceptor abnormalities. A number of inactivating mutations in both membrane and nuclear hormone receptors have been described (Table 2). In addition, the receptors may be occupied by autoantibodies, which prevent the normal hormone–receptor interaction from taking place. In contrast to the stimulatory effects of thyroid-stimulating immunoglobulins in patients with Graves' disease, blocking autoantibodies to the TSH receptor is a cause of goitrous hypothyroidism. Similarly, anti-insulin receptor antibodies may block the effect of insulin in some patients, whereas in others, the antibodies may mimic insulin effect and cause hypoglycemia. Normal receptors exposed to large quantities of its complementary hormone may be down regulated. Therapeutically, this is the mechanism by which large acting analogs of gonadotropin-releasing hormone (GnRH) lead to a loss of responsiveness by the gonadotrophs to endogenous GnRH, which in turn leads to a lower-

ing of LH and follicle-stimulating hormone (FSH) concentrations. Finally, hormone resistance may occur because of postreceptor defects involving the signal pathway. Albright's hereditary osteodystrophy, which is manifest by resistance to parathyroid hormone, TSH, and gonadotropins, results from inactivation of G$_s\alpha$ in a variety of tissues. Another type of postreceptor defect is homologous desensitization, which refers to the inability of a hormone to stimulate the signaling pathway after extensive interaction with its receptor at a time when other factors are able to continue to stimulate that pathway. Such homologous desensitization is seen in the corpus luteum during early pregnancy when human chorionic gonadotropin has completely occupied its receptors. Although early in pregnancy hCG is able to stimulate adenylyl cyclase activity after interaction with the hCG/LH receptor in the corpus luteum, once the receptors are occupied, adenylyl cyclase activity decreases, but it is still able to be stimulated by forskolin and phorbal esters, which act on the signaling mechanism at the postreceptor sites.

Certain disease states, drugs, and medications are known to alter the metabolism of hormones, and may result in underexpression of hormone action. Alcohol enhances the A-ring metabolism of testosterone, increasing its metabolism. Phenobarbital decreases the production of 25(OH)-vitamin D from its precursors by stimulating the formation of more polar metabolites by the liver.

3. EXAMPLES OF CLINICAL SYNDROMES WITH MULTIPLE PATHOPHYSIOLOGIC MECHANISMS

For virtually every hormone there exists a pathologic state of overexpression or underexpression of hormone action. In some instances, there may be no clinical manifestations because of physiological compensation by normal homeostatic mechanisms, or because the hormonal abnormality may have little or no relevance. Hypoprolactinemia in males is an example of the latter. In most cases, overexpression or underexpression of hormone action results in clinical manifestations. Although the predominant manifestations of hormone excess or deficiency will be the same no matter what the underlying pathologic lesion, there are usually unique clinical or biochemical findings present with each type of pathology that leads the clinician to the correct diag-

Table 4
Etiologies of Acromegaly/Gigantism

Excessive GHRH Secretion
  Eutopic
  Ectopic
Excessive GH secretion
  Eutopic
  Ectopic
Acromegaloidism

Abbreviation: GHRH, growth hormone-releasing hormone.

Table 5
Etiologies of GH Deficiency Syndromes

Hypothalamic GHRH deficiency
  Congenital
  Acquired
Stalk lesions
Pituitary
  Deletion of GH gene
  Biologically inactive GH
  Structural defects involving somatotrophs
    Congenital Pit-1 mutation
    Acquired
GH receptor defect (Laron dwarfism)
Postreceptor defect in IGF-1 generation (? Pygmies)
Resistance to IGF-1

Abbreviations: GHRH, growth hormone releasing hormone; GH, growth hormone; IGF-1, insulin-like growth factor-1.

nosis. This section will illustrate these concepts as well as the array of different pathophysiologic mechanisms that may result in the constellation of signs and symptoms that characterize some of the common endocrine syndromes.

3.1. Growth Hormone (GH)

3.1.1. ACROMEGALY/GIGANTISM

Acromegaly and gigantism are the result of excessive GH secretion. Gigantism occurs when GH is hypersecreted prior to fusion of the epiphysial plates of the long bones, resulting in excessive linear growth as well as growth of the bones of the jaw, supraorbital ridges, and spine. Once the long bones' epiphysial plates are fused, the occurrence of excessive GH secretion results only in overgrowth of soft tissues and bones that retain cartilaginous plates, such as the supraorbital ridges and the spine. Thus, these patients exhibit large beefy hands as well as a large tongue, coarsening of the facial features, skin tags, prognathism, dorsal kyphosis, enlargement of the heart and kidneys, colonic polyps, and osteoarthritis. Symptoms include excessive perspiration, lethargy or fatigue, weight gain, and if the pathology is owing to a large intracranial neoplasm, visual abnormalities and headaches. Glucose intolerance with hyperinsulinemia is often present. These manifestations are the result of the excessive secretion of GH and its primary mediator, insulin-like growth factor-1 (IGF-1).

Table 4 lists the various pathophysiologic mechanisms for acromegaly or gigantism. Excessive production of growth hormone-releasing hormone (GHRH) occurs eutopically in some patients with hypothalamic hamartomas or gangliocytomas that secrete the releasing factor in an autonomous fashion. Autonomous ectopic production of GHRH has

been described with pancreatic islet cell and carcinoid tumors. With both eutopic and ectopic GHRH secretion, the pituitary somatotrophs are stimulated to secrete excessive quantities of GH. Somatotroph hyperplasia is seen pathologically in these conditions. The majority of patients with acromegaly or gigantism harbor a somatotroph adenoma that secretes excessive quantities of GH eutopically. Rarely, GH may be secreted ectopically by tumors, such as pancreatic or lung carcinomas. In each of these situations, the clinical manifestations of acromegaly are similar, and it may be very difficult to distinguish the underlying pathology unless there are other local manifestations from the nonpituitary tumors that direct the attention to other areas. Of interest, similar clinical manifestations may be seen in a condition known as acromegaloidism, which is not the result of excessive secretion of GH, but is associated with another trophic hormone that can be measured in a bone marrow stem cell assay.

3.1.2 GROWTH HORMONE DEFICIENCY SYNDROMES

On the other end of the spectrum from acromegaly and gigantism are the clinical syndromes of GH deficiency. When present in childhood, profound growth retardation and often hypoglycemia are seen, whereas in adults weakness and deficiencies in skeletal muscle mass may be present.

A variety of different conditions may give rise to similar clinical findings of underexpression of GH action (Table 5). GHRH may be deficient because of congenital or acquired lesions of the hypothalamus. This in turn results in somatotroph atrophy and insufficient production of GH. A similar result can be found in lesions that destroy the hypothalamo-hypophyseal portal system through which GHRH is transported to the somatotrophs. Deficient production of GH may also occur if pituitary tissue is missing, as is found in pituitary aplasia or if somatotrophs are absent through a mutation of the Pit-1 gene. Complete deletion of the GH gene also results in absent GH production. Immunologically active, but biologically inactive forms of GH, presumably owing to point mutations in the GH gene or to post-translational processing abnormalities may also result in growth retardation.

Although GH does have intrinsic biologic activity, its growth-promoting activity is mediated through IGF-1 secreted by hepatocytes and other tissues that contain GH receptors. Mutations of the GH receptor result in Laron dwarfism, an autosomal-recessive disorder characterized by elevated serum GH concentrations, but low IGF-1 levels, which do not rise following the exogenous administration of GH. These patients have clinical findings, such as elfin facies, which distinguish them from other individuals with congenital GH deficiency. Pygmies also exhibit an inability to produce IGF-1, but have a normal concentration of GH and normal GH receptors. The low IGF-1 in this syndrome may represent a postreceptor abnormality in IGF-1 generation. Finally, growth retardation can be seen with resistance to the biologic effects of IGF-1, which may be the mechanism through which pharmacologic doses of glucocorticoids inhibit cartilaginous growth during childhood.

3.2. Adrenal Glucocorticoids

3.2.1. CUSHING'S SYNDROME

Long-standing glucocorticoid excess, whether owing to endogenous hypersecretion from the adrenal gland or exogenous intake, results in obesity, redistribution of body fat, hypertension, proximal muscle weakness, loss of connective tissue support with abdominal striae and easy bruisibility, emotional symptoms, osteopenia, and glucose intolerance. If gluocorticoid excess is present in childhood, significant growth retardation also is seen.

Glucocorticoid excess can be caused from autonomous production from a primary adrenal gland abnormality, or excessive stimulation of the

Table 6
Etiologies of Cushing's Syndrome

Excessive CRH secretion
  Eutopic
  Ectopic
Excessive autonomous ACTH secretion
  Eutopic
  Ectopic
Excessive autonomous cortisol secretion
  Adrenocortical adenoma
  Adrenocortical carcinoma
Exogenous glucocorticoids

Abbreviation: CRH, corticotropin-releasing hormone.

adrenal gland from increased quantities of ACTH from a pituitary adenoma or an ectopic tumor source, or through excessive pituitary stimulation by corticotropin-releasing hormone (CRH) from a hypothalamic lesion or nonhypothalamic tumor secreting CRH ectopically (Table 6). With all of these conditions, the patient will demonstrate clinical findings of glucocorticoid excess. However, each of the causes outlined in Table 6 have their own unique clinical manifestations. For instance, the onset of the clinical and metabolic abnormalities is more rapid in patients who have ectopic production of ACTH or adrenocortical carcinoma than with the other causes. Patients with adrenocortical carcinoma tend to secrete increased quantities of mineralocorticoids and adrenal androgens, in addition to the glucocorticoids resulting in hypokalemic alkalosis and virilization in women and feminization in men.

3.2.2. ADRENAL INSUFFICIENCY

Loss of adrenal glucocorticoid production is associated with weight loss, fatigue, weakness, anorexia, and postural hypotension. Pure glucocorticoid insufficiency may be found with hypothalamic or pituitary lesions. If the adrenal gland is absent or destroyed, then mineralocorticoid and adrenal androgen deficiency also may be present, as will hyperpigmentation from excessive secretion of proopiomelanocortin-derived peptides.

Adrenal insufficiency can occur on a congenital basis or through involvement with various acquired disease processes (Table 7). Normal glucocorticoid secretion requires a coordinated production of CRH, which stimulates pituitary ACTH release, which in turn stimulates cortisol production and release. Thus,

Table 7
Etiologies of Adrenal Insufficiency

Hypothalamic (CRH deficiency)
  Congenital
  Structural
  Functional
Pituitary (ACTH deficiency)
  Congenital
  Acquired
Adrenal
  Congenital adrenal hypoplasia
  Congenital adrenal hyperplasia
  ACTH receptor mutation
   (familial glucocorticoid deficiency)
  Adrenoleukodystrophy
  Acquired
   Structural
   ACTH receptor antibodies
   Drug-induced
Target tissues
  Glucocorticoid resistance

congenital deficiency of CRH or a processes that destroys hypothalamic CRH production will result in low ACTH and low cortisol, and clinical findings of glucocorticoid insufficiency. The most common functional abnormality of the hypothalamic–pituitary–adrenal axis is seen in patients who have received pharmacologic doses of exogenous glucocorticoids for long periods of time. Suppression of the hypothalamic–pituitary–adrenal axis following withdrawal of the steroids may be present for up to 1 yr, and during that time, patients may experience weakness, weight loss, and fatigue as well as develop acute adrenal insufficiency if physically stressed. Congenital and acquired structural lesions in the anterior pituitary also cause secondary adrenal insufficiency with inadequate adrenal stimulation and low cortisol levels. With both hypothalamic and pituitary adrenal insufficiency, the patients do not exhibit mineralocorticoid insufficiency, since the renin-angiotensin-aldosterone system generally remains intact. The other clinical manifestations of hypothalamic–pituitary diseases reflect the "neighborhood" neurologic findings.

Primary adrenocortical insufficiency is much more common than the secondary or tertiary causes, and is usually owing to autoimmune destruction, either as an isolated phenomenon or as part of a polyglandular autoimmune endocrine syndrome, or

to infectious destruction, especially from tuberculosis and fungal infections. Congenital causes include congenital adrenal hypoplasia, which has recently been found to be the result of a mutation in the DAX-1 nuclear receptor, which closely resembles the retinoic acid receptor member of the nuclear receptor superfamily. Mutations in the ACTH receptor are associated with familial congenital glucocorticoid deficiency, whereas antibodies that react and block the ACTH receptor have been found in some patients with an autoimmune diathesis. Enzyme defects in the glucocorticoid pathway in the adrenal lead to a combination of glucocorticoid insufficiency with evidence of defects in the mineralocorticoid and/or adrenal androgen pathways that result in combinations of adrenal insufficiency, ambiguous genitalia, and in some patients, precocious puberty and hypertension. In a similar fashion, drugs and some medications, such as ketoconazole, metapyrone, aminoglutethimide, and trilostane, also result in adrenal enzyme inhibition and in certain circumstances may lead to adrenal insufficiency. Finally, some patients have a rare familial syndrome associated with glucocorticoid resistance resulting from mutations in the nuclear glucocorticoid receptor. These individuals often exhibit precocious puberty, since pituitary ACTH levels are elevated and stimulate adrenal androgen production.

3.3. Gonadal Steroid Hormones

3.3.1. PRECOCIOUS PUBERTY

Precocious puberty is the appearance of secondary sexual characteristics prior to age nine in boys and eight in girls. Thus, development of axillary and pubic hair and rapid bone growth in both sexes, penile (and most often testicular) enlargement in males, and breast development and menarche in females are the major clinical manifestations.

Precocious puberty can be classified as occurring through gonadotropin-dependent or gonadotropin-independent mechanisms (Table 8). Among the former, the most common cause is premature activation of GnRH secretion either on a familial basis or owing to a structural or nonstructural (idopathic) central nervous system disorder. One of the more common central nervous system disorders associated with precocious puberty is a hypothalamic hamartoma involving the tuber cinereum, which contain GnRH-secreting cells. The GnRH stimulates the

Table 8
Etiologies of Precocious Puberty

Gonadotropin-dependent
 Premature activation of GnRH secretion
 hCG-secreting tumors
 Primary hypothyroidism
Gonadotropin-independent
 Constitutive activation of testicular LH/hCG receptors
  (testotoxicosis)
 Constitutive activation of gonadal adenylyl cyclase
  (McCune-Albright syndrome)
 Ovarian cysts
 Gonadal neoplasms
 Congenital adrenal hyperplasia
 Adrenal neoplasms
 Exogenous sex steroid exposure

gonadotrophs to secrete LH and FSH, which in turn stimulate the gonads to secrete the gonadal steroid hormones. hCG-secreting neoplasms in males, such as germ-cell tumors of testes or extragonadal tumors, including those located in the pineal region, and hepatoblastomas, are associated with gondotropin-dependent precocious puberty owing to direct interaction of hCG with the LH/hCG receptors present in the gonads. Another form of gonadotropin-dependent precocious puberty is seen in children with severe primary hypothyroidism, often in association with galactorrhea (Van Wyk-Grumbach syndrome). This is considered to be an example of a "hormonal-overlap" syndrome that may be associated with gonadotropin hypersecretion. Alternatively, the close similarity of TSH with the other glycoprotein hormones raises the possibility that the massively increased levels of TSH in children with primary hypothyroidism may actually interact with the LH/hCG receptors in the gonads.

Gonadotropin-independent precocious puberty is found in girls who are exposed to exogenous estrogens or who develop estrogen-secreting tumors of the ovary or follicular cysts. In males, androgen-secreting neoplasms or congenital adrenal hyperplasia with androgen excess may result in isosexual precocious puberty, whereas in girls virilization is found. Several point mutations in the seven-trans-membrane G-protein-linked LH/hCG receptor present in the testicular leydig cells have been described that result in constitutive activation of the receptor leading to autonomous overproduction of testos-

terone and precocious puberty (testotoxicosis). The McCune-Albright syndrome, which includes polyostotic fibrous dysplasia of the bones, cafe-au-lait spots along with precocious puberty have been found to be the result of a mutation present in the $G_s\alpha$ that leads to constitutive activation of gonadal adenylyl cyclase, which mimicks gonadotropin stimulation.

3.3.2. HYPOGONADISM

The manifestations of hypogonadism depend on the age at which the deficient production of sex steroid hormones occurs. In males, androgen deficiency occurring during the first 12 wk of fetal development will result in insufficient development of Wolffian duct structures and deficient conversion of testosterone to dihydrotestosterone in the genital ridge tissue, leading to a failure to fuse the labial-scrotal folds, which normally results in the development of a scrotum and penile urethra. Androgen deficiency at this time presents with male pseudo-hermaphroditism. Androgen deficiency late in gestation may only be manifest by cryptorchidism and micropenis. If androgen deficiency occurs postnatally but prepubertally, then secondary sexual characteristics including hair growth in the androgen-sensitive areas of the body, deepening of the voice, and increased muscle mass fail to develop. The epiphyses of the long bones do not close and continue to grow under the influence of growth hormone. Therefore, the individual develops eunuchoidal proportions. If the androgen deficiency is acquired and occurs post-pubertally, then there may develop testicular atrophy, muscle weakness, decreased libido, infertility, and impotence.

In girls, prenatal estrogen deficiency owing to ovarian dysgenesis or lack of appropriate pituitary gonadotropin stimulation does not result in anatomical abnormalities, since the female genital tract develops the same in the presence or absence of an ovary. Therefore, hypogonadism from congenital lesions or those acquired during childhood present much the same way with absence of pubertal development, including menarche. Postpubertal development of hypogonadism in women leads to amenorrhea, uterine atrophy, and regression of breast glandular tissue.

In males, hypogonadism can be divided into two groups: hypogonadotropic hypogonadism resulting from a lesion in the hypothalamic or pituitary region and hypergonadotropic hypogonadism resulting

Table 9
Etiologies of Male Hypogonadism

Hypogonadotropic hypogonadism
  Hypothalamic
    Kallmann's syndrome (KAL gene defect)
    Other complex genetic syndrome
    Structural defects
    Functional defects
  Stalk lesions
  Pituitary
    LH β mutation
    Structural lesions
Hypergonadotropic hypogonadism
  Testicular defects
    Genetic
      Gross structural lesions
      LH/hCG receptor defect
      Testosterone steroidogenic defects
    Acquired
  Androgen-insensitivity syndromes
  5α-Reductase deficiency

from defects in the testes or in the androgen target tissues (Table 9). Several complex genetic syndromes associated with hypothalamic-hypogonadism have been described. These include the Prader-Willi and Laurence-Moon-Bardet-Biedal syndromes. Isolated gonadotropin deficiency with anosmia of hyposmia characterizes Kallmann's syndrome. The most common form of this syndrome is X-linked and has been shown to the result of gene deletions as well as point mutations in the KAL gene, which as previously noted, encodes for an adhesion protein that resembles fibronectin and which is responsible for the migration of GnRH-secreting neurons from the olfactory placode to the hypothalamus. Lack of a normal KAL protein inhibits this migration resulting in a GnRH deficiency. Hypothalamic dysfunction can result from a variety of disease states associated with acute and chronic weight loss, as well as suppression of GnRH release by several medications. Interruption of the hypothalo-hypophyseal portal system leads to hypogonadotropic hypogonadism through inadequate stimulation of the pituitary gonadotrophs. Primary pituitary problems, especially large pituitary adenomas, are often associated with gonadotropin deficiency. An unusual congenital form of pituitary hypogonadism is owing to a mutation in the gene encoding the β subunit of LH, resulting in a biologi-

cally inactive, but immunologically active form of the hormone.

Hypergonadotropic hypogonadism in males is often the result of acquired testicular defects. It is quite common for serum-free testosterone levels to decrease with age, with a concomitant increase in LH, reflecting a mild hypogonadism. Klinefelter's syndrome, resulting from the XXY genotype, is the most prevalent genetic abnormality involving the testes and this results in hyalinization and fibrosis of the gonad at the time of puberty, hypogonadism, eunuchoidal skeletal proportions, and gynecomastia. Several inherited defects in the enzymes responsible for testosterone biosynthesis have been described (Table 2) and usually result in varying degrees of male pseudohermaphroditism, since the defect is present during embryogenesis. Leydig cell hypoplasia is a congenital lesion associated with an absent or mutated LH/hCG receptor in the gonad. Activation of the receptor is needed for the mesenchymal tissue present in the developing gonad to differentiate into leydig cells. Therefore, neither are leydig cells seen nor is testosterone production from the testes present with this syndrome. The androgen-insensitivity syndromes are another form of hypergonadotropic hypogonadism and run the gamut from mild androgen resistance in phenotypic men who have normal male genitalia and gynecomastia to the complete testicular feminization syndrome characterized by complete androgen resistance with a female phenotype and absence of pubic or axillary hair. All of the patients with these defects have a problem with the nuclear androgen receptor. A variety of lesions with the receptor have been characterized and include complete absence or truncation of the receptor, point mutations that cause inactivation or decreased ability of the receptor to be activated, as well as lesions that cause thermal instability of the receptor. The phenotypic manifestations of androgen resistance in these patients depend on the type of receptor lesion and severity of the lesion. Finally, male hypogonadism can result from a deficiency of the enzyme 5α-reductase in androgen target tissues. This enzyme is responsible for the conversion of testosterone to dihydrotestosterone, and with its absence, both testosterone and LH levels are elevated. Since this defect is present during embryogenesis, there is incomplete development of male external genitalia, resulting in the appearance of a bifid scrotum and "clitoromegaly." At puberty, either through mass

Table 10
Etiologies of Female Hypogonadism

Hypogonadotropic hypogonadism
  Hypothalamic
    Congenital
    Acquired
      Structural
      Functional
  Pituitary
    Congenital
    Acquired
Hypergonadotropic hypogonadism
  Ovary
    Gonadal dysgenesis
    17α-Hydroxylase deficiency
    Resistant ovary syndrome
    Acquired structural defects
    Aromatase enzyme deficiency

action resulting from an increase in testosterone or through other mechanisms, such as a direct action of testosterone, virilization occurs with an increase in muscle mass, enlargement of the phallus, and deepening of the voice.

Female hypogonadism can also be divided into hypogonadotropic and hypergonadotropic forms (Table 10). The hypothalamic and pituitary abnormalities described above may also present in women as primary amenorrhea with deficient secondary sexual characteristic development or secondary amenorrhea if a lesion develops following menarche. Gonadal dysgenesis, including XO Turner syndrome, and XX or XY pure gonadal dysgenesis, accounts for the majority of patients with hypergonadotropic hypogonadism with primary amenorrhea and lack of secondary sexual development. In addition to the streak ovaries and estrogen deficiency, patients with Turner syndrome have other physical stigmata, including short stature, webbed neck, lymphedema, micrognathia, low-set ears, epicanthal folds, shield-like chest, and renal and vascular abnormalities. In contrast, 46XX and 46XY gonadal dysgenesis patients only demonstrate sexual infantilism and develop eunuchoidal proportions because of the lack of estrogen-mediated epiphysial closure of the long bones. A rare form of congenital adrenal hyperplasia, 17α-hydroxylase deficiency, is also associated with sexual infantilism because of a block in the conversion of pregnenolone to proges-

terone. Another rare condition, the resistant ovary syndrome is associated with a defect in the ovarian FSH receptor, which in some patients may be overcome with pharmacologic concentrations of exogenous gonadotropins. A variety of acquired structural defects may destroy ovarian function and lead to premature ovarian failure. Recently, an aromatase deficiency syndrome in females has been described. Since the aromatase enzyme is required to convert androstenedione to estrone and testosterone to estradiol, lack of this enzyme will result in elevated concentrations of androgens and deficient levels of estrogens. Clinically, this is manifested by estrogen deficiency with virilization from unopposed androgen effect, as well as delayed epiphysial closure resulting in tall stature.

3.4. Antidiuretic Hormone

3.4.1. Syndrome of Inappropriate Secretion of Antidiuretic Hormone (SIADH)

SIADH is manifest by signs and symptoms of water intoxication resulting from enhanced reabsorption of free water by the kidney, which leads to hyponatremia, hypoosmolarity, and urine that is inappropriately concentrated with respect to the serum with continued sodium excretion despite the hyponatremia. In order to make the diagnosis of SIADH, there should be normal adrenal and thyroid function, since glucocorticoids and thyroid hormones are required for free water clearance. In addition, kidney function should be normal, and there should be no evidence of a secondary cause of appropriate ADH secretion, such as volume depletion, edema, or cardiac or hepatic disease. The signs and symptoms are the result of the degree of water intoxication and rate of fall of the sodium. When the serum sodium levels reach 115–120 meq/L, anorexia, nausea, vomiting, abdominal cramps, bloating, ileus, restlessness, confusion, withdrawal, hostility, headache, and muscle weakness may be prominent. If the serum sodium level falls below 110 meq/L, often there will be focal neurologic findings, including weakness, hemiparesis, ataxia, stupor, convulsions, or coma.

Both eutopic and ectopic sources of excessive antidiuretic hormone secretion have been identified (Table 11). Among the eutopic problems are a variety of central nervous system disorders that alter the intracranial pressure or involve the hypothalamus. Pulmonary disorders that alter the pressure dynamics

Table 11
Etiologies of SIADH

Eutopic production of ADH
    Central nervous system disorders
    Pulmonary disorders
    Drug-induced
    Reset osmostat
Ectopic production of ADH

Table 12
Etiologies of Diabetes Insipidus

Central (neurogenic)
    Neurophysin processing defect
    Structural hypothalamic/stalk/posterior
      pituitary lesions
Nephrogenic diabetes insipidus
    Vasopressin V2 receptor mutation
    Aquaporin-2 water channel mutation
    Acquired
Excessive vasopressinase activity in pregnancy

in the baroreceptors present in the left atrium and pulmonary veins may also result in inappropriate release of antidiuretic hormone from the hypothalamus and posterior pituitary. Several drugs stimulate vasopressin release, including chlorpropamide and clofibrate, whereas other drugs may stimulate antidiuretic hormone (ADH) release or enhance its activity at the renal level. Some patients appear to have developed a resetting of the osmostat present in the hypothalamus. These patients begin to release ADH at a lower level of serum osmolality than in normal individuals. In essence, the release of ADH parallels the normal curve, but the serum osmolality in the affected patients are lower than normals at any given plasma concentration of ADH. A number of tumors have been found to secrete ADH ectopically, especially oat cell carcinoma of the lung. Indeed, even the absence of clinical SIADH, many patients with lung carcinomas will demonstrate an inadequate urinary excretion of a water load.

3.4.2. DIABETES INSIPIDUS

Diabetes insipidus results from deficiency of ADH action leading to polyuria, polydipsia, and a urine osmolality that is low despite a high serum osmolality. From a pathophysiologic standpoint, diabetes insipidus can develop because of inadequate production of ADH from the hypothalamus and posterior pituitary (central or neurogenic diabetes insipidus), inability of ADH to act on the kidney to enhance resorption of free water (nephrogenic diabetes insipidus), or from excessive metabolism of ADH (Table 12).

Central diabetes insipidus may be present at birth from structural defects involving the hypothalamus, pituitary stalk, or posterior pituitary. In addition, a point mutation interfering with the processing of the neurophysin-ADH prohormone has been described that not only causes diabetes insipidus, but may also lead to neuronal degeneration in the hypothalamic

supraoptic and periventricular nuclei. Other structural defects affecting the region include tumors, cysts, infiltrative processes, and autoimmune destruction. Nephrogenic diabetes insipidus may occur congenitally from a mutation of the vasopressin V2 receptors in the renal-collecting duct epithelium, which are responsible for activation of G-proteins and the generation of cAMP. An additional genetic defect involving the aquaporin-2 water channel, which represents the terminal renal effect of ADH, may also cause congenital nephrogenic diabetes insipidus. Other causes of nephrogenic diabetes insipidus include chronic renal disease, hypercalcemia, hypokalemia, conditions that interrupt the renal medullary concentrating mechanism, and drugs, including lithium, demeclocycline, colchicine, and methoxyflurane anesthesia. ADH deficiency may also occur during pregnancy owing to the excessive secretion of placental vasopressinase that destroys the circulating ADH. This disorder remits following parturition as the vasopressinase concentrations rapidly disappear from the maternal circulation.

3.5. Thyroid Hormones

3.5.1. HYPERTHYROIDISM

Excessive circulating quantities of thyroid hormone bind to the widely distributed nuclear thyroid hormone receptor, and lead to an increase in metabolic rate and cell proliferation as well as increased tissue sensitivity to catecholamines. Thus, the signs and symptoms of hyperthyroidism include tachycardia, tremor, piloerection, increased perspiration, weight loss, elevation of cardiac output with a wide pulse pressure, nervousness, heat intolerance, hyperreflexia, proximal muscle weakness, and hyperdefecation.

Table 13
Etiologies of Thyrotoxicosis

TSH receptor and signaling pathway mediated
  TSH-producing pituitary tumors
  hCG-producing tumors
  Thyroid-stimulating immunoglobulin production
    (Graves' disease)
  Constitutive activation of TSH receptor
  Constitutive activation of $G_s\alpha$
Release of preformed thyroid hormone (thyroiditis)
Autonomous production
  Toxic nodule
  Thyroid carcinoma
Exogenous thyroid hormone intake

Several different mechanisms and pathologic states have been identified that lead to similar signs and symptoms of thyrotoxicosis (Table 13). Activation of the TSH receptor or TSH receptor-coupled signal pathway is the most common endogenous cause of hyperthyroidism. The rare TSH-producing pituitary adenoma leads to the presence of hyperthyroidism and goiter because of excessive autonomous secretion of TSH by the pituitary tumor. TSH stimulates growth of the thyroid follicular cells as well as stimulation of thyroid hormone synthesis and release. Receptor crossreaction is the mechanism by which hCG-secreting tumors account for hyperthyroidism. Although this may occasionally be seen in a patient with choriocarcinoma of the testes or ovary, most patients who have hCG-induced hyperthyroidism harbor a hydatidiform mole that secretes enormous quantities of the placental glycoprotein hormone. Since the α subunit of each of the glycoprotein hormones is virtually identical and the β subunits share some degree of homology, it is not surprising that hCG has intrinsic TSH-like activity. The most common cause of endogenous hyperthyroidism is Graves' disease, an autoimmune process associated with the production of thyroid-stimulating immunoglobulins. These immunoglobulins bind with the TSH receptor and mimic the action of TSH, causing growth of the thyroid and synthesis and release of thyroid hormones. Constitutive activation of the TSH receptor owing to a mutation leads to continuous stimulation of its G-protein and adenylyl cyclase. This type of lesion has been shown to cause congenital hyperthyroidism in neonates without a maternal history of Graves' disease. The congenital

form is the result of a germ-line mutation in the receptor. Activating somatic mutations in the thyrotropin receptor gene have also been noted in some patients with autonomously functioning adenomas associated with hyperthyroidism (hot nodules). Similarly, constitutive activation of the $G_s\alpha$ subunit has been found in the some patients with toxic thyroid adenomas.

Another mechanism of hyperthyroidism is release of preformed thyroid hormone from the thyroid gland. This is found in various inflammatory conditions involving the thyroid gland. It is perhaps most prominent in patients with subacute thyroiditis in which a viral inflammation of the thyroid gland leads to disruption of the normal follicles and release of thyroid hormone. This is a self-limited condition and once all of the thyroid hormone is released, the patients usually go through a period of hypothyroidism before the thyroid recovers and the thyroid hormone levels return to normal. Acute release of thyroid hormone can also be seen in some patients with autoimmune (Hashimoto's) thyroiditis and in the postpartum state in women who develop a self-limited autoimmune thyroiditis. Thyroid hormone may be produced autonomously by toxic adenomas without a known defect in the TSH receptor or signal pathway, as well as in patients with large body burden of thyroid carcinoma. In the latter situation, although individual thyroid carcinoma cells are relatively inefficient in production of thyroid hormone, a large mass of well-differentiated thyroid cancer may produce sufficient quantities of thyroxine and triiodothyronine to cause hyperthyroidism.

3.5.2. HYPOTHYROIDISM

The clinical manifestations of hypothyroidism depend on the age of onset. Untreated congenital hypothyroidism results in cretinism associated with diffuse puffiness, short stature, mental retardation, and neurologic abnormalities. In children and adolescents, growth retardation, decrease in mental concentrating ability and school performance, and precocious puberty may be found. In adults, periorbital and peripheral puffiness, cold intolerance, weight gain, constipation, muscle cramps, decreased mental concentrating ability, and easy fatigability are common.

Table 14 lists the etiologies of hypothyroidism according to the level of the defect. Tertiary or hypothalamic hypothyroidism may accompany multiple tropic hormone deficiencies in patients with panhy-

Table 14
Causes of Hypothyroidism

Tertiary (hypothalamic) hypothyroidism
  TRH deficiency
  Drug-induced
Secondary (pituitary) hypothyroidism
  Thyrotroph destruction
    Congenital Pit-1 mutation
    Acquired
  TSH β subunit mutation
  Altered TSH glycosylation
Primary (thyroidal) hypothyroidism
  Congenital
    Thyroid dysgenesis
    TSH receptor defects
      Congenital owing to receptor mutation
      Autoimmune blocking antibodies
    TSH postreceptor $G_s\alpha$ mutation
    Iodide transport defect
    Biosynthetic enzyme defects
    Thyroglobulin mutation
  Acquired
    Destruction
    Iodine deficiency
    Drug-induced
  Thyroid hormone nuclear receptor defect (thyroid
    hormone resistance syndromes)

popituitarism or may occur as a monotropic deficiency in the secretion of thyrotropin-releasing hormone (TRH). It is not known whether this is the result of mutation in the TRH gene processing or secretory abnormality. Drugs, including thyroid hormones and α-adrenergic blockers, decrease hypothalamic TRH production. Secondary or pituitary hypothyroidism may be seen in patients with structural abnormalities of the thyrotroph because of replacement by tumor, infiltrative processes or vascular compromise, or congenital absence of the thyrotroph because of a mutation in the Pit-1 gene, which is a pituitary-specific intranuclear transcription factor necessary for the development and function of somatotrophs, lactotrophs, and thyrotrophs. Point mutations in the TSH-β subunit gene may cause congenital hypothyroidism. A form of TSH with reduced biologic activity because of altered glycosylation has been found in some patients with hypothalamic hypothyroidism who exhibit slightly increased levels of immunoreactive TSH activity despite profound central hypothyroidism.

Congenital primary hypothyroidism is found in patients who have dysgenesis of the thyroid gland. Goitrous congenital primary hypothyroidism may occur with inactivating point mutations of the TSH receptor or the G-protein that couples the receptor to adenylyl cyclase. A more common cause of a TSH receptor problem is the presence of TSH receptor-blocking antibodies produced in women with autoimmune thyroid disease, which cross the placenta, enter the fetal circulation, and bind to the fetal thyroid TSH receptors. Deficiencies of thyroid peroxidase enzyme, iodotyrosine deiodinase, or with the follicular cell iodide transport (trapping mechanism) also result in hypothyroidism. Mutations in the thyroglobulin gene have been found to result in a thyroglobulin molecule that is incapable of functioning properly for the formation of thyroxine or triiodothyronine. Iodine deficiency, the ingestion of goitrogens, and thyroiditis are acquired causes of primary hypothyroidism.

Defects in the thyroid hormone nuclear receptors lead to resistance to the effect of thyroid hormones. The defects are owing to mutations in the thyroid hormone receptor β-gene, and the clinical manifestations depend on whether there is generalized resistance to thyroid hormones or selective pituitary resistance. There is a great deal of phenotypic variability in different families with generalized resistance to thyroid hormone. Some individuals demonstrate marked hypothyroidism, whereas others have very mild degrees of hypothyroidism that are compensated for by an increased secretion of TSH, resulting in thyroid growth and production of normal quantities of thyroid hormones. Patients with pituitary resistance to thyroid hormones secrete increased quantities of TSH, which results in goiter and hyperthyroidism since the peripheral tissues are not resistant to the effects of the thyroid hormone.

3.6. Calcium Abnormalities

3.6.1. Hypercalcemia

An elevation of serum calcium concentration leads to depression of central nervous system function, increased gastrin secretion and gastric acid production, a decreased renal response to ADH, increased peripheral vascular resistance, increased ionotrophic effect on the myocardium, and decreased contractility of smooth and skeletal muscles. Hence, patients with hypercalcemia often complain of weakness, anorexia, nausea, vomiting, abdominal pain,

Table 15
Etiologies of Hypercalcemia

Hyperparathyroidism
Malignancy-associated
   PTH-related protein production
   Cytokine production
   Prostaglandin-secretion
   25 (OH)-vitamin D-1α-hydroxylase dysregulation
Granulomatous disease
Other endocrine disease
   Hyperthyroidism
   Hypothyroidism
   Adrenal insufficiency
Metabolic bone disease with immobilization
Drug-induced
Familial hypocalciuric hypercalcemia

constipation, polyuria, and thirst. They may exhibit confusion, personality disturbances, obtundation, and coma.

There are multiple pathophysiologic mechanisms responsible for the development of hypercalcemia (Table 15). Overproduction of parathyroid hormone (PTH) from a parathyroid adenoma or hyperplastic parathyroid glands results in hyperparathyroidism, which stimulates osteoclastic bone resorption with release of calcium and phosphorus into the circulation. The elevated PTH also stimulates the renal 1α-hydroxylation of 25(OH)-vitamin D converting it to 1,25(OH)$_2$-vitamin D, which enhances the absorption of calcium from the gastrointestinal tract. In a similar manner, the overproduction of PTH-related protein that binds to the PTH receptor may also cause hypercalcemia through similar mechanisms. A number of cytokines, including the interleukins, as well as prostaglandins produced locally by tumors present in the bone, may stimulate osteoclastic bone resorption, releasing calcium into the circulation. If the calcium load exceeds the ability of the kidneys to excrete it, then hypercalcemia results. Some tumors, such as lymphomas, cause hypercalcemia through the presence of a 25(OH)-vitamin D-1α-hydroxylase enzyme, which converts 25(OH)-vitamin D to 1,25(OH)$_2$-vitamin D, causing a hypervitaminosis D syndrome. A similar mechanism of hypercalcemia is found in patients with granulomatous diseases. Mild hypercalcemia can be found in patients with hyperthyroidism presumably because of the rapid turnover of bone during the hypermetabolic state.

Hypercalcemia is also associated with hypothyroidism and adrenal insufficiency through mechanisms that are presently unclear. Patients with metabolic bone disease associated with rapid bone turnover who are immobilized lose the pizoelectric effect, which stimulates osteoblastic bone formation, and therefore, there can be at least transient uncoupling of bone resorption and bone formation favoring resorption. A number of drugs are associated with hypercalcemia, including vitamin D and vitamin A excess and lithium carbonate. Familial hypocalciuric hypercalcemia is found in patients who have a mutation in the calcium-sensing receptor. This results in an increase in the feedback regulatory set point of serum calcium on parathyroid gland PTH secretion. Thus, a higher level of serum calcium is needed to inhibit PTH secretion in patients with this syndrome. Such patients generally demonstrate mild hypercalcemia and hypocalciuria, and may have parathyroid hyperplasia. The PTH effects on the kidney increase the reabsorption of calcium; hence, for a given level of serum calcium, these patients have hypocalciuria in contrast to normal individuals or those with non-PTH-mediated hypercalcemia.

3.6.2. HYPOCALCEMIA

A decrease in the serum ionized calcium concentration results in central nervous system depression and muscular irritability. Patients usually complain of lethargy, confusion, irritability, dry skin, and muscle cramps, and often demonstrate emotional lability and confusion. Neuromuscular irritability can be demonstrated on physical examination.

Since calcium is regulated by both parathyroid hormone and vitamin D, disorders of these hormonal systems may result in hypocalcemia (Table 16). Decreased parathyroid hormone secretion can be found in patients born with structural defects in the parathyroid gland as well as in individuals who have mutations involving parathyroid hormone processing. Structural defects of the parathyroid gland can occasionally occur with infiltrative disorders, but the most common acquired structural problem results from thyroid or parathyroid surgery with extirpation of the parathyroid glands or compromise of their vascular supply. A functional defect in the secretion of parathyroid hormone is found in patients who have magnesium deficiency, which also results in decreased responsiveness of the bone

Table 16
Etiologies of Hypocalcemia

Decreased PTH secretion
  Congenital structural defects of parathyroids
  PTH hormone-processing defect
  Acquired structural defects
  Acquired functional defects
PTH resistance
  Defective PTH receptor (pseudohypoparathyroidism
    Type IB)
  PTH $G_s\alpha$ mutation (pseudohypoparathyroidism
    Type IA)
  Renal insufficiency
  Magnesium deficiency
Active vitamin D production abnormalities
  Deficient intake or sunlight
  Vitamin D malabsorption
  Abnormal metabolism
  Congenital renal 1α-hydroxylase deficiency (vitamin
    D-dependent Rickets Type I)
Vitamin D receptor abnormalities
  1,25 $(OH)_2$-vitamin D-resistant Rickets
  Renal insufficiency
Excessive tissue deposition
  Hyperphosphatemia
  Acute hemorrhagic pancreatitis
  Osteoblastic metastases
Drug-induced

Table 17
Etiologies of Hypoglycemia

Excessive insulin receptor stimulation
  Increased insulin secretion
    Islet cell tumor
    Islet hyperplasia
    Alimentary
  Ectopic IGF-2 production
  Anti-insulin receptor antibodies
  Anti-insulin antibodies
Deficiency of glucose contraregulatory hormones
  GH
  ACTH
  Cortisol
  Thyroid hormone
  Catecholamines
  Glucagon
Defective hepatic glucose production
  Liver disease
  Gluconeogenic substrate deficiency
Drug-induced

to parathyroid hormone. Other causes of parathyroid hormone resistance are defective parathyroid hormone receptors resulting from a mutation to the receptor itself (pseudohypoparathyroidism Type IB) or from an inactivating $G_s\alpha$ mutation in the PTH receptor-signaling pathway (Albright hereditary osteodystrophy; pseudohypoparathyroidism Type 1A). PTH resistance is also found in patients who have renal insufficiency.

Abnormalities in vitamin D production, absorption, or metabolism result in a decrease absorption of calcium and phosphorus from the gastrointestinal tract. Mutations of the vitamin D nuclear receptor also result in decreased absorption of calcium and phosphorus from the diet, and are responsible for the syndrome of 1,25$(OH)_2$-vitamin D-resistant rickets. Hypocalcemia may also occur because of chelation with phosphate, which leads to deposition of calcium phosphate in soft tissues, and from saponification of fat in patients with fulminant acute hemorrhagic pancreatitis. Rarely, osteoblastic metastases may be so

extensive that hypocalcemia is found. Finally, a variety of drugs may also bring about hypocalcemia through inhibition of osteoclastic bone resorption, chelation, or alterations in vitamin D metabolism.

3.7. Glucose Abnormalities

3.7.1. HYPOGLYCEMIA

Hypoglycemia results in two types of symptoms: those resulting from a rapid rate of fall of the blood glucose resulting in stimulation of the sympathoadrenal system and those reflecting the low level of blood sugar on central nervous system function (neuroglycopenic systems). When the sympathetic nervous system and adrenal medulla are activated, patients develop tachycardia, piloerection, anxiety, tremulousness, diaphoresis, and hunger. Levels of plasma glucose below 36 mg/L lead to concentrating difficulties, fatigue, headache, confusion, seizures, and coma.

A simple classification scheme of causes of hypoglycemia based on pathophysiology is presented in Table 17. Excessive stimulation of the insulin receptor can occur when the pancreatic islet of Langerhans secretes excessive quantities of insulin. Islet cell hyperplasia from adenomatosis or nesidioblastosis, as well as autonomously functioning benign or malignant islet cell neoplasms secrete insulin regardless of the blood sugar concentration. The hyperstimulation of the insulin receptor leads to increase glucose uptake by a multitude of tissues while inhibiting hepatic glucose production. Similarly, increased insulin secretion is found in patients who have an alimentary form of hypoglycemia following gastric surgery. The rapid transit and absorption of carbohydrate leads to stimulation of insulin secretion and elevation of insulin levels at a time when the plasma glucose has decreased. The hyperinsulinemia reduces the glucose further leading to hypoglycemic symptoms. Insulin-like growth factor-2 (IGF-2) is produced ectopically by nonislet cell tumors associated with hypoglycemia. Many of these tumors are derived from mesenchymal tissues, such as retroperitoneal fibrosarcomas and mesotheliomas. The hypoglycemia associated with ectopic IGF-2 production may be the result of IGF-2 acting through the insulin receptor or the IGF-1 receptor. Although the majority of patients with the Kahn Type B insulin resistance syndrome associated with anti-insulin receptor antibodies have hyperglycemia, some will develop intermittent hypoglycemia. The syndrome occurs in individuals with other abnormalities of the immune system, including elevated levels of antinuclear and and anti-DNA antibodies, elevated IgG, IgM, and IgA concentrations, leukopenia, decreased serum complement levels, proteinuria, alopecia, and vitiligo. This condition has also been found in patients with systemic lupus erythematosus, thrombocytopenia, primary biliary cirrhosis, and scleroderma. Another rare immune-mediated cause of hypoglycemia is the appearance of anti-insulin antibodies in individuals who have not been exposed to exogenous insulin. These antibodies bind endogenous insulin, and at times, the insulin will disassociate from the antibody, resulting in hypoglycemia. This phenomenon has been found in patients with Graves' disease, and such conditions as multiple myeloma and lymphoma.

GH ACTH, cortisol, thyroid hormones, catecholamines, and glucagon are all required for glucose homeostasis. Congenital or acquired deficiencies of one or more of these hormones may be associated with hypoglycemia. In the absence of food intake, plasma glucose concentrations are maintained initially through glycogenolysis and then gluconeogenesis. Patients who have liver disease or are unable to generate sufficient quantities of gluconeogenic amino acids develop hypoglycemia. Finally, several drugs are associated with hypoglycemia either through induction of hyperinsuline-

Table 18
Etiologies of Hyperglycemia

Inadequate insulin production
  Type I and II diabetes mellitus
  Mutation of proinsulin/insulin gene
    Proinsulin-processing defect
    Insulin gene point mutations
  Pancreatic disease
  Drug-induced
Insulin receptor defect
  Mutation of insulin receptor gene
  Receptor downregulation
  Antireceptor antibody
Excessive production of glucose contraregulatory
    hormones
    GH
    Cortisol
    Catecholamines
    Glucagon

mia (sulfonylureas, pentamidine) or without hyperinsulinemia (alcohol).

3.7.2. HYPERGLYCEMIA

Hyperglycemia whether resulting from insulin-dependent Type I or noninsulin-dependent Type II diabetes mellitus or to secondary diabetes results in osmostic diuresis with loss of water and electrolytes. Patients therefore develop polyuria, polydipsia, polyphagia, weight loss, weakness, and fatigue. If the serum hyperosmolality is very high and the degree of dehydration severe, then obtundation and coma may be present. With severe insulin deficiency, ketoacidosis may develop resulting in dehydration, rapid, deep respirations, stupor, and coma. Patients with long-standing, poorly controlled diabetes may also exhibit retinopathy, neuropathy, and nephropathy.

From a pathophysiologic standpoint, hyperglycemia may be caused by inadequate insulin production, insulin receptor defects, or excessive production of glucose contraregulatory hormones (Table 18). Both Type I and II diabetes mellitus are associated with inadequate insulin production with Type I showing a more profound defect. Inadequate biologically active insulin production is also seen with point mutations of the proinsulin/insulin gene, resulting in either a proinsulin processing defect with hyperproinsulinemia or in an abnormal circulating insulin. Pancreatic diseases, such as acute pancreatitis or pentamidine-induced β-cell destruction, are associated with inadequate insulin production, as is also seen with a variety of drugs, such as diazoxide, thiazide diuretics, or phenytoin, which reduce the release of insulin from the pancreas. Several different mutations affecting the insulin receptor gene have been found. Some of these mutations are associated with decreased insulin binding to the receptor, whereas others result in impaired transport of insulin to the cell surface, a decrease in the receptor-associated tyrosine kinase activity, or in some instances, accelerate receptor degradation. Occupation of the insulin receptor by anti-insulin receptor antibodies is associated with insulin resistance in Kahn Type B insulin resistance. Patients who exhibit marked insulin resistance because of mutations or antireceptor antibodies also may have acanthosis nigricans. In women with this syndrome, polycystic ovaries are often present and are associated with increased ovarian production of testosterone, hirsutism, and virilization. Several conditions that are associated with hyperinsulinemia also lead to a insulin receptor downregulation. This is commonly seen in patients with Type II diabetes as well as obesity. Excessive production of the glucose contraregulatory hormones, growth hormone, cortisol, catecholamines, or glucagon is also associated with hyperglycemia generally through a postreceptor antagonism of insulin action.

4. CONCLUSIONS

The study of each of the endocrine disorders listed in Tables 4–18 nicely illustrates the progression of our knowledge from bedside to bench and back to the patient. The initial descriptions of diseases, such as precocious puberty, hypogonadism, hyperthyroidism, and hypothyroidism, were confined to clinical and then biochemical observations on patients presenting with the disorders. As more patients were studied, it became clear that although the predominant clinical findings were similar, differences existed with some of the clinical manifestations. For instance, boys who have central, gonadotropin-dependent precocious puberty exhibit enlargement of their testicles, whereas those who develop precocious puberty because of an androgen-secreting adrenal neoplasm retain small testicles. In a similar fashion, a patient presenting with a secondary hypothyroidism will have a small thyroid gland,

whereas an individual with primary hypothyroidism may have a goiter. As bioassays and immunoassays became available to measure the hormones involved, patients presenting with similar signs and symptoms could be subclassified and different pathophysiologic mechanisms to explain the findings formulated. The explosion of knowledge in cellular and molecular biology has allowed us to understand further the diversity of mechanisms that give rise to endocrine diseases and allows us to understand the differences in clinical manifestations of our patients. Just as advances in our understanding of endocrine diseases provide insight into the target tissue response to hormonal action, the advances in our understanding of hormonal action provide insight into the mechanisms of endocrine disease.

One of the lessons that we have learned from clinical medicine, which is being reinforced by our advances in understanding of the molecular mechanisms for the various disease states, is that although a patient may present with signs and symptoms of a certain endocrine disease, the therapies used to treat one patient with the disease may not be appropriate for another patient presenting with a similar disease owing to a different hormonal or molecular pathologic abnormality. Thus, using methimazole or propylthiouracil to treat a patient with hyperthyroidism from Graves' disease is appropriate since the hyperthyroxinemia in that disease is the result of enhanced synthesis and release of thyroid hormones. However, those drugs are inappropriate for a patient who has hyperthyroidism from subacute thyroiditis, since the hyperthyroxinemia in that situation is owing to disruption of the normal integrity of the thyroid with release of preformed thyroid hormones into the circulation. Once we are able to understand the specific pathophysiology for an endocrine disease presenting in a particular patient, we should be able to design more specific therapies for treating that patient.

REFERENCES

Jameson JL. Applications of molecular biology in endocrinology. In: DeGroot et al., eds. *Endocrinology*, 3rd ed. Philadelphia: W.B. Saunders, 1995: 119.

SUGGESTED READINGS

Bell GI, Froguel P, Nishi S, et al. Mutations of the human glucokinase gene and diabetes mellitus. *Trends Endocrinol Metab* 1993; 4:86.

Braunstein GD. Ectopic hormone production. In: Felig P, Baxter JD, Frohman LA, eds. *Endocrinology and Metabolism*, 3rd ed. New York: McGraw-Hill, 1995:1733.

Brent GA. The molecular basis of thyroid hormone action. *N Engl J Med* 1994; 331:847.

Clapham DE. Why testicles are cool. *Nature* 1994; 371:109.

Clark AJL, Weber A. Molecular insights into inherited ACTH resistance syndromes. *Trends Endocrinol Metab* 1994; 5:209.

Garvey WT, Birnbaum MJ. Cellular insulin action and insulin resistance. *Clin Endocrinol Metab* 1993; 7:785.

Haavisto A-M, Pettersson K, Bergendahl M, Virkamaki A, Huhtaniemi I. Occurrence and biological properties of a common genetic variant of luteinizing hormone. *J Clin Endocrinol Metab* 1995; 80:1257.

Haugen BR, Ridgway EC. Transcription factor Pit-1 and its clinical implications: From bench to bedside. *Endocrinologist* 1995; 5:132.

Herman-Bonert V, Fagin JA. Molecular pathogenesis of pituitary tumors. *Clin Endocrinol Metab* 1995; 9:203.

Knoers N VAM. Molecular characterization of nephrogenic diabetes insipidus. *Trends Endocrinol Metab* 1994; 10:422.

Kopp R, van Sande J, Parma J, et al. Brief report: Congenital hyperthyroidism caused by a mutation in the thyrotropin-receptor gene. *N Engl J Med* 1995; 332:150.

Ludgate ME, Vassart G. The thyrotropin receptor as a model to illustrate receptor and receptor antibody diseases. *Clin Endocrinol Metab* 1995; 9:95.

Schwindinger WF, Levine MA. McCune-Albright syndrome. *Trends Endocrinol Metab* 1993; 4:238.

Shenker A, Laue L, Kosugi S, Merendine JJ, Minegishi T, Cutler GB. A constitutively activating mutation of the luteinizing hormone receptor in familial male precocious puberty. *Nature* 1993; 365:652.

Smith EP, Boyd J, Frank GR et al. Estrogen resistance caused by a mutation in the estrogen-receptor gene in a man. *N Engl J Med* 1994; 331:1056.

Sunthornthepvarakul T, Gottschalk ME, Hayashi Y, Refetoff S. Brief report: resistance to thyrotropin caused by mutations in the thyrotropin-receptor gene. *N Engl J Med* 1995; 332:155.

Taylor SI, Cama A, Kadowaki H, Kadowaki T, Accili D. Mutations of the human isnulin receptor gene. *Trends Endocrinol Metab* 1990; 1:134.

17

Oncogenes and Tumor Suppressor Genes in Tumorigenesis of the Endocrine System

Lin Pei, MD, PhD, and Shlomo Melmed, MD

CONTENTS

INTRODUCTION
ONCOGENES
TUMOR SUPPRESSOR GENES
PROTO-ONCOGENES AND TUMOR SUPPRESSOR GENES IN ENDOCRINE TUMORS
PITUITARY TUMORS
THYROID TUMORS
PARATHYROID NEOPLASIA
CLINICAL IMPLICATIONS

1. INTRODUCTION

Tumor formation is a multistep process that involves uncoupling of the interdependent mechanisms of cell proliferation and differentiation. Mutations of either proto-oncogenes or tumor suppressor genes may confer growth advantage to mutant cells, enabling them to proliferate more rapidly than normal cells and to alter their interaction with their surroundings, resulting in local invasion and or distant metastases. Studies of cellular proto-oncogenes and tumor suppressor genes during the past decade have yielded major advances in the understanding of the molecular basis of tumorigenesis. This chapter focuses on the role of these genes in development of tumors of the endocrine system.

From: *Endocrinology: Basic and Clinical Principles* (P. M. Conn and S. Melmed, eds.), Humana Press Inc., Totowa, NJ.

2. ONCOGENES

Oncogenes were initially discovered by studies of tumor viruses capable of infecting normal cells and transforming them into tumor cells. The discovery that the Rous sarcoma virus-associated oncogene, src, originated from the genome of normal chicken cells suggested the existence of a cellular gene (proto-oncogene) with oncogenic potential that could be activated by a virus. The compelling evidence that genetic alterations of cellular proto-oncogenes are involved in human tumor formation came from DNA transfection experiments. DNA from tumor cells was extracted and introduced to normal fibroblast cells. Some transfected cells grew in culture with similar characteristics to transformed cells and, when injected into nude mice, formed rapidly growing tumor masses. Subsequent isolation and molecular cloning of several oncogenes from

Table 1
Representative Oncogenes In Human Tumors

Oncogenes	Tumor	Mechanism of activation	Properties of gene product
erb-B	Mammary carcinoma glioblastoma	Amplification	Growth factor receptor
ret	Papillary thyroid carcinoma	Rearrangment	Cell-surface receptor
raf	Stomach carcinoma	Rearrangement	Cytoplasmic serine/ threonine kinase
H-ras	Stomach carcinoma	Point mutation	GDP/GTP binding
K-ras	Bladder carcinoma	Point mutation	Signal transducer
N-ras	Leukemia	Point mutation	Signal transducer
myc	Lymphomas, carcinomas	Amplification, chromosome translocation	Nuclear transcription factor
bcl-2	Follicular and undifferentiated lymphomas	Chromosome translocation	Cytoplasmic membrane protein
gsp	Pituitary tumors	Point mutation	GDP/GTP signal transducer

Adapted from Weinberg (1994).

transfected cells showed that they are structurally very similar to genes present in DNA of normal cells, but contain one or more somatic mutations that occurred during tumor pathogenesis. A subtle change in gene structure even at the single-base-pair level, appeared sufficient to convert a normal cellular proto-oncogene into a transforming oncogene.

Proto-oncogenes play important roles in regulating normal cell growth and differentiation, and to date, over 100 have been identified. The cellular functions of proto-oncogenes fall into several groups, including growth factor cell-surface receptors, cytoplasmic serine/threonine kinases, signal transducers, and nuclear transcription factors. Table 1 lists representative proto-oncogenes of these different groups associated with human tumors.

Activation of proto-oncogenes can result from either a point mutation in the structural region that encodes for amino acids of a protein, or from changes in the regulatory region that modulates gene expression in response to developmental or physiological stimuli. Point mutations that activate the Ras oncogene are the best-characterized mutations found in the former category. These mutations occur most frequently at codons 12, 13, and 61. The Ras protein is a guanine nucleotide-binding protein that acts as a proximal membrane-associated signal transducer resulting in a complex cascade transmitting growth-stimulatory signals. Binding to Guanine Triphosphate (GTP) results in Ras activation and signal transduction, whereas hydrolysis of bound GTP to

Guanine Diphosphate (GDP) by GTPase leads to inactivation of Ras and termination of signal transduction. The three-dimensional structure of Ras has revealed that the amino acid residues most commonly mutated in the Ras protein are directly involved in GTP binding and hydrolysis. Thus, mutations in these residues abolished the ability of the Ras protein to hydrolyze GTP to GDP, resulting in constitutively activated Ras protein, which leads to overexpression of growth-stimulatory signals.

Oncogenic conversion of the nuclear protein, myc, results from aberrant expression of the protein rather than a point mutation. A variety of genetic changes can increase the level of myc expression. In Burkitt's lymphoma, for example, a chromosome translocation occurs whereby the myc proto-oncogene is placed under the control of a regulatory sequence derived from an immunoglobulin gene, uncoupling myc from its normal physiological modulator and leading to continuous myc expression. In other types of tumor cells, the myc gene is amplified to multiple copies, resulting in a proportional increase in the level of myc protein. In both of these cases, deregulation of myc gene expression results in uncontrolled cell proliferation.

3. TUMOR SUPPRESSOR GENES

The notion that neoplastic transformation may involve alterations in genes whose products negatively regulate cell proliferation was originally derived from evidence obtained from cell hybrid experiments, stud-

Table 2
Representative Tumor Suppressor Genes In Human Tumors

Chromosomal localization	Name of locus	Tumors involved	Properties of gene product
5p	APC	Familial adenomatous polyposis, colotectal carcinoma	Cytoplasmic protein
10q	—	MEN 2, astrocytoma	—
11p	WT-1	Wilm's tumor, rhabdomyosarcoma, hepatoblastoma, bladder and lung carcinoma	DNA-binding protein
11q	—	MEN 1	—
13q	Rb-1	Retinoblastoma, osteosarcoma, breast and bladder carcinoma	DNA-binding protein
17q	p53	Small cell and squamous cell lung carcinoma, breast carcinoma, colorectal carcinoma, and other	DNA-binding protein
17q	NF-1	Neurofibromatosis type 1	Induces GTP hydrolysis of Ras protein
18q	DCC	Colorectal carcinoma	Cell-surface receptor

Adapted from Weinberg, (1994).

ies of familial neoplasms, and observed loss of allelic heterozygosity in tumors. These genes are termed tumor suppressor genes. In contrast to proto-oncogenes, which induce tumors when converted to oncogenes, tumor suppressor genes are present in tumor cells as an inactive or null allele. Since tumor suppressor genes act in normal cells to suppress proliferation, tumor cells lacking these genes exhibit unconstrained growth associated with malignancy.

Evidence from somatic cell hybrid experiments first suggested that genetic alterations underlying neoplastic transformation might result from the loss of function of normal alleles. Hybrid cells generated between tumorigenic and normal cells did not always give rise to tumors when injected into suitable hosts, unless specific chromosomes were lost from the hybrids. This phenomenon of tumor suppression suggested that recessive genetic changes were responsible for the tumorigenic phenotype. Although cell hybrid studies of tumor suppression provided very useful information on chromosomal assignment, this method could not lead to gene identification, and to date, no suppressor gene thus has been isolated.

The identification of tumor suppressor genes has been greatly facilitated through studies of familial cancers. This is best illustrated in the identification and isolation of the retinoblastoma susceptibility (RB) gene. The essential features of retinoblastoma are that in the familial forms of the tumor, the affected individual inherits a mutant, "loss of function" allele from an affected parent and a second somatic muta-

tion inactivates the normal allele derived from the unaffected parent. In contrast, the sporadic forms of the tumor involved two somatic mutational events. According to this recessive mutation model homozygous deletion of the RB gene would be expected in some tumors, and RB gene expression could be altered in retinoblastoma compared to normal tissue. Homozygous deletion of chromosome 13q14 was in fact detected in retinoblastomas, and using chromosomal walking to identify sequences conserved in evolution that were expressed in retinoblasts, but were absent or altered in retinoblastomas, the candidate gene for RB was isolated.

Another powerful strategy for discovering new tumor suppressor genes in human tumors is to identify specific genetic markers that are repeatedly reduced to homozygosity in many tumors of a given type. Loss of heterozygosity for this specific marker suggests the presence of a closely linked suppressor gene whose second allele has been eliminated from tumor cells during tumor pathogenesis. For example, allele losses on the long arm of chromosome 18 are a frequent occurrence in colorectal carcinomas, but not in adenomas, suggesting the presence of a suppressor gene on this chromosome whose loss frequently accompanies the conversion of benign adenomas to carcinomas. Based on this evidence, the responsible gene, termed DCC for "deleted in colon carcinoma" was identified and isolated. Similar methodology was used to identify other tumor suppressor genes, such as p53 and WT-1 (Table 2).

Table 3
Oncogenes and Tumor Suppressor Genes in Endocrine Tumors

Gene	Defect	Tumor phenotype
H-*ras*	Point mutation	Thyroid adenomas and carcinomas, pituitary carcinoma metastases
K-*ras*	Point mutation	Thyroid tumors
N-*ras*	Point mutation	Thyroid tumors
Ret	Chromosomal rearrangement point mutations	Papillary thyroid carcinoma MEN 2
trk	Chromosomal rearrangement	Papillary thyroid carcinoma
$G_s\alpha$	Point mutation	Pituitary tumors, thyroid adenomas
11q	LOH	MEN 1, pituitary tumors
13q	LOH	Parathyroid and pituitary carcinomas
p53	Point mutation	Anaplstic thyroid carcinoma
PRAD1	Chromosomal rearrangement	Parathyroid adenoma
c-*myc*	Overexpression	Thyroid carcinoma
c-*fos*	Overexpression	Thyroid carcinoma

4. PROTO-ONCOGENES AND TUMOR SUPPRESSOR GENES IN ENDOCRINE TUMORS

Like tumors in other tissues, tumors in the endocrine system arise as monoclonal expansions of a signal mutated cell. For most tumor types, multiple genes are involved and different combinations of gene mutations may result in similar phenotypes. Some genes contribute to tumors of only one cell type, whereas other genes are involved in different types of tumors. The role of proto-oncogenes and tumor suppressor genes in tumorigenesis of the endocrine system is presently being actively studied. Table 3 summarizes the oncogenes and tumor suppressor genes that have been implicated in endocrine tumor formation, and some of these genes are discussed in detail below.

4.1. Multiple Endocrine Neoplasia Type 1 (MEN 1)

MEN 1 is an autosomal-dominant disorder characterized by tumors of parathyroid gland, pancreatic islet, and anterior pituitary. Based on the assumption that tumorigenesis involves loss of function for a tumor suppressor gene (*see* Section 3.), and utilizing restriction-fragment-length polymorphisms (RFLP), the MEN 1 locus was mapped to chromosome 11q13. The candidate for the MEN1 gene has not yet been cloned. However, loss of heterozygosity at 11q13 has been detected in the majority of parathyroid tumors obtained from MEN 1 patients, in 25–30% of sporadic parathyroid adenomas, in islet tumors from MEN 1 patients, and in some pituitary tumors either associated with MEN 1 or sporadically occurring, suggesting that a tumor suppressor gene is likely to be present in this region (Table 4).

4.2. Multiple Endocrine Neoplasia Type 2 (MEN 2)

MEN 2 consists of three clinically distinct, dominantly inherited cancer syndromes. Patients with MEN 2A develop medullary thyroid carcinoma (MTC), pheochromocytoma, and primary hyperparathyroidism. Those with MEN 2B have MTC, pheochromocytoma, and in addition, skeletal abnormalities and ganglioneuromas of the gastrointestinal tract. In familial MTC, only the thyroid is affected. All three syndromes have been assigned to chromosome 10q11 region, where a proto-oncogene RET has also been assigned, suggesting that RET might be the candidate gene for MEN 2.

The RET gene was identified and cloned through rearrangements that occur in papillary thyroid carcinomas and in vitro during transfection studies. It consists of 21 exons and encodes a receptor kinase. RET mRNA is expressed in developing central and peripheral nervous system and during renogenesis in the mouse embryo. Mice homozygous for mutant RET fail to develop kidneys and enteric neurons, and die within 16–24 h after birth.

**Table 4
Chromosome 11 Deletions in Sporadic
Endocrine Tumors**

Tumor	Deletion present (%)
Nonfunctioning pituitary adenoma	20%
GH cell adenoma	16%
PRL cell adenoma	12%
ACTH cell adenoma	28%
Parathyroid adenoma	25%

RET proto-oncogene missense mutations have been detected in 95% of patients with MEN 2A. All MEN 2A mutations involve four conserved cysteins residues in the cystein-rich region of the cadherin-like ligand-binding domain. These mutations probably interfere with ligand binding. Missense mutations of RET in the same cystein residues were also identified in all families with familial MTC. Germ-line mutations in the RET proto-oncogene were found in over 93% of MEN 2B cases. Almost all cases have the same missense change (918T), resulting in a methionine to threonine change in the substrate-recognition pocket of the tyrosine kinase domain. The same (918T) mutation was also detected in about 30% of sporadically occurring MTC and phenochromocytomas. It has been suggested that this mutation is a dominant tyrosine kinase-activating mutation, perhaps altering target specificity, which would explain the tissue hyperplasia leading to both tumors and ganglioneuromas. In papillary thyroid cancer, the genetic defect in RET gene results from rearrangements rather than a point mutation. The exons that encode tyrosine kinase domain of RET are fused to 5′-regulatory sequences of other genes, leading to constitutive activation in this malignancy.

5. PITUITARY TUMORS

Tumors of the pituitary gland are mostly benign adenomas that are either hormonally functional or nonfunctional. Functional tumors are characterized by autonomous hormone secretion, leading to clinical hormone excess syndromes, such as acromegaly or Cushing's disease, whereas nonfunctioning pituitary adenomas often secrete clinically inactive glycoprotein hormones or their free subunits. Pituitary carcinomas are extremely rare, and to date, only about 40 cases have been documented.

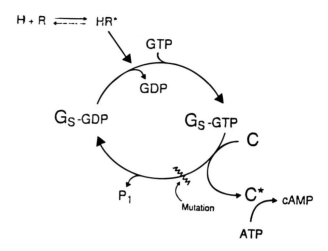

Fig. 1. Activation of G-protein upon hormone stimulation. Hormone binding to its cell-surface receptor results in GTP binding to the $G_s\alpha$ subunit, which activates adenylyl cyclase to increase intracellular cAMP levels. Hydrolysis of bound GTP to GDP by intrinsic GTPase activity of $G_s\alpha$ results in inactivation of $G_s\alpha$ and termination of signal transduction. Mutations in $G_s\alpha$ result in inhibition of GTP hydrolysis leading to constitutive activation of $G_s\alpha$. H: hormones, R: receptor, C: catalytic subunit of the G-protein.

The first point mutations detected in pituitary tumors were localized in the G-protein α subunit. Signal transduction of many peptide hormones and their cell-surface receptors are coupled with G-proteins that consist of three polypeptides: an α-chain that binds to guanine nucleotide, and a β- and a γ-chain. Activation of receptor accelerates the binding of GTP, which induces a conformational change in G-protein, releases α subunit from βγ, and allows it to interact with target proteins. Hydrolysis of bound GTP to GDP by the intrinsic GTPase activity of the α subunit terminates signal transduction (Fig. 1). Growth hormone-releasing hormone (GHRH) utilizes cAMP as a second messenger to stimulate growth hormone (GH) secretion and somatotrope proliferation. The GHRH receptor contains seven-transmembrane domains and is coupled to G-protein. Characterization of GH-secreting pituitary adenomas revealed that a subgroup of these tumors has elevated basal cAMP and GH secretion, and were no longer responsive to GHRH stimulation. The hormone-independent induction of cAMP synthesis in these tumors could occur as a result of the autonomous activation of GHRH receptor, the catalytic domain of adenylyl cyclase, or the stimulatory subunit of G-protein. Subsequently, point mutations of $G_s\alpha$ were identified in about a third of these tumors. These missense mutations occur either in Arg-201 or Gln-227, in a region of the $G_s\alpha$ that is involved in GTP hydrolysis. Thus, these mutations activate $G_s\alpha$ by inhibiting its intrinsic GTPase activity. The identification of GTPase-inhibiting mutations in pituitary tumors led to the hypothesis that in cells that proliferate in response to cAMP, $G_s\alpha$ can be converted into an activating oncogene, gsp. $G_s\alpha$ point mutations have also been found in other types of endocrine tumors (*see* Section 6).

Since the pituitary gland is under the control of multiple hormones and growth factors, signal transduction of these factors utilizes pathways other than those coupled to G-protein. The product of proto-oncogene Ras plays an important role in growth factor signal transduction. There are three functional Ras genes, H-, N-, and K-ras, that encode for a 21-kDa protein P^{21ras}. P^{21ras} is guanine nucleotide-binding protein, posesses intrinsic GTPase activity, and is associated with the plasma membrane. The similarities between P^{21ras} and G-proteins suggest that Ras protein is involved in signal transduction pathways regulating growth and differentiation. Recent evidence indicates that Ras is brought to close contact with tyrosine kinase receptors through interaction with other proteins. Signaling downstream of Ras involves cascade of protein kinases that transmit the incoming signal to the nucleus. Point mutations of the *Ras* gene can convert Ras to a constitutively active oncogene (*see* Section 2). Ras oncogenes have been implicated in the development of a variety of tumors and represent one of the most common mutations detected in human neoplasia. However, Ras gene mutations appear to be a rare event in pituitary tumors. To date, only one invasive prolactinoma was found to harbor a missense mutation of Ras. Mutations of Ras were also detected in metastatic deposits of pituitary carcinomas, but not in the primary pituitary tumors. These findings suggest that activation of Ras oncogene is not the initial event in pituitary tumorigenesis. However, point mutations of Ras may be important in the formation or growth of metastases originating from the rarely occuring pituitary carcinomas.

The first indication for a role of a tumor suppressor gene in pituitary tumorigenesis was derived from studies of the MEN 1 gene. Loss of heterozygosity of chromosome 11q13 was found not only in pituitary tumors associated with MEN 1, but also in up to 15%

of sporadically occurring pituitary adenomas of all cell types.

The RB gene, a well-characterized tumor suppressor gene, is inactivated on both alleles in a variety of human tumors. Individuals with germ-line mutations on one RB allele have a >90% chance to develop retinoblatoma during childhood. The RB gene maps to chromosome 13q14, and loss of heterozygosity at this locus was demonstrated in retinoblastoma cells. The RB gene product, pRB, is a major determinant of cell-cycle control and acts as a signal transducer interfacing the cell-cycle apparatus with the transcriptional machinery. pRB is phosphorylated in a cell-cycle-dependent manner, being maximal at the start of the S phase and low after mitosis and entry into G1, and its state of phosphorylation regulates its activity. pRB interacts with a variety of viral and cellular proteins, and through this interaction, pRB allows the cell-cycle "clock" to control genes that mediate the advance through a critical phase of the cell growth cycle. Thus, loss of pRB function deprives the cell of an important mechanisms for controlling cell proliferation through regulation of gene expression.

The role of the RB gene in pituitary tumor formation was initially suggested by studies in transgenic mice, in which one allele of the RB gene was disrupted. Embryos homozygous for the RB mutation die between 14 and 15 d of gestation, and exhibit neuronal cell death and defective erythropoiesis. Mice heterozygous for the RB gene mutation are not predisposed to retinoblastoma, but interestingly develop pituitary tumors at a high frequency. These tumors originate from the intermediate lobe of the pituitary, and are classified histopathologically as proopiomelanocortin (POMC) immunoreactive adenocarcinomas. DNA derived from these tumors shows the absence of the wild-type RB allele, and retention of the mutant allele. Pituitary tumor tissue in the mice also displays expression of a dysfunctional RB protein. In benign human pituitary tumors, however, loss of heterozygosity at the RB locus was not detected. However, in invasive pituitary adenomas and in pituitary carcinomas, allelic deletion of RB was observed. Therefore, loss of heterozygosity at the RB locus is unlikely to be the initiating event in pituitary tumorigenesis. Instead, it may play a role in progression of benign tumors to more invasive and malignant phenotypes. It is likely that another tumor suppressor gene on chromosome 13 located in close proximity to the RB locus might be involved in pituitary tumor formation. Interestingly, although p53 tumor suppressor gene mutations have been detected in a wide variety of human tumors, no such mutation has been found in comprehensive screening of pituitary tumors.

6. THYROID TUMORS

Thyroid neoplasia is comprised of benign follicular adenomas, differentiated carcinomas (follicular carcinomas and papillary carcinoma), and anaplastic or undifferentiated carcinomas.

The most common mutations found in thyroid tumors are point mutations of the Ras proto-oncogene. Mutations of all three Ras genes have been identified in follicular adenomas and thyroid carcinomas. In addition to activating point mutations of Ras, some thyroid tumors also exhibit Ras gene amplifications.

Thyrotropin (TSH) not only regulates differentiated function of thyroid cells, but also acts as a growth factor for thyrocytes. The growth-inducing function of TSH on thyrocyte growth is mediated by cAMP, which is induced after adenylyl cyclase activation by $G_s\alpha$ protein. As in growth-hormone-secreting pituitary tumors, point mutations that inhibit the intrinsic GTPase activities of $G_s\alpha$ have been detected in 25% of hyperfunctioning thyroid adenomas. Some hyperfunctioning adenomas have mutations in the third intracellular loop of the TSH receptor, resulting in a constitutively active receptor and inappropriate activation of adenylyl cyclase.

A novel oncogene, PTC-RET, is unique to papillary thyroid carcinomas. PTC-RET arises as the result of an intrachromosome inversion that juxtaposes unrelated gene sequences to the tyrosine kinase domain of the RET proto-oncogene (*see* Section 4.2). Other activating gene rearrangements found in this group of thyroid carcinomas include the nerve growth factor receptor (trk).

Anaplastic carcinoma is the most aggressive form of thyroid cancer and displays complete loss of thyroid differentiation. These tumors exhibit a high prevalence of p53 tumor suppressor gene missense mutations that are not present in differentiated thyroid carcinomas. p53 is a sequence-specific DNA-binding protein that binds to DNA as a tetramer and regulates transcription of genes that negatively control cell growth and invasion. p53 induces differentiation and acts as a checkpoint protein that arrests the cell cycle in response to DNA damage, allowing DNA repair to take place or to activate pathways for apoptosis. The p53 gene is the most frequently mutated locus in human neoplasia involved in 50% of human cancers. Typically, one allele of the p53 gene is lost, and point mutations occur in the remaining allele, resulting in production of a mutant protein. The majority of missense mutations occur within the evolutionarily conserved regions of the gene. Some mutants either lose the ability to bind to DNA or to transactivate target genes. Other mutations seem to affect p53 function by changing the global conformation of the protein. All mutant p53 proteins have lost the ability to suppress transformation, and some mutants can also act as dominant oncogenes in cooperation with Ras in transformation of primary cells. The presence of p53 point mutations in anaplastic carcinomas, but not in differentiated thyroid tumors suggests that inactivation of the p53 tumor suppressor gene may play a role in transition to the more malignant phenotype of thyroid carcinomas.

7. PARATHYROID NEOPLASIA

Parathyroid adenomas can occur either sporadically or in association with MEN 1. The majority of MEN 1-associated and about 25% of sporadic parathyroid adenomas show loss of heterozygosity at the MEN 1 locus on chromosome 11q13. A subgroup of parathyroid adenomas contains a chromosome 11 inversion in which the 5′-regulatory region of the parathyroid hormone (PTH) is fused to the coding region of the PRAD1 gene. This gene rearrangement leads to overexpression of the PRAD1 gene in tumor cells. Cloning of the PRAD1 cDNA revealed that it is structurally related to the cyclins, and it is now termed cyclin D1. Cyclins are a group of proteins that play important roles in controlling cell-cycle progression. Cell-cycle progression is regulated at two critical checkpoints, the G2/M border and the G1/S transition. Cyclin D1 is a "G1 cyclin" whose function is to push cells through the G1/S transition checkpoint. Cyclin D1 forms complexes with cyclin-dependent kinases (cdks), and also interacts directly with the product of RB gene to participate in cell-cycle regulation. Overexpression of cyclin D1 could lead to excessive cell proliferation. The implication of cyclin D1 as a parathyroid oncogene indicates that the cell-cycle machinery can be an important player in the induction of parathyroid

Table 5
Clinical Impact of Genetic Screening
in Endocrine Tumors

Early prediction of tumor behavior
Portends response to therapeutic interventions
Genetic screening for tumor prediction
Design of novel subcellular therapies

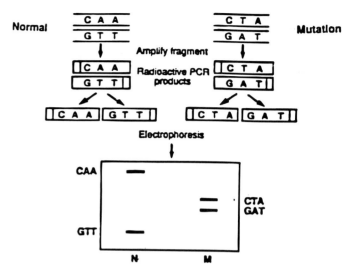

Fig. 2. Schematic presentation of PCR-SSCP detection of mutations. DNAs from normal and tumor tissues are amplified by PCR. The PCR products are separated on polyacrylamide gels. Mutations are identified by the altered conformation of the DNA patterns on the gel.

tumors, by regulating the biochemical pathways that control parathyroid cell proliferation. Most parathyroid carcinomas show loss of heterozygosity at the RB allele. As in pituitary tumors, inactivation of RB is only found in more aggressive tumors but not in benign parathyroid adenomas, suggesting that RB gene assessment could be used as a diagnostic or prognostic molecular marker for parathyroid carcinoma.

8. CLINICAL IMPLICATIONS

Genetic changes in proto-oncogenes and tumor suppressor genes appear to play important roles in the development and progression of various types of endocrine tumors. Identifying and studying the function of new tumor suppressor genes and oncogenes will not only provide important insights into normal growth regulation of endocrine cells and genetic alterations that lead to tumor formation, but may also provide diagnostic or prognostic tools for these lesions (Table 5).

For example, Ras proto-oncogene point mutations have been found in all types of thyroid tumors, but rarely in pituitary tumors. The development of polymerase chain reaction (PCR) coupled to single-stranded conformational polymorphism (SSCP) has made it possible to detect readily activating mutations of Ras from tumor tissues (Fig. 2). The presence of Ras gene point mutations in pituitary tumors indicates an aggressive phenotype, and may deterrmine more aggressive postoperative management and followup. Detection of loss of heterozygosity (LOH) on Rb alleles can be used as a prognostic indicator for pituitary and parathyroid tumors. LOH at the RB locus in these tumors indicates a malignant change. It is evident that oncogene and suppressor gene research will also provide insights into designing subcellular therapeutic modalities for managing endocrine neoplasia in the future (Table 6).

Table 6
Potential Endocrine Tumor-Targeted Gene Therapy

Replace functions of tumor suppressor gene	13q, 11q, 17p
Interrupt self-stimulatory autocrine loops	gsp, hypothalamic hormone receptor antagonists
Interrupt aberrant signal responsiveness	RET
Specific immunotherapy	Mutant receptors Growth factors

REFERENCES

Weinberg, R.A. Molecular mechanisms of carcinogenesis. *Sci. Am.* 1994; 253.

SELECTED READING

Bishop JM. Molecular themes in oncogenesis. *Cell* 1991; 64:235.
Bookstein R, Lee WH. Molecular genetics of the retinoblastoma suppressor gene. *Crit Rev. Oncogene* 1991; 2:221.
Bos JL. Ras genes in human cancer: A review. *Cancer Res* 1989; 49:4682.
Evan GI, Littlewood TD. The role of myc in cell growth. *Curr Opin Genet Dev* 1993; 3:44.
Fagin JA. Molecular pathogenesis of human thyroid neoplasms. *Thyroid Today* 1994; 97.
Harris CC. p53: at the crossroads of molecular carcinogenesis and risk assessment. *Science* 1993; 262:1980.

Knudson AD. All in the (cancer) family. *Nature Genet* 1993; 5:103.

Larsson C, Friedman E. Localization and identification of the multiple endocrine neoplasia type 1 disease gene. *Endocr Metabo Clin N Amer* 1994; 23:67.

Melmed S. Pathogenesis of pituitary tumors. In: *Molecular Genetics of Nervous System Tumors*. Wiley-Liss, New York, 1995: 255.

Motokura T, Arnold A. Cyclins and oncogenesis. *Biochem Biophy Acta* 1993; 155:63.

Santoro M, et al. Activation of RET as a dominant transforming gene by germline mutations in MEN2A and MEN2B. *Science* 1995; 267:381.

Weinberg RA. Tumor suppressor genes. *Science* 1991; 254:1138.

18 The Pineal Hormone—Melatonin

Irina V. Zhdanova, MD, PhD and
Richard J. Wurtman, MD

Contents

1. INTRODUCTION

The pineal gland or epiphysis cerebri (Fig. 1) is a neuroendocrine organ that exerts important regulatory influences in vertebrate animals by secreting its hormone, melatonin (Fig. 2), in variable amounts, depending on the animal's age, the time of day, and in some species, the time of year. The daily rhythm in plasma melatonin concentrations (Fig. 3), which is low during the day and high at night, is probably a significant factor in sleep initiation and maintenance. The decline in nocturnal melatonin levels during adolescence may be a factor in the onset of puberty; the further decline observed with advancing age (Fig. 4) may be a causal factor in age-related insomnia. In some mammalian species, seasonal changes in the number of daylight hours each day influence serum melatonin levels, and thereby seem to trigger the annual recrudescence and, later, atrophy of the gonads. Daily and annual rhythms in serum melatonin levels may also affect the timing of other biological rhythms, for example the day–night rhythm in body temperature and locomotor activity.

Lerner and his colleagues in 1958 traced the isolation of melatonin from bovine pineal glands using a bioassay technique based on the ability of melatonin to lighten isolated frog skin (by causing the melanin granules within the dermal melanophores to aggregate around the cell's nucleus). Initial studies on possible physiological roles of melatonin focused on its effects on pigmentation (a phenomenon that is not observed in mammals) and on gonadal maturation. Kitay and Altschule (1954) had demonstrated that pinealectomy accelerated gonadal maturation in rats and that administration of pineal extracts had the opposite effect. We (Wurtman et al., 1963) then showed that melatonin was the constituent of pineal extracts that were responsible for their antigonadal activity, and suggested that melatonin is a hormone. On the basis of evidence that either removing a rat's pineal or exposing the maturing animal to continuous illumination caused equivalent—but not additive—increases in gonadal weight, we further

From: *Endocrinology: Basic and Clinical Principles* (P. M. Conn and S. Melmed, eds.), Humana Press Inc., Totowa, NJ.

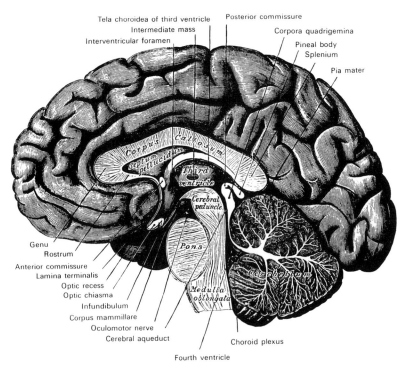

Tela choroidea of third ventricle
Intermediate mass
Interventricular foramen
Posterior commissure
Corpora quadrigemina
Pineal body
Splenium
Pia mater

Genu
Rostrum
Anterior commissure
Lamina terminalis
Optic recess
Optic chiasma
Infundibulum
Corpus mammillare
Oculomotor nerve
Cerebral aqueduct
Choroid plexus
Fourth ventricle

Fig. 1. Median sagittal section of brain (Clemente, 1985).

proposed that light exposure suppressed the formation of the pineal's antigonadal hormone. Later results confirmed that light indeed suppresses melatonin synthesis, and that the rhythm in melatonin synthesis parallels the natural diurnal rhythm in environmental illumination. Our laboratory also observed that serum melatonin levels in humans exhibit a characteristic daily pattern; levels are very low during the day (1–6 pg/mL) and can be as high as 200–300 pg/mL at night (Fig. 3).

The pineal and its hormone, melatonin, apparently play an important role in the organization of rhythmic biochemical, physiological, and behavioral processes in living systems. This chapter explores some of the fundamental mechanisms that control pineal function and mediate melatonin's effects. It also considers possible clinical implications of impaired pineal function.

2. THE PINEAL GLAND

The pineal gland is a small unpaired organ located approximately in the geometric center of the brain (Fig. 1) whose function has puzzled researchers for centuries. Postulates regarding the significance of

the pineal range from that of "a mere vestigial appendage of the brain" to Descartes' (1662) designation of the pineal as the "seat of the rational soul". Experimental investigation over the last half century has revealed that the pineal is indeed a biologically significant organ that has undergone profound changes in both form and cytological differentiation during the course of its phylogenetic expression, while retaining a functional role in the temporal organization of animal life.

Embryologically, the pineal organ arises as an evagination of the roof of the diencephalon. The diencephalon also gives rise to the lateral eyes and to the hypothalamus. This common embryological origin is reflected in a common physiological property—the capacity to respond to cyclic changes in environmental illumination. A fixed temporal pattern of photic input is a ubiquitous phenomenon, generated by the earth's daily rotation in reference to the sun. Viewed from an evolutionary perspective, the pineal is part of a sophisticated photoneuroendocrine system with photoreceptors represented both in the lateral eyes and, in some species (but not mammals), in the pineal organ itself. With development, this organ system has acquired a unique feature: an

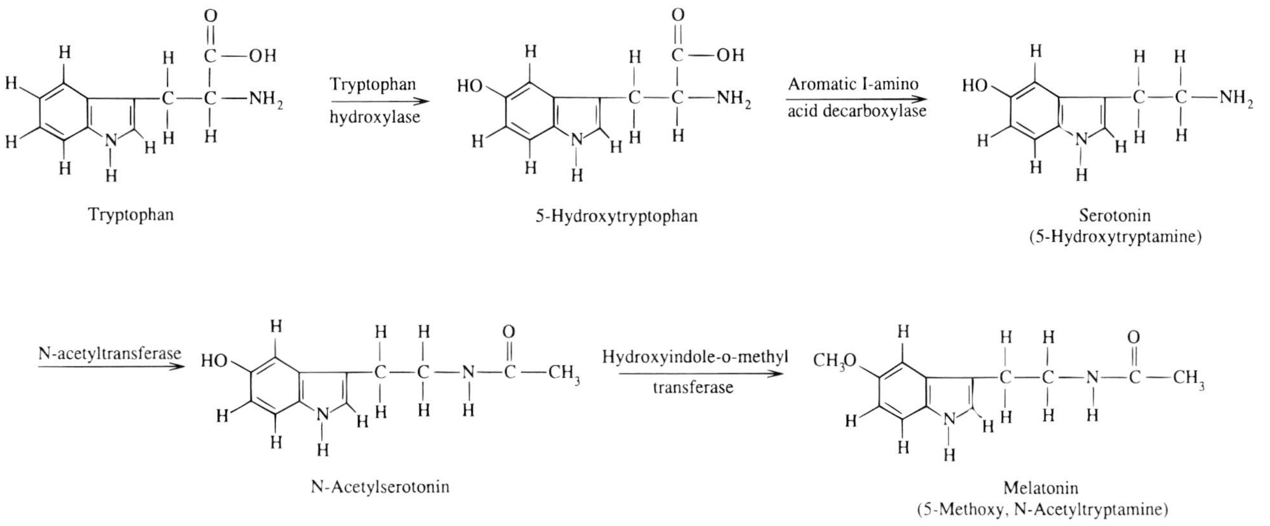

Fig. 2. Metabolism of tryptophan to melatonin in the pineal gland.

endogenous, circadian (circa—around, dian—day) rhythmic pattern in its metabolic and/or neural activity. In mammals, a neuronal component of this neuroendocrine complex, the suprachiasmatic nuclei (SCN) of hypothalamus, displays a regular pattern of spontaneous neuronal discharges, entrained to the cyclic photic input, with a higher frequency during the daylight hours. This physiologic counterpart of the environmental light–dark cycle has been shown to persist in the absence of a day–night cycle, and thereby facilitates the adaptive modulation of rhythmic behavioral and physiological processes. In phylogenetically more primitive vertebrate classes whose pineals possess true photoreceptors (e.g., birds and reptiles), the pineal organ itself manifests a sustained circadian oscillation in melatonin biosynthesis. In the mammalian pineal, the absence of true photoreceptors is accompanied by the loss of this endogenous pace-setting capacity. This class of vertebrate animals relies on the SCN for its autonomous circadian stimulation. Under natural conditions, the environmental light–dark cycle and the SCN's endogenous oscillator act in concert to produce the daily rhythm in melatonin production. A complex neural pathway has evolved that relays information regarding environmental illumination from the ganglion layer of the retina to pinealocytes via the optic nerve, the SCN, the lateral hypothalamus, and through the spinal cord by preganglionic fibers synapsing in the superior cervical ganglion. Finally, postganglionic fibers reach the pineal via the nervi

conarii. Norepinephrine, released from the postganglionic sympathetic fibers at night, activates the adenylate cyclase system, stimulating production of the second messenger cyclic adenosine monophosphate (cAMP), thereby driving melatonin synthesis in the pineal gland. Exposure to sufficiently bright light quickly suppresses melatonin synthesis; however, under conditions of constant darkness, a circadian rhythm in melatonin production persists, generated by the cyclic SCN output.

3. MELATONIN SYNTHESIS AND SECRETION

The circulating amino acid L-tryptophan (L-TRP) is the precursor of melatonin. Within cells in the pineal gland, it is converted to serotonin (5-HT) by a two-step process, catalyzed by the enzymes tryptophan hydroxylase (TH) and 5-hydroxytryptophan decarboxylase. Pineal 5–HT concentrations in mammals are high during the daily light phase and decrease during the dark phase, when melatonin is produced in greater amounts. This process, which occurs principally, but not exclusively in the pineal gland (e.g., also in retina), involves serotonin's N-acetylation, catalyzed by N-acetyltransferase (NAT), and then its methylation by hydroxyindole-O-methyltransferase (HIOMT) to produce melatonin (Fig. 2).

Since there is no evidence of melatonin storage in the pineal, the hormone is thought to be released directly into the bloodstream and/or the cerebrospinal

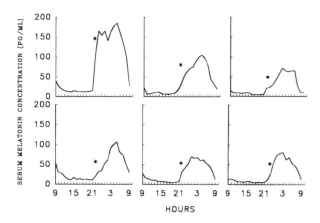

Fig. 3. Twenty-four hour serum melatonin profiles measured from 9 AM to 9 AM in a group of six young healthy males; * The time of the onset of habitual evening sleepiness.

fluid (CSF) as it is synthesized. The pattern of melatonin secretion in humans is characterized by a gradual nocturnal increase and morning decrease in serum concentrations of the hormone (Fig. 3). About 50–70% of circulating melatonin is reportedly bound to plasma albumin; the physiological significance of this binding is unknown. Inactivation of melatonin occurs in the liver, where it is converted to 6-hydroxymelatonin by the P-450-dependent microsomal mixed-function oxidase enzyme system. Most of the 6-hydroxymelatonin is excreted in the urine and feces as a sulfate conjugate (6-sulfatoxymelatonin), and a much smaller amount as a glucuronide. Some melatonin may be converted to *N*-acetyl-5-methoxykynurenamine in the central nervous system. About 2–3% of the melatonin produced is excreted unchanged in the urine.

4. MELATONIN EFFECTS ON CELLULAR METABOLISM

Melatonin is a highly lipophilic hormone. The extent to which this characteristic, by permitting its ready entrance into each body cell, plays a role in some of the effects exhibited by melatonin is still not clear. The development of radioiodinated melatonin, a ligand that preserves the biological activity of the hormone, has facilitated the demonstration of membrane receptors of high affinity and low density. In lower vertebrates, specific iodomelatonin binding occurs mainly in the visual, auditory, and limbic systems. In the brains of mammals, the most consistent melatonin binding is observed in the pars tuberalis

(PT) of the pituitary gland; such labeling is especially intensive in seasonal breeders. In humans, melatonin binding in this region is reportedly relatively low. The SCN is a second brain region that is clearly labeled with iodomelatonin in many species, including humans. Melatonin-binding sites have also been reported in various peripheral tissues of different species: retina, gonads, spleen, liver, thymus, the gastrointestinal tract, and several neoplastic tissues. Reppert and coworkers (1994) have succeed in isolating the cDNA for a high-affinity melatonin receptor initially from frog dermal melanophores and, later, from sheep and human brain tissues. The receptor cDNAs encode proteins that are members of a newly discovered group within the G-protein-coupled receptor family. The melatonin receptor accomplishes inhibition of adenylate cyclase activity and cAMP formation through a pertussis toxin-sensitive mechanism. The sheep and human melatonin receptor cDNAs encode proteins of 366 and 350 amino acids, respectively.

Inhibition of cAMP synthesis may be a primary action of the pineal hormone, though its possible effects on other second messengers cannot be excluded. Melatonin's effects seem to depend not only on the concentration of the hormone, but also on the duration of exposure of tissues and the sensitivity of melatonin receptors, which appear to vary as a function of the time of day. Although a direct effect of melatonin is inhibition of cAMP synthesis, an important study has revealed that when PT cells were exposed to a physiologic melatonin concentration for a period comparable in length to the normal duration of nighttime melatonin secretion, followed by a washout of the hormone, it provoked an increase in cAMP accumulation. Thus, the aftereffects of an increase in melatonin concentrations for a certain period of time may be of importance as well.

5. ONTOGENY OF MELATONIN SECRETION

It has been shown in work with several mammalian species, including humans, that the fetus and newborn infants do not produce their own melatonin, but rely on the hormone supplied via the placental blood, and, postnatally, via the mother's milk. The few studies on development of the circadian system in full-term human infants, including the melatonin secretory rhythm, the sleep–wake rhythm, and the

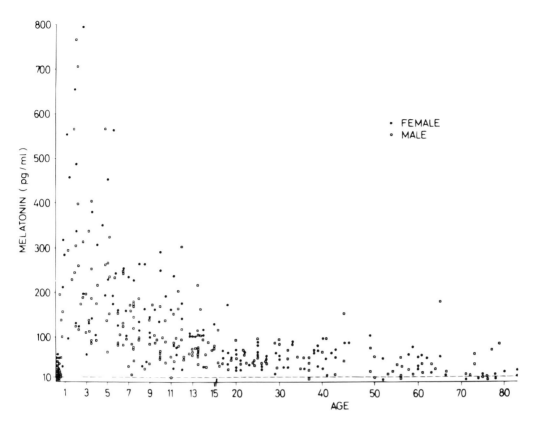

Fig. 4. Nighttime serum melatonin concentrations in 367 subjects (210 males and 157 females) aged 3 d to 90 yr (Waldhauser et al., 1988).

body temperature rhythm, reveal an absence of circadian variation in the neonatal stage until 9–12 wk. Preterm babies display a substantial delay in the appearance of rhythmic melatonin production. Total melatonin production rapidly increases during the first year of life. The highest nighttime melatonin levels have been observed in very young children, aged 1–3 yr, and start to fall around the time of onset of puberty. Thereafter, melatonin levels decrease substantially with physiologic aging (Fig. 4). Marked, unexplained interindividual variation in "normal" melatonin levels is observed in all age groups. Some elderly people do still exhibit relatively high serum melatonin levels. Several factors may explain the decline in melatonin concentration during the life-span: the increase in body mass from infancy to adulthood results in a greater distribution and, therefore, a decline in the melatonin concentration in body fluids, even if melatonin production is almost constant; the calcification of the pineal gland with advancing age may cause suppression of melatonin production; or a reduction in the sympathetic innervation of the pineal, which is essential for melatonin's nocturnal secretion, may result in diminished melatonin production. High variability

in melatonin production among individuals of the same age group may result from a combination of genetic predisposition, general health, and environmental conditions (e.g., light–dark cycle). These questions require further investigation.

6. INTERACTION WITH THE SCN

In mammals, whose pineals do not generate endogenous circadian rhythms, melatonin production is synchronized to the oscillatory activity of what is considered the major circadian pacemaker, the SCN. During the day, when the SCN metabolic and neuronal activity is high, pineal melatonin production is low. This pattern is reversed during night, when the SCN is relatively inactive and melatonin production is substantially increased. Acute exposure to light stimulation, mediated through the lateral eyes, has been shown to produce an excitatory response in the SCN neurons and an inhibition of melatonin production. On the other hand, melatonin itself exerts an inhibitory effect on both the neuronal firing rate and 2-deoxyglucose uptake by the SCN (Fig. 5). These experimental findings indicate that activation of the SCN and melatonin synthesis in the

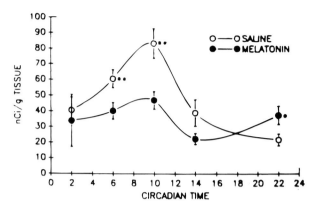

Fig. 5. Circadian rhythm in 2-DG uptake, expressed in nCi/g tissue, was observed in suprachiasmatic nuclei of saline-treated rats such that uptake was high during subjective day circadian time (CT2, CT6, and CT10) and low during subjective night (CT14 and CT22). Melatonin administration (1 mg/kg) significantly decreased 2-DG uptake at CT6 and CT10 ($P < 0.01$), significantly increased 2-DG uptake at CT22 ($P < 0.05$), and had no effect at either CT14 or CT22 (Cassone et al., 1988).

pineal have an inverse relationship. At the same time, the two components of the mammalian photoneuroendocrine system are mutually supportive. Ablation of the SCN in rams disrupts rhythmic secretion of melatonin and causes a significant decline in peak melatonin levels (Fig. 6A and B). Similarly, inhibition of melatonin production in hamsters, either by exposure to constant environmental illumination or by pinealectomy, leads to a suppression of the rhythmic increase in the firing rate of the SCN neurons (Fig. 7). Thus, the endocrine (melatonin) and the neuronal (SCN) components of the circadian neuroendocrine system exist in a complex relationship that involves positive- and negative-feedback elements, which remain to be fully elucidated. The interplay of stimulatory (photic) and inhibitory (melatonin) inputs to the SCN contributes to the dynamic homeostasis of circadian rhythmicity.

7. MELATONIN
AND PHYSIOLOGIC FUNCTIONS

Diversity in the adaptive strategies employed by different mammalian species may dictate specific responses to the circadian signal provided by melatonin release. Effects of melatonin on several physiologic functions, such as behavioral rhythmicity, sleep, reproduction, and thermoregulation, have been studied most extensively in both laboratory animals and

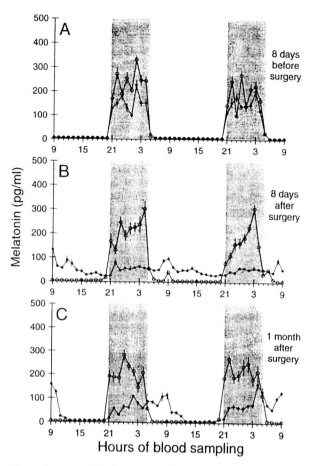

Fig. 6. Mean ± SEM plasma melatonin concentrations 8 d before surgery in sham ($-\circ-$; $n = 4$) and in SCN-lesioned rams ($-\bullet-$; $n = 6$) **(A)**, 8 d after surgery in sham rams ($-\circ-$; $n = 4$) and in SCN-lesioned rams ($-\bullet-$; $n = 6$) **(B)** and 1 mo after surgery in sham rams ($-\circ-$; $n = 4$) and in SCN-lesioned rams ($-\bullet-$; $n = 4$) **(C)**. The shaded area represents the dark phase (Tessonneaud et al., 1995).

humans, and will be discussed below. Observations on both the normal occurrence of melatonin in the blood and experimental manipulation of melatonin concentrations in vivo or in vitro have also implicated the pineal hormone in activation of the immune system, intracellular antioxidative processes, physiologic aging, tumor growth, and psychiatric disorders.

7.1. Sleep

The concurrence of melatonin release from the pineal gland and the habitual hours of sleep in diurnal mammals, including humans, has led to a long-standing suspicion that the former might be causally related to the later. Desynchronization of these two daily rhythms occurs as a result of:

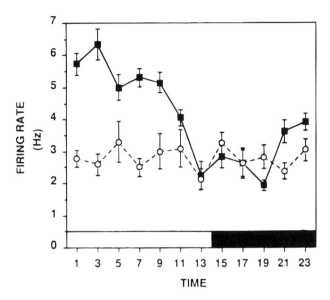

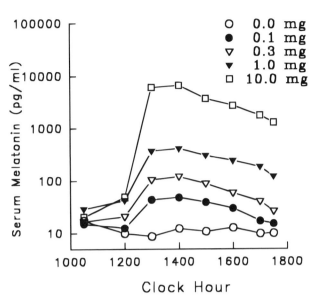

Fig. 7. Mean (±SEM) firing rates of SCN cells recorded in 2-h bins throughout the daily cycle in slices from hamsters housed in a lighting cycle (closed squares) or transferred to constant light for 48 h before slice preparation (open circles). The lighting cycle for animals is illustrated at the bottom (Guang-Di et al., 1993).

Fig. 8. Mean (±SEM) serum melatonin profiles of 20 subjects sampled at intervals after ingesting 0.1, 0.3, 1.0, and 10 mg of melatonin or placebo at 11:45 AM (Dollins et al., 1996).

1. Complete blindness, when the melatonin rhythm free-runs with a period usually longer than 24 hrs;
2. Pinealectomy or functional destruction of the pineal, resulting in a lack of melatonin production; and
3. Temporal displacement of the daylight period, as in transmeridian flight (the jet-lag syndrome) or shift work. Such desynchronization diminishes the quantity and quality of sleep, a condition that can be ameliorated by the timely administration of exogenous melatonin. These effects of exogenous melatonin in humans are generally attributed to the ability of the hormone to re-entrain an underlying pacemaker.

Initial studies regarding the acute effects of melatonin on sleep utilized pharmacological doses of the hormone (1 mg–1.2 g), which tended to induce sleepiness and sleep. The large doses of the hormone that were administered and details of the experimental designs were not consistent, and could explain differences in the results obtained. These effects of the pineal hormone were commonly considered to be "side effects" of the pharmacologic concentrations of melatonin induced. Recently, we found that low melatonin doses (0.1–0.3 mg), which induce serum

hormone concentrations comparable to typical nocturnal melatonin levels in adults (50–120 pg/mL) (Fig. 8), facilitate sleep induction in humans (Fig. 9). The response occurs within an hour following the administration of the hormone, independent of the time of the treatment; thus, phase-shift induction can be excluded as a possible explanation. Elevation of circulating melatonin within the physiologic range, although improving sleep in insomniacs, does not cause significant changes in nocturnal sleep structure in people with normal sleep and is without untoward side effects on the morning following treatment. These results support the idea that in humans daily melatonin secretion by the pineal gland may be physiologically related to the normal sleep process. This relationship would explain the high correlation between the onset of evening sleepiness or habitual bedtime in people and the onset of their melatonin release late in the evening. It may also partially explain the high incidence of insomnia in the elderly, whose circulating melatonin levels are, in general, significantly lower than those in young adults. Such an acute effect of "physiologic" doses of the hormone suggests a potential use of melatonin as a hypnotic agent with an extremely low probability of untoward side effects.

Melatonin administration has also been reported to influence sleep in various animal species. Implantation of crystalline melatonin into subcortical structures or

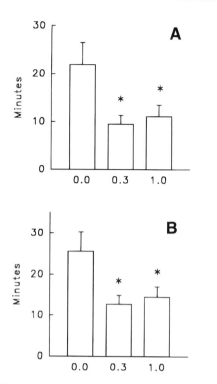

Fig. 9. Effects of melatonin (0.3 or 1.0 mg, po.) on average (±SEM) latency to: (A) sleep onset and (B) stage 2 sleep, relative to placebo (n = 11); * p < 0.05 (Zhdanova et al., 1996).

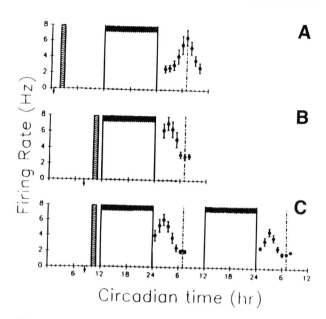

Fig. 10. Effects of melatonin on the time-of-peak in the SCN electrical activity rhythm depend on the circadian time of treatment. Results of three individual experiments are plotted as the running 2-h mean firing rates vs circadian time. (A) Melatonin applied at circadian time (CT) 2.0 had no detectable effect on the time of peak activity. (B) Melatonin treatment at CT 10.0 advanced the phase of the neuronal activity rhythm nearly 4 h, such that the peak on day 2 in vitro occurred at CT 3.0. (C) Recording on days 2 and 3 in vitro after melatonin treatment at CT 10.0 on day 1 revealed that the peak occurred at CT 3.0 on both days, indicating a permanent resetting of the clock. Dashed line indicates mean time-of-peak in untreated slices (CT 6.9 ± 0.2, $n = 8$), as well as EtOH controls (CT 7.0, $n = 2$). Horizontal bar indicates subjective night. Treatment period with 10^{-9} M melatonin is indicated with a vertical bar. Arrow indicates time of slice preparation (McArthur et al., 1991).

intraventricular injection of the hormone resulted, soon thereafter, in the initiation of sleep in cats. Inconsistent results have been reported in work with rats ranging from a minor somnogenic effect to reduced sleep following the administration of melatonin doses. Such diversity in observed effects could result from the high, pharmacologic doses of melatonin that were used, the time of melatonin administration, or the fact that the relation between the sleep–wake cycles of the animals studied (i.e., nocturnally active rats and crepuscular cats) and the serum melatonin rhythm is different from their relationship in diurnally active animals (i.e., their melatonin levels are high at times of the increased activity and low when they sleep). Thus, the melatonin signal may have a different biological meaning in nocturnal and diurnal species.

7.2. Behavioral Rhythmicity

Melatonin treatment can induce a phase shift in the circadian oscillation of SCN activity (Fig. 10), which, in turn, alters the physiological and behavioral rhythmicity of the entire organism. This relationship is likely to be responsible for the re-entrainment induced

by exogenous melatonin on circadian physiologic rhythms in vertebrates after their normal rhythmic pattern was disrupted by constant darkness, constant illumination, or changes in the timing of their light/dark exposure. This effect depends critically on the timing of melatonin administration. There is a relatively narrow window of time for accessing sensitivity to melatonin's shift-inducing effect, which varies from species to species. It has been shown that the human rest/activity cycle and endogenous melatonin rhythm are also sensitive to manipulation by exogenous melatonin, and can be shifted to some extent by judicious timing of melatonin administration (Fig. 11). This property of melatonin has found a useful application in treatment of the jet-lag syndrome

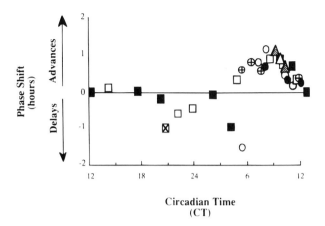

Fig. 11. Phase shifts of the dim light melatonin onset (DLMO) as a function of CT for all subjects' 30 trials, providing the first evidence of a human melatonin phase–response curve (PRC). Each of the nine subjects has a separate symbol. Exogenous melatonin was administered at various times with respect to the time of endogenous melatonin production (CT 14 = baseline DLMO for each trial). The time of administration appears as CT by convention (Lewy et al., 1992)

experienced by travelers after transmeridian flight and the sleep disruption experienced by workers on rotating shifts, whose endogenous rhythms are not synchronized with their rest–activity cycle.

Physiologic mechanisms that may involve the entraining capacity of endogenous melatonin are not entirely clear. Light, a primary environmental zeitgeber and a potent melatonin release inhibitor, does not seem to require melatonin as a messenger to entrain SCN activity. Information about environmental lighting conditions reaches the SCN directly from the retina via the retino-hypothalamic tract and only then indirectly influences activity of the pineal gland; pinealectomy does not prevent light-induced phase shift in SCN activity. Partial recovery of rhythmic melatonin production in SCN-lesioned animals (Fig. 6C) may indicate that other endogenous or exogenous factors (e.g., ambient temperature), or secondary oscillators may contribute to the secretory activity of the pineal gland.

7.3. Reproductive Physiology

The idea that pineal gland function in some way relates to gonadal expression originated in 1898 when Heubner (1898) described a 4-yr-old boy who exhibited both precocious puberty and a nonparenchymal

tumor that destroyed his pineal gland. The efficacy of the pineal hormone, melatonin, in modifying reproductive functions has been found to vary markedly, depending on the species and age of the animal tested, and the time of melatonin administration relative to the prevailing light–dark schedule. Animal studies show that in seasonal breeders, melatonin mediates the effects of changes in photoperiod and, thus, the season on reproductive physiology. Interestingly, the effects of experimentally manipulated melatonin levels in those animals that are adapted to fall–winter inhibition of reproductive activity (e.g., hamsters) appear to be opposite from those of animals that are reproductively passive in the spring–summer season (e.g., goats and sheep).

Whether pineal melatonin secretion influences, to some extent, reproductive physiology in nonseasonal mammals, including humans, is still not clear. It is hypothesized that melatonin may play a role during sexual maturation. However, observations regarding the relationship between circulating melatonin levels and the onset of puberty in humans are inconsistent, and the question requires further investigation. There are conflicting observations regarding serum melatonin levels during normal menstrual cycles in women. Some investigators report a transient decrease in nocturnal melatonin levels during the preovulatory phase; others failed to document any association between circulating melatonin and the phase of the menstrual cycle.

Certain reproductive disorders in humans are reportedly associated with an increase in melatonin production or its suppression. Some patients with tumors involving pinealocytes, which result in an increased secretion of melatonin, display delayed puberty; nonparenchymal tumors, which may destroy pinealocytes and suppress melatonin production, are associated with precocious puberty.

In women with amenorrhea whose estrogen levels are extremely low, melatonin concentrations are often substantially elevated. Exogenous estrogen has been shown to suppress nocturnal melatonin secretion in women with secondary amenorrhea significantly. Long-term experimental suppression of estrogen synthesis in healthy women leads to an elevation in their circulating melatonin. Interestingly, treatment with conjugated estrogen in women with normal menstrual cycles and initially normal estrogen levels did not suppress circulating melatonin. These findings support the idea that there is an inhibitory feedback control by estrogen on pineal function, but that it depends on the initial status of the organism.

Other dysfunctions of the reproductive system may also be associated with abnormal melatonin levels: girls with central idiopathic precocious puberty may show diminished levels of circulating melatonin; some cases of male primary hypogonadism are reportedly associated with elevated serum melatonin. However, it is still not clear whether a change in melatonin level is the cause or the consequence of these reproductive disorders.

Melatonin is a possible candidate for control of prolactin release. Several studies reveal a correlation between nocturnal melatonin secretion and an increase in circulating prolactin in humans. Modulation of melatonin levels may cause changes in serum prolactin content: suppression of melatonin production by bright light reportedly correlated with a decline in prolactin levels; supraphysiologic doses of melatonin induced significant elevation in prolactin secretion.

Further study of melatonin's modulatory role in human reproductive physiology may aid in the development of new therapeutic approaches, using either administration of the hormone or a melatonin antagonist.

7.4. Thermoregulation

The circadian system provides integrated signals for adaptive physiological and behavioral adjustments, including one of the most important adaptive mechanisms—the coordination of energy consumption and expenditure. Core body temperature, which reflects energy metabolism, has a clearly defined circadian oscillation in endothermic animals, exhibiting high levels during the day and lower levels at night. "Constant routine" studies in humans reveal that the daily decline in body temperature occurs 1–2 h prior to onset of the increased melatonin release from the pineal gland. Peak melatonin concentrations precede the temperature minimum by about 2 h (Fig. 12). Thus, though these two circadian rhythms have an inverse relationship, their extremes do not coincide and the decline in daytime temperature normally precedes the increase in melatonin production.

Animal studies reveal a hyperthermic effect of pinealectomy in some species (sparrows, chickens, rabbits, sheep), and an absence of effect or hypothermia in others (rats and hamsters). The administration of pharmacologic doses of mela-

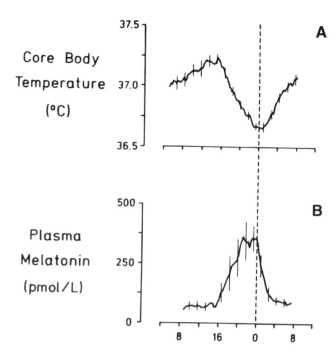

Fig. 12. Average ± SE waveforms of core body temperature and plasma melatonin during initial constant routines from eight subjects (**A** and **B**, respectively) (Shanahan and Czeisler, 1993).

tonin tends to lower body temperature. Human studies consistently show that pharmacologic doses of the hormone suppress daytime and nighttime core body temperature. Exposure to bright light or administration of a β-adrenergic antagonist at night, which blocks sympathetic input to the pineal, suppresses melatonin production and increases core body temperature. Melatonin is reported to be effective in re-establishing such experimentally modified temperature levels. In contrast, the administration of a physiologic melatonin dose (0.3 mg, po) to young healthy adults whose core body temperature was not experimentally altered left temperature values unchanged (Fig. 13).

8. CLINICAL IMPLICATIONS

The pineal gland, through the rhythmic secretion of its hormone melatonin, is part of a complex neuroendocrine mechanism that controls the temporal organization of physiological, biochemical, and behavioral processes within the organism, and synchronizes the pattern of their activity to that of environmental cycles. Melatonin may, for example, play

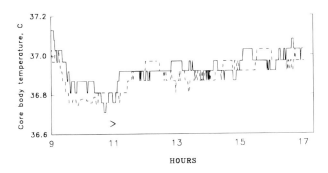

Fig. 13. Daytime core body (rectal) temperature in young healthy male after the administration of placebo (solid line) or 0.3 mg of melatonin (dashed line) at 11 AM (>) on two consecutive days.

a significant role in the establishment and synchronization of physiologic rhythms in infants. Underdevelopment of normal circadian rhythmicity, together with low circulating melatonin levels, might be a possible cause for Sudden Infant Death Syndrome. The characteristic time-course of nocturnal melatonin secretion, together with the somnogenic effect of exogenous melatonin in physiologic doses, implies its involvement in the normal daily sleep process and suggests its potential use as a treatment for insomnia, particularly in the elderly whose nocturnal serum melatonin levels tend to be diminished. The phase-shift-inducing effects of melatonin treatment on the activity pattern of the suprachiasmatic nucleus can bring about entrainment of other rhythmic functions to an altered time schedule. Thus, prudent administration of the pineal hormone has been shown to help ameliorate jet-lag symptoms and to assist shift workers in coping with their changing rest–activity schedule. Manipulation of circulating melatonin levels may also prove useful in the clinical management of pathological conditions of the reproductive system, like amenorrhea in women, or in the development of contraceptive agents. The results of clinical and experimental investigations indicate that, with further study, melatonin may become a useful therapeutic tool.

Available data suggest that, as with other hormones, an excess or a deficit in melatonin may be incompatible with normal, "healthy" functioning. Abnormal melatonin levels may negatively influence the delicate mechanism of the biological clock, resulting in dissociation of adaptive, mutu-

ally dependent circadian body rhythms, or they may acutely alter physiologic reactions in various tissues. Substantial increases in circulating melatonin may be related to the hypoactivity of the reproductive system both in men and women; a deficit during a critical period in childhood may be associated with precocious puberty. Some cases of insomnia in children, young adults, and especially in the elderly may be related to low circulating melatonin levels. Supraphysiologic levels of the hormone have been shown to interfere with temperature regulation, one of the most vital functions of endothermic organisms. Thus, in any attempt to exploit melatonin's modulatory effects, it is critically important to consider appropriate doses and treatment schedules that will preserve or promote adaptive physiologic harmony among rhythmic processes, which appears to be a key function of melatonin's daily secretion.

REFERENCES

Cassone VM, et al. Effects of melatonin on 2-deoxy—[1-14C] glucose uptake within rat suprachiasmatic nucleus. *Am J Physiol* 1988; 255:R332.

Clemente CD, ed. *Anatomy of the Human Body by Henry Gray.* 1985:989.

Descartes R. *De Homine; Figuris et Latinitate Donatus a Florentio Schuyl,* 1662.

Dollins AB, et al. Effect of inducing nocturnal serum melatonin concentrations in daytime on sleep, mood, body temperature, and performance. *Proc Natl Acad Sci USA* 1994; 91:1829.

Guang-Di Y, et al. Regulation of melatonin-sensitivity and firing-rate rhythms of hamster suprachiasmatic nucleus neurons: constant light effects. *Brain Res* 1993; 602:191.

Heubner O. Tumor der glandula pinealis. *Dtsch Med Wochenschr* 1898; 24:214.

Kitay JI, Altschule MD. The pineal gland—a review of the physiological literature. Cambridge, MA: Harvard University Press, 1954.

Lerner AB, Case JD, Takahashi Y, Lee TH, Mori W. Isolation of melatonin, the pineal gland factor that lightens melanocytes. *J Am Chem Soc* 1958; 80:2587.

Lewy, AJ. et al. Melatonin shifts human circadian rhythms according to a phase–response curve. *Chronobiol Int* 1992; 5: 380.

Lynch HJ, Wurtman RJ, Moskowitz MA, Archer MC, Ho MH. Daily rhythm in human urinary melatonin. *Science* 1975; 187:169.

McArthur AJ, et al. Melatonin directly resets the rat suprachiasmatic circadian clock in vitro. *Brain Res* 1991; 565:158.

Shanahan TL, Czeisler CA. Light exposure induces equivalent phase shifts of the endogenous circadian rhythms of circulating plasma melatonin and core body temperature in men. *J Clin Endocrinol Metabol* 1993; 73 no 2:227.

Tessonneaud, A., et al. Bilateral lesions of the suprachiasmatic nuclei alter the nocturnal melatonin secretion in sheep. *J Neuroendocrinol* 1995; 7:145.

Waldhauser, F., et al. Alterations in nocturnal serum melatonin levels in humans with growth and aging. *Clin Endocrinol Metab* 1988; 66, no 3:618.

Wurtman RJ, Axelrod J, Chu E. Melatonin, a pineal substance: effect on the rat ovary. *Science* 1963; 141:277.

Zhdanova IV, Wurtman RJ, Lynch HJ, Ives JR, Dollins AB, Morabito C, et al. Sleep-inducing effects of low doses of melatonin ingested in the evening. *Clin Pharmacol Ther* 1995; 57:552.

SELECTED READINGS

Blask DE. Melatonin in oncology. In Yu H-S, Reiter RJ, eds. *Melatonin: biosynthesis, Physiological Effects and Clinical Applications*. CRC 1993:447.

Goldman BD, Nelson RJ. Melatonin and seasonality in mammals. In Yu H-S, Reiter RJ, eds. Melatonin: *Biosynthesis, Physiological Effects, and Clinical Applications*. CRC: Boca Raton, FL, 1993:225.

Hastings MH, Vance G, Maywood E. Some reflections on the phylogeny and function of the pineal. *Experientia* 1989; 45:903.

Lewy AJ, Sack RL. Use of melatonin to assess and treat circadian phase disorders. In Y. Touitou Y, Arendt J. Pevet P, eds. Melatonin and the Pineal Gland—From Basic Science to Clinical Application. 1993:205.

Reiter RJ. The melatonin rhythm: both a clock and a calendar. *Experientia* 1993; 49:654.

Reppert SM, Weaver DR, Ebisawa T. Cloning and characterization of a mammalian melatonin receptor that mediates reproductive and circadian response. *Neuron* 1994; 13:1177.

Sugden D. Melatonin biosynthesis in the mammalian pineal gland. *Experientia* 1989; 45:922.

19 Thyroid Hormones (T_4, T_3)

Gregory Brent, MD

1. INTRODUCTION

Thyroid hormone is produced by all vertebrate. In mammals, the thyroid gland is derived embryologically from endoderm at the base of the tongue and develops into a bilobed structure lying anterior to the trachea. The structure and arrangement of thyroid tissue, however, vary significantly among species. The thyroid gland receives a rich blood supply, as well as sympathetic innervation, and is specialized to synthesize and secrete thyroxine (T_4) and triiodothyronine (T_3) into the circulation (Fig. 1). This process is regulated by thyroid-stimulating hormone (TSH) secreted from the pituitary, which is in turn stimulated by thyrotropin-releasing hormone (TRH) from the hypothalamus. Both TSH and TRH are regulated in a negative-feedback loop by circulating T_4 and T_3. Iodine and the trace element selenium are essential for normal thyroid hormone metabolism. Regulatory mechanisms within the thyroid gland allow for continuous production of thyroid hormone despite variation in the supply of dietary iodine. Thyroid hormone regulates a wide range of processes, including amphibian metamorphosis, development, reproduction, growth, and metabolism. The specific processes that are regulated differ among species, tissues, and developmental phase.

2. THYROID HORMONE SYNTHESIS

The synthesis of thyroid hormones requires; iodide, thyroid peroxidase, thyroglobulin, and hydrogen peroxide (H_2O_2). Iodine is transported into the thyroid in the inorganic form, is oxidized by the thyroid peroxidase-H_2O_2 system, and is then utilized to iodinate tyrosyl residues in thyroglobulin. Coupling of iodinated tyrosyl intermediates in the thyroid peroxidase-H_2O_2 system produces T_4 and T_3, which are hydrolyzed and then secreted into the circulation. These processes are closely linked, and defects in any of the components can lead to impairment of thyroid hormone production or secretion.

From: *Endocrinology: Basic and Clinical Principles* (P. M. Conn and S. Melmed, eds.), 1Humana Press Inc., Totowa, NJ.

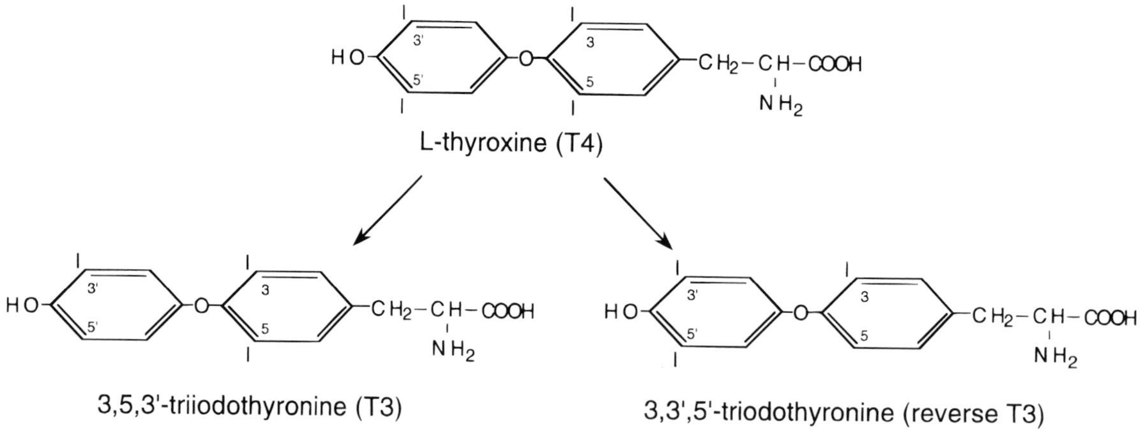

Fig. 1. Structure of L-thyroxine (T_4) and its major metabolites, triiodothyronine (T_3) and reverse triiodothyronine (rT_3).

2.1. Structure of the Thyroid Follicle

The functional unit for thyroid hormone synthesis and storage, common to all species, is the thyroid follicle (Fig. 2). The follicle consists of cells arranged in a spherical structure. The thyroid cell synthesizes thyroglobulin, which is secreted through the apical membrane into the follicle lumen. The secreted substance containing thyroglobulin, "colloid," serves as a storage form of iodine, and is resorbed to provide substrate for T_4 and T_3 synthesis. The amount of stored colloid varies as a result of a number of conditions, including the level of TSH stimulation and iodine availability. With TSH stimulation, colloid is resorbed to synthesize thyroid hormone, and with chronic stimulation, the size of the follicular lumen decreases. TSH also stimulates expression of elements of the cytoskeleton, which mediate changes in follicular cell shape that favor thyroid hormone production. Defects in thyroid hormone synthesis or release can result in increased colloid stores.

2.2. Thyroglobulin

Thyroglobulin is the major iodoprotein of the thyroid gland. It is a large dimeric glycoprotein (660 kDa) that serves as a substrate for efficient coupling of monoiodotyrosine and diiodotyrosine (MIT and DIT) by the thyroid peroxidase-H_2O_2 system, to produce T_4 and T_3, as well as providing a storage form of easily accessible thyroid hormone (Fig. 3). Because of this storage capacity, the thyroid gland can continue to secrete thyroid hormone despite transient deficiencies in environmental iodine. Thyroglobulin synthesized on the endoplasmic reticulum is trans-

ported to the Golgi, where carbohydrate moieties are added. The thyroglobulin is then localized at the apical membrane where internal tyrosyl residues are iodinated by thyroid peroxidase and H_2O_2.

The intracellular generation of H_2O_2 is essential for thyroglobulin iodination and coupling, and is generated by the thyroid follicular cell. TSH stimulates uptake of glucose, which is metabolized by the pentose monophosphate shunt, generating NADPH from NADP. The reduced adenosine nucleotide, NADPH, and NADPH oxidase are considered the major mechanisms for the reduction of molecular oxygen to H_2O_2.

Coupling between two DIT moieties forms T_4, and coupling of MIT and DIT produces T_3 (Fig. 3). The coupling reaction is catalyzed by thyroid peroxidase and involves the cleavage of a tyrosyl phenolic ring, which is joined to an iodinated tyrosine by an ether linkage. The structural integrity of the thyroglobulin protein matrix is essential for efficient coupling. The usual thyroidal secretion contains about 80% T_4 and 20% T_3; however, the ratio of secreted T_4:T_3 can be altered. Hyperstimulation of the TSH receptor by IgG in Graves' disease is associated with an increase in the relative fraction of T_3 secretion. This is owing to preferential MIT/DIT coupling as well as increased activity of the intrathyroidal Type I 5'-deiodinase that converts T_4 to T_3 (*see below*). Repletion of iodine after a period of iodine deficiency also results in an increase in the fraction of T_3 in the thyroidal secretion.

The process of thyroid hormone release and secretion begins with TSH-stimulated resorption of colloid (Fig. 3). Pseudopods and microvilli are formed at the apical membrane, and pinocytosis of colloid produces

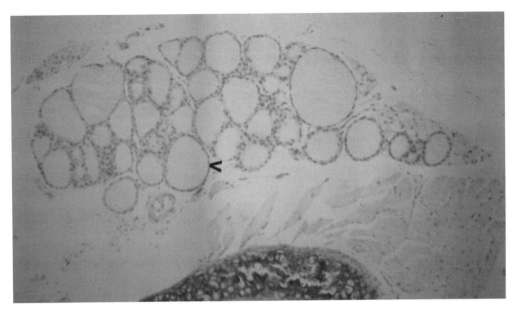

Fig. 2. A photomicrograph of thyroid follicles of varying sizes are shown. Each follicle consists of rings of cells filled with colloid (*see* arrow).

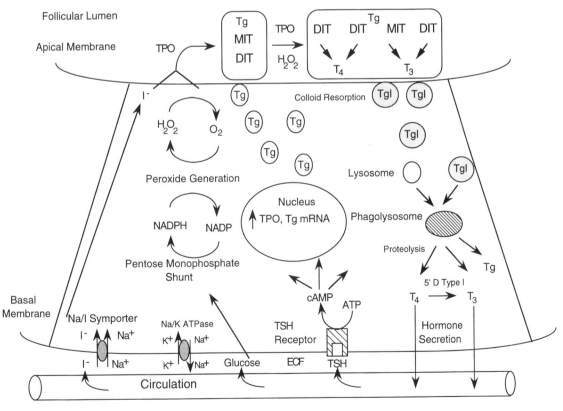

Fig. 3. Diagram of the major steps involved in thyroid hormone synthesis and secretion. Tg–thyroglobulin, DIT-diiodotyrosine, MIT-monoiodotyrosine, ECF-extracellular fluid, 5′D Type I—5′-iodothyronine deiodinase Type I, TPO-thyroid peroxidase, TSH-thyroid-stimulating hormone.

multiple colloid droplet vesicles. Lysosomes move from the basal to apical region of the cell and fuse with colloid droplets to form phagolysosomes. Proteolysis of thyroglobulin releases iodothyronines, free iodotyrosines, and free amino acids. T_4 and T_3 then diffuse across the cell and into the circulation.

2.3. Iodine Transport

The thyroid contains 70–80% of the total iodine in the body (15–20 mg). The thyroid gland must trap about 60 μg of iodine/day from the circulation to maintain adequate thyroid hormone production. The urinary excretion of iodine matches intake, and low levels indicate inadequate iodine intake. The Na^+/I^- symporter is a membrane-bound protein located in the basolateral portion of the thyroid follicular cell that passively transports 2 Na^+ and one I^- down the Na^+ ion gradient, resulting in an iodine concentration gradient from the thyroid cell to extracellular fluid of 100:1 (Fig. 3). The iodide gradient can be increased as high as 400:1 in conditions of iodine deficiency. Iodine transport is driven by the Na gradient generated from Na^+/K^+ ATPase. Iodine uptake is an active transport process that occurs against an iodide electrochemical gradient, is sensitive to competitive inhibition, and is induced by TSH via cAMP. The Na^+/I^- symporter cDNA has recently been isolated using expression cloning in *Xenopus* oocytes and is being characterized. Iodine transport is seen in other tissues including the salivary gland, gastric mucosa, lactating mammary gland, ciliary body of the eye, and the choroid plexus. Iodine is not organified in these tissues, and they are unresponsive to TSH.

Endemic goiter is the presence of thyroid enlargement in >10% of a population, a higher fraction than that owing to intrinsic thyroid disease alone, and indicates that the etiology is likely to be owing to dietary and/or environmental factors. Most endemic goiters are the result of reduced thyroidal iodine resulting from deficient dietary iodine. Mountainous areas, including the Andes and Himalayas, as well as central Africa, and portions of Europe remain relatively iodine-deficient. Reduced thyroidal iodine may also be the result of factors that inhibit the Na^+/I^- symporter. Inhibitors can be natural dietary "goitrogens," such as the cyanogenic glucosides found in cassava, a staple in parts of Africa and Asia. Cyanogenic glucosides are hydrolyzed in the gut by glucosidases to free cyanide that is then converted to

thiocyanate. Thiocyanate inhibits thyroid iodide transport and, at high concentrations, interferes with organification. Other inhibitors include perchlorate, chlorate, periodate, and even high concentrations of iodine, which cause transient inhibition of thyroid hormone synthesis (Wolff-Chaikoff effect). A wide range of heritable defects also result in impaired iodide transport or organification. Perchlorate causes release of nonorganified iodine and is used diagnostically, after radioiodine tracer uptake, to distinguish defects of iodine uptake from organification (radioiodine transported, but not organified will be released after perchlorate administration).

The Na^+/I^- symporter is utilized clinically for both diagnostic and therapeutic applications. Radioisotopes of iodine can be given orally and are taken up into thyroid tissue with high efficiency. Nonincorporated iodine is rapidly excreted by the kidneys. Short-half-life, low-energy isotopes, such as I^{123}, are used to make images of functional thyroid tissue. Longer-half-life, high-energy isotopes, such as I^{131}, are used therapeutically to destroy thyroid tissue in both hyperthyroidism and thyroid cancer. Less-differentiated thyroid cancers, however, either do not have or lose the ability to transport iodine. Stimulation of expression of the Na^+/I^- symporter or augmentation of its function, in these situations, may be useful therapeutically.

2.4. Thyroid Peroxidase

Thyroid peroxidase is a membrane-bound glycoprotein with a central role in thyroid hormone synthesis catalyzing iodine oxidation, iodination of tyrosine residues, and iodothyronine coupling. The human cDNA codes for a 933 amino acid protein with transmembrane domains at the carboxy-terminus. The extracellular region contains five potential glycosylation sites. The human thyroid peroxidase gene is found on chromosome 2 and spans approx 150 kb with 17 exons. The 5′-flanking sequence contains binding sites for a number of thyroid-specific transcription factors, including thyroid transcription factors 1 and 2. TSH stimulates thyroid peroxidase gene expression by an increase in intracellular cAMP, although the level of regulation (transcriptional vs posttranscriptional) varies by species.

IgG autoantibodies to thyroid peroxidase are pathogenic in a number of thyroid diseases. The predisposition to forming thyroid peroxidase autoantibodies is inherited as an autosomal-dominant trait in women, but has incomplete penetrance in men. This pattern of inheritance is consistent with the female preponderance of autoimmune thyroid disease. In addition to the diagnosis of autoimmune thyroid disease, the magnitude of elevation of these antibodies correlates with disease activity. Thyroid peroxidase antibodies are known to damage cells directly by activating the complement cascade. A number of epitopes for thyroid peroxidase autoantibodies have been defined. Clinically, thyroid destruction can be transient with temporary phases of increased and then decreased thyroid hormone levels (lymphocytic thyroiditis) or permanent hypothyroidism (Hashimoto's disease). Lymphocytic thyroiditis is often seen in the post partum period.

2.5. Influence of Thyrotropin on Thyroid Hormone Synthesis

The major stimulus to thyroid hormone production and thyroid growth is stimulation of the TSH receptor. Other factors that modify this response include neurotransmitters, cytokines, and growth factors. In addition to physiologic regulation via TSH, there are a number of clinical disorders of excess and reduced thyroid hormone production mediated by the TSH receptor (*see* Section 7.1.).

The human TSH receptor gene is on the long arm of chromosome 14 and consists of 10 exons spread over 60 kb. Analysis of the regulatory region of the gene has identified binding sites for thyroid transcription factors 1 and 2 as well as cAMP response elements. TSH is a G-protein-coupled receptor with a classic seven-transmembrane domain structure. The primary structure contains leucine-rich motifs and six potential *N*-glycosylation sites. Such motifs are similar to those that form amphipathic α-helices and may be involved in protein–protein interactions. The receptors for the pituitary glycoprotein hormones, TSH, follicle-stimulating hormone (FSH), and leutinizing hormone (LH)/chorionic gonadotropin (CG), are very similar in the transmembrane domain containing carboxy-terminal portion (70%), but have less similarity in the extracellular domain (about 40%). The similarity is clinically relevant in glycoprotein hormone "spillover" syndromes, where marked elevations in these hormones stimulate related receptors. Excess CG from trophoblastic disease can stimulate thyroid hormone production via the TSH receptor, and excess TSH in

prepubertal children with primary hypothyroidism can stimulate precocious puberty via stimulation of the FSH and/or LH/CG receptors. Gain of function mutations have been identified in the TSH receptor, resulting in constitutive activation (TSH independent) of thyroid hormone production. These mutations are manifest in the heterozygous state, produce thyroid growth as well as an increase in thyroid function, and have been found in the majority of hyperfunctioning thyroid nodules. Similar constitutive mutations in the germ line produce diffuse thyroid hyperfunction and growth. Inactivating TSH receptor gene mutations have also been reported. Characterization of these mutations has helped to map functional domains of the TSH receptor.

TSH stimulation of thyroid follicular cells promotes protein iodination, thyroid hormone synthesis and secretion. These effects can be reproduced by agents that enhance cAMP accumulation (theophylline, cholera toxin, forskolin, cAMP analogs). At high concentrations of TSH, there is activation of the CA^{2+} phosphotidylinositol 1,4,5-phosphate (PIP_2) cascade. The relative influence of the cAMP and PIP_2 pathways appears to differ by species, e.g., dog has only the cAMP pathway and humans have both. TSH acting via cAMP generation stimulates the expression of a number of genes involved in thyroid hormone synthesis and secretion, including thyroglobulin and thyroid peroxidase. In many species (e.g., human, rat, and dog), TSH is mitogenic and promotes thyroid growth.

2.6. Interference of Thyroid Hormone Synthesis by Antithyroid Drugs

The thionamides were first observed in the 1940s to produce goiters in laboratory animals. Propylthiouracil and methimazole are the most commonly used of these compounds, and both have intrathyroidal and extrathyroidal actions. They reduce thyroid hormone production by interfering with the actions of thyroid peroxidase, which include the oxidation and organification of iodine, and the coupling of MIT and DIT to form T_4 and T_3. The thionamides compete with thyroglobulin tyrosyl residues for oxidized iodine. These medications are primarily used in patients with hyperthyroidism resulting from Graves' disease, but are effective in any form of hyperthyroidism owing to overproduction of thyroid hormone. Propylthiouracil has an additional effect of reducing T_4 to T_3 conversion by inhibiting the Type I

5'-deiodinase. Both agents are thought to have additional immunosuppresive actions that may help in the treatment of autoimmune hyperthyroidism.

3. IODOTHYRONINE DEIODINATION

The thyroid gland secretes primarily T_4, which must be converted to the active form, T_3, by 5'-iodothyronine deiodinase (Fig. 1). The various pathways of thyroid hormone metabolism allow for regulation of hormone activation at the target tissue level as well as adaptation for times of reduced thyroid hormone production. There are a large number of iodothyronine metabolites that are degradation products of T_4, in addition to T_3, including reverse T_3 (3,3',5'-triiodothyronine), T_2s, 3'-T_1, and T_0. The levels of these products vary in a number of thyroid states and, in some situations, have been used diagnostically. Reverse T_3, for example, is metabolically inactive, but is elevated in illness and fasting. The liver solubilizes, T_4 metabolites by sulfation or glucuronide formation for excretion by the kidney or in the bile. The process allows for the conservation of body iodine stores. Deiodinase enzymes have distinctive characteristics based on tissue distribution, substrate preference, kinetics, and sensitivity to inhibitors, such as propylthiouracil and iopanoic acid. Deiodinases can be separated into phenolic (outer ring) 5'-deiodinases or tyrosyl (inner ring) 5-deiodinases (Table 1, Fig. 1).

3.1. Type I 5'-Deiodinase

The primary source of T_3 in the peripheral tissues is the 5'-monodeiodination of T_4 by the Type I deiodinase (Fig. 1). This enzyme is found predominantly in thyroid, liver, and kidney. T_3, TSH, and cAMP all increase expression of Type I deiodinase in FRTL5 thyroid cell cultures. Consistent with this observation are the in vivo findings of increased Type I deiodinase activity in hyperthyroidism and reduced activity in hypothyroidism. The biochemical properties of Type I deiodinase include a preference for reverse T_3 as a substrate over T_4. Type I requires reduced thiol as a cofactor and is sensitive to inhibition by propylthiouracil and gold. Other inhibitors of Type I 5'-deiodinase include illness, starvation, glucocorticoids, and propranalol.

3.2. Type II 5'-Deiodinase

Type II is a related 5'-deiodinase with distinct tissue distribution, biochemical properties, and physiologic function. Type II 5'-deiodinase is found primarily in the pituitary, brain, and brown fat. This enzyme functions to regulate intracellular T_3 levels in tissue where an adequate concentration is critical. The biochemical properties include a preference for T_4 over rT_3 as a substrate and insensitivity to inhibition by PTU. The activity of the Type II deiodinase increases in hypothyroidism, apparently to sustain intracellular T_3 levels despite falling levels of T_4, especially in the brain. Both Type I and Type II are inhibited by the iodine contrast agent, iopanoic acid.

3.3. 5-Deiodinase (Type III)

The Type III deiodinase is found in the developing brain, placenta, and skin and inactivates T_3 by removal of a tyrosyl ring iodide. The activity of the enzyme, like the Type I deiodinase, is regulated by thyroid hormone with less enzyme activity when thyroid hormone levels are low. This deiodinase may play a role in regulating T_4/T_3 availability, especially during development.

3.4. Selenium and Deiodination

The role of selenium in thyroid hormone metabolism was suggested by studies of rats fed a selenium-deficient diet. Compared with control animals, those with selenium deficiency had elevated serum T_4 and reduced serum T_3 concentrations associated with reduced hepatic Type I deiodinase activity. Analysis of the Type I deiodinase cDNA identified a TGA codon, usually indicating a stop codon, which codes for the amino acid selenocysteine (an analog of cysteine with selenium in place of sulfur). Substitution of cysteine for selenocysteine completely altered the activity and properties of the enzyme. A number of other glutathione requiring enzymes contain a selenocyteine and share properties with the deiodinase. A common stem loop structure that is present in the 3'-untranslated region of the Type I deiodinase mRNA directs insertion of a selenocysteine rather than terminating translation at the TGA codon.

Epidemiological studies have also demonstrated the importance of selenium for thyroid hormone metabolism. Groups in Africa and China with selenium-deficient diets have been studied, and have a high incidence of goiter and reduced serum T_3 concentrations. In some of these areas, selenium deficiency coexists with iodine deficiency. In these situations, it is harmful to replace selenium without

Table 1
Properties of Iodothyronine Deiodinases

	Type I 5′-deiodinase	Type II 5′-deiodinase	5-deiodinase (Type III)
Tissue distribution	Thyroid, liver, kidney	Brain, pituitary, brown fat	Placenta, developing brain, skin
Preferred substrate	$rT_3 \gg T_4 > T_3$	$T_4 > rT_3$	T_3 (sulfate) $> T_4$
Target	Outer ring	Outer ring	Inner ring
Response to T_4	Increase	Decrease	Increase
Inhibition by PTU	Yes	No	No
Inhibition by ipodate	Yes	Yes	Yes
Physiologic role	Extracellular T_3 production	Intracellular T_3 production	Inactivation of T_4 and T_3

T_4—thyroxine, T_3—triiodothyronine, rT_3—reverse T_3, PTU—propylthiouracil.

iodine, since this activates the Type I deiodinase and accelerates degradation of T_4, the primary source of T_3 to the brain. The slowed metabolism of T_4 from selenium deficiency may be partially protective for the reduced T_4 production in iodine deficiency.

4. THYROID HORMONE-BINDING PROTEINS AND MEASUREMENT OF THYROID HORMONE LEVELS

4.1. Serum Proteins That Bind Thyroid Hormones

The thyroid hormones are hydrophobic and circulate predominantly bound to serum proteins. The free fraction, which represents the metabolically active form of hormone, comprises only .02% of the total T_4 concentration and .30% of the total T_3 concentration. The predominant serum protein that binds thyroid hormone is thyroxine-binding globulin (TBG), which carries approx 70% of serum T_4 and T_3. TBG is synthesized in the liver and is a 54-kDa glycoprotein with approx 20% of its weight from carbohydrates. The extent of sialylation directly influences the clearance of TBG from the serum. Desialylated TBG has a circulating half-life of only 15 min, whereas fully sialylated TBG has a circulating half-life as long as 3 d. The variation in the carbohydrate component is likely to be responsible for microheterogeneity on isoelectric focusing. However, it causes little effect on ligand affinity or immunogenic properties. The remainder of thyroid hormone is bound to transthyretin (previously called thyroid-binding prealbumin) and albumin. Transthyretin is a 55-kDa protein consisting of 4 identical subunits of

127 amino acids each, and is synthesized in the liver and choroid plexus. In addition to binding thyroid hormone, transthyretin transports retinol by forming a complex with retinol-binding protein.

Owing to the large fraction of circulating thyroid hormone bound to protein, alterations in binding significantly change total hormone measurements. Mutations of the TBG gene, located on the X chromosome, produce abnormalities that range from partial or complete deficiency to excess. Abnormalities of T_4 binding have also been reported as a result of transthyretin and albumin mutations. The most common thyroid hormone-binding disorder, dysalbuminemic hyperthyroxenemia, is the result of a mutation in the albumin gene, which produces a mutant albumin with increased affinity for T_4, but not T_3. Affected individuals have elevated total T_4, normal total T_3, and a normal TSH.

In addition to inherited defects in thyroid hormone-binding proteins, there are a number of conditions and medicines that can alter serum-binding protein concentrations and thyroid hormone-binding affinity. The most common cause of TBG excess is the result of estrogen, either exogenous (oral contraceptives or postmenopausal replacement) or pregnancy. Rather than increased TBG synthesis, this is the result of estrogen-stimulated increase in sialylation, prolonging the circulating half-life. TBG is also increased in acute hepatitis and by medications, including methadone, 5-fluorouracil, perphenazine, and clofibrate. Reduced TBG has been reported in cirrhosis of the liver, from excess urinary loss in nephrotic syndrome, and from medications, including, androgens, glucocorticoids, and L-asparaginase.

In the majority of cases, individuals with abnormalities of binding proteins have normal serum concentrations of thyrotropin and free T_4 and free T_3. The identification of these abnormalities is important, so that affected individuals are not inappropriately treated for thyroid hormone excess or deficiency.

4.2. Measurement of T_4, T_3 and TSH

Total serum T_4 and T_3 are measured by radioimmunoassay (RIA). The free fraction, however, is relatively small, and changes in binding proteins can significantly affect total hormone levels, even when the free fraction is normal. The free fraction can be measured directly by RIA or ultrafiltration. An estimate of binding site saturation can be obtained by adding a tracer amount of radioiodine and a binding resin to a serum sample. Available binding sites are inversely proportional to the resin uptake of radioiodine. The free fraction of hormone is estimated by adjusting the total hormone measurement based on the estimate of binding site saturation. The concentration of TBG can also be measured directly by RIA.

TSH is currently measured by a double-antibody "sandwich" method, which allows for precise measurement of very low levels of hormone. Previous assay techniques could determine only abnormally elevated levels associated with an underactive thyroid, but not the abnormally low levels associated with hyperthyroidism. Since TSH, in most cases, is regulated based on the concentration of free hormone, this is the most useful way to assess thyroid hormone action.

4.3 Conditions that Alter Thyroid Hormone Measurements

Measurement of thyroid hormones can be influenced by a variety of factors, including illness and medications. Severe illnesses are associated with an elevation in the free fraction measured relative to the total hormone concentrations. Medications, such as salicylates, diphenyl hydantoin, and furosemide, may impair thyroid hormone binding and artificially elevate measurements of free hormone concentration. Serum TSH can be reduced in severe illness or by medications, such as dopamine and glucocorticoids. TSH can remain suppressed below normal levels for several months after treatment of long-standing hyperthyroidism, even when circulating thyroid hormone levels are normal or low, presumably owing to impairment of TSH synthesis.

5. MOLECULAR ACTION OF THYROID HORMONE

5.1. Thyroid Hormone Receptor (TR) α- and β-Genes

TR is a member of the superfamily of nuclear receptors that are ligand-modulated transcription factors (Fig. 4). Within the superfamily, TR is most closely related to the all-trans (RAR) and 9-cis (RXR) retinoic acid receptors. The DNA-binding domain is the most highly conserved region among the members of the family and consists of a pair of "zinc fingers," which interact with target DNA sequences. The DNA sequence that these nuclear receptors recognize is determined by a few amino acid residues at the base of the first zinc finger, termed the P box. More recently, sequences in the amino-terminus have been shown to influence DNA-binding site recognition. A unique carboxy-terminal domain mediates ligand binding.

There are two TR genes, α and β, which are cellular homologs of the viral oncogene v-erbA, one of the two oncogenes carried by avian erythroblastosis virus. TRα and TRβ are coded on chromosomes 17 and 3, respectively, and each gene has at least two alternative mRNA and protein products. The TRβ isoforms, TRβ1 and TRβ2, contain identical DNA- and ligand-binding domains, but differ in their amino-termini. The β-2-specific exon is regulated separately from the β-1-specific exon, leading to differential expression of TRβ1 and TRβ2. By contrast, the TRα variants have identical transcription initiation sites, but diverge after the DNA-binding domain. TRα2 differs from TRα1 at the 3′-end, and has a unique carboxy-terminus that does not bind T_3. TRα2 antagonizes T_3 action in a transient transfection assay.

5.2. Developmental and Tissue-Specific Expression of TR Isoforms

TR isoforms have both developmental and tissue-specific patterns of expression, suggesting unique functions of the different isoforms. Expression of TRβ2 was originally thought to be restricted to the pituitary, but has subsequently been shown in a number of other brain areas and the retina. A recent study using a variety of TRβ2-specific antibodies

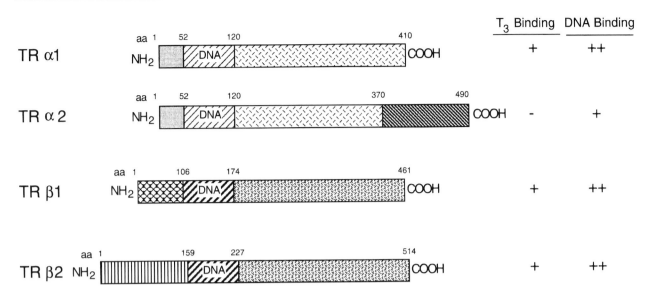

Fig. 4. The deduced protein structure of the major products of the two thyroid hormone receptors (TR) genes, α and β. The relative ability of the receptor isoform to bind T₃ and DNA is indicated. Domains with identical amino acid (aa) sequence are shown by common shading patterns.

concluded that TRβ2 represents as much as 10–20% of T₃-binding capacity in the adult brain, liver, kidney, and heart. The other TR isoforms are found in virtually all other cells, although the proportion varies among tissues and cell types. In the heart, levels of TRα1 and TRβ1 are nearly equal, whereas in liver TRβ1 is the predominant species. In brain, TRα1 and TRα2 are predominantly expressed. The finding that TRβ1 and TRβ2 are expressed in rat embryonic cochlear tissue supports the hypothesis that TRβ has a specific function in the development of hearing. Several investigators have studied the spatial and temporal expression of TR isoforms during development. TRα2 is the first isoform to be expressed during CNS development and is expressed at high levels throughout all locations in the developing brain. TRβ1 is expressed later, predominantly in regions of cortical proliferation, whereas TRα1 is found predominantly in regions of cortical differentiation. Several genes expressed in the brain have been shown to be preferentially regulated by the TRβ isoform, including a Purkinje cell gene (PCP-2), thyrotropin-releasing hormone, and myelin basic protein. Within the pituitary, TRβ2 is expressed at the highest level in thyrotropes and somatotropes. Expression increases further in hypothyroidism. T₃ stimulation of TRβ1 mRNA levels has been shown, and an element that confers this response has been identified in the 5′-flanking region.

5.3. Mechanism of Gene Regulation by Thyroid Hormone

TR interacts with specific DNA sequences, T₃-response elements (TREs), that positively or negatively regulate gene expression (Fig. 5A). Mutational analysis of TREs from a number of T₃-regulated genes have identified a consensus hexamer-binding nucleotide sequence, A/G GGT C/A A. Most elements that confer positive regulation consist of two such elements arranged as a direct repeat with a 4-bp gap. A number of other arrangements are seen, including inverted repeats and palindromes. Flanking sequences are important with a marked increase in affinity by addition of AT to the 5′-end of the hexamer. Elements that confer negative regulation are often single hexamers and are located adjacent to the transcriptional start site. Although receptor monomers and homodimers can bind to a TRE and transactivate a gene, TR heterodimers (with such partners as RXR) bind DNA with higher affinity to most elements (Fig. 5B). There are a number of potential functional TR complexes that confer T₃ regulation. Receptor dimers can consist of homodimers (α/α, α/β or β/β), and also heterodimers with RXR, RAR, or other nuclear receptor partners. Regions of the TR ligand-binding domain that are highly conserved among members of the nuclear receptor superfamily, are important for TR

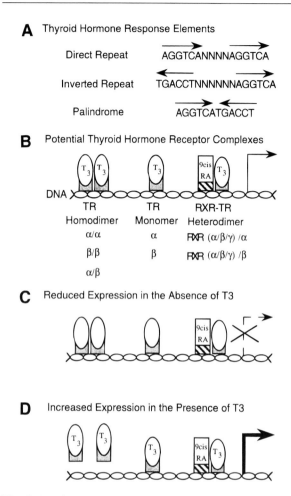

A Thyroid Hormone Response Elements

Direct Repeat   AGGTCANNNNAGGTCA

Inverted Repeat   TGACCTNNNNNNAGGTCA

Palindrome   AGGTCATGACCT

B Potential Thyroid Hormone Receptor Complexes

DNA

TR   TR   RXR-TR
Homodimer   Monomer   Heterodimer

α/α α RXR $(\alpha/\beta/\gamma)$ /α

β/β β RXR $(\alpha/\beta/\gamma)$ /β

α/β

C Reduced Expression in the Absence of T3

D Increased Expression in the Presence of T3

Fig. 5. A series of diagrams depict thyroid hormone receptor (TR)–DNA interactions. **A.** A variety of DNA sequence arrangements are found in thyroid hormone response elements. Arrows indicate the orientation of the consensus hexamer sequence AGGTCA. **B.** There are a number of potential complexes among TR isoforms and the 9-cis-retinoic acid receptor (RXR). **C.** In the absence of T_3, unliganded receptors bind to response elements and reduce the activity of genes that are normally positively regulated. **D.** Addition of T_3 disrupts TR homodimer, but not TR-RXR heterodimer binding on most thyroid hormone response elements.

dimerization. There is polarity to the heterodimer–DNA interactions with RXR occupying the upstream hexamer. T_3 action is further complicated by the observations that unliganded TR reduces expression from positively regulated genes (Fig. 5C) and that T_3 disrupts TR homodimers bound to DNA, but not TR-RXR heterodimers (Fig. 5D). The complexity of the ligand–receptor–DNA interaction suggests that the specific TRE, as well as tissue level concentrations of ligand, TR, and nuclear cofactors, dictate the functional complex.

5.4. Specific Genes Positively Regulated by Thyroid Hormone

Transcriptional regulation by T_3 has been shown for a number of genes. In the liver, these include α-glycerol phosphate dehydrogenase, malic dehydrogenase, and the lipogenic enzyme "spot 14." T_3 stimulates α-myosin heavy-chain expression in cardiac muscle, as well as cardiac and skeletal muscle forms of sarcoplasmic reticulum CaATPase. A complex response element that confers T_3 responsiveness has been identified in the 5′-flanking region of the Type I deiodinase gene. Growth hormone expression in rats is transcriptionally regulated by T_3. Growth and thermogenesis are highly dependent on the presence of thyroid hormone, although a number of these effects are likely to be permissive and not the result of direct transcriptional regulation. In rodent brown fat, thyroid hormone is required for facultative thermogenesis. T_3 stimulates heat production by increasing expression of the uncoupling protein (which generates heat by uncoupling oxidative phosphorylation), and by stimulating CaATPase.

Thyroid hormone is an absolute requirement for amphibian metamorphosis. TRβ and TRα are expressed at the earliest developmental phase, before thyroid hormone is available. Unliganded TR may function to modulate retinoic acid action. Thyroid hormone acts initially to increase the expression of TR in all tissues, which corresponds with the onset of metamorphosis. Prolactin antagonizes the action of thyroid hormone and, if administered at the time of metamorphosis, can completely halt the process. A number of thyroid hormone-responsive genes that may mediate this process have been identified and are being characterized.

5.5. Specific Genes Negatively Regulated by Thyroid Hormone

The most potent examples of negative regulation of gene expression by thyroid hormone are the TSH β and α subunit genes and the TRH gene. These are transcriptionally regulated by T_3, mediated by specific TR-binding elements identified within the gene. Interactions with *Fos* and *Jun* as well as the cAMP-stimulated CREB protein may be important for negative gene regulation. The importance of accessory factors is demonstrated by the observation that negative regulation of TRH gene expression by T_3 varies by tissue (e.g., regulated in paraventricular nucleus of the hypothalamus and prostate, but not in other brain areas or gut), despite the presence of nuclear TR in all of these tissues.

5.6. Extranuclear Effects of Thyroid Hormone

Both T_3 and T_4 have documented extranuclear actions that include stimulation of ion pumps, CaATPase, and Na/K ATPase, mediated by specific membrane-binding sites. Cellular uptake of amino acids and 2-deoxy glucose is rapidly stimulated by T_3. A direct effect of thyroid hormone on relaxation of vascular smooth muscle has been shown. Thyroid hormone stimulates ADP uptake and oxygen consumption by mitochondria. These actions of thyroid hormone are rapid (within seconds), and are not blocked by inhibitors of transcription or translation.

6. CLINICAL MANIFESTATIONS OF REDUCED THYROID HORMONE LEVELS

6.1. Clinical Settings in Which Thyroid Hormone Levels Are Reduced

The most common causes of primary thyroid failure are autoimmune destruction caused by Hashimoto's thyroiditis or as a sequela of radioiodine or surgical ablation for hyperthyroidism (Table 2). Hypothyroidism as a result of pituitary/hypothalamic dysfunction is rare. Congenital hypothyroidism affects about 1 in 4500 live births and is part of routine neonatal screening in most countries. A variety of defects of thyroid growth and function have been identified as causes. When adequate amounts of thyroxine replacement are given to hypothyroid infants within the first few months after delivery, growth and neurologic function are normal. Effects of maternal hypothyroidism on fetal development are thought to be minimal, since the fetal thyroid functions at 10–12 wk. Maternal hypothyroidism from iodine deficiency, however, results in maternal and fetal hypothyroidism. Some offspring of severely iodine-deficient mothers have permanent and severe neurologic deficiencies, including mental deficiency, deaf/mutism, and motor rigidity. This condition, neurologic cretinism, is part of the spectrum of

endemic cretinism in iodine-deficient areas. Iodine supplementation in the first trimester, but not later in pregnancy, largely prevents these abnormalities. Rare, but informative cases of hypothyroidism have been reported from defects in the Pit 1 pituitary-specific transcription factor reducing TSH expression, from defects in thyroid transcription factor 1 associated with deficient thyroglobulin expression, and from germ-line TSH receptor gene-inactivating mutations.

6.2. Clinical Findings

Mild hypothyroidism is associated with relatively nonspecific symptoms, including weight gain, low energy level, amenorrhea, and mood disorders (especially depression). More severe hypothyroidism is associated with hypothermia, hypoventilation, hyponatremia, and eventually coma. Other findings include constipation, hair loss, and dry skin. The characteristic puffy facial appearance and nonpitting edema of arms and legs are the result of increased glycosaminoglycans, such as hyaluronic acid. This deposition is the result of reduced degradation by hyaluronidase. Changes in serum chemistries include elevations in cholesterol, creatine kinase from skeletal muscle, and carotene.

6.3. Treatment

Thyroid hormone deficiency can, in most cases, be easily treated with oral supplementation of thyroxine. Historically, thyroid extracts were used to replace patients with hypothyroidism. Such combinations of T_4 and T_3 were either animal thyroid extracts or synthetic combinations, and were used because they simulated normal thyroidal secretion. The disadvantages, however, include the rapid absorption and short half-life of T_3 as well as variation in tablet content. The observation was convincingly made that the majority of circulating T_3 (80%) was generated from peripheral conversion of T_4. Thyroxine alone could, therefore, replicate the normal function of the thyroid gland and is recommended for thyroid hormone replacement. Thyroxine has a long half-life of 7–10 d, which means that once steady-state levels are achieved, levels are quite stable despite variation in timing of doses, and so on. The adequacy of replacement is primarily determined by the measurement of the serum concentration of TSH. Owing to the availability of the sensitive TSH assay, it is possible

Table 2
Conditions Associated with Reduced Serum Concentrations of T_4/T_3

Diagnosis	Etiology	Thyroid gland	TSH	Anti-bodies	Outcome/treatment
Hashimoto's thyroiditis	Mediated by IgG to TPO	Often enlarged initially, ultimately becomes atrophic	Elevated	TPO-positive	Usually permanent, although small subset (perhaps 5–10%) may be owing to TSH receptor blocking antibodies and reverse
Postablative therapy	Usually after radioiodine or surgical treatment for hyper-thyroidism	Absent or atrophic	Elevated	Negative	Permanent
Congenital hypothyro-dism (sporadic cretinism)	Thyroid agenesis, genetic defect in thyroglobulin synthesis, iodine transport, or organification	Usually absent	High	Negative	Most cases are permanent, can be reversible with the result of maternal TSH receptor blocking antibodies; sequelae are reversible if treatment is started promptly
Central hypothyroidism	Pituitary or hypothalamic dysfunction, TSH β gene defect	Atrophic	Low bioactivity, can be low/normal immunoactive	Negative	Depends on reversibility of pituitary/hypothalamic defect
Lymphocytic thyroiditis	Usually immune-mediated, often seen postpartum	Often slightly enlarged	Initially low, then mildly elevated during the hypo-thyroid phase	TPO-positive	Usually reverts to normal, can be permanent (5–10%); if postpartum, will recur in subsequent pregnancies
Pit-1 deficiency	Defect in the Pit-1 transcription factor gene	Atrophic	Low	Negative	Permanent

T_4—thyroxine, T_3—triiodothyronine, TSH—thyroid-stimulating hormone, TPO—thyroid peroxidase.

to determine when the thyroxine dose is too large or small. Even moderate excessive replacement has been associated with cardiac complications of left ventricular enlargement and an increased risk of atrial fibrillation in the elderly. Postmenopausal women on excessive doses of thyroxine, according to some studies, are at risk for accelerated reduction in bone density.

7. CLINICAL MANIFESTATIONS OF EXCESS THYROID HORMONE LEVELS

7.1. Clinical Settings in Which Thyroid Hormone Levels Are Increased

The most common etiology of excess thyroid hormone production is Graves' disease, associated with circulating autoantibodies that stimulate TSH receptors (Table 3). Stimulation of these receptors results in thyroid growth and an increase in thyroid hormone production. The relative concentration of T_3 in the thyroidal secretion increases and is, in general, proportional to the severity of the disease. The cloning of the TSH receptor has allowed for the mapping of the specific epitopes for Graves-associated antibody. The eye manifestations of Graves' disease include periorbital swelling, infiltration of the extraocular muscles, and protrusion of the eye globe outside of the orbit, and are mediated by the same or related antibodies.

The thyroid gland can make thyroid hormone autonomously, independent of the usual regulation by TSH. The underlying pathology can be an autonomously functioning nodule or a diffusely hyperfunctioning goiter. A large fraction of autonomous nodules studied have a somatic mutation of the TSH receptor gene, which results in constitutive activation of the TSH receptor, and, therefore thyroid hormone production and thyroid cell growth. Approximately 1 in 100 infants born to mothers with Graves' disease will have transient (several weeks to months) hyperthyroidism owing to transplacental passage of maternal IgG. An infant with a germ-line TSH receptor-activating mutation was identified with severe neonatal hyperthyroidism.

7.2. Tissue-Specific Manifestations

A large fraction of hyperthyroid symptoms—nervousness, tachycardia, excess perspiration, and tremulousness—are a manifestation of increased sensitivity to stimulation from the adrenergic ner-

vous system. The molecular basis of this sensitivity is not known, but the effect is thought to be mediated by adrenergic receptors. Longer-term effects of thyroid hormone include weakness, muscle wasting and weight loss owing to acceleration of the basal metabolic rate.

7.3. Treatment

The treatments available for hyperthyroidism include antithyroid drugs, radioiodine, and surgery. The choice of treatment varies by the clinical situation and even geographically. For example, radioiodine is used to a much greater extent in the US compared with Asia or Europe, where antithyroid drugs are more commonly used.

8. THYROID HORMONE RESISTANCE

8.1. Clinical Presentation

Resistance to thyroid hormone (RTH) is a syndrome characterized by the presence of a diffuse goiter, elevated serum T_4 and T_3 concentrations, inappropriately "normal" (given elevated serum T_4 and T_3 concentrations) or elevated serum TSH concentration, and varying manifestations of hypothyroidism, including growth retardation, mental retardation, dysmorphisms, and deafness. Although most manifestations are consistent with reduced thyroid hormone action, an elevated heart rate in many patient indicates retained sensitivity to thyroid hormone effects on the heart. Attention deficit disorder is a frequent finding, seen in as many as 60% of RTH patients. Most patients are identified based on finding a goiter, elevated thyroid hormone levels, or as a result of family screening after an affected individual is identified.

8.2. Associated TR Mutations

All reported cases of RTH in which a defect has been found have been associated with mutations in the TRβ gene. Over 20 different mutations have been described, all located in the terminal 2 exons of the TRβ gene, which encode the carboxy-terminus of the protein (Fig. 4). Reduced affinity for T_3 is seen in all of the mutant receptors, and they function as dominant negative inhibitors of wild-type receptor. In most kindreds, RTH is inherited as an autosomal-dominant trait. In the original kindred described, however, the trait was autosomal-recessive, and individuals heterozygous for the defect had no

Table 3
Conditions Associated with Elevated Serum T_4 and T_3 Concentrations

Diagnosis	Etiology	Thyroid gland	TSH	Antibodies	Outcome/treatment
Graves' disease	Circulating antibodies that stimulate the TSH receptor	Usually symmetrically enlarged	Suppressed	TSI-Positive	Usually characterized by exacerbations and remissions, rarely resolves completely without treatment
Neonatal Graves' disease	Result of transplacental transfer of maternal thyroid-stimulating immunoglobulin, rarely the result of a germ-line-activating mutation of the TSH receptor	Enlarged	Suppressed	Maternal TSI crosses placenta	Self-limited, although may require temporary antithyroid drug treatment, TSH receptor mutation requires antithyroid drug treatment/thyroidectomy
Toxic nodule	Independent hormone production in nodule(s), many associated with constitutive mutations of the TSH receptor	Focal/nodular enlargement	Suppressed	Negative	Hormone production generally proportional to size, can be treated with medicine, radioiodine, or surgery
Toxic goiter	Areas of autonomy throughout thyroid	Diffuse irregular enlargement	Suppressed	Negative	Usually progresses slowly, can be treated with medications, surgery, or radioiodine
TSH-secreting pituitary adenoma	Excess TSH unresponsive to negative feedback from T_4/T_3	Diffusely enlarged	Inappropriately "normal" or elevated	Negative	Requires resection of pituitary adenoma; if unresectable or unresponsive may require thyroidectomy
Resistance to thyroid hormone	All reported cases are TRβ receptor mutations or deletions	Usually enlarged	Inappropriately "normal" or elevated	Negative	Not progressive; some recommend thyroxine treatment

T_4—thyroxine, T_3—triiodothyronine, TSH—thyroid-stimulating hormone, TSI—thyroid-stimulating immunoglobulin.

Table 4
Molecular Classification of Resistance to Thyroid Hormone

TRβ gene	Serum TSH concentration	Serum thyroxine concentration
β/β Wild-type	Normal	Normal
β*/β Heterozygous dominant negative	"Normal" to +	+
β*/β* Homozygous dominant negative	+++	+++
β⁻/β Heterozygous deletion	Normal	Normal
β⁻/β⁻ Homozygous deletion	"Normal" to +	+

+ Above normal.
+++ Very high.
TR—thyroid hormone receptor, TSH—thyroid-stimulating hormone.

abnormal phenotype. The affected individuals from this kindred were later found to have complete deletion of the coding region of the TRβ gene. Only one patient, the product of consanguineous parents, has been described who was homozygous for a dominant negative TRβ mutation. This child was severely affected with very high serum thyroid hormone concentrations, profound neurologic abnormalities, and died after a few years of life. A classification of RTH based on TRβ deletion/mutations and clinical findings is shown (Table 4). TRα mutations have not been identified in patients with RTH, although analogous TRα mutants studied in vitro can function as a dominant-negative receptor. TRα may be redundant or alternatively may be essential for life.

8.3. Mechanisms of Mutant Receptor Inhibition of Thyroid Hormone Action

The heterogeneity of clinical manifestations of RTH support the hypothesis that tissues differ in their ability to compensate for an absent or mutant TR isoform. There are a number of proposed mechanisms for inhibition of T_3 action by mutant TRβ receptors. It is known that there is a correlation between mutations or deletions that interfere with T_3 binding and inhibition of wild-type receptor. Examples of naturally occurring mutants that have this property include the oncogene-v*erb* A and the α2 variant of TRα. Several studies have demonstrated the importance of an intact DNA-binding domain for inhibition. Mutant receptors can heterodimerize with the wild-type receptor and may form inactive complexes. The mutant receptor may compete with wild-type receptor for some limiting cofactor that is required for a response.

Mutant receptors vary in their ability to have normal function restored by high concentrations of T_3. Furthermore, this normalization of function varies by the specific response element used, implying that a specific gene may be differentially affected. This may explain why tissues vary in their response to thyroid hormone, for example, some kindreds have primarily resistance to thyroid hormone action in the pituitary. Differential expression of the mutant and wild-type allele may occur during development or in specific tissues. The majority of studies have shown equal transcription, although a single study showed greater transcription from the mutant allele during a period of delayed linear growth.

SELECTED READINGS

Bartalena L. Recent achievements in studies on thyroid hormone-binding proteins. *Endocr Rev* 1990; 11:47.

Berry MJ, Larsen PR. The role of selenium in thyroid hormone action. *Endocr Rev* 1992; 13:207.

Brent GA, Moore DD, Larsen PR. Thyroid hormone regulation of gene expression. *Ann Rev Physiol* 1991; 53:17.

Brent GA. The molecular basis of thyroid hormone action. *N Engl J Med* 1994; 331:847.

Carrasco N. Iodine transport in the thyroid gland. *Biochim Biophys Acta* 1993; 1154:65.

Chatterjee VKK, Tata JR. Thyroid hormone receptors and their role in development. *Cancer Surveys* 1992; 14:147.

Glass CK. Differential recognition of target genes by nuclear receptor monomer, dimers, and heterodimers. *Endocr Rev* 1994; 15:391.

Lazar MA. Thyroid hormone receptors: multiple forms, multiple possibilities. *Endocr Rev* 1993; 14:184.

Medeiros-Neto G, Targovnik HM, Vassart G. Defective thyroglobulin synthesis and secretion causing goiter and hypothyroidism. *Endocr Rev* 1993; 14:165.

McLachlan SM, Rapoport B. The molecular biology of thyroid peroxidase: cloning, expression and role as autoantigen in autoimmune thyroid disease. *Endocr Rev* 1992; 13:192.

Refetoff S. Inherited thyroxine-binding globulin abnormalities in man. *Endocr Rev* 1989; 10:275.

Refetoff S, Weiss RE, Usala SJ. The syndromes of resistance to thyroid hormone. *Endocr Rev* 1993; 14:348.

Vassart G, Dumont JE. The thyrotropin receptor and the regulation of thyrocyte function and growth. *Endocr Rev* 1992; 13:596.

Williams GR, Brent GA. Thyroid hormone response elements. In Weintraub B, ed. *Molecular Endocrinology: Basic Concepts and Clinical Correlations*. New York: Raven, 1995; 217.

Yen PM, Chin WW. New advances in understanding the molecular mechanisms of thyroid hormone action. *Trends Endocrinol Metab* 1994; 5:65.

20 Calcium-Regulating Hormones

Vitamin D and Parathyroid Hormone

Geoffrey N. Hendy, PhD

Contents

INTRODUCTION

This chapter will describe the structure and actions of vitamin D, which is essential for maintaining a positive calcium balance and skeletal integrity, and the parathyroid hormone (PTH) responsible for minute-to-minute maintenance of calcium homeostasis, which is critical for neuromuscular activity.

1. VITAMIN D

Vitamin D originally came to attention by virtue of its antirachitic properties. It is now appreciated to be a natural product of the body and is the precursor of the calcium-regulating hormone, 1,25-dihydroxyvitamin D(1,25[OH]$_2$D$_3$). This is produced in the kidney, released into the circulation, and exerts its effects on mineral homeostasis by acting on intestine, bone, kidney, and the parathyroid gland. The hormone acts like a steroid hormone in the nuclei of target cells and its production is subject to feedback regulation. Vitamin D and its metabolites form the basis of an endocrine system that interacts with the parathyroid glands and is of fundamental importance in the hormonal control of mineral metabolism.

From: *Endocrinology: Basic and Clinical Principles* (P. M. Conn and S. Melmed, eds.), Humana Press Inc., Totowa, NJ.

1.1. Production and Metabolism of Vitamin D

1.1.1. Chemical Structure

Vitamin D is a 9–10 secosterol with the A-ring rotated into the cis configuration. Although it is related to a C$_{21}$ steroid, it differs in structure by disruption of the bond between C-9 and C-10, opening the B-ring, and thus forms a conjugated triene structure. It also has an elongated side chain (Fig. 1). Cholecalciferol (vitamin D$_3$) is the natural form of the vitamin. This C$_{27}$ compound is produced by irradiation of the precursor, 7-dehydrocholesterol. Ergocalciferol (vitamin D$_2$) is a synthetic C$_{28}$ compound originally produced by irradiation of the plant sterol, ergosterol. The side chain of vitamin D$_2$ differs from that of vitamin D$_3$ by having a double bond between C-22 and C-23 and a methyl group at C-24. Vitamins D$_2$ and D$_3$ are metabolized along the same pathways to produce active metabolites with equivalent effects. Vitamin D written without a subscript can refer to either form of the vitamin.

1.1.2. Photoproduction

Normally, synthesis of vitamin D$_3$ in the skin can provide the body's full requirement unless exposure to sunlight is restricted. Production of vitamin D$_3$ occurs by nonenzymatic photolysis of 7-

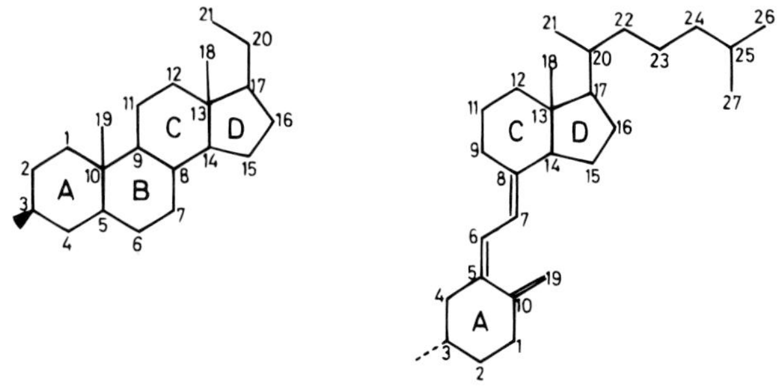

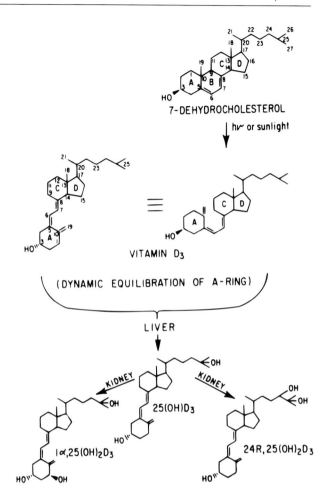

Fig. 1. Structure of a C_{21} steroid (left) compared with a C_{27} secosterol (right), such as vitamin D_3 (Papapoulos et al., 1979).

dehydrocholesterol (provitamin D) in the epidermis (Fig. 2). Near-UV light of wavelength 290–315 nm opens the B-ring by cleaving the bond between C-9 and C-10 of 7-dehydrocholesterol, forming previtamin D_3, and rearrangement of the molecule, which is temperature-dependent and is favored at body temperature, yields vitamin D_3. Two other biologically inert products, lumisterol and tachysterol, are produced by photolysis of previtamin D. The skin pigment melanin can also absorb UV light and, when present in large amounts, competes with 7-dehydrocholesterol for this energy source. Given the same UV exposure, heavily pigmented individuals produce less vitamin D_3 than lightly pigmented people.

Vitamin D can also be obtained from the diet either as vitamin D_3 from foods that contain it naturally (e.g., livers of fatty fish) or from milk and dairy products, which are frequently fortified with either vitamin D_2 or D_3.

1.1.3. METABOLIC ACTIVATION OF VITAMIN D

Biological responses to vitamin D_3 after its administration to animals are apparent only after a significant time lag. Vitamin D must undergo two hydroxylation steps before it assumes the physiologically active form, 1,25-dihydroxyvitamin D ($1,25[OH]_2D_3$). This allows it to bind to intracellular receptors in target tissues.

1.1.3.1. 25-Hydroxylation in the Liver. Vitamin D_3 produced either in the skin or absorbed from the small intestine rapidly accumulates in the liver, where it is hydroxylated at C-25 of the side chain to form 25-hydroxycholecalciferol ($25[OH]D_3$), the most abundant form of the vitamin (Fig. 2). Vitamin D_2 is similarly metabolized to 25-hydroxyergocalciferol

Fig. 2. Metabolic pathway of vitamin D_3 production and activation beginning with synthesis of previtamin D_3 by UV irradiation of 7-dehydrocholesterol in the skin. Rearrangement of previtamin D_3 yields vitamin D_3, which is metabolized to $25(OH)D_3$ in the liver. In the kidney, $25(OH)D_3$ is either metabolized to the hormonally active $1,25(OH)_2D_3$ or catabolized to $24,25(OH)_2D_3$. (Adapted from Minghetti and Norman, 1988).

($25[OH]D_2$). This step is obligatory for further metabolism of the sterol. The liver is the principal site of production in vivo, and total hepatectomy causes the virtual disappearance of 25(OH)D from the circulation. Hepatic 25-hydroxylase activity is associated with mitochondrial and microsomal fractions, and both activities are the result of cytochrome P-450 enzymes. Although a mitochondrial cytochrome P-450 (CYP27) has been cloned, it is not specific for vitamin D and will hydroxylate cholesterol. The enzyme(s) responsible for the high-specificity, low-capacity 25-hydroxylase activity remains to be identified and characterized.

25(OH)D$_3$ is more effective than vitamin D$_3$ in curing rickets, and acts more rapidly in stimulating both intestinal calcium absorption and calcium mobilization from bone. At one time it was believed to be the final active metabolite of vitamin D$_3$. However, although it is not biologically active at physiological concentrations in vivo, it is active in binding the intestinal vitamin D receptor (VDR) and stimulating calcium transport at high concentrations. The hypercalcemia produced by vitamin D intoxication is mediated by 25(OH)D.

1.1.3.2. 1α-Hydroxylation in the Kidney. Further metabolism of 25(OH)D occurs in mitochondria of renal proximal tubules to the most biologically active metabolite of vitamin D known, 1,25(OH)$_2$D (Fig. 2). Although other tissues and cultured cells can produce 1,25(OH)D, these sources do not normally contribute significantly to the circulating 1,25(OH)$_2$D concentration. 1,25(OH)D$_2$ is absent from the serum of anephric animals and humans. In pregnancy, additional hormone is supplied to the circulation by placental production of 1,25(OH)$_2$D. Hypercalcemia associated with granulomatous diseases, such as sarcoidosis and tuberculosis, and certain lymphomas, is also the result of extrarenal synthesis of 1,25(OH)$_2$D.

The renal 1α-hydroxylase is of the P-450 mixed-function type, and requires a ferrodoxin and NADPH, which is generated in the mitochondria by an energy-dependent transhydrogenase. Although all components have been isolated and reconstituted to form an active 1α-hydroxylase system, and a ferrodoxin characterized, the nature of the cytochrome P-450 component remains to be elucidated.

1.1.3.3. 24-Hydroxylation. Hydroxylation of 25(OH)D at C-24 produces 24,25(OH)$_2$D (Fig. 2), the second most abundant circulating metabolite of vitamin D. It circulates at concentrations 10-fold lower than those of 25(OH)D. Most circulating 24,25(OH)$_2$D is derived from the kidney, but many other tissues can also produce this metabolite. The renal tubular 24-hydroxylase enzyme is located in mitochondria, but is distinct from the renal 1α-hydroxylase. The P-450 component of this enzyme has been cloned and characterized in human and other species. Its main substrate is 25(OH)D, but the enzyme also hydroxylates 1,25(OH)$_2$D to form 1,24,25(OH)$_3$D. 24,25(OH)$_2$D is far less active than 1,25(OH)$_2$D in bioassays, and a clear physiological role has been difficult to ascribe. 24-Hydroxylation renders the vitamin D molecule susceptible to side-chain cleavage and oxidation, and 24,25(OH)$_2$D represents the first metabolic step in hormonal inactivation.

1.1.3.4. Further Metabolism of Vitamin D. Other forms of vitamin D have been identified in the circulation. 25,26-Dihydroxyvitamin D(25,26[OH]$_2$D), which is produced in the kidney and liver, circulates at a concentration slightly lower than that of 24,25(OH)$_2$D. 1,25(OH)D can be catabolized by two pathways to either the C$_{23}$ calcitroic acid (1[OH])-24,25,26,27-tetranor-23-COOH-D) or 1,25(OH)$_2$-26,23-lactone. 24,25(OH)$_2$D can also be metabolized by two pathways leading to either 25,26,27-trinor-24-COOH-D or 24,25,26,27-tetranor-23-COOH-D.

1.1.4. REGULATION OF VITAMIN D METABOLISM

Dietary intake and endogenous synthesis of vitamin D are variable, and there is a need for regulation of the production of the more active metabolites. Potentially, this is feasible at the stages of hepatic and renal hydroxylation. Hepatic 25-hydroxylation is not regulated by serum calcium or phosphate. Although it is more efficient at low levels of substrate, it is not tightly regulated, since suppression of the enzyme can be overcome by large amounts of vitamin D. This has practical application in the clinical administration of a synthetic form of vitamin D$_3$, 1α-hydroxycholecalciferol (1α[OH]D$_3$), which requires hepatic hydroxylation at C-25 to become active. This might give a safety factor if there was product inhibition of 25-hydroxylase, but in fact, hypercalcemia can be produced with 1α(OH)D$_3$ even in microgram doses, and careful monitoring of treatment with this drug is needed.

More important is the control of 1α- and 24-hydroxylases in the kidney. There is a switching mechanism that determines the relative activity of these two enzymes. Normally, serum concentrations of 1,25(OH)$_2$D change little in response to vitamin D administration. Several circulating factors modulate the fine control of the 1α-hydroxylase, the most important being PTH, calcium, phosphate, and 1,25(OH)$_2$D$_3$ (Fig. 3).

1.1.4.1. Calcium and PTH. In hypocalcemia, 25(OH)D is preferentially converted to 1,25(OH)$_2$D, whereas in normo- and hypercalcemia, it is mainly

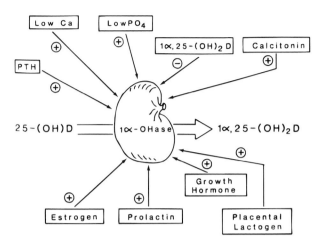

Fig. 3. 1,25(OH)$_2$D is produced in the kidney by metabolism of 25(OH)D. The renal 1α-hydroxylase is modulated both positively (+) and negatively (−) by several regulators (shown in boxes) including mineral ions, hormones, and 1,25(OH)$_2$D itself (Pike, 1992).

metabolized to 24,25(OH)$_2$D. This effect is achieved largely by hypocalcemia stimulating the parathyroid gland to secrete PTH, which enhances renal proximal tubular 1α-hydroxylase activity and raises serum 1,25(OH)$_2$D$_3$. This enhances intestinal calcium absorption, and the increased serum calcium concentration inhibits PTH secretion, closing the feedback loop. Some studies have suggested that the circulating calcium concentration can also directly modulate the renal 1α-hydroxylase (Fig. 3).

1.1.4.2. Phosphate. Low-serum phosphate concentrations stimulate and high-phosphate concentrations inhibit renal 1α-hydroxylase activity (Fig. 3). These effects are independent of PTH.

1.1.4.3. 1,25-(OH)$_2$D. 1,25(OH)$_2$D controls its own synthesis (Fig. 3) by decreasing 1α-hydroxylase activity and stimulating 24-hydroxylase activity. When large doses of 1,25(OH)$_2$D$_3$ are given to vitamin D-deficient chicks, the switch in enzyme activity occurs rapidly, and this can be prevented by actinomycin D. This suggests that 1,25(OH)$_2$D regulates its own production by the synthesis of new protein. Indirect regulation may also occur via the effect of 1,25(OH)$_2$D on the parathyroid glands, and the consequent changes in serum calcium and phosphate.

1.1.4.4. Other Regulators. Calcium requirements are increased in physiological states, such as growth, pregnancy, lactation, and egg-laying, and hormonal changes occurring during these conditions influence vitamin D metabolism. In mammals, prolactin, insulin, growth hormone, and calcitonin all stimulate 1α-hydroxylase activity (Fig. 3). In birds, enhanced estrogen and progesterone secretion during egg-laying enhance 1α-hydroxylation and increase serum 1,25(OH)$_2$D levels.

1.2. Absorption, Transport, and Excretion

After absorption from the duodenum and distal ileum, vitamin D is incorporated into chylomicrons. Disruption of this process, as in steatorrhea, can lead to vitamin D malabsorption. Normally, as much as half of the absorbed vitamin is stored in body fats.

Vitamin D derived from either diet or epidermis is bound in the circulation by the vitamin D-binding protein (DBP), an α-globulin of 55,000 Dalton, previously known as group-specific component (Gc). This has a single high-affinity binding site that binds vitamin D and all its metabolites, although it has higher affinity for 25(OH)D, 24,25(OH)$_2$D, and 25,26(OH)$_2$D than for vitamin D or 1,25(OH)$_2$D. This facilitates partitioning of vitamin D in lipid stores and favors entry of 1,25(OH)$_2$D into target cells. The serum DBP concentration greatly exceeds the concentration of all vitamin metabolites, such that only 3–5% of available binding sites are occupied. Hepatic synthesis of the protein is increased in pregnancy and decreased in chronic liver disease, and serum concentrations are also reduced in the nephrotic syndrome. DBP concentrations are not influenced by vitamin D status; they are unaltered in disorders of mineral homeostasis.

There is little urinary excretion of vitamin D and its metabolites. After 1,25(OH)$_2$D has performed its function in target tissues, it is converted to inactive metabolites, such as calcitroic acid, via a 24-oxidation pathway and excreted in bile. Anticonvulsant drug administration increases the biliary excretion of vitamin D metabolites.

1.3. Biological Actions of Vitamin D

1.3.1. INTESTINE

In the small intestine, 1,25(OH)$_2$D$_3$ actively stimulates calcium transport, and this is accompanied by passive movement of phosphate. In addition, an independent active phosphate transport system is also stimulated throughout the small and large bowels. The calcium transport response to a dose of $1,25(OH)_2D_3$ is biphasic, with the first phase peaking at 6 h and the second phase maintaining elevated calcium transport for several days. In vitro $1,25(OH)_2D_3$ and $25(OH)_3D_3$ can both increase calcium absorption by a direct action on the gut, whereas vitamin D_3 cannot.

The synthesis of several intestinal epithelial cell proteins that may function in the calcium transport process is induced by $1,25(OH)_2D_3$. In particular, production of a calcium-binding protein (calbindinD28K in chick and calbindin9K in mammals) is dependent on vitamin D in the intestine, and its appearance in villus enterocytes is induced within a few hours of administration of $1,25(OH)_2D_3$. However, despite extensive study, defining a role for calbindins or other intestinal proteins in the calcium transport process has remained elusive.

$1,25(OH)_2D$ induces changes in plasma membrane phospholipase activity in intestinal epithelial cells with a similar time-course to the $1,25(OH)_2D$-stimulated uptake of calcium into brush border membrane vesicles. It has been suggested that $1,25(OH)_2D$-induced alteration in membrane lipids initiates the calcium transport process.

1.3.2. Skeleton

The antirachitic effects of vitamin D are mainly indirect, relying more on increasing serum calcium and phosphate through its actions on intestinal absorption than a direct action on bone formation. Intravenous infusion of calcium and phosphate in vitamin D-deficient rats can cure rickets in the absence of circulating $1,25(OH)_2D$. However, $1,25(OH)_2D$ does act directly on bone-forming cells. In cultured osteoblast-like cells, $1,25(OH)_2D$ regulates the expression of several genes. It decreases synthesis of citrate decarboxylase, either increases or decreases alkaline phosphatase and type I collagen production, and increases synthesis of osteopontin, osteocalcin, and matrix-Gla protein. The precise effect of the seco-sterol may depend on the growth and differentiation state of the cells.

$1,25(OH)_2D$ also increases bone mineral resorption as shown in vitro in neonatal calvaria or long bones prelabeled with ^{45}Ca. PTH and vitamin D metabolites potentiate each other's osteolytic activity. $1,25(OH)_2D$ plays an important role in the formation of mature osteoclasts—multinuclear bone- resorbing cells—from mononuclear cell precursors. It stimulates monocytic differentiation of immature hematopoietic cells and the differentiation of mononuclear phagocytes into osteoclasts in cooperation with osteoblastic cells. Overall, $1,25(OH)_2D$ facilitates bone remodeling.

1.3.3. Kidney

As it does in other tissues, $1,25(OH)_2D$ induces the transcriptional activity of the 24-hydroxylase gene in the kidney. $1,25(OH)_2D$ causes a decrease in both calcium and phosphate excretion by increasing renal proximal tubular reabsorption, although the phosphate-conserving action may in part be indirect via PTH.

1.3.4. Other Tissues

$1,25(OH)_2D$ inhibits PTH synthesis and secretion as part of an important feedback loop in regulating mineral ion homeostasis. This has led to the use of iv $1,25(OH)_2D_3$ and its analogs in the treatment of the secondary hyperparathyroidism of chronic renal failure.

In addition to the classic actions of vitamin D on mineral metabolism, $1,25(OH)_2D$ has pleiotropic actions in many tissues that are not necessarily related to its role as a calcium-regulating hormone. These often involve the sterol acting as an antiproliferative, prodifferentiation agent in both normal and cancer cells. For example, $1,25(OH)_2D_3$ induces maturation of basal epidermal skin cells into keratinocytes and stimulates mouse myeloid leukemic cells to differentiate into macrophages.

1.3.4.1. Nonhypercalcemic Vitamin D Analogs. Because of its antiproliferative effects, $1,25(OH)_2D_3$ is potentially useful clinically in the control of secondary hyperparathyroidism, various cancers, and in the treatment of the common, benign hyperproliferative skin disorder, psoriasis. However, hypercalcemia results from $1,25(OH)_2D_3$ treatment. Recently, synthetic $1,25(OH)_2D_3$ analogs have been developed that display reduced calcemic activity (Fig. 4). Many of these carry side-chain modifications that reduce affinity for the serum vitamin D-binding protein, alter tissue distribution, and accelerate metabolic degradation. Several of these derivatives have been shown to be highly effective in controlling cellular differentiation and maintain a

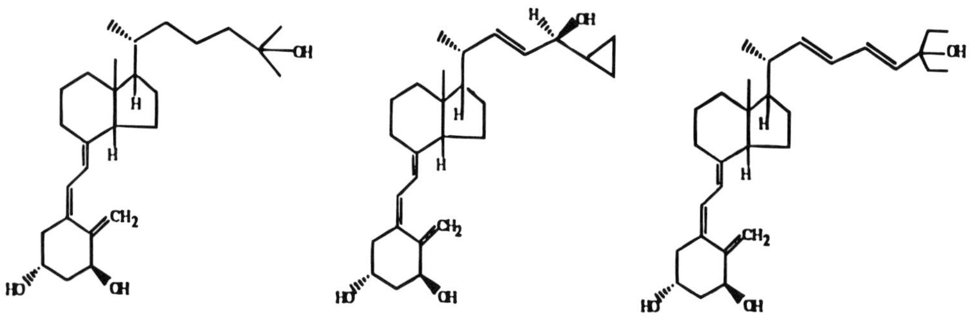

Fig. 4. Structure of 1,25(OH)$_2$D$_3$ and its "noncalcemic" analogs, MC903 and EB1089. MC903 and EB1089 differ only in the side chain as compared with 1,25(OH)$_2$D$_3$, and demonstrate reduced calcemic activity, but are equipotent or more potent than 1,25(OH)$_2$D$_3$ in inhibiting cell proliferation (Yu et al., 1995).

high affinity for the VDR. One of these compounds, Calciotriol (MC903), is currently available for treatment of psoriasis.

1.4. Biochemical Mechanism of Action

1.4.1. GENOMIC ACTIONS

Tissues responsive to vitamin D contain a specific, high-affinity intracellular receptor (VDR) that mediates the ability of 1,25(OH)$_2$D to regulate gene expression by binding vitamin D-responsive elements (VDREs). Free 1,25(OH)$_2$D (that fraction of circulating 1,25[OH]$_2$D not bound to the serum vitamin D-binding protein) diffuses across the cell membrane and binds the VDR. It is not clear whether this binding initially takes place in the cytoplasm followed by ligand-bound VDR translocation to the nucleus or whether the VDR is located solely in the nucleus. The VDR is closely related structurally to the thyroid hormone and retinoic acid receptors, which all function as ligand-activated transcription factors.

The VDREs in positively controlled genes are direct hexanucleotide repeats with a spacer of three nucleotides. The VDR associates with the VDRE as a heterodimer with a retinoid X receptor (RXR). The VDR has several functional domains: an NH$_2$-terminal zinc finger DNA-binding domain, a hinge region, and a COOH-terminal hormone-binding domain that also contains regions responsible for heterodimerization with the RXR (Fig. 5). Binding of 1,25(OH)$_2$D to the VDR alters the conformation of the VDR, facilitating dimerization with RXR enhancing association with the VDRE. RXR binds the 5'-VDRE repeat, and the VDR binds the 3'-VDRE repeat.

After heterodimerization with RXR, the VDR directly binds transcription factor IIB (TFIIB), a key component of the basal RNA polymerase II transcription machinary. Positive vitamin D-responsive elements have been identified in several genes, including those for osteocalcin, osteopontin, 24-hydroxylase, and β$_3$ integrin. Negative vitamin D-responsive elements have been described in the PTH and bone sialoprotein genes, although it remains less clear how 1,25(OH)$_2$D negatively modulates gene transcription. Other coregulatory proteins than RXR are likely to interact with the VDR and modulate its effect on gene transcription.

1.4.2. NONGENOMIC ACTIONS

1,25(OH)$_2$D can also act on target cells via nongenomic mechanisms. Unlike genomic events, which take several hours or days to be apparent, nongenomic effects take place in minutes or less after hormonal treatment. The nongenomic effects include stimulation of Ca^{2+} influx, release of Ca^{2+} from intracellular stores, protein phosphorylation, and phospholipid turnover. An important finding is that genomic and nongenomic effects are pharmacologically separable. Thus, it has been speculated that a distinct membrane vitamin D receptor exists, possibly coupled to a phospholipase, which mediates these nongenomic actions. It should be emphasized, however, that such a receptor has yet to be identified. Some of the nonhypercalcemic analogs discussed above retain the genomic activities of 1,25(OH)$_2$D, and decrease cellular proliferation and promote differentiation, but lack the nongenomic

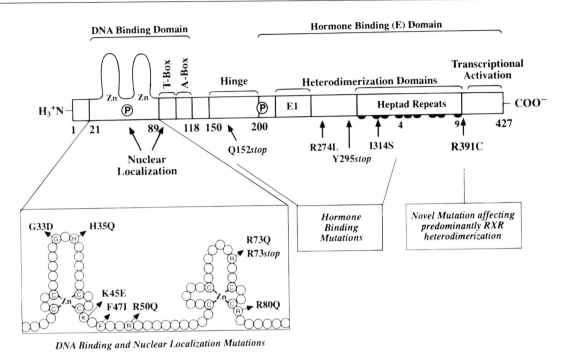

Fig. 5. Structure/function map of the human vitamin D receptor showing the naturally occurring mutations causing hereditary vitamin D-dependent rickets type II. P indicates a phosphorylation site (Haussler et al., 1995).

effects that stimulate calcium mobilization. These compounds have the greatest therapeutic potential for the treatment of hyperproliferative disorders while minimizing hypercalcemic side effects.

1.5. Pathophysiology of Hypervitaminosis D and Hypovitaminosis D, Receptor Defects

1.5.1. ASSESSMENT OF VITAMIN D STATUS

Assays for vitamin D and its metabolites in serum use radioligand-binding techniques—radioreceptor or radioimmunoassay—most of which require prior chromatography to separate the metabolite to be measured. The circulating concentration of 25(OH)D is the best index of overall vitamin D status. There is a seasonal fluctuation in serum 25(OH)D concentrations, with highest values occurring in late summer and lowest values in late winter. The physiological status of an individual should be considered in interpreting serum $1,25(OH)_2D$ levels, which may be increased during growth, pregnancy, or lactation. The frequently encountered clinical conditions that may present with an abnormal serum concentration of 25(OH)D or $1,25(OH)_2D$ are listed in Table 1. Insufficient dietary intake or cutaneous synthesis of vitamin D can lead to inadequate production of

25(OH)D substrate for conversion to $1,25(OH)_2D$. Disturbances in vitamin D metabolism at the level of liver or kidney can cause reduced production of $1,25(OH)_2D$. In renal failure, a decline in functional renal mass, with increased phosphate retention, reduces or eliminates 1α-hydroxylase activity. Hypoparathyroidism and pseudohypoparathyroidism are associated with low circulating $1,25(OH)_2D$ concentrations. In vitamin D-dependent rickets type I, serum $1,25(OH)_2D$ levels are low because of an inherited defect in the renal 1α-hydroxylase enzyme. In contrast, in vitamin D-dependent rickets type II, resulting from an inherited defect in the VDR, the end organ resistance can lead to grossly elevated serum $1,25(OH)_2D$ concentrations.

Clinical deficiency of vitamin D can result from perturbations at several different levels—synthesis, metabolism, or action. Because of this, for accurate assessment of the pathophysiology, it may be necessary to consider both 25(OH)D and $1,25(OH)_2D$ concentrations. For example, low $1,25(OH)_2D$ levels need not necessarily indicate defective renal production of the metabolite. They could result from insufficient vitamin D intake, and this would be indicated by a low serum 25(OH)D concentration. However, if $1,25(OH)_2D$ values are low in the presence of a

Table 1
Vitamin D Metabolite Concentrations
in Patients with Disordered Calcium Homeostasis

	25(OH)D	*1,25(OH)$_2$D*
Hypocalcemia		
Vitamin D deficiency	↓	↓ or ↑ or →
Severe hepatocellular disease	↓	↓ or →
Nephrotic syndrome	↓	↓ or →
Renal failure	→	↓
Hyperphosphatemia	→	↓
Hypoparathyroidism	→	↓ or →
Pseudohypoparathyroidism	→	↓ or →
Hypomagnesemia	→	↓ or →
Vitamin D-dependent rickets, type I	→ or ↑	↓
Vitamin D-dependent rickets, type II	→ or ↑	↑
Hypercalcemia/hypercalciuria:		
Vitamin D, 25(OH)D intoxication	↑	→ or ↓
1,25(OH)$_2$D Intoxication	→	↑
Granuloma-forming diseases	→	↑
Lymphoma	→	↓ or ↑
Hyperparathyroidism	→	↓ or ↑
Williams syndrome	→	↑
Idiopathic hypercalciuria	→	↑
Idiopathic osteoporosis	→	→ or ↑
PTHrP-associated	→	↓

↓ = decreased; ↑ = increased; → = normal
Adapted from Clemens and Adams (1993).

normal 25(OH)D value, decreased renal synthesis of 1,25(OH)$_2$D is likely.

1.5.2. RECEPTOR DEFECTS

Vitamin D-dependent rickets type II is a rare, autosomal recessive disorder in which severe hypocalcemia and rickets develop in early childhood. The disease is unresponsive to all forms of vitamin D, including high doses of 1,25(OH)$_2$D$_3$. In affected individuals, a number of naturally occurring mutations in the VDR gene have been identified (Fig. 5), which disrupt either DNA binding and/or nuclear localization, ligand binding, or RXR heterodimerization.

1.6. Summary

A recent provocative and controversial finding has suggested that the VDR gene, as marked by allelic variants, is a predictor of bone mass in some populations. Whether this involves the VDR itself or another gene at the same chromosomal locus

(12q13–14) is to be established. 1,25(OH)$_2$D exhibits pleiotropic actions, not only playing a key role in mineral metabolism, but also influencing cell differentiation. These effects are achieved through genomic mechanisms involving the widely expressed VDR and nongenomic mechanisms.

2. PTH

PTH is essential for the maintenance of calcium homeostasis, and an excess or deficiency can cause severe and potentially fatal illness. PTH is synthesized in the parathyroid glands in the neck, and after secretion, exerts its effects directly on the skeleton and kidneys.

2.1. Hormone Gene

2.1.1. STRUCTURE

PTH is the product of a single-copy gene and, in mammals, has 84 amino acids. The gene, which

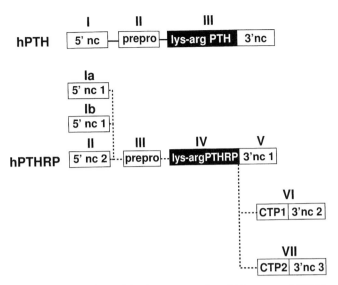

Fig. 6. Comparison of the structural organization of the human parathyroid hormone (hPTH) and parathyroid hormone-related protein (hPTHrP). Nc denotes noncoding region and CTP carboxyl-terminal peptide. Roman numerals denote exons (Goltzman and Hendy, 1995).

encodes a larger precursor molecule of 115 amino acids, prepro-PTH, is organized into three exons. Exon I encodes the 5′-untranslated region of the messenger RNA, exon II encodes the NH_2-terminal pre- or signal peptide and part of the short propeptide, and exon III encodes the Lys^{-2}-Arg^{-1} of the prohormone cleavage site, the 84 amino acids of the mature hormone, and the 3′-untranslated region of the mRNA (Fig. 6).

This general organization is shared by the PTH-related peptide (PTHrP) gene, in which the same functional domains—the untranslated region, prepro-sequence of the precursor peptide, and the prohormone cleavage site and most or all of the mature peptide—are encoded by single exons (Fig. 6). For the PTHrP gene, exons encoding alternative 5′-untranslated regions, carboxyl-terminal peptides, and 3′-untranslated regions may also be present, depending on the species.

The PTH and PTHrP genes map to chromosome 11p15 and chromosome 12p12.1–11.2, respectively. These two human chromosomes are thought to have been derived by an ancient duplication of a single chromosome, and the PTH and PTHrP genes and their respective gene clusters have been maintained as syntenic groups in the human, rat, and mouse genomes. Because of the similarity in NH_2-terminal sequence of their mature peptides, their gene organization, and chromosomal locations, it is likely that the PTH and PTHrP genes evolved from a single ancestral gene, with PTHrP being the more ancient gene, and form part of a single gene family.

2.1.2. REGULATION

Transcription of the PTH gene occurs almost exclusively in the endocrine cells of the parathyroid gland, and is subject to strong repressor activity in all other cells. Ectopic PTH synthesis (i.e., synthesis outside parathyroid tissue) has been documented in only a very few cases of malignancies associated with hypercalcemia. In the majority of instances of hypercalcemia associated with malignancies, PTHrP is the responsible causal factor.

Activation of genes in particular tissues is often related to demethylation of cytosine residues, and the PTH gene in parathyroid cells is hypomethylated at CpG residues relative to other tissues. The human PTH gene has two functional TATA transcriptional start sites, a cyclic AMP (cAMP) response element (CRE), and a VDRE in its proximal promoter. Distally, several kilobase pairs upstream of the transcription start site a calcium response element (CaRE), and sequences that function to repress transcription in nonparathyroid cells are present. PTH gene transcription is negatively regulated by both extracellular calcium and the hormonally active metabolite of vitamin D, 1,25-dihydroxyvitamin D.

PARATHYROID HORMONE

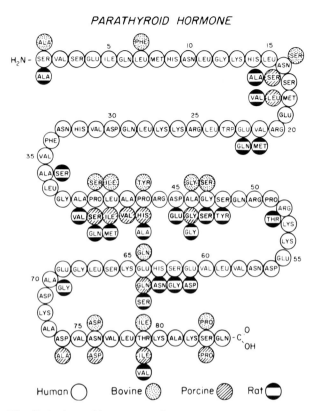

Fig. 7. Amino acid sequence of mammalian PTH. The backbone is that of the human sequence, and substitutions in the bovine, porcine, and rat hormones are shown (Goltzman and Hendy 1995).

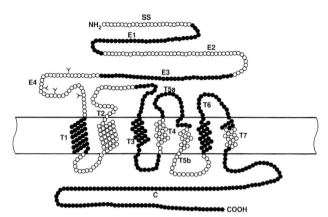

Fig. 8. Schematic representation of the PTH/PTHrP receptor. The gene contains 17 exons. The first three encode portions of two different 5'-untranslated regions of the mRNA. The portions of the receptor encoded by the remaining 14 exons are schematically represented by the alternate blocks of unfilled and filled circles. Exons are depicted as follows: SS; putative signal sequence; E1–E4; extracellular sequences; T1–T7; transmembrane sequences; C; cytoplasmic sequence (Goltzman and Hendy, 1995).

2.1.3. Species Comparison

The primary structure of the major glandular form of PTH, PTH (1–84), has been determined in several mammalian species, including human, bovine, porcine, and rat (Fig. 7). In the chicken, the PTH polypeptide contains 88 rather than 84 amino acids. The NH_2-terminal 34 amino acids are the most well-conserved portion of the molecule, and structure and function studies have emphasized the importance of the NH_2-terminal region to bioactivity in all species. Considerable deletion of the middle and COOH-terminal region of the intact polypeptide can be tolerated without apparent loss of biological activity.

2.1.4. Ultrastructure

The conformation assumed by the PTH molecule in the presence of its receptor is unknown. In aqueous solution, PTH-(1-34) and PTHrP-(1-34) have little secondary structure. In the presence of organic solvents or lipids, there is a dramatic increase in the α-helical content of the peptides. A common three-

dimensional model has been proposed for both PTH-(1-34) and PTHrP-(1-34) in which amino- and carboxy-terminal α-helical domains align side by side in antiparallel fashion with inwardly facing hydrophobic residues forming a core. Hydrophilic residues comprise a loop connecting the helices and also line their outer surfaces.

2.2. PTH Receptor Gene

Like other peptide hormones, PTH and PTHrP bind receptors on the plasma membrane of target cells. The PTH/PTHrP receptor belongs to a new subgroup of the G-protein-coupled seven-transmembrane-spanning receptor superfamily that, by virtue of their structural similarities, also includes the receptors binding secretin, calcitonin, vasoactive intestinal peptide, glucagon, glucagon-like peptide I, and growth hormone-releasing hormone.

2.2.1. Structure

The rat, mouse, and human PTH/PTHrP receptor genes have a similar complex organization and possess at least 17 exons. The first three exons encode two different 5'-untranslated regions of the mRNA, and the remaining 14 exons encode the receptor (Fig. 8). This has 585–593 amino acids depending on species. Four exons encode portions of the extracellular domain, and eight exons encode the seven predicted transmembrane domain. This arrangement is not only well conserved within species, but is also very similar to that of related subgroup family members, such as the growth hormone-releasing factor receptor, calcitonin receptor, and glucagon receptor genes. This suggests that these receptor genes evolved from a common precursor.

Both promoters in the PTH/PTHrP receptor gene lack a consensus TATA element, and the downstream promoter is (G + C)-rich, containing several Sp-1 sites. In contrast, the upstream promoter is not (G + C)-rich, but does possess a CCAAT box. Whereas transcripts derived from the downstream promoter are widely expressed in many tissues, the upstream promoter is highly tissue-specific, being strongly active in kidney and weakly active in liver, but not expressed at all in other tissues. The regulatory regions responsible for this tissue-specific expression are unknown.

The PTH/PTHrP receptor gene maps to human chromosome 3p21.1–p22 and to mouse chromosome 9 and rat chromosome 8, which are highly homologous and show synteny conservation with human chromosome 3.

2.2.2. REGULATION

Homologous downregulation of PTH/PTHrP receptors by PTH is observed in bone and kidney cells. This may explain, in part, the well-recognized resistance to PTH action in primary and secondary hyperparathyroidism. Posttranscriptional mechanisms, such as receptor–ligand recycling and membrane reinsertion, are most likely involved, since the steady-state levels of PTH/PTHrP receptor mRNA are unaltered by PTH exposure. Heterologous regulation of the PTH receptor also occurs. For example, glucocorticoids increase and decrease PTH/PTHrP receptors in bone cells and kidney cells, respectively. $1,25(OH)_2D$ and retinoic acid decrease PTH receptors in bone cells. In these cases of heterologous regulation, parallel changes in the steady-state receptor mRNA levels have been observed, implicating direct effects on gene transcription and/or mRNA stability. The elements in the PTH/PTHrP receptor gene responsive to nuclear receptors, which mediate the actions of these ligands, remain to be identified.

2.2.3. SPECIES COMPARISON

The primary structure of the PTH/PTHrP receptor has been elucidated for several mammalian species including human, rat, mouse, and opossum. There is a high degree of conservation with the greatest divergence between rat and opossum whose sequences are 78% identical. The most striking differences in sequence are in parts of the amino-terminal extracellular region, and the first intracellular loop and the intracellular carboxy-terminal domain. Other parts of the amino-terminal extracellular region and the membrane-spanning regions are especially well conserved. Cysteine residues in the amino-terminal extension and in each of the first two putative extracellular loops, as well as potential asparagine-linked glycosylation sites in the extracellular domain, are highly conserved not only in the PTH/PTHrP receptor among species, but also in other members of the subgroup of G-protein-coupled receptors described above.

2.3. Embryology, Cytogenesis

Humans have two pairs of parathyroid glands lying in the anterior cervical region, which are of endodermal origin, being derived from the third and fourth pharyngeal pouches. Rats have a single pair of glands embedded in the cranial part of the thyroid. The chief cell is the predominant cell type in human with some oxyphil cells, which have an acidophilic cytoplasm and mitochondria, also present. The chief cell only is present in rat. Parathyroid cells have limited numbers of secretory granules containing PTH, indicating that relatively little hormone is stored in the gland. Parathyroid cells normally divide at an extremely slow rate—mitoses are rarely observed.

2.4. PTH Secretion

The NH_2-terminal 25-residue portion of prepro-PTH, characterized by its hydrophobicity, is called the signal or presequence, and facilitates entry of the nascent hormone into the cisternae of the endoplasmic reticulum to begin its journey through the regulated secretory pathway. After removal of the signal sequence, the resultant pro-PTH molecule—extended at the NH_2-terminus of PTH-(1-84) by six amino acids—is transported to the Golgi apparatus. In the trans-Golgi, pro-PTH is converted to PTH by the action of furin, one of the recently described mammalian proprotein convertases that are related to bacterial subtilisins. Little pro-PTH is stored within the gland, and the mature 84-amino acid form of the hormone is packaged in secretory granules. The hormone is released by exocytosis in response to the principal stimulus to secretion, hypocalcemia.

2.4.1. CALCIUM

In the absence of a stimulus for release, intraglandular metabolism of PTH occurs, causing complete degradation to its constituent amino acids or partial degradation to fragments through a calcium-regulated enzymatic mechanism. In the case of hypercalcemia, the predominant hormonal entities released from the gland are biologically inactive fragments composed of mid-region and COOH-terminal sequences. In response to hypocalcemia, degradation of PTH within the parathyroid cell is minimized, and the major hormonal entity released is the bioactive PTH-(1-84) molecule. Thus, in the presence of hypocalcemia, increased amounts of bioactive PTH are secreted even in the absence of immediate additional synthesis of hormone. Hormone stores are insufficient, however, to maintain secretion for more than a few hours, and other mechanisms—transcriptional and posttranscriptional—come into play to increase hormone production. In the presence of a sustained severe hypocalcemic stimulus, additional PTH secretion depends on an increase in the number of parathyroid cells. Such an increase may also be stimulated by the reduction in circulating 1,25-dihydroxyvitamin D that often accompanies hypocalcemia. Normally, the sterol inhibits parathyroid cell proliferation by inhibiting expression of early immediate response genes, such as the *MYC* proto-oncogene.

There is an inverse relationship between ambient calcium levels and PTH release that is curvilinear rather than proportional. This relationship between PTH and extracellular calcium is in stark contrast to the influence of the calcium ion as a secretagogue in most other secretory systems in which elevations in this ion enhance release of the secretory product. This distinction between the parathyroid cell and other secretory cells is maintained intracellularly, where elevations rather than decreases in cytosol calcium correlate with decreased PTH release. Alterations in extracellular fluid calcium levels are transmitted through a parathyroid plasma membrane calcium-sensing receptor that couples through a G-protein complex to phospholipase C. Increases in extracellular calcium lead to increases in inositol 1,4,5-trisphosphate (IP_3) and mobilization of intracellular calcium stores. The manner in which this inhibits hormone secretion is not understood.

2.4.2. 1,25-DIHYDROXYVITAMIN D

Vitamin D metabolites modulate PTH release. There is a feedback loop between PTH-induced increase in 1,25-dihydroxyvitamin D and vitamin D metabolite-induced decrease of PTH levels. Although 1,25-dihydroxyvitamin D is of uncertain importance in influencing immediate hormone release, it plays a role in modulating hormone synthesis within the gland, by direct action on prepro-PTH gene transcription, thus altering the quantities of hormone available for immediate release by secretagogues.

2.4.3. OTHER FACTORS

In addition to calcium and vitamin D metabolites, several other factors influence the release of PTH from parathyroid glands. The cation magnesium affects PTH release like calcium, although with reduced efficacy. High concentrations of aluminum also suppress PTH release. Hyperphosphatemia is associated with increased circulating levels of PTH, an effect that is almost certainly indirect and a result of the hypocalcemia that accompanies the rise in serum phosphate. However, the issue of a direct action of the anion on PTH secretion continues to be actively debated. Glucocorticoids increase PTH secretion Such agents as biogenic amines, which increase parathyroid gland cAMP levels, induce PTH secretion, and those that lower cAMP levels within the parathyroid gland decrease PTH secretion. Peptides derived from chromogranin A (CgA), inhibit low-calcium-stimulated PTH release from parathyroid cells in culture. The physiological significance of these observations is unclear.

2.5. PTH Action

The major function of PTH is the maintenance of a normal level of extracellular fluid calcium. The hormone exerts direct effects on bone and kidney, and indirectly influences the gastrointestinal tract. In response to a fall in the extracellular fluid ionized calcium concentration, PTH is released from the parathyroid cell, and acts on the kidney to enhance renal calcium reabsorption and promote the conversion of 25-hydroxyvitamin D to 1,25-dihydroxyvitamin D. This active metabolite increases gastrointestinal absorption of calcium and with PTH, induces skeletal resorption, causing the restoration of extracellular fluid calcium and the neutralization of the signal initi-

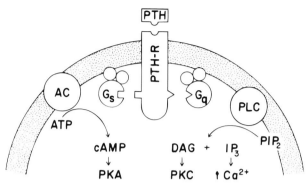

Fig. 9. PTH/PTHrP receptors can activate two intracellular signaling pathways. G$_s$ couples to adenyl cyclase (AC) and stimulates production of cAMP, which activates protein kinase A (PKA). G$_q$ couples to phospholipase C (PLC) to form inositol-(1,4,5)-triphosphate (IP$_3$) and diacylglycerol (DAG) from phosphatidylinositol-(4,5)-biphosphate (PIP$_2$). IP$_3$ releases calcium (Ca^{2+}) from intracellular stores, and DAG stimulates protein kinase C (PKC) activity. Each heterotrimeric G-protein comprises a unique α subunit and βγ-dimer (Levine et al., 1994).

ating PTH release. PTH also perturbs the extracellular concentration of other ions, the most important of which is phosphate. As a consequence of PTH-enhanced 1,25-dihydroxyvitamin D production, the gastrointestinal absorption of phosphate is increased to some extent, and with PTH-induced skeletal lysis, extracellular phosphate as well as calcium levels are increased. PTH acts to inhibit renal phosphate reabsorption producing phosphaturia and a net decrease in extracellular fluid phosphate concentration. The phosphaturic action of PTH is a classic manifestation of renal PTH responsiveness.

In target tissues, the result of interaction of PTH with the plasma membrane PTH/PTHrP receptor has classically been appreciated to be the stimulation of the enzyme adenylate cyclase on the inner surface of the plasma membrane, although the same receptor can couple to phosphatidylinositol turnover as well (Fig. 9). The product of this adenylate cyclase activity, cellular cAMP, and the products of phospholipase activity, IP$_3$, diacylglycerol, and intracellular Ca^{2+}, initiate a cascade of events leading to the final cellular response to the hormone. Whether the PTH/PTHrP receptor activates both these intracellular signaling pathways equivalently in all target tissues or acts preferentially by means of one or other pathway in different cells is unknown.

2.5.1. BONE

The best-documented effect of PTH is a catabolic one, which results in the breakdown of mineral constituents and bone matrix, as manifested by the release of calcium and phosphate, by increases in plasma and urinary hydroxyproline, and other indices of bone resorption. This process is mediated by osteoclastic osteolysis, but the mechanism is unclear, since PTH does not apparently bind directly to multinucleated osteoclasts. However, the PTH/PTHrP receptor is expressed on osteoblasts, and PTH stimulates second messenger accumulation in osteoblast-enriched populations of cells from skeletal tissues and in osteosarcoma cells of the osteoblast lineage. It is suggested that PTH-induced stimulation of multinucleated osteoclasts occurs through the action of PTH-stimulated osteoblast activity via intermediary factors.

The consequences of the effects of PTH on osteoblast activity are complex. The examination of bone after in vivo PTH administration has demonstrated an increase in osteoblasts and new bone formation, indicating that PTH may also play an anabolic role under some circumstances. Whether the anabolic and catabolic effects of PTH on osteoblasts represent direct and indirect effects, effects of different domains of the PTH molecule, discrete functions of morphologically similar, but functionally distinct osteoblasts, or differences in hormonal effects based on different times of exposure or different hormone concentrations remains to be determined.

2.5.2. KIDNEY

PTH has diverse actions on the renal tubule, most of which can be mimicked by infusion of cAMP onto the luminal aspect of tubular cells. This is consistent with cAMP's postulated role as a second messenger for many renal responses. Nevertheless, it is evident that inositol phosphates and intracellular calcium also play an important role in the renal action of PTH.

PTH-induced inhibition of phosphate reabsorption is localized to the proximal convoluted tubule and the pars recta. The proximal tubule is the major site of action of PTH in stimulating the 1α-hydroxylase and increasing the production of 1,25-dihydroxy vitamin D. The important site of PTH action to increase calcium and magnesium transport is the thick ascending limb of the loop of Henle, and the distal convoluted tubule and earliest portion of the cortical collecting duct.

2.5.3. OTHER TARGET TISSUES

Hepatocyte binding of PTH has been associated with adenylate cyclase stimulation and may reflect PTH-enhanced gluconeogenesis. Other actions of PTH include effects on vascular tone, stimulation or inhibition of mitosis of various cells in vitro, promoting increased concentrations of calcium in mammary and in salivary glands, and enhancing lipolysis in isolated fat cells. The widespread expression of the PTHrP gene and the equally broad expression of the PTH/PTHrP receptor gene suggest that many of the noncalcemic actions ascribed to PTH may be carried out by PTHrP acting in an autocrine or paracrine manner.

2.6. Pathophysiology of Hypersecretion/ Hyposecretion/Receptor Defects

2.6.1. HYPERPARATHYROIDISM

Abnormally increased parathyroid gland activity may be primary or secondary. Primary hyperparathyroidism is associated with hyperplasia and neoplasia, with the latter being predominantly the result of adenomas—parathyroid carcinoma is extremely rare. Parathyroid adenomas are monoclonal involving molecular genetic derangements, such as loss of the multiple endocrine neoplasia (MEN) Type I gene locus on chromosome 11q13 thought to encode a tumor suppressor gene, loss of another putative tumor suppressor gene on chromosome 1p, or overexpression of the cyclin D1 gene on chromosome 11q. Hyperparathyroidism may occur as part of rare familial syndromes, which include MEN Type 1, MEN type 2A, Familial Hypocalciuric Hypercalcemia (FHH), and Neonatal Severe Hyperparathyroidism (NSHPT).

Almost 20 inactivating mutations scattered throughout the parathyroid calcium-sensing receptor gene (CASR) located on chromosome 3q13.3–21 have been described in FHH and NSHPT. These might disrupt biosynthesis of the protein or its targeting to the plasma membrane. Mutations within the extracellular domain could modify the ligand-binding properties of the receptor, and those within transmembrane and cytoplasmic domains could disrupt coupling with G-proteins and subsequent activation of signal transduction pathways. Mutations in

the CASR gene itself do not contribute to sporadic parathyroid tumorigenesis. However, it is likely that mutations in other genes important in determining the calcium set point will be implicated in abnormal parathyroid cell proliferation.

Mice heterozygous for deletion of the CASR gene demonstrate a phenotype analogous to that of humans with FHH, and homozygous animals, like humans with NSHPT, demonstrate more markedly elevated serum calcium and PTH levels, parathyroid hyperplasia, bone abnormalities, and premature death.

Excess circulating parathyroid hormone leads to altered function of bone cells, renal tubules, and gastrointestinal mucosa. This may result in kidney stones and calcium deposits in renal tubules, and decalcification of bone, resulting in bone pain and tenderness and spontaneous fractures. The hypercalcemia may also lead to muscle weakness and gastrointestinal symptoms.

Secondary hyperparathyroidism occurs when the extracellular fluid calcium and/or 1,25-dihydroxy vitamin D levels fall below normal, as in chronic renal disease or vitamin D deficiency. Tertiary hyperparathyroidism refers to the condition that ensues when a parathyroid adenoma arises from the secondary hyperplasia caused by chronic renal failure.

2.6.2. HYPOPARATHYROIDISM

There are a variety of causes of hypoparathyroidism in which the deficiency of PTH secretion results in hypocalcemia and hyperphosphatemia. Isolated or idiopathic hypoparathyroidism develops as a solitary endocrinopathy: familial forms occur with either autosomal-dominant, autosomal-recessive, or X-linked recessive modes of inheritance. In some cases of familial autosomal hypoparathyroidism, inactivating mutations in the PTH gene have been identified, and in other cases, activating mutations in the parathyroid calcium-sensing receptor have been documented. Hypoparathyroidism may also occur as a part of a pluriglandular autoimmune disorder or as a complex congenital defect, including the DiGeorge, Kenny-Caffey, or Barakat syndromes, among others.

2.6.3. PSEUDOHYPOPARATHYROIDISM

This term describes a heterogeneous collection of conditions characterized by biochemical hypoparathyroidism—hypocalcemia and hyperphosphatemia—but increased circulating PTH levels and target tissue unresponsiveness to PTH. Patients with pseudohypoparathyroidism (PHP) Type 1a exhibit a distinctive physical appearance, referred to as Albright's hereditary osteodystrophy (AHO) characterized by distinctive skeletal and development defects. The urinary cAMP and phosphorous response to PTH is defective, and serum calcium levels are low. There is a generalized hormone resistance. However, within families, some affected members may show all the above features, whereas others manifest only the features of AHO with no evidence of biochemical abnormalities—so-called pseudo-pseudohypoparathyroidism (pseudo-PHP). The trait is inherited in an autosomal-dominant fashion, and affected individuals demonstrate reduced $G_s\alpha$ activity, and carry mutations in the $G_s\alpha$ gene. In contrast, PHP Type 1b patients have a normal appearance, and the hormone resistance is limited to PTH target tissues. Despite extensive analysis, mutations in the PTH/PTHrP receptor gene have not been identified in patients with PHP Type 1b. Therefore, mutations in genes for other proteins involved in the PTH/PTHrP signaling pathway are most likely responsible for the defects.

2.6.4. RECEPTOR DEFECTS

Ablation of the PTHrP gene in mice is lethal with death occurring in the perinatal period. Likewise, knockout of the PTH/PTHrP receptor gene leads to an even more severe phenotype with few fetuses surviving to term. These animals manifest extensive skeletal abnormalities owing to impaired endochondral ossification, which is the highly organized process responsible for longitudinal growth of bones during embryogenesis and early postnatal life. Both PTHrP and the PTH/PTHrP receptor are expressed in proliferating chondrocytes, but not by terminally differentiated chondrocytes. In PTHrP-less mice, the chondroplastic phenotype results from disruption of multiple stages of chondrogenesis, from reduced cellular proliferation to premature terminal differentiation and programmed cell death. This results in premature ossification of the developing skeleton. Thus, PTHrP normally maintains chondrocytic cells in a dedifferentiated state and protects them from apoptosis. This latter property may be the result in part of PTHrP's ability to localize to the nucleolus, which is mediated by a func-

tional nucleolar targeting signal sequence located in the midregion of the molecule.

In contrast to the PTHrP-less mice, patients with Jansen-Type metaphyseal chondrodysplasia (JMC) with short-limbed dwarfism demonstrate little ossification at the chondro-osseous junctions of their long bones. They also manifest features of hyperparathyroidism, such as severe hypercalcemia and hypophosphatemia, despite normal or undetectable levels of circulating PTH and PTHrP. Recently, JMC patients have been found to be heterozygous for "activating" missense mutations in either the first intracellular loop (H223R) or the sixth transmembrane domain (T410P) of the PTH/PTHrP receptor. This provides evidence that the PTH/PTHrP receptor does indeed mediate both the endocrine actions of PTH, and the autocrine or paracrine actions of PTHrP necessary for orderly endochondral bone formation.

2.7. PTH Measurement

Circulating PTH is heterogeneous. The major circulating bioactive moiety is similar or identical to intact PTH-(1–84). This is metabolized by the liver, which releases midregion and COOH-terminal fragments into the circulation for subsequent clearance by the kidney. These biologically inert moieties generated by metabolism and secretion from the parathyroid gland are cleared more slowly than intact PTH, and comprise the majority of the circulating immunoreactive PTH. Circulating bioactive PTH is best measured by sensitive immunometric assays that simultaneously recognize NH_2 and COOH epitopes on the PTH molecule, and detect only intact PTH-(1–84). This is the method of choice for the accurate diagnosis of patients with hypercalcemia, especially in distinguishing patients with primary hyperparathyroidism from those with hypercalcemia of malignancy (Fig. 10).

2.8. Summary

PTH is the key polypeptide hormone responsible for minute-to-minute maintenance of calcium homeostasis. PTHrP plays a critical role in development, especially skeletogenesis, but is not involved in normal calcium homeostatic control in the adult. Both factors act through the PTH/PTHrP receptor, which is widely expressed, and signals through multiple second messenger pathways. Recently, a related receptor that responds only to PTH has been identified that has a very restricted tissue distribution—it

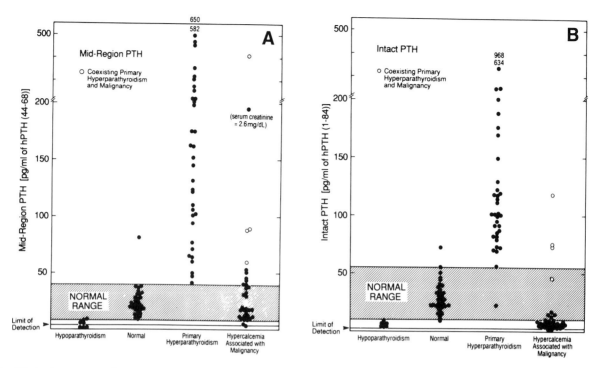

Fig. 10. An immunometric two-site assay measuring intact PTH (right panel) is the method of choice in differentiating patients with primary hyperparathyroidism from those with hypercalcemia associated with malignancy. This type of assay does not register circulating mid- and COOH-terminal bioinactive PTH fragments as do other types of assay (e.g., the midregion assay—left panel). Four patients (open circles) had coexisting hyperparathyroidism and cancer (Nussbaum and Potts, 1994).

is expressed in brain, but not bone or kidney and, therefore, cannot mediate the calcemic actions of PTH. However, it is likely that other receptors exist that specifically mediate the actions of PTH or PTHrP.

REFERENCES

Clemens TL, Adams JS. Vitamin D and metabolites. In: Favus MJ ed. *Primer on the Metabolic Bone Diseases and Disorders of Mineral Metabolism*. 2nd ed., New York: Raven Press, 1993:103.

Goltzman D, Hendy GN. Parathyroid hormone. In: Becker KL, ed. *Principles and Practice of Endocrinology and Metabolism*, 2nd ed. Philadelphia: JB Lippincott, 1995:455.

Haussler MR, Jurutka PW, Hsieh J-C, Thompson PD, Selznick SH, Haussler CA, Whitfield GK. New understanding of the molecular mechanism of receptor-mediated genomic actions of the vitamin D hormone. *Bone* 1995; 17 suppl:33S.

Levine MA, Schwindinger WF, Downs RW Jr, Moses AM. Pseudohypoparathyroidism. Clinical, biochemical, and molecular features. In: Bilezikian JP, Marcus R, Levine MA, eds. *The Parathyroids. Basic and Clinical Concepts*. New York: Raven, 1994:781.

Minghetti PP, Norman AW. 1,25(OH)$_2$-Vitamin D$_3$ receptors: gene regulation and genetic circuitry. *FASEB J* 1988; 2:3043.

Nussbaum SR, Potts JT Jr. Advances in immunoassays for parathyroid hormone. Clinical applications to skeletal disor-

ders of bone and mineral metabolism. In: Bilezikian JP, Marcus R, Levine MA, eds. *The Parathyroids. Basic and Clinical Concepts*. New York: Raven, 1994:157.

Papapoulos SE, Lewin IG, Clemens TL, Hendy GN, O'Riordan JLH. Vitamin D. In: Gray CH, James VHT, eds. *Hormones in Blood*. 3rd ed., vol 3. London: Academic, 1979:53.

Pike JW. Molecular mechanisms of cellular response to the vitamin D$_3$ hormone. In: Coe FL, Favus MJ, eds. *Disorders of Bone and Mineral Metabolism*. New York: Raven, 1992:163.

Yu J, Papavasiliou V, Rhim J, Goltzman D, Kremer R. Vitamin D analogs: new therapeutic agents for the treatment of squamous cancer and its associated hypercalcemia. *Anti-Cancer Drugs* 1995; 6:101

SELECTED READINGS

Bassett JHD, Thakker RV. Molecular genetics of calcium homeostasis. In: Thakker RV, ed. *Genetic and Molecular Biological Aspects of Endocrine Disease. Baillière's Clinical Endocrinology and Metabolism*. London: Baillière Tindall, 1995:581.

Bilezikian JP, Marcus R, Levine MA, eds. *The Parathyroids. Basic and Clinical Concepts*. New York: Raven, 1994.

Bouillon R, Okamura WH, Norman AW. Structure–function relationships in the vitamin D endocrine system. *Endocr Rev* 1995; 16:200.

Brown EM, Pollak M, Seidman CE, Seidman JG, Chou Y-HC, Riccardi D, Hebert SC. Calcium-sensing cell-surface receptors. *N Engl J Med* 1995; 333:234.

Favus MJ, ed. *Primer on Metabolic Bone Diseases and Disorders of Mineral Metabolism*, 3rd ed. New York: Raven, 1996.

Halloran BP, Nissenson RA, eds. *Parathyroid Hormone-Related Peptide: Normal Physiology and Its Role in Cancer*. Boca Raton: CRC, 1992.

Hendy GN, Arnold A. Molecular basis of PTH overexpression. In: Bilezikian JP, Raisz LG, Rodan GA, eds. *Principles of Bone Biology*. San Diego: Academic, 1996:757.

Holick MF. Noncalcemic actions of 1,25-dihydroxyvitamin D_3 and clinical applications. *Bone* 1995; 17 suppl:107S.

Orloff JF, Stewart AF. Editorial: The carboxy-terminus of parathyroid hormone—inert or invaluable? *Endocrinology* 1995; 136:4729.

Ross TK, Darwish HM, Deluca HF. Molecular biology of vitamin D action. *Vitam Horm* 1994; 49:281.

21 The Endocrine System of the Gastrointestinal Tract

Gary A. Wittert, MB, BCh, MD, Robert Fraser, MB, BS, PhD, and John E. Morley, MB, BCh

CONTENTS

1. INTRODUCTION

The movement of food through the gastrointestinal tract requires coordination with the processes of digestion and absorption. Integration is also achieved with energy balance, fat storage, appetite regulation, and memory. The gut is exposed to the exterior, and mucosal integrity must be maintained. In order to accomplish this, a complex control system has evolved. The complexities of this system have led to it being characterized as the little brain. This involves a specialized enteric nervous system and an enteroendocrine system, which are integrated with each other and have a bidirectional communication with the central nervous system. This integration may at least in part be the result of the evolution of a common pool of messenger peptides and receptors.

2. THE ENTEROENDOCRINE CELL SYSTEM

Enteroendocrine cells make up <1% of intestinal epithelial cells, but comprise the largest and most complex endocrine organ of the mammalian body.

From: *Endocrinology: Basic and Clinical Principles* (P. M. Conn and S. Melmed, eds.), Humana Press Inc., Totowa, NJ.

There are at least 16 subpopulations of enteroendocrine cells based on major peptide and/or amine products (Table 1). Enteroendocrine cells differentiate from pluripotent stem cells, which are of endodermal origin. These cells are distinguished by their ability to produce peptide hormones from amine precursors. Some of the endocrine cells are oriented with their apices exposed to the gut lumen and may function to detect luminal stimuli, such as nutrients, hormones released into the lumen, or those present in food, for example, exorphins. These cells are referred to as "open." Others are "closed." The peptides released from enteroendocrine cells may function in a classic endocrine (for example, gastrin, secretin, and cholecystokinin) or, alternatively, a paracrine fashion (for example, somatostatin). Some peptides function in an autocrine fashion, for example, to modulate their own release (Fig. 1).

3. THE ENTERIC NERVOUS SYSTEM (ENS)

The (ENS) is a network of neurons and supporting cells embryologically derived from neural crest, which is found in the intestine, gallbladder, and pancreas. Neuroblasts, from the neural crest,

Table 1
Hormones of the Gastrointestinal Tract

Hormone	Chromosomal location	Cellular site	Released by	Functions
Gastrin/CCK family				
Gastrin	17	G (gastric antrum)	Aromatic amino Small peptides Calcium	Gastric acid Secretion
Cholecystokinin	3	I (small intestine)	Fat Protein	Inhibits gastric emptying Pancreatic enzyme secretion Gallbladder emptying Satiation Memory enhancement
Secretin family				
Secretin		S (proximal small intestine)	Acid Bile Fatty acids Peptides	Pancreatic bicarbonate and enzyme secretion Stimulates hepatic bile secretion
Vasoactive intestinal peptide	6	Enteric nerves		Lower esophageal sphincter relaxation Adaptive relaxation of the fundus Decending relaxation of the intestine Stimulates water and electrolyte secretion from colon Stimulates biliary and pancreatic secretion Promotes lipolysis
Gastric-inhibitory polypeptide	17	K (duodenum and upper jejunium)	Glucose Proteins Amino acids Fatty acids Fatty acids	Stimulates insulin secretion Inhibits gastric acid secretion
Glucagon-like peptide	2	L (intestine, colon, rectum) A (pancreatic)	Glucose Amino acids	Insulinotropic effect Inhibitor of gastric motility
The pancreatic polypeptide family				
Pancreatic polypeptide	17	D and F (pancreas)	Fat Protein	Inhibits pancreatic excretion
Peptide YY	17	L (distal small intestine, colon, rectum, pancreas)	Fatty acids Bile acids Amino acids	Inhibits acid and pepsin and secretion from stomach, water, and chloride from jejunum Slows small intestinal transit time Inhibits pancreatic exocrine secretion

(continued)

Table 1 *(continued)*

Hormone	Chromosomal location	Cellular site	Released by	Functions
Neuropeptide Y	7	Submucosal enteric nerves		Inhibits colonic motor activity weight loss NPY inhibits gastric and small intestinal motility and secretion Centrally is a potent enhancer of food intake
Miscellaneous Neurotensin	20	N (ileum and jejunum)	Fat	Inhibits gastric and pancreatic secretion Stimulates colonic motility
Galanin	11	Enteric nerves	Intestinal distension	Inhibits gastric emptying Slows colonic transit time Increases food intake (centrally)
Gastrin-releasing peptide	18	Enteric nerves	Cholinergic stimulation	Stimulates gastrin release Contracts lower esophageal sphincter
Motilin	6	M (duodenum)	Acidification of duodenum Gastric distension	Regulates phase III migratory motor complexes Gall Bladder contraction Releases pepsinogen
Thyrotropin-releasing hormone	3	B (pancreas) G (stomach) Enteric nerves		Inhibits gastric acid Inhibits amylase and lipase Stimulates intestinal smooth muscle Inhibits cholesterol synthesis in intestinal mucosa
Calcitonin gene-related hormone	12	Sensory nerves Enteric nerves	Glucose	Vasodilation
Somatostatin	3	D (stomach, pancreas) Enteric nerves	Acid Exorphins	Inhibition of peptide hormone, fluid, and electrolyte secretion Pancreatic enzyme secretion and gut motility

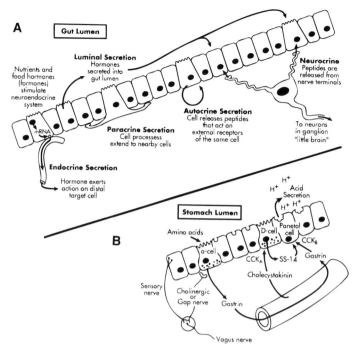

Figure 1. A. Examples of the different mechanisms by which gut peptides effect cells. **B**. Mechanisms involved in regulation of gastric acid secretion from the stomach lumen. CCK_A = cholecystokinin, CCK_B = cholecystokinin, SS = somatostatin, H^+ = hydrogen ion.

migrate from proximal to distal in the gut during fetal life, and develop interconnected neuronal networks or plexuses. Two major types of plexuses are present in the intestinal tract: myenteric, which control peristaltic activity, and submucosal, which are mainly responsible for controlling secretion and absorption.

Based on neurotransmitter content, six different types of enteric neurons have been identified: cholinergic (acetylcholine), adrenergic (norepinephrine), serotonergic (5HT), GABAergic, peptidergic, and those containing nitric oxide (NO). NO is predominantly colocalized with peptide neurotransmitters, such as vasoactive intestinal peptide (VIP). This type of communication has been characterized as neurocrine. The neuropetides of the ENS are summarized in Table 2. The neuropeptides are released from the nerve terminals and reach their target cells by crossing a short synaptic gap.

4. THE GASTROINTESTINAL PEPTIDES AND THEIR FUNCTIONS

The gastrointestinal peptides are grouped into families, based on structural homology and mechanisms of

release and action. Members of a family may function as neurotransmitters, hormones, or both. Five identifiable families include those related to gastrin, secretin, pancreatic polypeptide, tachykinin (Chapter 7), and Opioids (Chapter 5). A miscellaneous group includes motilin, galanin, neurotensin, gastrin-releasing peptide (GRP), thryrotropin-releasing peptide, and a group of novel lumenal peptides.

4.1. The Gastrin/ Cholecystokinin (CCK) Family

Gastrin and CCK are synthesized in the G- and L-cells of the gut, respectively. The gastrin and CCK genes both consist of three exons that are intervened by two introns at almost identical positions. Gastrin and CCK have probably evolved by gene duplication of a primordial transcription unit. The α-amidated carboxyl-terminal pentapeptide sequence of CCK is identical to that of gastrin and is crucial for biological activity. The unique CCK-like activity depends on the position and posttranslational sulfation of a tyrosine residue toward the amino-terminus of this pentapeptide. In birds, unlike mammals, the amino sequences of gastrin and CCK have evolved in differ-

Table 2
Substances that Act Principally
as Neuropeptides of the ENS

Tachykinins	*Endogenous opioids*
Substance P	Enkephalins
Substance K	Dynorphin
Neuromedin K	β-Endorphin
Secretin family	*Other*
VIP	Galanin
PHI/PHM	GRP
PP family	CGRP
Neuro NPY	TRH

ent ways. The structure of chicken gastrin is similar to mammalian CCK rather than to mammalian gastrin.

4.1.1. GASTRIN

Gastrin was the first gastrointestinal hormone to have its sequence determined. Gastrin is mainly expressed in G-cells, which are "open" neuroedocrine cells scattered throughout the mucosa of the gastric antrum.

4.1.2. GENE

The human gene encoding gastrin spans 4.1 kb, consists of 3 exons, and is located on chromosome 17. The mouse gastrin gene is 2.6 kb. The rat gastrin gene is comparable in size to the mouse. The overall organization of the gene across species is similar, and the difference relates to the size of the first intron. The first exon is noncoding, the second exon encodes the signal peptide and propeptide sequence, and the third exon encodes the bioactive hexadecapeptide and carboxyl-terminal extension peptide. Gastrin mRNA is 0.6 kb in size and encodes a pre-progastrin precursor of 101 amino acids in the human, mouse, and rat. Gastrin exists in several biologically active molecular forms, G34, G17, and G14. Sites of processing are highly conserved between species. In humans, big gastrin (G34) and little gastrin (G17) are the most abundant circulating forms of gastrin.

The promoter region of the gastrin gene contains sequences known to bind AP2 and a mammalian homolog of the yeast transcription factor RAP1. There is also an element responsible for induction by epidermal growth factor (EGF) in the human, but not the mouse or rat gene. Nevertheless, the mouse promoter is responsive to EGF. The gastrin gene promoter also has a negative element (the gastrin-negative element), which is adjacent to an E-box element. Developmental changes in the pattern of gastrin gene expression have been demonstrated in the stomach, colon, and pancreas. In the rat fetus, the pancreas is the major site of gastrin gene expression. A similar phenomenon is noted for Peptide YY (PYY). RAP1 and the CACC-binding protein may be important in pancreas-specific gastrin gene expression.

Achlorhydria results in a four-fold increase in gastrin mRNA, via an effect both at the level of transcription and stability of mRNA. Somatostatin directly inhibits gastrin mRNA accumulation. The constant inhibitory effect of somatostatin on the G-cell includes an action at the level of gene expression. The effect of cAMP to upregulate gastrin gene expression is inhibited by somatostatin.

4.1.3. RELEASE

Gastrin is released from antral G-cells in response to partially digested food. Aromatic amino acids, small peptides, and calcium are potent stimulants for gastrin release. Coffee, wine, and beer also stimulate gastrin release, an effect unrelated to the presence of alcohol or caffeine. Fat and glucose do not stimulate gastrin release. Stimulation by cholinegic, β-adrenergic, GRPergic, and GABA neurons also results in gastrin release. Somatostatin released from neighboring D-cells in response to acidification is a major inhibitor of gastrin release.

4.1.4. RECEPTOR

The gastrin receptor has been cloned and is identical to the CCK-B receptor, which is discussed below.

4.1.5. ACTIONS

The most important physiological action of gastrin is to stimulate gastric acid secretion in response to a meal. Gastrin also plays a role in mediating the acid secretory response to gastric distension, but only a minor role in mediating the cephalic phase of gastric secretion. Gastrin exerts a trophic effect on gastric mucosa. Pharmacologic actions of gastrin include an increase in contractility of the lower esophageal sphincter, gastric antrum, small intestine, and colon. Whether gastrin has any physiological role as a mediator of gut motility is unclear. Gastrin may also have a role in the development and growth of the gastrointestinal tract.

4.2. CCK

CCK was first demonstrated to exist when duodenal extracts were shown to stimulate gallbladder contractility. Subsequently, hormonal activity from extracts of jejunal mucosa was shown to increase pancreatic secretion.

4.2.1. GENE

The CCK gene was first cloned from a rat medullary thyroid carcinoma. The human CCK gene spans 7 kb, is located on chromosome 3, and is expressed in both the brain and the gut of all vertebrate classes. The CCK gene encodes a 94 amino acid residue prohormone. The amino acid sequence of prepro-CCK is highly homologous in the rat, pig, dog, and human. The most highly conserved portion, CCK-33, which includes the residues necessary for biological activity, is encoded by exon 3. Exon 2 encodes the signal peptide and the prohormone portion. The 5′-untranslated region is coded for by exon 1. CCK is processed to CCK-83, 58, 39, 33, 22, 8, and 5, all sharing identical carboxyltermini. The processing of prepro-CCK occurs in a tissue-specific fashion. The major active form of the hormone is an octopeptide containing a sulfated tyrosine and an amidated carboxyl-terminal phenylalanine.

Activation of both the cAMP/protein kinase A (pKA), and the protein kinase C (pKC) second messenger pathways results, in increased CCK mRNA levels in vitro. In rats, CCK mRNA levels ad peptide release increase in the intestine in response to antagonism of the CCK-A receptor. Bile/pancreatic juice diversion stimulates gene expression of both CCK, and secretin and both CCK and secretin are involved in luminal feedback regulation. CCK mRNA levels increase in response to cytotoxic injury of the intestine in rats.

CCK is found in the I-cells of the proximal small intestine. CCK is also found in nerve fibers branching to gastric and colonic myenteric ganglia, submucosal ganglia, and smooth muscle. In the brain, CCK is present in high levels in the cerebral cortex and limbic system.

4.2.2. SECRETION

CCK is released from I-cells in the small intestine in response to the presence of intraluminal nutrients, specifically fat and protein. GRP and bombesin also stimulate CCK release.

4.2.3. RECEPTORS

Two forms of CCK receptors have been identified, the CCK-A (alimentary) receptor and the CCK-B (brain) receptor. The CCK-A and CCK-B receptors share 48% homology at the amino acid level, and have both been cloned from the rat, guinea pig, and human. Each receptor is highly conserved between species. They are both seven-transmembrane domain G-protein-coupled receptors. The parietal cell gastrin receptor has recently been cloned and is identical to the CCK-B receptor. The CCK-B gene has been cloned from the human and consists of five exons interrupted by four introns. The gene appears to be alternately spliced to yield two different receptor isoforms which differ by five amino acids in the putative third intracellular loop. The human CCK-A and CCK-B receptors are located on chromosomes 4 and 11, respectively. In the mouse, the CCK-A receptor has been mapped to chromosome 5 and the CCK-B receptor has been mapped to chromosome 7, in the same region as the obesity mutation *tub*, which identifies this gene as a candidate gene for the tubby mutation. Both the CCK-A and CCK-B/gastrin receptor couple to phosopholipase c (PLC) activation.

Little is known about the regulation of CCK receptor gene expression. However glucocorticoids transiently stimulate an increase in CCK-A receptor mRNA-stability without affecting the receptor transcription rate.

Although the CCK-A receptor is expressed predominantly in the periphery, expression has also been detected in the vagus nerve, pituitary, mesolimbic neurons, nucleus tractus solitarius, area postrema, and hypothalamus. The CCK-B receptor is widely distributed throughout the brain. The CCK-B/gastrin receptor has also been found on smooth muscle cells and cells of the immune system, an addition to the parietal cell. The nucleotide sequence of the receptor is identical in each of these sites.

4.2.4. FUNCTIONS

4.2.4.1. Stomach. CCK is a physiologically important inhibitor of gastric emptying in both animals and humans. CCK inhibits proximal gastric motility, but increases the force of antral and pyloric contractions. These effects are mediated via the Type A receptor, which is present on smooth muscle as well as on afferent vagus nerve fibers. The current hypothesis is that the effect of CCK in decreasing

gastric emptying is mediated by sensory nerve endings of the vagus in the stomach and duodenum.

4.2.4.2. Pancreas. CCK plays a role in meal-induced pancreatic enzyme secretion, which is dependent on neural mechanisms, but has no role in pancreatic fluid secretion. CCK has a trophic effect on pancreatic acini.

4.2.4.3. Gallbladder. CCK is responsible for meal-induced gallbladder emptying, an effect mediated via the CCK-A receptor. Gallbladder motor activity is also subjected to neuronal regulation.

4.2.4.4. Appetite. CCK enhances satiation and reduces food consumption. The effects are mediated by both direct effects on vagal afferents in the stomach and/or duodenum, as well as a centrally mediated effect via the CCK-A receptor.

4.2.4.5. Other Actions. CCK stimulates somatostatin and pancreatic polypeptide release. CCK enhances memory through a direct effect on vagal afferents. The memory-enhancing pathway passes up the vagus, through the nucleus tractus solitarius, to the amygdala, and then to the hippocampus.

4.3. VIP/Secretin/Glucagon

A family of structurally related peptides comprise VIP, peptide histidine isoleucine/methionine (PHI, PHM), secretin, glucagon, gastric-inhibitory polypeptide (GIP), glucagon-like peptide-1 (GLP 1), growth hormone-releasing hormone (GHRH), and pituitary-adenylate-activating polypeptide (PACAP). The receptors for these peptides are also structurally related and are seven-transmembrane domain G-protein-coupled receptors.

4.4. VIP

VIP is a highly basic-28 amino acid linear peptide, originally isolated from small intestine. The sequences of VIP are identical in the human, rabbit, dog, rat, pig, sheep, and goat. Carboxyamidation of VIP is not critical for biological activity. The largest amounts of VIP are found in the gut, where it functions as a neuropeptide. VIP-containing neurons innervate epthelial cells, exocrine glands, smooth muscle cells, and other neurons.

4.4.1. Gene

In the human, VIP gene is located on chromosome 6. The VIP gene spans approx 8.8 and 7.4 kb in the human and rat, respectively, and consists of 7 exons, separated by 6 introns. The difference in size of the two genes is owing to differences in intron length. The organization of the VIP gene is conserved in humans, rodents, and chickens. A 5′-noncoding exon is followed by 5 exons, which encode prepro-VIP and a 3′-noncoding exon. The VIP precursor, prepro-VIP, consists of 170 in addition to amino acids. The precursor contains, VIP, another biologically active peptide PHM/PHI, which each consist of 27 amino acids in its sequence. PHM is the human equivalent of PHI. The VIP and PHI/M peptides are encoded for by exons 4 and 5, respectively. PHM/PHI is structurally related to VIP and shares many of its biological activities, although it is less potent. A number of other peptide sequences are found during the proteolytic cleavage of the precursor, the significance of which is uncertain. However, the processing of prepro-VIP can follow an alternative pathway in which the dibasic cleaved site after PHM is uncleaved, resulting in a C-terminally extended form of PHM. This peptide, PHV-42, is just as potent as VIP in relaxing smooth muscle. A tissue-specific expression of prepro-VIP-derived peptides has been found, which most likely is the result of variations in posttranslational processing.

The VIP gene is expressed in neurons of the gastrointestinal, respiratory, and urogenital tracts, and also in the central nervous system in the hypothalamus, hippocampus, and cortex. In mammals, the mRNA transcribed from this gene contains both VIP/PHI/M coding sequences, and alternative splicing does not occur. The VIP gene in the chicken and turkey is alternatively spliced in the hypothalamus. At least three second messenger systems, cAMP, pKC, and Ca^{2+}, have been shown to regulate VIP gene expression. A 17-nucleotide enhancer element within the human VIP gene, distinct from AP-2, mediates transcriptional activation by both phorbol esthers and forskolin. Outside the gastrointestinal tract, tissue-specific regulation by estrogens, glucocorticoids, thyroid hormones, retinoic acid, and insulin-like growth factor I has also been demonstrated. There is evidence for a role of the 3′-untranslated region of VIP RNA in the regulation of mRNA stability in the rat pituitary.

4.4.2. Receptors

The VIP receptor belongs to a family of receptors, the PACAP and VIP receptors, which have recently been cloned. The PACAP/VIP receptors show homology with the secretin, GLP-1, PTH, GHRH, and calcitonin receptors. These receptors, which are glycoproteins, are all seven transmembrane domain G-protein-coupled receptors. PACAP Type I receptors recognize PACAP 1–27 and PACAP 1–38 with the same affinity, but do not recognize VIP. The PACAP Type I receptor has been cloned from the rat and human, and they have 93% homology over their common sequence. The PACAP Type II receptor is of two types, VIP$_1$ (HVR1) (based on affinity for VIP) and VIP$_2$ (based on affinity for helodermin). There is marked species variation in the specificity of the peptide–receptor interactions. The HVR1 receptor has been cloned in the rat and human, and is found in the gut and central nervous system. In the human, the HVR1 receptor, cloned from a colon cancer cell line and from human small intestinal epithelium differ by three amino acids, which are deleted in the colon cancer cell line. The human genome contains only one HVR1 receptor gene, which spans 22 kb, consists of 13 exons, and is located on chromosome 3. The promoter region of this receptor contains binding sites for Sp1, AP2, ATF, interferon-regulatory factor 1, NF-IL6, and NKκB. The HVR1 gene is expressed most abundantly in lung, but also in prostate, peripheral blood leukocytes, liver, brain, small intestine, large intestine, colon, heart, spleen, placenta, kidney, thymus, and testis.

The HVR1 receptor is linked to stimulation of adenylate cyclase activity. The production of cAMP in target cells of VIP probably accounts for most of its biological effects. In some cells of the central nervous system, VIP has been shown to induce the generation of inositol triphosphate, activate pKC, and mobilize calcium.

In the intestine, the VIP receptor emerges early in differentiation of epithelial cells from stem cells. The epithelial VIP receptor is included in the program of gene expression leading to different phenotypes, i.e., hydroelectric or mucous-secreting. VIP receptors have been identified on muscle cells of the stomach, intestine, and gallbladder. The VIP2 receptor has been cloned from the rat olfactory bulb and the human SUP-T1 lymphoblast cell line, and is found in the central nervous system and certain human immune cells lines, as well as NCI-H345 lung carcinoma cells.

4.4.3. FUNCTIONS

The main actions of VIP are relaxation of vascular and nonvascular smooth muscle and secretion. VIP

gene expression is higher in sphincteric than nonsphincteric regions of the gut. VIP has a role in the relaxation of gut smooth muscle sphincters in response to the appropriate reflexes. VIP gene expression is greater in the myenteric plexus than in smooth muscle cells.

4.4.3.1. Pancreas. VIP stimulates water, electrolyte, and enzyme secretion, and probably plays a role in regulating the secretory functions of pancreatic islets.

4.4.3.2. Esophagus. VIP effects smooth muscle, and may cause either contraction or relaxation. Although VIP can cause contraction of the body of the esophagus, it is likely to be responsible for the relaxation of the esophageal sphincter, which occurs in advance of a bolus in the esophagus. Patients with achalasia of the esophagus have a reduced number of VIP neurons and fibers in the affected areas.

4.4.3.3. Stomach. VIP is present in intrinsic neurons of the stomach innervating the smooth muscle layer. VIP is most likely the neuropeptide (acting in concert with NO *vide infra*) involved in the nonadrenergic, noncholinergic neuronal mediation of adapative relaxation of the fundus of the stomach. In the pyloric region, VIP also mediates relaxation of smooth muscle and prolongs transpyloric passage time.

4.4.3.4. Intestine. VIP may have a role as a mediator of the descending relaxation that occurs during the peristaltic reflex. VIP increases intestinal blood flow, and stimulates water, electrolyte, and mucus secretion. In humans, in the iloecaecal junction and cecocolonic junction, the muscle wall is devoid of, and the myenteric plexus extremely poor in, VIP-positive nerve fibers and cells, suggesting that VIP is not an important modulator of motility at these gut junctions, unlike its role at other gut junctions.

4.4.3.5. Colon. VIP mediates smooth muscle relaxation, stimulates water and chloride secretion, and inhibits absorbtion.

4.4.3.6. Gallbladder. VIP produces relaxation of smooth muscle.

4.4.3.7. Liver. VIP stimulates biliary secretion. In rodents, VIP has been shown to promote glycogenolysis and gluconeogenesis.

4.4.3.8. Other Functions. In adipose tissue, VIP promotes lipolysis. VIP also plays an important role in penile erection and has an effect on memory that is purely amnestic.

4.5. Relationship Between VIP and NO in Gastrointestinal Function

VIP and NO are colocalized in the same population of neurons in the myenteric plexuses of the gut. Like VIP, NO also serves as an inhibitory neurotransmitter in the gut. The distribution of nitric oxide synthase (NOS)-containing nerves is compatible with a major role for NO in the regulation of gut motility and sphincter tone. A role in the regulation of blood flow and secretion is also likely. The weight of evidence suggests that NO and VIP are cotransmitters, released in parallel from inhibitory enteric nerves.

4.5.1. SECRETIN

Secretin, identified by Baylis and Starling in aqueous extracts of dog upper intestine in 1902 was the first hormone to be discovered. Secretin is a 27 amino acid peptide that which exhibits close structural homology to glucagon and only differs by two amino acids.

4.5.2. GENE

The mouse secretin gene spans 751 bp and consists of 4 exons separated by 3 introns. The rat and porcine secretin precursor consists of a 134 amino acid residues (133 in the mouse) and consists of a signal sequence, encoded by exon 1, an N-terminal peptide and secretin, encoded by exon 2, and a C-terminal peptide encoded by the third and fourth exons.

Secretin is produced in S-cells located in the proximal small intestine. In the rat, the secretin gene is also expressed in the brain (hypothalamus, pituitary, medulla, pons, cortex, and brainstem), heart, lung, kidney, and testis. However, secretin-like immunoreactivity can only be detected in the brain and intestine. The secretin gene is expressed in the pancreatic β-cell during development. A specific sequence CAGCTG within the secretin enhancer resembles that of the core of the β-cell-specific enhancer of the insulin gene. Upregulation of secretin gene expression occurs in rat cholangiocytes after bile duct ligation.

4.5.3. RELEASE

Secretin is released from S-cells of the duodenum in response to acid or bile in the lumen. Fatty acids and peptides can also cause the release of secretin.

4.5.4. RECEPTOR

The secretin receptor has been cloned in the human and rat. The human secretin receptor cDNA, isolated from a pancreatic adenocarcinoma cell line, is 1717 bp in length and encodes a 440 amino acid polypeptide. A 1.8-kb transcript is detectable on Northern blot analysis. The human secretin receptor gene has been mapped to chromosome 2. There is a high degree of homology between the cDNA and the amino acid sequence of the human and rat secretin receptor. The receptor couples functionally to the stimulation of adenylate cyclase. In the rat, secretin receptor mRNA is expressed in the liver, and ligation of the bile duct leads to upregulation of secretin gene expression. A 1616-bp cDNA has also been cloned from human lung tissue that also encodes a 440 amino acid polypeptide. A 2.1-kb transcript is detectable on Northern blot analysis. This receptor couples to stimulation of intracellular cAMP and calcium and phosphatidylinositol hydrolysis. The amino acid sequences of these two receptors are identical.

Messenger RNA for the secretin receptor has been detected in the human pancreas and intestine by Northern blot analysis. Low-level expression has also been detected in the human colon, kidney, lung, and liver. Trace amounts have been detected in the brain, heart, and ovary.

4.5.5. FUNCTIONS

Secretin potently stimulates the secretion of bicarbonate-rich fluid, potassium ion, and enzymes from the pancreas. Secretin inhibits lower esophageal sphincter tone, gastric emptying, gastrin release, and acid secretion. Secretin also stimulates secretion of hepatic bile.

4.6. GIP and GLP-1

Glucagon-like peptide (GLP) and GIP are part of the glucagon-secretin-VIP family of peptide hormones. The receptors for GIP and GLP-1 peptides share 25–50% homology at the amino acid level.

4.7. GIP

GIP, one of the largest members of the secretin family, is a 42 amino acid peptide originally isolated as a contaminant of partially purified CCK by Brown in 1970. It was identified on the basis of its action to inhibit gastric acid.

4.7.1. GENE

The gene for pro-GIP has been been cloned in the rat and human, and consists of six exons and five introns. The human gene spans 10 kb and is located on the long arm of chromosome 17, where it is tightly linked to the PPY gene. Exons 2, 3, and 4 contain the sequences that code for a 153 amino acid precursor protein, and most of the mature GIP peptide (GIP 1–42) is coded for by exon 3. Human GIP differs from rat and porcine GIP by only one and two amino acids, respectively. The N-terminal region of the peptide is important for biological activity. There is no evidence for the existence of any other physiologically relevant forms of GIP in the peripheral circulation.

In rats, the gene for GIP is exclusively expressed in neuroendocrine K-cells (in the duodenum, upper jejunum, and the ileum) and in the submandibular gland. In humans, GIP expression in the submandibular gland has not been described, and it occurs predominantly in the duodenum and upper jejunum. The GIP gene is not found to be colocalized with any other hormones in intestinal neuroendocrine cells. The GIP gene is regulated by the cAMP/pKA second messenger pathway. In rats, intraduodenal infusion of fat increases GIP mRNA.

4.7.2. RELEASE

GIP is released from K-cells, which are located exclusively in the proximal small intestine. GIP release after nutrient intake is dependent on the rate of nutrient absorption, rather than simply the presence of nutrients in the small intestine. Glucose, sucrose, and galactose are secretagogs for GIP. Oral ingestion of fructose does not result in the release of GIP. Proteins and amino acids are also GIP secretagogs, but higher amounts are required. Long-chain fatty acids can release GIP. Glucose, but not fatty acid-stimulated GIP release is accompanied by an increase in insulin secretion. In vitro, GIP cells are responsive to activation of adenylate cyclase, increases in intracellular calcium, depolarization by potassium, GRP, and β-adrenergic stimulation.

4.7.3. RECEPTORS

The human GIP receptor (GIPR) gene is about 13 kb long, consists of 14 exons, and is located on chromosome 19. The human GIPR cDNA encodes a protein of 466 amino acids that is about 81% homologous to the hamster and rat GIPR. The receptor is a seven-transmembrane domain G-protein-coupled receptor. The receptor activates adenylate cyclase, and also increases intracellular calcium accumulation. The receptor undergoes a rapid and reversable homologous receptor desensitization. The gene for GIPR is expressed on pancreatic β-cells. The mRNA expression for the rat GIP receptor has also been detected in pancreas, stomach, duodenum, proximal small intestine, adipose tissue, adrenal cortex, brain, and pituitary. The regulation of GIP receptor expression is unknown. Nodular adrenal hyperplasia or Cushing's syndrome may occur as a result of ectopic expression of GIP receptors on adrenal cells.

4.7.4. FUNCTIONS

4.7.4.1. Pancreas. GIP has a well-established insulinotropic action. GIP stimulates insulin secretion in the presence of elevated glucose levels and increases proinsulin gene expression at a transcriptional level. This effect is inhibited by galanin. Glucose metabolism of the β-cell is a prerequisite for GIP-stimulated insulin secretion to occur. GIP is a weak stimulator of somatostatin secretion in the perfused rat pancreas.

4.7.4.2. Stomach. At supraphysiological concentrations, GIP inhibits gastric acid secretion in humans.

4.7.4.3. Other functions. GIP reduces glucagon-stimulated hepatic glucose production. In adipocytes, GIP stimulates glucose uptake, inhibits glucagon-induced lipolysis, and increases insulin affinity binding. In addition, GIP stimulates the synthesis and release of lipoprotein lipase from mouse 3T3 preadipocytes, augments insulin-stimulated triglyceride synthesis in rat epidydimal adipose tissue, and stimulates fatty acid synthesis.

4.8. GLP-1

Glucagon-like activity in the gut was first detected by Sutherland and deDuve in 1948. A single precursor, preproglucagon, codes for glucagon and related peptides.

4.8.1. GENE

The human proglucagon gene spans 10 kb and is located on the long arm of chromosome 2. The gene for proglucagon consists of six exons and five introns in the rat, hamster, guinea pig, and human. Exons 3,

4, and 5 code for glucagon, GLP-1, and GLP-2. The amino acid sequence of GLP-1(7–37) is identical in all mammals studied so far. The sequence encoding GLP-2 is absent in fish and chicken proglucagon. Preproglucagon mRNA is expressed in the pancreas and brain, as well as the intestine from the same gene, and encodes for a 180 amino acid proglucagon precursor. GLP (7–37) (proglucagon 78–107) is produced in intestinal L-cells by limited proteolysis. C-terminal truncation and amidation yield GLP (7–36) amide, which accounts for 80% of circulating GLP-1 in humans. The N-terminal part of the peptide is responsible for receptor binding and activation. Amidation does not appear to affect either biological activity or clearance.

After a meal, almost all GLP-1 immunoreactivity in the peripheral circulation represents the mature GLP-1 peptide, released from the L-cells of the intestine. Infusion of L-arginine, which is a potent secretagog for pancreatic A-cells, results in an increase in a higher-mol-wt form (proglucagon 72–158).

The GLP-1 gene sequence is found to be expressed in the L-cells of the small intestine, colon, rectum, pancreatic A-cells, and several brainstem nuclei. The GLP-1 gene products in L-cells are found to be colocalized with other proglucagon-derived peptides (enteroglucagon) and to some extent with peptide YY. Enteroglucagon is the term used to describe two peptides glicentin (1–69) and its product oxytomodulin (33–69), which are derived from alternative processing of proglucagon. The biological significance of this is unknown.

A cAMP-responsive element has been identified in the promoter of the rat proglucagon gene. To date, the regulatory sequences that confer tissue-specific expression have not yet been identified. There is little information about nutrient-specific regulation of proglucagon mRNA levels. The levels of proglucagon mRNA increase after massive small bowel resection, and this effect is independent of the presence of nutrients. There is no evidence for an effect of insulin on either pro-GIP or proglucagon gene expression.

4.8.2. SECRETION

GLP-1 is released from L-cells, which are mainly in the distal portion of the small intestine. In humans, GLP-2 is promptly released into the circulation after oral ingestion of glucose or mixed meals. Intravenous glucose is without effect. Oral galactose, oral (but not intravenous) arginine, and mixtures of amino acids are also good stimulators of GLP-1 release. After a mixed meal, GLP-1 levels increase rapidly and return to basal in 90 min. In rats, the autonomic nervous system and other humoral mediators also play a role in GLP-1 release, but to date there is no evidence that this is so in humans.

4.8.3. RECEPTORS

Receptors for GLP-1 have been detected on several insulinoma cell lines and on human insulinoma cell membranes, as well as somatostatin-secreting cells. GLP-1 binds to this receptor with high specificity. After binding, GLP-1 is internalized into the β-cell. cDNAs for the human and rat GLP-1 receptor have been cloned. The gene for the human receptor is located on the long arm of chromosome 6. Using Northern blot analysis with rat RNA, the receptor has been found to be predominantly expressed in pancreatic islets and lung, with low-level expression in brain, liver, skeletal muscle, and kidney. Although the sequences of the lung and pancreatic receptors are almost identical, the molecular weights of the receptors expressed in the two sites are different, suggesting tissue-specific posttranslational modification. Glycosylation is a prerequisite for GLP-1 receptor function.

The GLP-1 receptor couples via a stimulatory G-protein to adenylate cyclase. The effects of GLP-1 on insulin gene expression are mediated mainly via the cAMP/pKA second messenger pathway. GLP-1 also activates a voltage-dependent calcium channel in β-cells, which is necessary for GLP-1 to potentiate glucose-induced insulin release. There is also evidence that the GLP-1 receptor can couple to phospholipase C. Dexamethasone downregulates expression of the GLP-1 receptor in vitro. Steady-state mRNA levels are also decreased by activation of both the cAMP/pKA and pKC second messenger pathways.

4.8.4. FUNCTIONS

4.8.4.1. Pancreas. GLP-1 has a potent insulinotropic effect, which is dependent on blood glucose concentrations. GLP-1 increases proinsulin gene transcription, as well as proinsulin biosynthesis. This effect is inhibited by galanin. In humans, GLP-1 lowers basal plasma glucose levels by about 20% before it loses its insulinotropic effect. GLP-1 has been shown to increase glucose turnover in humans. GLP-1 increases the release of somatostatin from pancreatic D-cells, an effect independent of increases in blood glucose levels. GLP-1 inhibits glucagon secretion, although this effect may be indirect. Amylin is coreleased with insulin after stimulation by GLP-1. Infusion of GLP-1 into normal humans increases in insulin levels, an effect that is pronounced at higher glucose levels. Glucagon concentrations were decreased, but this effect was not glucose-dependent. The insulinotropic effects of GIP and GLP-1 are additive, and together are able to account for the full incretin effect.

4.8.4.2. Stomach. GLP-1 exerts a histamine-like effect on gastric parietal cells. GLP-1 strongly inhibits pentagastrin-stimulated acid secretion as well as the cephalic phase of acid secretion in humans. GLP-1 inhibits gastric motility. The exact mechanism by which these effects occur and whether they are of physiological importance are not clear.

4.8.4.3. Other Functions. Enteroglucagons have been proposed to have a role in intestinal mucosal development and adaptation to intestinal resection. The exact component responsible for this is unknown. GLP-1 stimulates mucus secretion from isolated rat trachea and relaxes preconstricted vessels in isolated rings of pulmonary arteries. In the brain, GLP-1 acts as a neurotransmitter involved in autonomic and neuroendocrine regulation. It was recently demonstrated to inhibit food intake potently in rats.

4.9. The Pancreatic Polypeptide (PP) Family

The PP family consists of three peptides—PP isolated in 1975, and PYY and neuropeptide Y (NPY), both of which were isolated in 1982. Examination of the structure of each peptide reveals that residues at key sites are conserved and provide hydrophobic interactions, which result in a characteristic PP-fold motif consisting of a polyproline-like helix and an antiparellel α-helix joined by a Type I β-turn. A unique tyrosine amide is present at the C-terminus, but both ends of the peptide are required for receptor binding.

The cDNA-encoding precursors of all three peptides demonstrate a conserved structure consisting of a 28–29 amino acid signal protein, a 36 amino acid mature hormone, and a C-terminal residue of 30 amino acids. These marked similarities suggest that each of these peptides is derived from a single ancestral gene possibly by a gene-duplication event.

4.10. PP

PP was isolated in 1975 by Kimmel and coworkers from chicken pancreatic extracts as a byproduct of insulin purification. PP is a 36 amino acid residue peptide with the typical tyrosine amide at the carboxy-terminal residue. The tertiary structure is highly conserved and characterized by a globular appearance created by an α-helix in the center of the molecule with a terminal tyrosine residue. Only one active form of pancreatic polypeptide exists.

4.10.1. GENE

The human pancreatic polypeptide gene spans 2.8 kb and is located on chromosome 17. The gene is composed of four exons and three introns. Exon 1 encodes for the 5′-untranslated region of mRNA, exon 2 encodes the signal sequence and the sequence of pancreatic polypeptide, exon 3 encodes the icosapeptide, and exon 4 encodes a carboxy-terminal heptapeptide and the 3′-untranslated region of mRNA. The structural organization of the gene is similar between mammalian species, but divergent in avian species.

The mRNA-encoding human pancreatic polypeptide encodes for a 95 amino acid precursor. Following cotranslational removal of a 29 amino acid signal sequence, a 66 amino acid prohormonal form is further cleaved to produce the 36 amino acid PP.

The promoter region of the PP gene contains an AP2-CS4 transcription factor-binding site. This element is common to the PYY and NPY genes. An MAL T box is present in the PP and PYY gene promoters.

The major expression (93%) of PP is in the duodenal part of the pancreas (head and uncinate process). PP secreting cells are seen in clumps between acinar cells and occasionally in the periphery. Elevated levels of PP are seen in gastrointestinal endocrine tumors, including gastrinomas, glucagonomas, insulinomas, and carcinoids, and their metastases where PP is secreted in addition to other hormones. Although a small amount of immunoreactivity for PP can be see in the gastrointestinal tract, following total pancreatectomy, circulating PP cannot be detected.

4.10.2. RELEASE

PP is released by pancreatic D- and F-cells in the fasted state in a cyclical pattern. The major stimulus for release of PP is related to meals containing lipids and proteins. PP release occurs in a biphasic pattern with an initial rapid peak within 5 min owing to cephalic mechanisms, followed by a sustained gastrointestinal phase. Cephalic release can be initiated by the sight and smell of food. It is vagally mediated, and can be abolished by vagotomy or intravenous atropine. The prolonged plateau phase, which persists for several hours, represents an integrated response to neural and hormonal stimulation modified by the effects of circulating nutrients. PP is also released by gastric distension, hypoglycemia, and electrical stimulation of the vagus nerves. CCK is important in postprandial PP secretion, and administration of the CCK-A antagonist, loxiglumide, reduces both early and plateau phases of PP release. PP release is stimulated by gastrin, gastrin-releasing polypeptide, secretin, CGRP, substance P, and neuromedin B and C. Hyperglycemia, somatostatin, and bombesin reduce pancreatic polypeptide levels.

4.10.3. Receptors

A 67–kb protein receptor specific for PP has been identified on the basolateral membrane of small intestinal cells and on central and peripheral neural tissue. In view of its putative action on pancreatic secretion, it is noteworthy that PP receptors have not been described on pancreatic exocrine cells. The PP receptor has a greater affinity for PP than PYY or NPY.

4.10.4. Functions

The biological role of PP remains unclear, in part because of the lack of a suitable antagonist.

4.10.4.1. Pancreas. PP inhibits postprandial pancreatic exocrine secretion. Exogenous administration of PP to produce physiological levels of PP inhibits pancreatic enzyme output. Immunoneutralization of PP also increases pancreatic secretion. This potential inhibitory effect is indirect probably via vagally mediated cholinergic pathways. During embryonic development, PP-expressing genes appear to be essential for differentiation of pancreatic islet cells.

4.10.4.2. Central Nervous System. PP may also have an important vagal regulatory effect, since circulating PP crosses the leaky blood–brain barrier in the region of the area postrema and may bind to specific PP receptors in the brainstem. Intracisternal microinjection of PP causes vagally mediated

increases in gastric acid secretion, gastric motility, and reduces pancreatic secretion. The lack of an early increase in PP following sham feeding has been used as an indicator of autonomic neuropathy.

4.11. PYY

PYY was initially isolated by Tatemoto (1982) from porcine duodenal mucosa while screening for C-terminally amidated peptides. The name is based on the presence of a tyrosine residue (Y is the single-letter abbreviation for tyrosine) at both the amino- and carboxy-termini. Porcine, rat, and canine PYY have an identical primary sequence, but in the human, PYY has two-conservative substitutions at positions 3 (Ile for Ala) and 18 (Gly for Ser). Human PYY shows 50% homology with pancreatic polypeptide. PYY is regarded as prodigestive proabsorptive agent. Two molecular variants are secreted—the full 36 amino acid hormone and a PYY3-36 form identified from colonic extracts.

4.11.1. Gene

The gene for human PYY has been localized on chromosome 17 within 10 kb of that for pancreatic polypeptide. The gene spans 1.2 kb and is composed of 4 exons and 3 introns. The cDNA precursor for rat PYY encodes a preprohormone of 98 residues composed of a signal peptide, the 36-residue PYY followed by the cleavage amidation sequence Gly-Lys-A and a 31-residue carboxy-terminal extension peptide of unknown function.

The promoter of the rat PYY gene has been shown to be responsive to both forskolin and *O*-tetradecanoyl-phorbol-13 acetate (TPA) when transfected into HeLa cells. The promoter region of the human PYY gene contains an MAL-T box, three AP2-CS4-binding sites, which overlap with an NFB site, and a CTF-NF1- and an AP4-binding site.

The PYY gene has a complex pattern of tissue-specific expression during development. In the adult, the peptide is expressed in open-type L-cells (colocalized with preproglucagon), which have a luminal projection in the distal small intestine, colon, and rectum. PYY is also present to a lesser extent in pancreas. PYY immunoreactivity has also been reported in the canine ENS.

4.11.2. Release

PYY fulfills the criteria for a true gastrointestinal hormone. It is regulated by luminal stimulants, paracrine factors, and vagal influences. The peptide is released in response to ingestion of a meal. The concentration rises within 15–30 min of meal ingestion, but does not peak for several hours. The initial increase may reflect neural or hormonal regulation, whereas the later increments may be owing to direct stimulation of L-cells by nutrients. Intestinal infusions of fatty acids (e.g., oleic acid) and bile acids are very potent stimulants of PYY secretion, as are intracolonic infusions of amino acids. PYY is also released in response to enteric neural stimulation. Both GRP and CCK also lead to PYY secretion.

4.11.3. Receptors

PYY mimics NPY in most models with a potency similar to or slightly greater than NPY. The receptor subtypes are considered below under NPY receptors.

4.11.4. Functions

In the gastrointestinal tract, the effects of PYY on secretion, motility, and blood flow are all inhibitory. In view of major effects of ileal lipids on PYY release, the peptide has been proposed as a possible candidate mediator for the ileal brake—the negative-feedback mechanism responsible for slowing gastrointestinal transit by nutrients in the distal small bowel.

4.11.5. Stomach

PYY inhibits secretion of both acid and pepsin. In addition, the peptide decreases gastric emptying, reducing nutrient transport to the small intestine. A reduction in gastric contractility occurs via inhibition of acetylcholine. The effects of PYY on the stomach are owing to PYY1-36, and PYY3-36 has less activity.

4.11.6. Small Intestine and Colon

PYY reduces jejunal contractility and increases small intestinal transit times. Furthermore, PYY is a potent inhibitor of water and chloride ion secretion from jejunal crypt cells. PYY is a trophic hormone and may be important in both the development of the intestinal mucosa and dietary adaptation. PYY inhibits colonic motor activity.

4.11.7. Pancreas

PYY is a powerful inhibitor of pancreatic exocrine secretion during stimulation by secretin and cholecystokinin. PYY 1-36 and PYY 3-36 are equipotent in this regard.

4.11.8. Others

PYY is a potent vasoconstrictor and, like NPY, leads to a marked reduction in both mesenteric and pancreatic vascular blood flow. Injection of PYY into the dorsal vagal centers in the brainstem leads to inhibition of thyrotropin-releasing hormone (TRH)-stimulated gastric motility.

4.12. NPY

NPY is a 36 amino acid peptide discovered by Tatemoto and Mutt while searching for C-terminally amidated peptides in extracts of porcine brain. The amino acid composition of the peptide is well conserved during evolution and between mammalian species, with sequence identity among humans, rats, guinea pigs, and rabbits, and a single replacement of methionine by leucine at position 17 in pigs. It has approx 50 and 70% homology with PP and PPY, respectively. Posttranslational processing of NPY is very efficient, and the full-length amidated biologically active molecule is the predominant form in different tissues.

4.12.1. Gene

The human NPY gene is located on chromosome 7, spans approx 8 kb, and is composed of 4 exons and 3 introns. The first exon encodes the 5′-untranslated sequence. The second exon codes for the signal protein and the mature NPY hormone. The third exon codes for a 27 amino acid sequence, and the fourth exon encodes for the terminal heptapeptide and the 3′-nontranslated DNA. The amino acid sequence for human prepro-NPY has been deduced from a clone harboring NPY cDNA derived from human pheochromocytome cells. The cDNA encodes a preprohormone of 97 amino acids, which consists of a signal peptide, the NPY sequence, and a 27 amino acid sequence.

The human NPY gene has an SP1-binding site, an AP2-CS4-binding site, and an AP2-like element. NPY is found in very high concentrations throughout the central nervous system with NPY-containing neurons in the cortex, hippocampus, basal forebrain striation, limbic structures, such as the amygdala, the hypothalamus, and the brainstem. In these neurons, NPY is usually colocalized with other neurotransmitters, such as somatostatin, and catecholamines. NPY-containing neurons are also widely represented in the peripheral nervous system. In perivascular sympathetic neurons, NPY is colocalized with noradrenaline. NPY is also found in the myenteric and submucous plexuses of the ENS throughout the gut. NPY release into the circulation is only seen in patients with pheochromocytomas or neuroblastomas or during extreme sympathetic stress.

4.12.2. RECEPTORS

With one exception, NPY and PYY use the same subtypes of receptors with similar affinities, and the receptors for both are therefore considered together. Multiple receptor subtypes exist, and these have been distinguished on the basis of their specificity for NPY, PYY, a long COOH-terminal NPY fragment, such as NPY_{13-36}, and NPY analogs, such as $[Leu^{31} Pro^{34}]$ NPY and $[Pro^{34}]$ NPY. Only the Y-1 receptor has been cloned. It is a glycoprotein comprising 384 amino acids and has seven putative transmembrane domains like other members of the G-protein-coupled superfamily of receptors. The receptor is negatively coupled to adenyl cyclase and associated with mobilization of calcium ions. The gene is a located on chromosome 4 and has three exons. The Y-1 receptor binds NPY, PYY, and $[Pro^{34}]$ NPY with similar affinities, but C-terminal fragments, such as NPY_{13-36}, bind poorly. The Y-2 receptor has been purified and is a monomeric glycoprotein probably of the G-protein class with a mol wt of approx 60 kDa. It is defined on the basis of a preferential binding to NPY_{13-36} over analogs, such as $[Pro^{34}]$ NPY. The receptor is negatively coupled to adenyl cyclase and also inhibits N-type calcium ion channels. In central nervous system, Y-2 receptors are found in the hippocampus, substantia nigra, thalamus, hypothalamus, and brainstem, whereas in the periphery, Y-2 receptors exist on sympathetic, parasympathetic, and sensory neurons. Y-3 receptors are the newest and least studied of the established NPY receptors subtypes. It is best characterized in the nucleus tract solitarius of the rat brainstem. Although NPY is fully effective, PYY has only a weak affinity for the receptor. The Y-3 receptor is coupled to the influx of calcium, but does not appear to affect adenyl cyclase. A fourth receptor with a modest preference for PYY over NPY has been described in the crypts of the rat small intestine, and subsequently the adipocyte and proximal kidney of the kidney. The receptor that has some similarities to Y-2 receptors is a 44-kDa glycoprotein. It is coupled in a negative manner to adenyl cyclase and is sensitive to pertussis toxin.

4.12.3. FUNCTIONS

4.12.3.1. Gastrointestinal. NPY has potent effects on fluid and electrolyte secretion by the intestine, and inhibits gastric and small intestinal motility in a similar fashion to PYY. In the ENS, NPY may serve as a neuromodulator, releasing noradrenaline to adrenoreceptors on cholinergic nerves. The concomitant inhibition of VIP may be important in the potent inhibition of intestinal secretion by NPY.

4.12.3.2. Central Nervous System. The wide distribution of NPY in the brain suggests a variety of roles in central nervous system function. NPY, expressed in the paraventricular nucleus of the hypothalamus, has a role in appetite and satiety. A decrease in NPY concentrations has been associated with psychiatric disorders. NPY may also enhance lutenizing hormone release via stimulation of gonadotrophin-releasing hormone (GnRH). Injection of NPY into the brainstem leads to a reduction in blood pressure, heart rate, and respiratory rate.

4.12.3.3. Cardiovascular. Intravenous administration of NPY leads to prolonged vasoconstriction with a decrease in blood flow to gastrointestinal, mesenterio, and pancreatic vascular beds. This effect is not blocked by α- or β-adrenergic antagonists. A second phase in which the blood pressure falls appears to be owing to histamine release.

4.13. Motilin

Motilin is a 22 amino acid polypeptide originally isolated from porcine intestine.

4.13.1. GENE

The motilin gene spans 9 kb The human motilin gene is located on chromosome 6 and is tightly linked to the HLA-DQ α-locus. The 0.7-kb motilin mRNA is encoded by 5 exons. Exon 2 and 3 encode for motilin. The primary sequence of human motilin, deduced from its cDNA clone, is identical to porcine motilin. The porcine prohormone is 199 amino acids, and consists of a 25 amino acid N-terminal signal peptide, motilin itself, and a 70 amino acid residue C-terminal peptide. In the human, the N-terminus is similar to porcine, but the C-terminal peptide consists of 68 residues, and the amino acid sequence is markedly different. The biological activity of motilin resides in the first seven amino acids. The first six amino acids are highly conserved among different species. The binding of the peptide to its receptor is facilitated by a

C-terminal α-helical structure initiated from the middle portion of the molecule. This middle portion provides protection from enzymatic degradation.

The motilin gene is expressed in the duodenum, and by Northern analysis, motilin expression has been found in the brain, broncoepithelial cells, and an adenocarcinoma cell line.

4.13.2. Secretion

Motilin is periodically released from M-cells in the duodenum in the fasted state and is involved in the regulation of gastrointestinal motor activity during fasting. Physiological release of motilin occurs toward the end of phase II and during the phase III of the migrating motor complex (MMC). Acidification of the duodenum causes release of motilin in humans. Motilin release is inhibited after a meal. Motilin is also released in response to sham feeding, gastric distension, and stimulation by opioid agonists.

4.13.3. Receptor

The motilin receptor is present on smooth muscle cells of the proximal gastrointestinal tract and gallbladder. Motilin receptors have also been detected in colonic smooth muscle, but their role is uncertain. Chronic exposure to erythromycin, a motilin receptor agonist, leads to motilin receptor downregulation.

4.13.4. Functions

Motilin is beleived to be responsible for the onset of phase III MMCs. The increase in plasma motilin levels is synchronous with phasic and tonic contractile activity of the lower esophageal shincter (LES) and of the stomach. The current hypothesis is that in the human, motilin agonists act on the LES by stimulating cholinergic nerves, but could also modify gastric motility by direct muscle stimulation. Motilin enhances food intake, possibly secondary to its ability to increase gastric emptying. Motilin has also been shown to stimulate pepsinogen secretion in humans, dogs, and guinea pigs. In the guinea pig stomach, this has been shown to be a direct effect of motilin on chief cells. The motilin receptor mediates PP release. This effect is dependent on an intact antrum and on intact long vagal cholinergic pathways. Motilin induces contractions of the gallbladder during the interdigestive state. In vivo, the action of motilin occurs via cholinergic nerves. Duodenojejunal anatomical integrity is essential for gallbladder contraction via the motilin receptor. A direct effect on gallbladder smooth muscle is also possible.

4.14. Neurotensin (NT) and Neuromedin N (NmN)

NT is a tridecapeptide originally isolated from bovine hypothalamus. NT is present in N-cells of the gut, with greatest abundance in the ileum in all species so far examined.

NmN is a structurally related six amino acid peptide, originally isolated from porcine spinal cord and shows close structural homology to the carboxyl-terminal biologically active part of NT. These peptides are not amidated at the carboxyl-terminal.

4.14.1. Gene

The structure of the gene encoding NT has been determined in rats and humans. In the human, the NT gene is located on chromosome 20. The rat NT-NmN gene spans 10.2 kb and is composed of 4 exons. Exon 4 encodes for both NT and NmN. In the brain, mRNAs of 1.0 and 1.5 kb are expressed, whereas in the intestine, only a 1-kb mRNA species is found. In each species, a highly conserved precursor protein of 169–170 amino acid residues encodes both NT and NmN.

The NT/NmN promoter contains a cAMP response element, AP-1-binding site, and a glucocorticoid response element. Glucocorticoids and forskolin act synergistically to enhance NT production in hypothalamic neurons. Activation of the NT gene promoter involves synergistic interactions between specific AP-1 complexes and ligand-activated glucocorticoid receptor. NT/NmN mRNA in the hypothalamus increases in response to stress. Expression of the NT gene in the intestine of the rat increases with aging, unaccounted for by significant changes in the number of N-cells. *Ras* enhances the expression NT/NmN gene in the gut-derived CaCo2 cell line.

NT is expressed in the central (predominantly the hypothalamus) and peripheral nervous system, heart, adrenal gland, pancreas, and respiratory tract. In the gut, NT expression occurs in the jejunum as well as the ileum. Tissue-specific posttranslational processing occurs.

4.14.2. Secretion

NT is released by the N-cells of the distal ileum in response to intraluminal fat, but not amino acid or glucose solutions. Stimulation by bombesin and GRP also induces NT release.

4.14.3. RECEPTORS

The interaction of NT with its receptors triggers an increase of cyclic GMP levels, inhibition of pres-timulated cAMP formation, and activation of phos-phatidylinositol turnover. At least three different high-affinity forms of NT receptor have been postu-lated. A high-affinity NT receptor cloned from rat brain encodes a 424 amino acid protein exhibiting the structural properties of G-protein-coupled recep-tors. A human counterpart of this receptor that exhibits 85% identity with the rat receptor has also been cloned from the HT-29 colonic adenocarci-noma cell line. This receptor is internalized after binding, couples to phosphatidylinositol hydrolysis and intracellular calcium accumulation, but does not modulate intracellular levels of cyclic nucleotides. This receptor has been found to be expressed on human pancreatic cancer cells.

4.14.4. FUNCTIONS

NT exerts a trophic effect on pancreas and gut mucosa that is more pronounced in aged compared to young animals. Other physiological effects of NT that have been described in the gut include inhibition of postprandial gastric acid and pancreatic secretion, stimulation of colonic motility, and inhibition of small intestinal and gastric motility. NT facilitates translocation of fatty acids in the proximal small intestine. NT is a potent stimulant of PP release and also of histamine release from mast cells.

4.15. Galanin

Galanin was originally isolated from porcine intestine on the basis of its C-terminal amidation of alanine. Rat, porcine, and bovine galanin are all 29 amino acid C-terminal-amidated peptides, with a high degree of homology. In the human, two molec-ular forms of galanin exist (19 and 30 amino acids) that share the sequence of the N-terminal 15 residues with other mammalian galanins, but exhibit charac-teristic differences in other portions of the molecule and are not C-terminal amidated.

4.15.1. GENE

The human galanin gene is located on chromo-some 11, spans 6.5 kb, and is composed of 6 exons. The first exon encodes only the 5′-untranslated sequence. The second exon encodes for the signal peptide. The first 13 amino acids of galanin are encoded on exon 3. Exon 4 codes for the rest of galanin, and combines with exons 5 and 6 to encode galanin message-associated polypeptide (GMAP) and the 3′-untranslated region. The overall structure of the galanin gene is similar between species. The mRNA encoding porcine galanin has been isolated from the adrenal medulla and encodes for a 123 amino acid prohormone, preprogalanin. This precur-sor consists of a signal peptide, the galanin sequence, and a 59 amino acid sequence, GMAP. A similar structure has been described for the prohormones of rat, bovine, and human galanin.

The promoter region of the human galanin gene contains potential binding sites for transcription fac-tors, such as SP1, AP2, and NFκB. Three half-palin-dromic estrogen response elements (EREs) are also found. In rodents, estrogen markedly stimulates galanin gene expression in the anterior pituitary gland and also in specific hypothalamic cell nuclei. Galanin gene expression can also be induced by pKA, pKC, and calcium-mediated pathways.

Galanin is expressed in the gut, pancreas, adrenal medulla, pituitary, and central and peripheral nervous system of several mammalian species, including the human. However, there is major species variation in the expression of galanin. In the gastrointestinal tract, galanin immunoreactivity is present only in enteric nerves, predominantly in myenteric and submucosal plexi. The exact distribution varies according to species and region of the gut studied. Nerve fibers containing galanin project into the smooth muscle layers and the mucosa in a caudad direction.

4.15.2. RELEASE

In the pig, galanin is released from enteric nerves in response to distension, chemical stimulation of the mucosa, or electrical stimulation of mixed periarter-ial nerves. Intrinsic galanin-storing neurons receive an inhibitory noradrenergic and an excitatory cholin-ergic input from the extrinsic nerves.

4.15.3. RECEPTOR

The galanin receptor is a seven-transmembrane domain G-protein-coupled receptor. Binding sites for galanin have been recognized in the pancreas, central nervous system, and intestinal and gastric smooth muscle. At least two and possibly three sub-types of galanin receptor have been identified.

4.15.4. FUNCTIONS

4.15.4.1. Pancreas. In the dog, galanin is an important pancreatic neurotransmitter, mediating the inhibition of insulin secretion seen during sympathetic nerve stimulation. In rats, there are few galanin-containing nerve fibers associated with islets, although galanin inhibits cAMP production in the rat insulinoma cell line RIN m5F and inhibits glucose-induced insulin release in vivo. In humans, there are similarly few galanin-containing nerve fibers associated with islets. Infusion of galanin has no effect on plasma insulin levels in either humans or baboons. Galanin inhibits GIP and GLP-1 stimualtion of proinsulin gene transcription.

4.15.4.2. Gut. Galanin is a neurotransmitter in the ENS. Galanin's effect on gastrointestinal smooth muscle varies in different species. Stimulation of contraction, relaxation, and neuromodulation has been described. Effects on smooth muscle may be neurally mediated or direct. In humans, galanin inhibits gastric emptying and slows colonic transit time.

4.15.4.3. Other Actions. Galanin also has effects on the hypothalamus, pituitary, and adrenal. In rodents, galanin has been shown to increase food intake after central administration.

4.16. Bombesin/GRP and Neuromedin B

The bombesin-like peptides are a diverse family of peptides originally characterized in frog skin. The family includes bombesin from *Bombina orientalis* and ranatensin from *Rana pipiens*. GRP is a mammalian homolog of bombesin, and neuromedin B (NMB) is the mammalian homolog of ranatensin. A third member of the family, phyllotorin, does not have a mammalian homolog. GRP was first isolated from porcine stomach. The carboxy-terminal α-amidated heptapeptide of bombesin, GRP, and neuromedin B are identical.

4.16.1. Gene

The human, GRP gene consists of three exons and is mapped to chromosome 18. Alternative splicing of primary transcripts has been described. In the human, a GRP prohormone of 145 amino acid residues consists of a 23-residue signal peptide, 27-residue GRP, and a 95-residue carboxyl-terminal extension. Different molecular forms of GRP-like immunoreactivity have been shown to exist, including GRP 14–27 and GRP 18–27 (alternatively known as neuromedin C). A cAMP response element is present in the promoter of the GRP gene. The neuromedin B gene is mapped to chromosome

15. A 76 amino acid prohormone codes for a signal peptide, which is immediately followed by NMB-22 and a 17-amino acid residue carboxyl-terminal extension peptide. Two NMB mRNA species each of approx 800 bp are widely distributed in the brain and gastrointestinal tract. GRP is widely distributed in the brain, gastrointestinal tract, reproductive tract, and lung of most mammalian species. In the brain and gut, GRP is located in neurons, whereas in the lung, it is located in endocrine cells. GRP and neuromedin B are found predominantly in the submucosal and myenteric plexus of the gut, including the stomach, small intestine, and colon. There is an abundant presence of GRP-containing nerves in the human pancreas.

4.16.2. Release

GRP is released in response to cholinergic stimulation.

4.16.3. Receptors

Discrete binding sites for these peptides are located in the gut, central nervous system, and various tumor cells. In the gut, receptors are present on smooth muscle cells and neurons of the myenteric plexus. Three receptors for mammalian bombesin-like peptides have been cloned to date a GRP-preferring subtype (GRP-R), an NMB-preferring subtype (NMB-R), and a third subtype designated bombesin receptor subtype 3 (BRS-3) for which the ligand is unknown, but which preferentially binds GRP compared with NMB. These receptors are all seven-transmembrane domain G-protein-coupled receptors. The GRP-R and BRS-3 are located on the X chromosome, and the NMB-R on chromosome 6. After activation of these receptors, an increase in phospholipase C activity, increased intracellular calcium, and increased phosphoinositol production have all been described. GRP-R is found throughout the gut, whereas NMB-R is found in esophageal and intestinal muscularis. BRS-3 is found in the testes and lung carcinoma cells.

4.16.4. Functions

4.16.4.1. Gastrointestinal Tract. Within the gut, GRP acts to stimulate secretion of gastrin via a direct effect on the G-cell. This effect is independent of gastric distention, but may be responsive to the presence of intraluminal nutrients. GRP stimulates the release of somatostatin, CCK, VIP, GIP, neurotensin, and glucagon, as well as pancreatic enzymes (an effect that may be dependent on intra-pancreatic CCK release). GRP has effects on gut motility, for example, lower esophageal sphincter contraction. GRP induces the release of substance P from nerve endings in colonic mucosa and may also have a role in the maintenance of mucosal immunity. GRP may regulate a variety of functions in the pancreas. GRP acts as a growth factor and stimulates the growth of normal cells of the gut and pancreas.

4.16.4.2. Other Actions.
In humans, the highest levels of GRP are found in fetal lung and small-cell lung-carcinoma. GRP has been shown to be a growth factor for both normal and neoplastic lung, and may act as autocrine growth factors in small-cell lung cancer. Central actions of GRP include regulation of appetite and meal-associated processes, such as memory, blood sugar, cardiac function, and thermoregulation. Centrally administered GRP inhibits gastric acidity. GRP markedly suppresses food intake in a range of species, when infused either centrally or systemically.

4.17. Calcitonin Gene-Related Peptide (CGRP)

The human calcitonin/CGRP genes CALC-A, CALC-B, and the pseudogene CALC-P are local-ized to a 220-kb SacII fragment on chromosome 11. The related amylin gene occurs on chromosome 12. The gene comprises six exons with the first three exons being spliced to the 5th and 6th exons in the brain and enteric nervous system to generate the mRNA encoding for the precursor of the 37 amino acid peptide, α-CGRP. A second CGRP gene pro-duces β-CGRP, a 37 amino acid peptide with a lys substitution for glu in position 35. This second gene does not contain the sequence for calcitonin. α-CGRP is present in the gut in primary afferent fibers coming from the spinal cord. β-CGRP is present in enteric neurons. CGRP fibers are also closely con-nected to the splanchnic vasculature.

Two forms of CGRP receptors have been identi-fied in peripheral organs a 70–86 kDa glycosylated receptor that activates adenylate cyclase and a 44-kDa receptor that is not glycosylated. Amylin at high concentrations binds to the CGRP receptor, but a separate high-affinity receptor for amylin has also been identified.

CGRP is a mediator of gastric mucosal vasodila-tion. This effect appears to be mediated through NO release, stimulating cGMP to produce arteriolar dilatation. CGRP produces splanchnic and periph-eral vasodilatation. Since CGRP is released by glu-cose, a role for CGRP in producing postprandial hypotension has been suggested. CGRP regulates food intake at both peripheral sites and within the central nervous system. CGRP release is also stimu-lated by acid in the gastric mucosa. This CGRP released from primary afferent sensory nerves stimu-lates the release of somatostatin, thus decreasing gas-tric acid secretion.

4.15. TRH

TRH is widely distributed throughout the gas-trointestinal tract with high concentrations in the pancreas, stomach, and colon. The TRH metabo-lite histidylproline diketopiperazine is also distrib-uted throughout the gastrointestinal tract. TRH levels in the pancreas increase during the peri- and postnatal period and then decrease into adulthood. This is most probably owing to a marked increase in TRH-degrading activity in the pancreas in adult-hood. TRH is synthesized in the B-cells of the Islets of Langerhans from a prohormone contain-ing the TRH progenitor sequence and six cryptic sequences separated by paired basic amino acid residues. Pro-TRH has also been identified in the stomach and the intestine. TRH-like immunoreac-tivity has been observed in gastrin cells of the stomach and the myenteric plexus of the esopha-gus, stomach, and intestine. TRH levels in the stomach decrease during cold stress, which is suffi-cient to produce ulcers.

TRH has been shown to have numerous periph-eral effects on the gut. TRH suppressed gastric acid secretion stimulated by pentagastrin, as well as in patients with Zollinger-Ellison syndrome and sys-temic mastocytosis. Both histamine (H_2 receptor) and serotonin stimulate TRH release from the stom-ach, whereas endogenous opioids inhibit TRH release. Chronic TRH administration induces pan-creatic hyperplasia with a decrease in the pancreatic content of amylase, trypsin, and lipase. TRH inhibits amylase release from the pancreas. TRH slows the rate of gallbladder emptying in response to CCK. TRH stimulates smooth muscle of the intestine. TRH and histidylproline diketopiperazine inhibit cholesterol synthesis in intestinal mucosa by a direct action on 3-hydroxy 3-methylglutaryl coenzyme-A reductase.

4.19. Lumenal Hormones

A number of hormones are released directly into the gastrointestinal lumen. They appear to modulate gastrointestinal secretion and hormone release from other gut endocrine cells. Guanylin is a 22 amino acid peptide that is derived from a 115 amino acid precursor protein in the jejunum, ileum, and colon. Its gene spans 2.6 kb and has 3 exons. Binding to its intestinal receptor increases cGMP levels and inhibits fluid and salt absorption, leading to diarrhea when it is activated in excess, eg, by *Escherichia coli* entertoxin. Other luminal hormones include sorbin (153 amino acid peptide that monitors fluid fluxes in the gallbladder), monitor peptide (61 amino acid peptide that releases CCK), and cryptins (Paneth cell peptides that have antibacterial properties). Trefoil peptides are highly resistant to protease digestion owing to a cloverleaf three-loop structure joined by disulfide bonds. Spasmolyte polypeptide is an example of a trefoil peptide that has high concentrations in the mucosal layer and increased expression in the mucosa of patients with regional ileitis.

5. ENDOCRINE TUMORS OF THE GASTROINTESTINAL TRACT

Tumors of the endocrine cells of the gut are uncommon (<10/million population). The peptides and amines secreted by these tumors produce distinct clinical syndromes related to the hormone excess. A dominant peptide secreted may give rise to a recognizable clinical syndrome, but many tumors secrete multiple peptide products. These tumors can in many instances be localized using radiolabeled octreotide, a long-acting somatostatin analog, and VIP. Tumors may occur in sporadic form or as part of the multiple endocrine neoplasia (MEN) 1 syndrome.

5.1. Carcinoid Syndrome

Carcinoids are tumors of the APUD cell system and can be classified by their site of occurrence into foregut, midgut, and hindgut. However, 95% of carcinoids occur in the appendix, rectum, or ileum. Usually the peptide products of these tumors are metabolized by the liver. The carcinoid syndrome, characterized by flushing and diarrhea, occurs in the face of metastatic disease or with a bronchial or ovarian primary. Associated features include pellagra, valvular heart disease, and asthma. A number of peptides are released by the

tumor. Flushing may be the result of bradykinin, NT, and substance P. Serotinin, which increases intestinal transit, is probably responsible for the diarrhea. The diagnosis is made by measurement of the serotonin metabolite 5-hydroxyindoleacetic acid (5-HIAA) in urine. Surgical resection is the treatment of choice where possible. Octreotide is of benefit to relieve symptoms.

5.2. Gastrinoma

Tumors that secrete gastrin lead to a syndrome of severe peptic ulceration and gastric acid hypersecretion first recognized by Zollinger and Ellison in 1955. Clinical features include abdominal pain, diarrhea, steatorrhea, and esophageal symptoms. The tumor is located either in the pancreas (60%), duodenum (30%), or elsewhere in the proximal gastrointestinal tract (10%). Surgical treatment where possible is the treatment of choice. The "proton pump" inhibitors, such as omeprazole or lansoprazole, are effective in blocking acid secretion from parietal cells.

5.3. Vipoma

The syndrome described by Verner and Morrison is also known as the watery diarrhea, hypokalemia, and achlorhydria (WDHA) syndrome and is the result of a VIP-secreting tumor. These tumors occur in the pancreas (90%), or neural, adrenal, or periganglionic tissue (10%). About 60% of these tumors are malignant. Tumors that secrete VIP present with secretory diarrhea. Other clinical features in decreasing frequency of occurrence include hypokalemia, hypochlohydria, hyperglycemia, hypercalcemia, flushing, and a dilated atonic gallbladder. These tumors may also secrete GIP, secretin, PP, prostaglandins, and PHM, which may contribute to the clinical features. The diagnosis can be made by finding elevated plasma levels of VIP. Surgical excision is the treatment of choice where possible. Octreotide is effective in controlling the diarrhea.

5.4. Somatostatinoma

Tumors that secrete somatostatin are very rare. Clinical features may vary depending whether the tumor is in the pancreas or intestine. With pancreatic somatostatinomas, diabetes mellitus, gallbladder disease, diarrhea, steatorrhea, hypochlorhydria, and weight loss occur in most cases. With intestinal tumors, weight loss is most common (69%), and diabetes mellitus, steatorrhea, and hypochlorhydria occur in 21, 12, and 17%, respectively. These tumors are usually found incidentally and about 80% have metastasized by the time of diagnosis. Diagnosis can be made by finding elevated somatostatin levels in peripheral blood. Treatment is primarily surgical.

5.5. Other Gut Endocrine Tumors

Tumors that occur exclusively in the pancreas include insulinomas and glucagonomas, which virtually never occur outside the pancreas. Tumors that secrete pancreatic polypeptide are very rare. There is no known syndrome resulting from pancreatic polypeptide hypersecretion and the presentation is usually owing to the effects of the mass itself. Plasma levels of PP may be useful to monitor progress. Tumors that secrete GHRH, causing acromegaly and ACTH, causing Cushing's syndrome, have also been described. Amylin-secreting tumors can result in hyperglycemia.

6. NEUROENDOCRINE DISORDERS OF THE GASTROINTESTINAL TRACT

A number of disorders of gut function are now known to have, as an underlying basis, abnormalities of the enteric neuroendocrine system. In achalasia, the lower esophageal sphincter does not relax normally with swallowing, and normal esophageal peristalsis does not occur. Defects in the ENS regulation of motility and in particular a loss of inhibitory neurons have been demonstrated. A paradoxical increase in lower esophageal pressure occurs in response to CCK. A decreased number of VIP- and NO-containing neurons occur, and the lower esophageal sphincter is supersensitive to VIP. A total lack of NO inhibitory innervation may also be of pathogenetic importance in congential esophageal stenosis.

A number of disorders are characterized by gastric dysmotility in which abnormal patterns of gastric electrical activity have been noted, including diabetic gastroparesis, postoperative ileus, and motion sickness. Metochlopramide, which acts as a cholinomimetic in the antrum, cisapride, which enhances acetylcholine relesease from gut enteric nerves, and erythromycin, a motilin agonist, are all promotility agents that may be of benefit. Although the underlying basis for hypertrophic pyloric stenosis is unknown, the pylorus of affected infants does not contain NOS. Mice, homozygous for a deletion in the NOS gene develop a disorder resembling human pyloric stenosis.

In scleroderma, a multisystem connective tissue disorder that leads to obliterative vasculitis and proliferation of connective tissue, any part of the gastrointestinal tract may be involved. Phase III activity of the MMC is reduced in both frequency and amplitude, and serum motilin levels are elevated. The somatostatin analog octreotide increases the frequency of the MMC, and reduces malabsorption and symptoms in severely affected patients. A toxin produced by the parasite *Trypanosoma cruzi* damages the submucosal myenteric neural plexus and causes Chaga's disease. This results in failure of the lower esophageal sphincter to relax, and loss of peristalsis in the small intestine and colon, leading to dilatation. Hirschsprung's disease is the result of an absence of intramural ganglion cells in the colon and rectum. The neuroblast from neural crest is thought to be arrested in its caudal migration to the distal gut during development. The internal anal sphincter is always involved, and the extension proximally is variable. There is an absence of relaxant neurons containing VIP and NO. Patients present in infancy with intestinal obstruction or as adults with chronic constipation.

The ENS not only modulates gut secretomotor function, but also modulates gut immune responsiveness. A number of alterations in ENS function in inflammatory bowel disease have been defined. Heightened sensitvity of visceral afferent neurons to normal endogenous stimuli may play a role in functional bowel diseases, such as irritable bowel syndrome and nonulcer dyspepsia.

REFERENCES

Aratan-Spire S, Scharfmann R, Lechan RM, Tashjian AM Jr. Pro TRH gene expression by fetal pancreatic islets in culture. *Biochem Biophys Res Commun* 1990; 168:952.

Backlund BM, Wikander G, Peeters TL, Grasland A. Induction of secondary structure in the peptide hormone motilin by interaction with phospholipid vesicles. *Biochem Biophys Acta* 1994; 1190:337.

Baldwin GS. The role of gastrin and cholecystokinin in normal and neoplastic gastrointestinal growth. *J Gastro Enterol Hepatology* 1995; 10:215.

Beglinger C. Effect of cholecystokinin on gastric motility in humans. *Ann NY Acad Sci* 1994; 713:219.

Beuno L, Fioramonti J. Neurohormonal control of intestinal transit. *Reprod Nutr Dev* 1994; 34:513.

Bold RJ, Istizuka J, Townsend CM, Thompson JC. Biomolecular advances in gastrointestinal hormones. *Arch Surg* 1993; 128:1268.

Bologna SD, Hasler WL, Owyang C. Down-regulation of motilin receptors on rabbit colon myocytes by chronic oral erythromycin. *J Pharm Exp Ther* 1993; 266:852.

Brand SJ, Schmidt WE. Gastrointestinal hormones. In: Yamada T ed. *Textbook of Gastroenterology* Philadelphia: Lippincott 1995; 25.

Bredkjaer HE, Ronnov-Jessen D, Fahrenkrug L, Ekblad E, Fahrenkrug E. Expression of prepro VIP derived peptides in the human gastrointestinal tract: a biochemical and immuno-cytochemical study. *Regul Pep* 1991; 33:145.

Brookes SJH. Neuronal nitric oxide in the gut. *J Gastroenterol Hepatology* 1993; 8:590.

Bruley Des Varannes S, Parys V, Ropert A, Chayvialle JA, Roze C, Galmiche JP. Erythromycin enhances fasting and post-prandial proximal gastric tone in humans. *Gastroenterology* 1995; 109:32.

Chabry J, Labbé-Jullié C, Gully D, Kitabgi P, Vincent J-P, Mazella J. Stable expression of the cloned rat brain neurotensin receptor into fibroblasts: Binding properties, photoaffinity labelling, transduction mechanisms and internalization. *J Neurochem* 1994; 63:19.

Chabry J, Botto J-M, Nouel D, Beaudet A, Vincent J-P, Mazilla J. Thr-422 and Tyr-424 residues in the carboxyl terminus are critical for the internalisation of the rat neurotension receptor. *J Biol Chem* 1995; 270:2439.

Chaussade S, Michopoulos S, Sogni P, Guerre J, Couturier D. Motilin agonist erythromycin increases human lower esophageal sphincter pressure by stimulation of cholinergic nerves. *Dig Dis Sci* 1994; 39:381.

Chew L-J, Murphy D, Carter DA. Alternatively polyadenylated vasoactive intestinal peptide mRNA are differentially regulated at the level of stability. *Mol Endocrinol* 1994; 8:603.

Chow BKC. Molecular cloning and functional characterization of a human secretin receptor. *Biochem Biophys Res Commun* 1995; 212:204.

Christophe J. Type I receptors for PACAP (a neuropeptide even more importent than VIP?) *Biochem Biophys Acta* 1993; 1154:183.

Chu KU, Evers BM, Ishizuka J. Townsend CM, Thompson JC. Role of Bombesin on gut mucosal growth. *Ann Surg* 1995; 222:94.

D'Amato M, Curro D, Montuschi M, Ciabattoni E, Ragazzoni E, Lefebvre RA. Release of vasoactive intestinal polypeptide from the rat gastric fundus. *Br J Pharmacol* 1992; 105:691.

Daikh D, Douglass J, Adelman J. Structure and expression of the human motilin gene. *DNA* 1989; 8:615.

Deschenes RJ, Haun RS, Funckes CL, Dixon JE. A gene encoding rate cholecystokinin. *J Biol Chem* 1985; 260:1280.

deWeerth A, Pisegna JR, Huppi K, Wank SA. Molecular cloning, functional expression and chromosomal localization of the human cholecystokinin type A receptor. *Biochem Biophys Res Comm* 1993; 194:811.

Evans H, Baumgartner M, Shine J, Herzog H. Genomic organization and localization of the gene encoding human prepro-galanin. *Genomics* 1993; 18:473.

Evers BM, Zhou Z, Celano P, Li K. The neurotension gene is a downstream target for Ras activation. *J Clin Invest* 1995; 95:2822.

Fahrenkrug J. Transmitter role for vasoactive intestinal peptide. *Pharmacol Toxicol* 1993; 72:364.

Fathi Z, Corjay MH, Shapira H, Wada F, Benya R, Jensen R, Viallet J, Sausville EA, Battey JF. BRS-3: a novel bombesin receptor subtype selectively expressed in testis and lung carcinoma cells. *J Biol Chem* 1993; 268:5979.

Faussone-Pellegrini MS, Bacci S, Pantalone D, Cortesini C. Distribution of VIP-immnoreactive nerve cells and fibres in the human ileocaecal region. *Neurosci Lett* 1993; 157:135.

Fehmann H-C, Göke R, Göke B. Cell and molecular biology of the incretin hormones glucagon-like peptide-I and glucose dependent insulin releasing polypeptide. *Endocr Rev* 1995; 16:390.

Fink SJ, Vertave M, Walton K, Mandel G, Goodman RH. Cyclic AMP and phorbol esther-induced transcriptional activation are mediated by the same enhancer eleanert in the human vasoactive intestinal peptide gene. *J Biol Chem* 1991; 266:3882.

Friedman J, Schneider BS, Powell D. Differential expression of the mouse cholecystokinin gene during brain and gut development. *Proc Natl Acad Sci USA* 1985; 82:5593.

Giladi E, Shani Y, Gozes I. The complete structure of the rat VIP gene. *Mol Brain Res* 1990; 7:261.

Giladi E, Nagalla ER, Spindel ER. Molecular cloning and characterization of receptors for the mammalian bombesin-like peptides. *J Mol Neurosci* 1993; 4:41.

Gomez G, Zhang T, Rajaraman S, Thakore KN, Yanaihara N, Townsend CM, Thompson JC, Greeley GH. Intestinal peptide YY—ontogeny of gene expression in rat bowel and trophic actions on rat and mouse bowel. *Am J Physiol* 1995; 268:G71.

Gozes I, Bodmer M, Shani Y, Fridkin M. Structure and expression of the vasoactive intestinal peptide (VIP) gene in human tumor. *Peptides* 1986; 7:1.

Gozes I, Shani Y, Rostene WH. Developmental expression of the VIP-gene in brain and intestine. *Mol Brain Res* 1987; 2:137.

Grandt D, Schimiczek M, Beglinger C, Layer P, Goebell H, Eysselein VE, Reeve J, Jr. Two molecular forms of peptide YY (PYY) are abundant in human blood: characterization of a radioimmunoassay recognizing PYY 1-36 and PYY 3-36. *Regul Pept* 1994; 51:151.

Harling H. Galanin: a candidate neurotransmitter in the porcine gastrointestinal tract. *Dan Med Bull* 1993; 40:511.

Herrera PL, Huarte J, Zufferey R, Nichols A, Mermillod B, Philippe J. Muniesa P, Sanvito F, Orci L, Vassalli JD. Ablation of islet endocrine cells by targeted expression of hormone-promoter-driven toxigenes. *Proc Natl Acad Sci USA* 1994; 91:12,999.

Hörsch D, Fink T, Göke B, Arnold R, Büchler M, Weihe E. Distribution and chemical phenotypes of neuroendocrine cells in the human anal canal. *Reg Pep* 1994; 54:527.

Hort Y, Baker E, Sutherland GR, Shine J, Herzog H. Gene duplication of the human peptide YY (PYY) generated the pancreatic polypeptide gene (PPY) on chromosome 17q21.1. *Genomics* 1995; 261:77.

Huang PL, Dawson TM, Bredt DS, Snyder SH, Fishman SC. Targeted disruption of the neuronal nitric oxide synthase gene. *Cell* 1993; 75:1273.

Kato I, Suzuki Y, Akabane A, Yonekura H, Tanaka O, Kondo H, Takasawa S, Yoshimoto T, Okamoto H. Transgenic mice overexpressing human vasoactive intestinal peptide (VIP) gene in pancreatic β cells. *J Biol Chem* 1994; 269:21,223.

Keef KD, Shuttleworth WR, Xue C, Bayguinov O, Publicover NG, Sanders KM. Relationship between nitric oxide and vasoactive intestinal polypeptide in enteric inhibitory neurotransmission. *Neuropharmacology* 1994; 33:1303.

Kimmel JR, Hayden LJ, Pollock HG. Isolation and characterization of a new pancreatic polypeptide hormone. *J Biol Chem* 1975; 250:9369.

Kofler B, Evans H, Liu M, Falls ML, Iismaa TP, Shine J, Herzog H. Characterization of the 5′-flanking region of the human preprogalanin gene. *DNA Cell Biol* 1995; 14:321.

Koh TJ, Wang TC. Molecular cloning and sequencing of the murine gastrin gene. *Biochem Biophys Res Commun* 1995; 216:34.

Krane IM, Naylor SL, Chin WW, Spindel ER. Molecular cloning of cDNA's encoding the human bombesin-like peptide neuromedin B. Chromosomal localisation and comparison to cDNA's encoding its amphibian homolog ranatensin. *J Biol Chem* 1988; 263:13,317.

Krasinski SD, Wheeler MB, Kopin AS, Leiter AB. Pancreatic polypeptide and peptide YY gene expression. *Ann NY Acad Sci* 1990; 611:73.

Laburthe M, Couvineau A, Amiranoff B, Voisin T. Receptors for gut regulatory peptides. *Baillieres Clin Endocrinol Metab* 1994; 8:77.

Lamberts SWJ, Bakker WH, Reubi JC, Krenning EP. Somatostatin receptor imaging in the localisation of endocrine tumors. *N Engl J Med* 1990; 323:1246.

Lan MS, Kajiyama W, Donadel G, Lu J, Notkins AL. cDNA sequence and genomic organization of mouse secretin. *Biochem Biophy Res Commun* 1994; 200:1066.

Lerchen RA, Yum DY, Krajcik R, Minth-Worby CA. Transcriptional vs posttranscriptional control of neuropeptide Y gene expression. *Endocrinology* 1995; 136:833.

Malfertheimer P, Starr MG, Nebon OK, DiMagno EP. Role of the duodenum in postprandial release of pancreatic and gastrointestinal hormones. *Pancreas* 1994; 9:13.

McTigue DM, Rogers RC. Pancreatic polypeptide stimulates gastric motility through a vagal-dependent mechanism in rats. *Neurosci Lett* 1995; 188:93.

Miyake A, Mochizuki S, Dawashima H. Characterization of cloned human cholecystokinin-B receptor as a gastrin receptor. *Biochem Pharmacol* 1994; 47:1339.

Miyasaka K, Kanai S, Ohta M, Kawanami T, Kuno A, Funakoshi A. Lack of satiety effect of cholecystokinin (CCK) in a new rat model not expressing the CCK-A receptor gene. *Neurosci Lett* 1994; 180:143.

Morley JE, Garvin TJ, Pekary AE, Hershman JM. Thyrotropin releasing hormone in the gastrointestinal tract. *Biochem Biophys Res Commun* 1977; 79:314.

Muff R, Born W, Fischer JA. Receptors for calcitonin, calcitonin, gene related peptide, amylin and adrenomedullin. *Can J Physiol Pharmacol* 1995; 73:963.

Nagalla SR, Spindel E. Functional analysis of the 5′-Flanking region of the human gastrin-releasing peptide gene in small cell lung carcinoma cell lines. *Cancer Res* 1994; 54:4461.

Noh MJ, Kim SJ, Kang YK, Yoo OJ. Sequences responsible for transcription termination of the mouse gastrin gene. *Biochem Mol Biol Int* 1995; 35:1205.

Ohta M, Funakoshi S, Kawasaki T, Itoh N. Tisuue specific expression of that rat secretin preursor gene. *Biochem Biophys Res Commun* 1992; 183:390.

Okumura T, Pappas TN, Taylor IL. Pancreatic polypeptide microinjection into the dorsal motor nucleus inhibits pancreatic secretion in rats. *Gastroenterology* 1995; 108:1517.

Patel DR, Kong Y, Sreedharan SP. Molecular cloning and expression of a human secretin receptor. *Mol Pharmacol* 1995; 47:467.

Reubi JC. In vitro identification of vasoactive intestinal peptide receptors in human tumors: Implications for tumor imaging. *J Nucl Med* 1995; 36:1846.

Rosenfeld MG, Emeson RB, Yeakley JM, Menillat M, Hedjran F, Penz TS, Delsert C. Calcitonin gene related peptide: A neuropeptide generated as a consequence of tissue specific developmental regulated alternative RNA processing events. *Ann NY Acad Sci* 1992; 657:1.

Rosselin G. The receptors of VIP family peptides. Specificity and identity. *Peptides* 1986; 7(suppl 1):89.

Samuelson LC, Isakoff MS, Lacourse KA. Localization of the murine cholecystokinin A and B receptor genes. *Mammalian Genome* 1995; 6:242–246.

Sheikh SP. Neuropeptide Y and peptide YY: major modulators of gastrointestinal blood flow and function. *Am J Physiol* 1991; 261:G701.

Shimosegawa T, Asakura T, Kashimura J, Yoshida K, Meguro T, Koizumi M, Mochizuki T, Yanaihara N, Toyota T. Neurons containing gastrin releasing peptide-like immunoreactivity in the human pancreas. *Pancreas* 1993; 8:403.

Simon B, Tillotson L, Brand SJ. Activation of gastrin gene transcription in islet cells by a RAP1-like Cis-acting promoter element. *FEBS Letter* 1994; 351:340.

Singaram C, Sweet MA, Gaumnetz EA, Cameron AJ, Camilleri M. Peptidergic and nitrinergic denervation in congenital esophageal stenosis. *Gastroenterology* 1995; 109:275.

Song I, Brown DR, Wiltshire RN, Gantz I, Trent JM, Yamada T. The human gastrin/cholecystokinin type B receptor gene: alternative splice donor site in exon 4 generates two variant mRNAs. *Proc Natl Acad Sci USA* 1993; 90:9085.

Spindel ER, Zilberg MD, Chin WW. Analysis of the gene and multiple messenger ribonucleic acids (mRNA's) encoding human gastric-releasing peptide: alternate RNA splicing occurs in neural and endocrine tissue. *Mol Endocrinol* 1987; 1:224.

Sreedharan SP, Huang JX, Cheung MC, Goetzl EJ. Structure, expression and chromosomal localization of the type I human vasoactive intestinal peptide receptor gene. *Proc Natl Acad Sci USA* 1995; 92:2939.

Tamaka K, Masu M, Nakanishi S. Structure and functional expression of the cloned rat neurotensin receptor. *Neuron* 1990; 4:847.

Tatemoto K, Carlquist M, Mutt V. Neuropeptide Y—a novel brain peptide with structural similarities to peptide YY and pancreatic polypeptide. *Nature* 1982; 296:659.

Tatemoto K. Isolation and chracterisation of peptide YY (PYY) a candidate gut hormone that inhibits pancreatic endocrine secretion. *Proc Natl Acad Sci USA* 1982; 79:2514.

Tillotson LG, Wang TC, Brand SJ. Activation of Gastrin transcription in pancreatic insulinoma cells by a CACC Promoter element and a 70-KDa sequence specific DNA-binding protiein. *J Biol Chem* 1994; 269:2234.

Verchere CB, Kowalyk S, Shen GH, Brown MR, Schwartz MW, Baskin DG, Taborsky GJ. Major species variation in the expression of galanin messenger ribonucleic acid in mammalian celiac ganglion. *Endocrinology* 1994; 135:1052.

Virgolini I, Raderer M, Kurtasan A, et al. Vasoactive intestinal peptide-receptor imaging for the localisation of intestinal adenocarcinomas and endocrine tumors. *N Engl J Med* 1994; 331:1116.

Vita N, Laurent P, Lefort S, Cholon P, Dumont X, Kaghad M, Gully D, Lefort G, Ferrara P, Caput D. Cloning and functional expression of a complementary DNA encoding a high affinity human neurotensin receptor. *FEBS Lett* 1993; 317:139.

Vrontakis ME, Torsello A, Friesen GH. Galanin. *J Endocrinol Invest* 1991; 14:785.

Walli R, Schafer H, Morys-Wortmann C, Paetzold G, Nustede R, Schmidt WE. Identification and biochemical characterization of the human brain galanin receptor. *J Mol Endocrinol* 1994; 13:347.

Wang TC, Babyatsky MW, Oates PS, Zhang Z, Tillotson L, Chulak M, Brand SJ, Schmidt EV. A rat gastrin-human gastrin chimeric transgene directs antral G cell-specific expression in trasgenic mice. *Am J Physiol* 1995; 268:G1025.

Wank SA, Pisigna JR, deWeerth A. Brain and gastrointestinal cholecystokinin receptor family: Structure and functional expression. *Proc Natl Acad Sci USA* 1992; 89:8691.

Wettstein JG, Earley B, Junien JL. Central nervous system pharmacology of neuropeptide Y. *Pharmacol Ther* 1995; 65:397.

Whitcomb DC, Taylor IL, Vigna SR. Characterization of saturable binding sites for circulating pancreatic polypeptide in rat brain. *Am J Physiol* 1990; 259:G687.

Williams BY, Schonbrunn A. Bombesin receptors in a duodenal tumor cell line: Binding properties and function. *Cancer Res* 1994; 54:818.

Witteman BJM, Edwards Teunissen K, Hopman WPM, Jansen JBMJ. Effect of erythromycin on pancreatic polypeptide release: Role of the vagal nerve. *Neuroendocrinology* 1994; 60:452.

Yamada Y, Hayami T, Nakamura K, Kaisaki P, Someya Y, Wang C-Z, Seino S, Seino Y. Human gastric inhibitory polypeptide receptor: cloning of the gene (GIPR) and cDNA. *Genomics* 1995; 29:773

Yamasaki T, Chijiiwa K, Chijiiwa Y. Direct contractile effect of motilin on isolated smooth muscle cells from human gallbladder. *J Surg Res* 1994; 56:89.

Yano H, Seino Y, Fujita Y, Yamada Y, Inagaki N, Takeda J, Bell G, Eddy R, Fan Y, Byers M, Shows T, Imura H. Exonintron organisation, expression and chromosomal localization of the human motilin gene. *FEBS Letter* 1989; 249:248.

Yee LF, Mulvihill SJ. Neuroendocrine disorders of the gut. *West J Med* 1995; 163:454.

You S, Silsby JL, Farris J, Foster DN, Halawani ME. Tissue-specific alternative splicing of turkey preprovasoactive intestinal peptide messenger ribonucleic acid, its regulation, and correlation with prolactin secretion. *Endocrinology* 1995; 136:2602.

Zhou W, Povoski S, Bell RH. Characterization of cholecystokinin receptors and messenger RNA expression in rat pancreas: Evidence for expression of cholecystokinin A receptors but not cholecystokinin B (Gastrin) receptors. *J Surg Res* 1995; 58:281.

22 The Endocrine Pancreas

Insulin and Glucagon

Donald A. McClain, MD, PhD

CONTENTS

1. THE ISLETS OF LANGERHANS AND THE ENDOCRINE FUNCTION OF THE PANCREAS

The islets were morphologically identified by Paul Langerhans in 1869. Later in the century, Minkowski and von Mering established the endocrine function of the pancreas by showing that pancreatectomy resulted in diabetes. This laid the groundwork for the momentous purification of insulin by Banting and colleagues in the early 1920s. Since then, insulin has played an important role not only in the management of diabetes, but also in the development of the tools of basic science, such as protein sequencing, crystallization, radioimmunoassay, and molecular biology.

From: *Endocrinology: Basic and Clinical Principles* (P. M. Conn and S. Melmed, eds.), Humana Press Inc., Totowa, NJ.

1.1. Functional Organization of Cells Within the Islet

There are roughly two million islets in the pancreas, each consisting of hundreds to thousands of cells with features typical for their function of peptide secretion. Four cell types can be identified histologically, the α- or A-cells that secrete glucagon, the β- or B-cells that secrete insulin, the δ- or D-cells that secrete somatostatin, and the PP-cells that produce pancreatic polypeptide. The β-cells are most numerous, constituting ~80%, with most of the remainder being α-cells. The cells are intermixed, but β-cells tend to lie more centrally in the islet. The blood flow to the islet is through arterioles that branch into fenestrated capillaries in the central portion of the islet. There is some evidence that blood passes the nonsecretory pole of the β-cell first, then the secretory pole, and then courses more peripherally to pass the α- and δ-cells (Fig. 1). Thus, the non-β-cells are exposed to relatively high concentrations of secreted insulin and have the opportunity to respond to insulin in an endocrine fashion. Indeed, there is evidence that this highly localized endocrine control of glucagon by insulin, and possibly by somatostatin as well, is physiologically important: The loss of the normal inhibitory effect of insulin on glucagon secretion may account for the hyperglucagonemia of Type I diabetes, for example. The β-cells, on the other hand, probably are exposed to the same concentrations of glucagon and somatostatin that are in peripheral blood. B-cells are stimulated by glucagon and inhibited by somatostatin.

1.2. Modulation of Islet Cell Function by Neuronal and Possibly Paracrine Mechanisms

The most important regulators of insulin and glucagon release are glucose and amino acids, and as described above, the polarized blood supply of the islets also makes possible endocrine regulation of hormone release. In addition to these major regulatory mechanisms, there is opportunity for paracrine activity and direct crosstalk among the cell types by virtue of their shared extracellular space and the presence of gap junctions; current evidence suggest that endocrine control from circulating levels of other islet hormones is, however, the dominant means of hormonal control of islet cell function. Function of the cells of the islet may also be modulated by neuronal mechanisms. Both parasympathetic and sympathetic fibers have nonsynaptic release sites near islet cells, and acetylcholine, norepinephrine, and epinephrine all influence insulin secretion. The sympathetic nervous system has an important role in suppressing insulin and activating glucagon release during exercise, whereas parasympathetic innervation may be important in mediating insulin release during food intake. Finally, a variety of neuropeptides (galanin and vasoactive intestinal peptide (VIP), for example) also modulate insulin secretion.

2. INSULIN, THE CHIEF HORMONE INVOLVED IN CARBOHYDRATE AND LIPID HOMEOSTASIS

Insulin secretion in response to a meal results in the regulation of several enzyme and transport systems leading to the storage of carbohydrate as glyco-

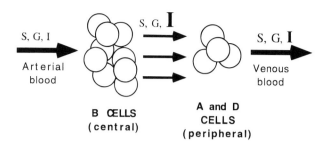

Fig. 1. Schematic diagram of blood circulation to the islets of Langerhans. Capillary blood with peripheral concentrations of somatostatin (S), glucagon (G), and insulin (I) first encounters the β-cells, located more centrally in the islet, which secrete insulin. The more peripheral α- and δ-cells are thus exposed to high concentrations of insulin, whereas the β-cells are not exposed to high concentrations of somatostatin and glucagon.

gen in muscle and liver (Table 1). Glucose production through glycogenolysis and gluconeogenesis by the liver, responsible for providing energy to tissues in the fasted state, is inhibited by insulin. Insulin also mediates the conversion of the adipocyte from an energy-releasing cell to an energy-storing cell. Insulin also has general effects on protein synthesis as well as specific transcriptional effects on several key enzymes involved in carbohydrate and lipid metabolism. The mechanism by which insulin exerts these effects has been the subject of intense study since the discovery of insulin earlier in this century.

2.1. Insulin and Its Family of Related Peptides

Insulin-related peptides have been identified in insects and molluscs, and vertebrate insulins are highly conserved; porcine insulin, for example, differs from human insulin at a single amino acid and has full biologic activity when given to humans. The primitive chordate amphioxus has a single gene for an insulin-like peptide homologous both to insulin and the insulin-like growth factor-1 (IGF-1). Successive gene duplications have resulted in three related genes in humans for insulin, IGF-1, and IGF-2 (Fig. 2). In rodents, an additional duplication of the insulin gene has occurred. IGF-1, the main mediator of skeletal growth, is structurally highly homologous to insulin, as is its receptor to the insulin receptor. In fact, each hormone can bind to the other's receptor with approx 1% of its normal

Table 1
Chief Actions of Insulin on Metabolic Pathways

Organ	Net effect	Chief mechanism
Liver	⇓ Glycogenolysis ⇓ Gluconeogenesis ⇓ Ketogenesis ⇑ Glycogen synthesis ⇑ Fatty acid synthesis	⇓ Phosphorylase (glucose-dependent enzyme dephosphorylation) ⇓ PEPCK (transcriptional regulation) ⇓ FDPase-2 (enzyme dephosphorylation) ⇓ Substrate (alanine) delivery from muscle ⇓ Substrate (free fatty acid) delivery from fat ⇑ Glycogen synthase (enzyme dephosphorylation) ⇑ Acetyl CoA carboxylase (transcription) ⇑ Fatty acid synthase
Muscle	⇓ Proteolysis ⇑ Protein synthesis ⇑ Glucose uptake ⇑ Glycogen synthesis	Multiple mechanisms ⇑ Activity at multiple steps ⇑ Recruitment of glucose transporters to cell surface ⇑ Glucose uptake ⇑ Glycogen synthase (enzyme dephosphorylation)
Fat	⇓ Lipolysis ⇑ Triglyceride synthesis	⇓ Hormone-sensitive lipase (enzyme dephosphorylation) ⇑ Delivery of triglycerides from liver ⇑ Lipoprotein lipase

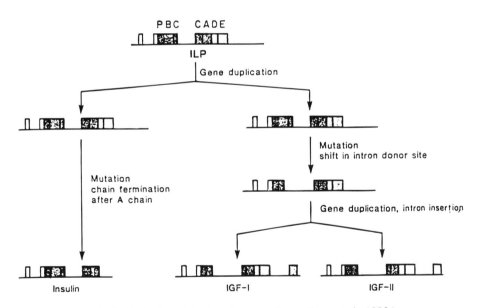

Fig. 2. Evolution of the insulin gene. (From Chan et al., 1992.)

affinity. This crossover can be clinically significant in cases of extreme hyperinsulinemia. Further complicating this picture of hormonal promiscuity is the existence of hybrid receptors, half insulin receptor and half IGF-1 receptor. Recently, another insulin-related receptor has been cloned, although its ligand is still not known.

2.2. Transcriptional Regulation of the Insulin Gene

The insulin gene is organized into three exons, with exon 1 encoding the 5′-untranslated sequence, exon 2 the signal peptide, B-chain, and part of the C-peptide (*see* Fig. 3), and exon 3 the rest of the mole-

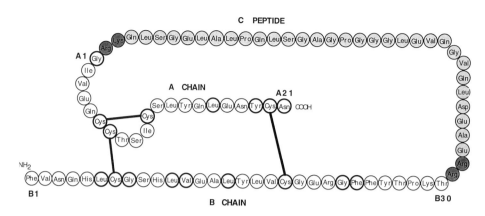

Fig. 3. Proinsulin. In light gray are the residues of the C-peptide that is cleaved from the molecule and cosecreted with insulin. The dibasic residues recognized by the insulin-processing enzyme are in dark gray. Bold circles identify residues in the mature insulin molecule that are evolutionarily conserved from hagfish through humans.

cule. The elements that confer tissue-specific and regulated gene expression are not yet completely elucidated. Two elements, the NIR and FAR boxes, confer basal and β-cell-specific transcription by interacting with members of the helix-loop-helix family of DNA-binding proteins; negative elements repress transcription and negatively acting trans-activators, such as the Id helix-loop-helix protein, may dimerize with and inactivate positively acting factors in non-β-cells. A cAMP response element also exists in the gene; it and/or other elements may be responsible for the observed regulation of insulin transcription by glucose.

2.3. Insulin Synthesis

Insulin is synthesized as a single polypeptide pre-prohormone in the rough endoplasmic reticulum. Cleavage of the signal sequence yields proinsulin, an 86 amino acid peptide with two intrachain disulfide bonds and limited biologic activity (Fig. 3). Conversion of proinsulin to insulin occurs in clathrin-coated prosecretory vesicles (Fig. 4). This involves proteolytic cleavage at two dibasic sites by a specific processing enzyme, resulting in excision of the bio-logically inactive C-peptide. The two Arg residues at the cleavage site of the B-chain are subsequently removed. Mature insulin is thus secreted as a molecule of two peptide chains linked by two disulfide bond residues and an additional intrachain disulfide; the B-chain has 30 amino acids, the A-chain 21. Naturally occurring mutations that prevent normal processing of proinsulin or that affect binding of insulin to its receptor have been described in humans, but are rare.

2.4. Insulin Secretion

The mature secretory vesicle in the β-cell contains equimolar amounts of insulin and C-peptide as well as small amounts of unprocessed proinsulin and zinc ions that are required for crystallization of insulin. Other peptides are also cosecreted with insulin. One of these, amylin, accumulates in the islets of subjects with Type II diabetes and has been hypothesized to play a role in the abnormalities of insulin secretion in that disease, as well as to serve a role in modulating insulin action.

2.5. Regulation of Insulin Secretion

The chief secretagogs of insulin are glucose and amino acids; glucose-stimulated secretion is better understood. It is known that the sensing of extracel-lular glucose by the β-cell requires metabolism of the sugar to and beyond glucose-6-phosphate (G6P). The relatively low affinities of the β-cell glucose transporter and glucokinase for their substrates allow the cell to respond in a graded fashion to a wide range of physiologic glucose concentrations. The precise nature of the metabolic signal beyond G6P is less clear; one current hypothesis is that glycolytic metabolism of the G6P results in a change in the cel-lular ATP/ADP ratio. ATP-sensitive K^+ channels close, depolarizing the cell and activating voltage-gated Ca^{2+} channels. Glucose also increases the pro-duction of diacylglycerol and inositol triphosphate. The latter mobilizes Ca^{2+} from stores in the endo-plasmic reticulum, and the former, in the presence of Ca^{2+}, activates protein kinase C. The precise link

INSULIN BIOSYNTHESIS

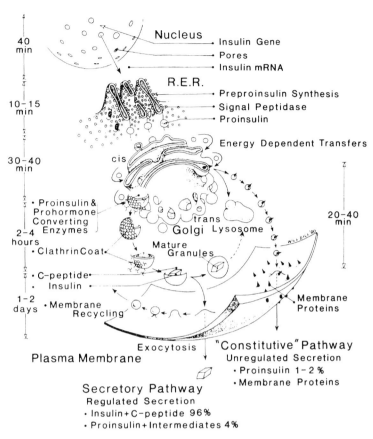

Fig. 4. Insulin biosynthesis and secretion. (From Steiner, 1994)

between these events and exocytosis remains poorly understood. Several other pathways modulate insulin secretion: cAMP and protein kinase A activate exocytosis, whereas activation of α-adrenergic and somatostatin receptors inhibits secretion.

2.6. Basal and Stimulated Insulin Secretion

At normal fasting glucose concentrations (4.5–5.5 m*M*), insulin is secreted in a basal fashion with some neuronally mediated periodicity. These basal levels are important in maintaining inhibition of lipolysis, while still not inhibiting fasting hepatic glucose production that is utilized for fuel by noninsulin-dependent tissues like the brain. With a meal, there is a rapid rise in insulin levels (the first phase response lasting roughly 5 min) followed by a more sustained rise (the second phase lasting roughly 1 h) that stimulates glucose uptake into the insulin-dependent tissues muscle and fat. The insulin is secreted into the portal circulation, and 50–60% of the insulin is

cleared by the liver. The portal concentration of insulin is therefore higher than that of peripheral blood by approximately threefold.

3. MEDIATION OF INSULIN ACTION BY ITS TRANSMEMBRANE RECEPTOR WITH PROTEIN TYROSINE KINASE ACTIVITY

3.1. The Insulin Receptor

Insulin's pleiotropic effects on metabolism and gene regulation are mediated by its binding to the insulin receptor α subunit (Fig. 5). The receptor is a heterotetrameric structure composed of two extracellular α-subunits and two transmembrane β subunits. The α and β subunits are encoded by a single gene; the precursor is subsequently proteolytically cleaved, but the α and β subunits remain disulfide-linked. The α subunits are also disulfide-linked, creating a stable heterotetrameric structure that

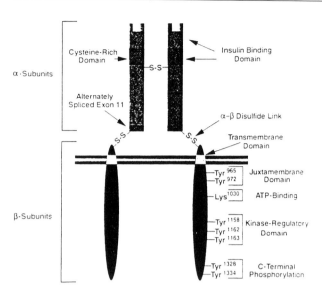

Fig. 5. A schematic model of the insulin receptor. (From Cheatham and Kahn, 1995.)

distinguishes the insulin and homologous IGF-1 receptors from most other monomeric growth factor receptors. The α subunits bind insulin, with the N-terminal and cysteine-rich domains contributing to binding specificity, affinity, and the property of negative cooperativity of binding. At physiologic insulin concentrations, only one insulin molecule is bound to the heterotetrameric receptor and that single insulin is capable of full activation of the receptor. Because the insulin monomer has no symmetry of its structure, and because it is known that a single α subunit is insufficient for high-affinity binding, it is likely that one insulin molecule contacts both α subunits at distinct sites, a situation analogous to growth hormone binding to its receptor.

One exon at the carboxyl end of the α subunit is alternatively spliced, yielding receptors of different affinity that are expressed in a tissue-specific fashion. Some studies also suggest that this alternate splicing is regulated by insulin, glucose, and/or glucocorticoids. Although most current evidence suggests that the receptor isoforms are equivalent in their signaling potential once insulin is bound, changes in the relative amounts of the two receptor isoforms could still play a role in insulin resistance and modulating insulin action. For example, the relatively high levels of the lower-affinity receptor in liver may allow that organ to respond in a measured fashion to the higher concentrations of insulin in the portal vein.

3.2. The Insulin Receptor β Subunit

The receptor β subunit is largely cytoplasmic and contains the enzymatic activity of the protein. This tyrosine-specific protein kinase is essential for all of the receptor's biologic activities, as demonstrated by the lack of effects on metabolism, cell division, and endocytosis of receptors with mutations that inhibit kinase activity. On insulin binding, one receptor β subunit autophosphorylates the other in a trans-fashion at several tyrosine residues. Additionally, the recent elucidation of the crystal structure of the insulin receptor kinase domain reveals one key tyrosine residue in the active site of the enzyme. It would appear likely that this tyrosine might function to inhibit the enzyme when unphosphorylated; on insulin binding, the residue might be cis-phosphorylated and move out of the active site to allow access of other tyrosine-containing substrates. Once activated, the receptor functions as a kinase toward exogenous proteins and initiates signal transduction. Other structural features of the β subunit include a C-terminal domain that serves an incompletely understood regulatory function in signal transduction. This region is the most poorly conserved between the insulin and IGF-1 receptors, and may play a role in differentiating the cellular responses elicited by those two hormones. Indeed, deletion of that portion of the receptor or mutation of its two tyrosines that undergo autophosphorylation results in changes in the relative efficiencies of signaling mitogenesis vs glucose transport, and thus, dissociates those aspects of insulin action. The carboxyl-terminus can bind signal transduction proteins independently of the usual mechanism that employs a docking protein, IRS-1, as described below.

One and possibly two β-turns in the juxtamembrane domain are involved in bnding IRS-1 and other members of the signal transduction complex (*see* Fig. 6) and in recognition of the receptor by the cell's endocytotic machinery. The receptor undergoes endocytosis only on ligand binding and activation of the tyrosine kinase; insulin is delivered to lysosomes for degradation while the receptor is dephosphorylated and recycles intact to the cell surface.

3.3. Insulin Signal Transduction

Activation of the tyrosine kinase activity of the receptor triggers a cascade of phosphorylation and

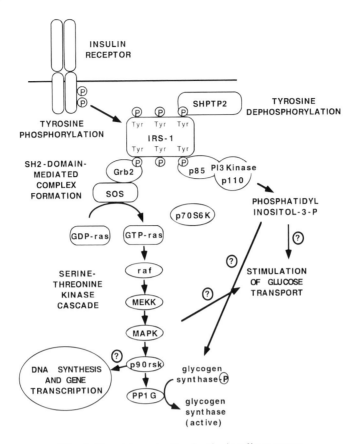

Fig. 6. Signal transduction by the insulin receptor.

dephosphorylation reactions, largely on serine and threonine residues, that modulate activity of multiple enzymes (Fig. 6). Recent studies of signal transduction have focused on the noncovalent association of signaling molecules into activated assemblies. These interactions are primarily mediated by src-homology 2 (SH2) domains in the signaling molecule that bind to specific phosphotyrosine residues. Unlike the case for other growth factor receptors, however, these signaling molecules do not as a rule bind directly to the insulin receptor. Rather, the insulin receptor phosphorylates a docking protein, IRS-1, that associates with the insulin receptor juxtamembrane domain. IRS-1, in turn, contains nine YXXM motifs that when phosphorylated, bind to the SH2 domains of signaling molecules, such as SHPTP2 (a phosphotyrosine phosphatase), Grb2 (an adapter protein that results in the activation of $p21^{ras}$, through the recruitment of a nucleotide exchange factor Sos), and the regulatory subunit of phosphatidylinositol 3′-kinase (P13K). In addition to SH2-dependent interactions, IRS-1 also associ-

ates with members of its signal transduction complexes through other mechanisms. These include a sequence in IRS-1 responsible for the phosphotyrosine-dependent, but SH2-independent association with the juxtamembrane domain of the insulin receptor and a pleckstrin homology domain in the amino-terminus that may serve to stabilize protein–protein interactions in the signal transduction complex.

There are in vitro experiments that directly implicate IRS-1 in both mitogenic and metabolic signaling mediated by the insulin receptor. It was therefore somewhat surprising that mice with both alleles of IRS-1 inactivated had only mild glucose intolerance and insulin resistance. This paradox is probably accounted for by the existence of other IRS-1-related proteins that may function analogously to IRS-1. For example, a protein designated IRS-2 was recently purified and cloned that has extensive homology to IRS-1. This protein can function interchangably with IRS-1 in mediating insulin action. These docking proteins are also utilized for signal transduction by a number of other receptors including IGF-I and several interleukins and cytokines.

The precise details of the involvement of the IRS proteins and other members of the signal transduction complexes in specific aspects of insulin action remain unknown. It is currently believed that the activation of the p21^{ras} pathway leads ultimately to the stimulation of mitogen-activated protein kinase (MAPK), which is an intermediate in the activation of protein phosphatase-1 that stimulates glycogen synthase. Other Ser-Thr kinases in this pathway may also be directly involved in the activation of nuclear transcription factors. The role of the P13K pathway is less well understood, although pharmacologic inhibition of this pathway affects both insulin-stimulated cell growth and the stimulation of glucose transport. Still not understood is the mechanism by which multiple receptors seem to activate many of these same signaling pathways and yet trigger diverse biologic effects.

3.4. Insulin Stimulation of Glucose Uptake into Cells

Hexose uptake is mediated by a family of proteins, GLUT 1–5, that differ in their affinities for glucose and in their distribution in tissues and subcellularly. GLUT 1 functions in the constitutive uptake of glucose in most tissues. Its activity is largely unaffected by insulin, and its relatively high affinity for glucose causes it to be near saturation at physiological glucose concentrations, guaranteeing a constant supply of fuel to such dependent organs as the brain. GLUT 2, expressed in the pancreatic β-cells and liver, has a lower affinity for glucose. Thus, glucose uptake into tissues expressing GLUT 2 is graded across the physiologic range of glucose concentrations, and allows the β-cells and the liver to "sense" the extracellular glucose concentration. GLUT 4 is responsible for insulin-stimulated uptake of glucose into muscle and adipose tissue. In the resting state, GLUT 4 is distributed in intracellular vesicles that on insulin stimulation, are translocated to the plasma membrane. The GLUT 4 at the cell surface can then function to augment tissue glucose uptake. The GLUT 4 subsequently undergoes endocytosis and is recycled to the intracellular compartment.

4. COUNTERREGULATORS OF INSULIN ACTION

Glucagon is the chief counterregulatory hormone, with catecholamines and cortisol also acting in this fashion.

4.1. Glucagon Synthesis by the Pancreatic α-Cells

Glucagon is a 29 amino acid polypeptide that is a member of a family of related hormones, including VIP, glucose-dependent insulinotropic peptide (GIP), and secretin.

Glucagon is the primary hormone determining the blood glucose concentration in the postabsorptive state through its stimulation of hepatic glycogenolysis and, after more prolonged fasting, gluconeogenesis (Table 2). Basal glucagon secretion accounts for approx 75% of hepatic glucose output, with most of the rest dependent on catecholamines. With prolonged fasting, glucagon also facilitates the utilization of fatty acids for oxidation by the liver. Glucose, insulin, and somatostatin inhibit glucagon release, whereas amino acids, exercise, and catecholamines stimulate glucagon secretion. Insulin and glucagon are therefore both stimulated by amino acids, but they are oppositely regulated by glucose, and this pattern of regulation has important physiologic consequences. In the face of a carbohydrate-rich meal, glucagon decreases and causes hepatic glucose production to decrease in the face of the incoming carbohydrate load. A protein meal without carbohydrate, on the other hand, will stimulate both glucagon and insulin; the insulin will result in enhanced glucose disposal, but in this case, glucagon will increase hepatic glucose production to prevent hypoglycemia. Although glucagon secretion is regulated, the levels of glucagon in blood do not fluctuate nearly to the degree that insulin does.

4.2. Glucagon Gene Expression

The glucagon gene is restricted in its expression to the α-cells of the islets of Langerhans. The enhancer elements, but not trans-acting factors conferring this specificity have been identified. Gene expression is negatively regulated by insulin. The gene contains six exons, three of which encode homologous sequences corresponding to the separate hormones glucagon and glucagon-like peptides 1 and 2 (Fig. 7). Glucagon is initially synthesized as a preprohormone. Cleavage of

Table 2
Chief Actions of Glucagon on Metabolic Pathways

Organ	Net effect	Chief mechanism
Liver	⇑ Glycogenolysis	⇑ Phosphorylase (cAMP-dependent phosphorylation)
	⇓ Glycogenesis	⇓ Glycogen synthase (phosphorylation)
	⇑ Gluconeogenesis	⇓ FDPase (phosphorylation)
	⇓ Glycolysis	⇓ Pyruvate kinase (phosphorylation)
	⇑ Ketogenesis	⇓ Substrate delivery, releasing inhibition of carnitine palmitoyl transferase, allowing mitochondrial transfer and oxidation of fatty acids

the signal peptide results in proglucagon, a 160 amino acid peptide that contains glucagon (residues 33–61), glucagon-like peptide (GLP)-1 (72–108), and GLP-2 (126–158), flanked by pairs of basic amino acids. Further tissue-specific proteolytic processing leads to different peptides in different tissues. In the islets, glucagon but relatively little active GLP is generated; conversely, in intestinal L-cells, mainly incompletely processed glucagon peptides (e.g., glicentin), but active GLP-1 are generated.

4.3. Glucagon Action

Glucagon action is initiated by its binding to a specific receptor that is expressed in the liver as well as in islet cells. It, like the GLP-1 receptor, has seven-transmembrane domains and is linked through GTP-binding (G)-proteins to the activation of adenylate cyclase. cAMP-dependent phosphorylation cascades lead to the inhibition of glycogen synthase, stimulation of glycogen phosphorylase (stimulating glycogenolysis), the phosphorylation of pyruvate kinase, and induction of phosphoenol pyruvate carboxykinase (stimulating gluconeogenesis). Insulin antagonism of glucagon effects is through insulin's stimulation of cAMP phosphodiesterase and its inhibition of cAMP-dependent protein kinase.

5. AUGMENTATION OF INSULIN RELEASE BY GLP-1 AND OTHER HORMONES

5.1 The Incretin Concept

In addition to glucose and amino acids, insulin secretion is influenced by a number of peptide hormones from the GI tract. GIP, originally named gastric inhibitory polypeptide, but recently renamed glucose-dependent insulinotropic polypeptide, is a so-called incretin, a hormone that stimulates insulin release in a glucose-dependent fashion. A quantita-

tively more important incretin is GLP-1. It is rapidly secreted from endocrine (L)-cells in the intestinal mucosa in response to a mixed meal or intraluminal glucose. The regulation of secretion is not completely understood; there is evidence for neuronal control, endocrine regulation, and direct control by nutrient sensing.

5.2. GLP-1 Synthesis

GLP-1 is derived from posttranslational processing of proglucagon (see Fig. 7). The prohormone is cleaved in the α-cells of the islet cells in the pancreas into glucagon and several other products, most of them biologically inactive. In the intestinal L-cells, processing generates a novel peptide (78–107 amide) with most of the biologic activity of GLP-1. The amino acid sequence of GLP-1 is conserved across several mammalian species.

5.3. GLP-1 Action

The action of GLP-1 is to augment insulin secretion in a glucose-dependent manner. At glucose concentrations less than approx 4 mM, GLP-1 does not result in further insulin secretion, so its administration is not associated with hypoglycemia. Recently, a component of Gila monster venom, exendin-4, has been found to be a receptor antagonist that blocks the incretin actions of GLP-1.

5.4. The GLP-1 Receptor

GLP-1, like glucagon, acts by binding with nanomolar affinity to a seven-transmembrane receptor on the β-cells. The receptor is a member of the G-protein-coupled superfamily, and binding of GLP-1 to the β-cell results in activation of adenylate cyclase. The precise interactions of GLP-1 signal transduction pathways with those of glucose to regulate insulin secretion have not been elucidated. The

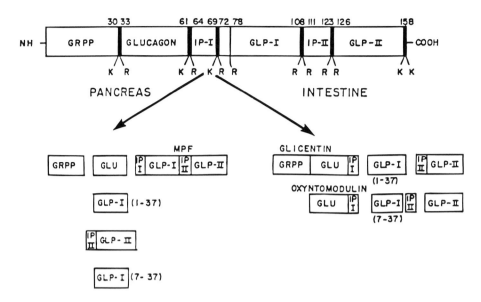

Fig. 7. Posttranslational processing of proglucagon. The pancreas produces mainly glucagon, glicentin-related pancreatic polypeptide (GRPP), and a large C-terminal fragment (MPF) that is not processed further. In the intestine glicentin, oxyntomodulin, GLP-1 and II-GLP-2, and intervening peptide (IP) II are the major end products of proglucagon processing. GLP-1(1–37)(PG72-108) is further cleaved to GLP-1(7–37); to some extent the C-terminal amino acid is removed and the new C-terminal residue is amidated, resulting in GLP-1(7–37)amide. (From Fehmann and Habener 1992.)

demonstration of the GLP-1 receptor on other islet cell types as well as in liver, fat, muscle, and the gastrointestinal (GI) tract opens up the possibility that the hormone may have significant effects beyond the β-cell as well.

6. OTHER HORMONES PRODUCED BY ISLET AND NONISLET CELLS IN THE PANCREAS WITH ENDOCRINE EFFECTS ON THE GI TRACT

6.1. Pancreatic Polypeptide

Pancreatic polypeptide (PP) release is largely neurally mediated. Sensing of food in the CNS causes vagal nerve-mediated secretion, and presence of food in the proximal GI tract also stimulates release. Whether the latter is directly mediated by food or indirectly by other endocrine hormones is not clear. PP affects GI motility, secretory activity of the stomach, intestine, and pancreas, and in some species, affects the release of other hormones, such as somatostatin.

6.2. Somatostatin

Somatostatin is produced by the δ-cells. This hormone inhibits a wide variety of endocrine and

exocrine secretory activity in the pituitary, GI tract, and pituitary gland. In the pancreas, it inhibits insulin, glucagon, PP, and exocrine secretion.

6.3. Other Hormones

A variety of endocrine hormones including gastrin and VIP are also produced by cells distributed in the pancreatic parenchyma. The properties of these are discussed in the chapter on gastrointestinal hormones (Chapter 21).

7. DIABETES MELLITUS AND OTHER DISEASES OF ISLET FUNCTION

7.1. Diseases Involving Insulin Secretion and Insulin Action

Numerous clinical syndromes exist involving hypersecretion of insulin, hyposecretion of insulin, and defects in insulin action or insulin resistance. The former results in hypoglycemia, and the latter two in diabetes mellitus. Hypersecretion of insulin occurs with insulinomas, tumors of the β-cells of the islets of Langerhans. These lead to hypoglycemia in the fasted state, manifest clinically through its two chief consequences: Activation of the adrenergic system tends to correct the hypoglycemia and results in the symptoms of tremulousness and rapid heart rate; at lower levels of glycemia, brain function that requires glucose for metabolic energy, begins to deteriorate, resulting in confusion and eventually coma. Other syndromes of pancreatic endocrine hypersecretion are rarer. In addition to insulinomas, a number of non-β-cell tumors can occur in isolation as part of the multiple endocrine neoplasia (MEN) Type I syndrome, including those that produce gastrin (causing peptic ulcers and diarrhea), VIP (watery diarrhea and hypokalemia), glucagon (migratory rash, diarrhea, and diabetes), and PP (occasional diarrhea).

7.2. Diabetes Mellitus

The hallmark of insulin hyposecretion and insulin resistance is hyperglycemia. At a somewhat arbitrary level of fasting blood glucose, 7.8 mM, this hyperglycemia is categorized as diabetes. The hyperglycemia causes excessive renal filtration of glucose, and results in polyuria (excessive urination) and polydipsia (excessive thirst) that can be the presenting symptoms of diabetes. In fact, the word diabetes is from the Greek word for siphon or faucet. (Mellitus means honey, referring to the sweetness of the urine.) In the longer term, hyperglycemia also results in the complications of diabetes. The precise mechanism for the deleterious effects of high glucose is not known. Whether from the nonenzymatic glycation of proteins or from regulatory effects of excess glucose, blood vessels are damaged, resulting in turn in damage to the retina and kidney, and compromise of the circulation to the heart, brain, and extremities. Thus, the chief morbidities of diabetes are blindness, renal failure, heart attack, stroke, and amputation.

7.3. Distinct Syndromes of Diabetes

There are several distinct syndromes of diabetes, the chief ones being insulin-dependent diabetes mellitus (IDDM or Type I diabetes) and noninsulin-dependent diabetes mellitus (NIDDM or Type II diabetes). Although there is some clinical overlap, Type I diabetes generally strikes younger individuals with peak onset in the first and second decades. This disease results from destruction of the β-cells by the immune system; it is speculated that this destruction may be triggered by a viral infection. The autoimmune nature of the disease accounts for its linkage to the major histocompatibility locus and the 35–40% concordance rate in identical twins. The lack of insulin results not only in hyperglycemia, but also ketoacidosis owing to excess lipolysis and fatty acid oxidation that is normally inhibited by insulin. Treatment currently involves subcutaneous administration of insulin, although transplantation of islets or β-cells may become feasible in the future. The availability of devices to monitor blood glucose levels easily at home has made near normalization of glycemia an achievable goal for many diabetics.

7.4. Type II Diabetes

Type II diabetes or NIDDM is a much more common disease that affects 5–10% of Americans. It typically attacks individuals in the fifth decade and beyond. It is more genetically determined than Type I, with concordance rates in identical twins approaching 100%. The disease is believed to be polygenic and is associated with other abnormalities, such as obesity and hypertension. Currently, the gene(s) that cause all but a few percent of cases of NIDDM remains unidentified. The pathophysiology of NIDDM is complex. The hallmark of the disease is insulin resistance, that is, defective action of insulin at its target tissues. This results in hyperglycemia secondary to impaired peripheral uptake and utilization of glucose by muscle and fat cells, as well as to uninhibited hepatic glucose output. In addition, a defect in insulin secretion eventually develops, but whether this is a primary defect or is secondary to damage from hyperglycemia or chronic hypersecretion in the face of insulin resistance is debated. Because the lack of insulin is not absolute and because tissues are more sensitive to the antilipolytic effects of insulin, ketoacidosis does not develop as frequently in NIDDM as in IDDM. More typically, untreated NIDDM progresses to a hyperosmolar state characterized by extremely high levels of blood glucose, dehydration, and stupor. NIDDM is treated with diet and weight loss (which improve insulin sensitivity), sulfonylureas (which augment endogenous insulin secretion by binding to potassium channels in the β-cell), biguanides (whose precise modes of action are unknown, but do inhibit glucose output from the liver), and, if these fail, insulin. (The term noninsulin-dependent diabetes is thus somewhat misleading in that many people with NIDDM do take insulin for control of their chronic hyperglycemia; the terminology relates to the lack of an acute requirement of insulin for continued life.)

7.5. Other Genetic Diabetes Syndromes

Genetic defects that cause a minority of cases of NIDDM have been identified. Mutations in the insulin receptor are frequently found in rare syndromes of severe insulin resistance, often associated with developmental abnormalities. These mutations can be associated with defective synthesis, processing, ligand binding, or tyrosine kinase activity of the receptor. Somewhat more common is the syndrome of maturity-onset diabetes of the young, or MODY. As its name implies, this is a noninsulin-dependent syndrome that is often mild and that becomes manifest much earlier in life than garden-variety NIDDM. Most MODY has been recently determined to result from mutations in the enzyme glucokinase that render it less active in generating glucose-6-phosphate (G6P). Glucose sensing by the β-cell requires metabolism of the sugar beyond G6P. Defects in the production of G6P therefore result in the β-cell "seeing" less glucose and secreting less insulin, even in the face of extracellular hyperglycemia.

REFERENCES

Chan SJ, Nagamatsu S, Cao Q-P, Steiner DF. Structure and evolution of insulin and insulin-like growth factors in chordates. *Prog Brain Res* 1992; 92:15.

Cheatham B, Kahn CR. Insulin action and the insulin signaling network. *Endocr Rev* 1995; 16:177.

Fehmann HC, Habener JF. Insulinotropic glucagonlike peptide-I(7–37)/(7–36)amide: A new incretin hormone. *Trends Endocr Metab* 1992; 3:158.

SELECTED READINGS

Bach JF. Insulin-dependent diabetes mellitus as an autoimmune disease. *Endocr Rev* 1994; 15:516.

Rifkin H, Porte D. *Diabetes Mellitus: Theory and Practice.* New York: Elsevier, 1993.

Matschinsky F, Liang Y, Kesavan P, et al. Glucokinase as pancreatic beta cell glucose sensor and diabetes gene. *J Clin Invest* 1993; 92:2092.

Mueckler M. Facilitative glucose transporters. *Eur J Biochem* 1994; 219:713.

Myers MG, Sun, X, White MF. The IRS-1 signalling system. *Trends Biochem Sci* 1994; 19:289.

Orci L. The insulin factory: A tour of the plant surroundings and a visit to the assembly line. *Diabetologia* 1985; 28:528.

Steiner DF. Chemistry and biosynthesis of the islet hormones. In: *Endocrinology* (L. DeGroot, ed.), Saunders: Philadelphia, 1994.

White MF, Kahn CR. The insulin signaling system. *J Biol Chem* 1994; 269:1.

23 Cardiovascular Hormones

Willis K. Samson, PhD

CONTENTS

VASOACTIVE HORMONE FAMILIES
THE NATRIURETIC PEPTIDE FAMILY
THE ENDOTHELINS
ADRENOMEDULLIN: A NOVEL VASOACTIVE PEPTIDE
INTERACTIVE EFFECTS OF THE CARDIOVASCULAR HORMONES

1. VASOACTIVE HORMONE FAMILIES

1.1. The Heart as an Endocrine Organ

Although the heart had long been considered merely a muscular pump that performed the physical labor of the circulation, it has been recognized for over five decades that in addition to the contractile ultrastructure, a secretory function was evidenced by the presence of dense-core granules in the myocytes. In the past decade, the endocrine nature of the heart has been established, and the physiology and pathophysiology of the cardiac hormones have been extensively characterized. The myocyte produces both constitutively and in a regulated fashion two members of a class of hormones designated natriuretic peptides on the basis of their abilities to stimulate salt and water excretion by direct renal actions and indirect effects on other tissues, including endocrine organs, responsible for the control of fluid and electrolyte homeostasis. Two members of the natriuretic peptide family, atrial natriuretic peptide (A-type natriuretic peptide, ANP) and brain natriuretic peptide (BNP, actually a misnomer, since although cloned from a brain library, little of this

isoform is present in brain) are produced in the heart and released in response to a variety of cues, all typical of plasma volume overload or hyperosmolality. Although numerous biological actions have been characterized, their hallmark effects are to unload the vascular tree via a combination of central nervous system, pituitary, adrenal, vascular, and renal actions (Fig. 1). This results in decreased venous return to the pump as a consequence of increased renal excretion of water and solute, vasorelaxation in certain vascular beds, increased capillary permeability, and decreased cardiac output. The third member of this family of hormones, although exerting many of the same actions as ANP and BNP, is unique in that it is predominantly produced in the vascular endothelium, not the heart, and is thought to act more in a paracrine fashion, regulating primarily vascular tone and growth. Additionally, this hormone, designated C-type natriuretic peptide (CNP), exerts several central nervous system actions that oppose those of ANP and BNP. For years, the major focus of vascular endocrinology was the renin-angiotensin system (see Chapter 25); however, with the discovery of the cardiac hormones and the realization that at least some of their actions were expressed by a functional antagonism of the actions of angiotensin, a broader view of the

From: *Endocrinology: Basic and Clinical Principles* (P. M. Conn and S. Melmed, eds.), Humana Press Inc., Totowa, NJ.

361

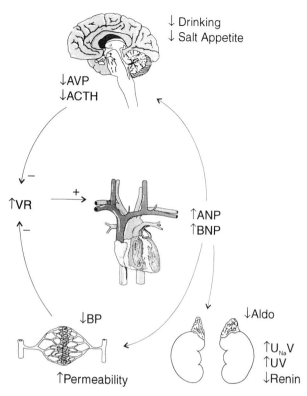

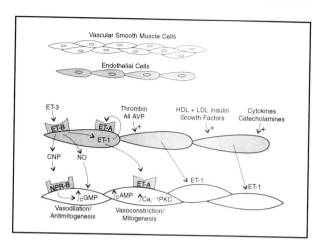

Fig. 1. Schematic representation of the volume-regulatory mechanisms of natriuretic peptide function. Both ANP and to a lesser extent under normal physiologic conditions, BNP are released (+) in response to increased venous return (VR). ANP and BNP act to unload the overexpanded vascular system by inhibiting vasopressin (AVP) and corticotropin (ACTH) secretion from the pituitary gland, inhibiting fluid and electrolyte intake by actions in brain, decreasing aldosterone (Aldo) secretion from the adrenal gland, increasing salt and water excretion into the urine ($U_{Na}V$, natriuresis; UV, diuresis), inhibiting renin secretion, increasing vascular permeability, and vasodilation. All of these effects reduce blood pressure and decrease (−) venous return, removing the stimulus for ANP and BNP secretion.

Fig. 2. Interactions at the endothelial cell–vascular smooth muscle cell interface. Circulating ET-3 acts via the endothelin type B receptor on the endothelial cell to stimulate (+) the release of the vasodilatory/antimitogenic factors CNP and NO. CNP activates natriuretic peptide type B receptors on the VSMC, and NO diffuses into the cells, both stimulating formation of cGMP. ET-3 also stimulates ET-1 secretion from the endothelial cell, which acts in an autocrine and paracrine fashion via ET-1 receptors to stimulate more ET-1 release and cause vasoconstriction and/or mitogeniesis, respectively, by elevating intracellular levels of cAMP and calcium and activation of protein kinase C (pKC). A variety of circulating factors can also stimulate ET-1 release into the interface, including angiotensin II (A II), vasopressin (AVP), and high- and low-density lipoproteins (HDL and LDL).

1.2. Hormones of the Endothelium

The vascular endothelium controls access of blood-borne factors not only to the interstitium, but also to the contractile and proliferative elements of the the vascular tree, the vascular smooth muscle cells (VSMC). Additionally, the endothelial cells are positioned optimally to respond themselves to circulating factors and to transduce those messages to the the VSMC. Many hormonal messages are in fact delivered to the contractile elements via factors produced in the endothelium (Fig. 2). Much attention has been focused on the ability of the endothelium to cause vasorelaxation via the generation of a soluble gas, nitric oxide (NO); however, peptidergic factors originating in these cells control VSMC function as well. Here the role of CNP as a paracrine factor has been established, and the endothelial–VSMC interface was the setting for the discovery and characterization of two additional, potent vasoactive hormones, endothelin and adrenomedullin. The endothelins are a family of hypertensive agents that exert their effects

importance of circulating hormones controlling vascular and renal function took shape. Then this doctrine of the endocrine regulation of cardiovascular and renal function was challenged and expanded by the realization that perhaps the largest endocrine organ in the body was the vasculature itself in the person of the endothelium. Not only was there a member of the natriuretic peptide family produced in and released from this tissue, but it became apparent that numerous peptidergic, as well as nonpeptidergic factors originating in the endothelium controlled vascular tone and proliferation.

directly on the VSMC and via recruitment of additional family members from the endothelium. Adrenomedullin, on the other hand, appears to be an important paracrine and perhaps even autocrine regulator of VSMC function. Thus, both circulating and locally produced vasoactive hormones can control regional blood flow, and this cellular interface has provided a model for the paracrine and autocrine effects of the peptides in other tissues as well. Most promising in a therapeutic sense has been the elucidation of the roles played by these locally produced hormones in the control of mitogenesis and their potential use in the clinical management of vascular remodeling.

2. THE NATRIURETIC PEPTIDE FAMILY

2.1. Gene Structure and Regulation

The members of the natriuretic peptide family share structural homology, but are products of unique genes. Expression of the separate genes and posttranslational processing of the nascent hormones is very similar. The genes for ANP and BNP have been localized to the same chromosome, whereas that for CNP resides in a separate chromosome, providing additional suggestive evidence for the similarity of the A- and B-type peptides and the uniqueness of CNP. Cloning of cDNA complementary to atrial mRNA revealed the presence of three exons in the ANP gene and the transcription of a prepro-ANP mRNA, which encoded a 151–152 amino acid preprohormone, depending on species. Removal of the N-terminal signal peptide results in a prohormone of 126 amino acids, which demonstrates extensive homology across species. This 126 amino acid prohormone is the major storage form of the peptide in secretory granules, except in the central nervous system, where further posttranslational modification results in the production of the mature peptide, which exists in storage as the 24 or 25 amino acid form. In the nonneural production sites, stored pro-ANP is processed at secretion to a variety of smaller, biologically active forms, primarily the mature 28 amino acid, C-terminal fragment. An additional form of ANP, extended at the N-terminus by four amino acids, is produced and released in the kidney. This isoform, designated urodilatin, is thought to act as a paracrine regulator of tubular function. Expression of the BNP gene differs in that the resultant mRNA is less stable and the final posttranslational product is 32

amino acids in length. Finally, CNP processing is quite similar to that of ANP, with the exception that the final posttranslational product lacks the C-terminal extension distal to the shared 17-membered disulfide loop, consisting then of only 22 amino acids (Fig. 3). In humans owing to the presence of an arginine in the prohormone at position 73, a second form of CNP is present, this being N-terminally extended consisting of 53 amino acids. Both CNP-22 and CNP-53 have similar biological profiles in many systems.

Although to date little is known of the regulation of CNP gene transcription, mechanisms for activation of ANP gene transcription have been extensively studied. Gene transcription is induced by glucocorticoids, α-adrenergic agents, growth factors, and calcium, and recent evidence suggests that BNP gene transcription is similarly regulated. In the adult, there exists a regional mismatch in gene expression of the two peptides with ANP expressed primarily in the atria and BNP in the ventricles. Indeed, induction of gene expression by cardiac overload results in increased expression of both genes and the appearance of ANP in the ventricle. Most striking, however, is the level of induction of BNP in the ventricle, resulting in remarkable increases in circulating levels of the hormone. At the molecular level, ANP gene transcription is regulated by numerous members of the activator protein 1 (AP 1) complex, being induced by c-*jun* and in most cases suppressed by c-*fos*. A close relative of c-*fos*, fra-1, exerts biphasic effects, reducing the magnitude of c-*jun* induction of ANP gene expression in atriocytes while amplifying the induction of expression by c-*jun* in ventriculocytes. Thus, the response of the ANP promotor to these early response elements may vary under unique physiologic conditions, permitting a wider repertoire of control of gene expression.

2.2. Hormone Secretion
2.2.1. PHYSIOLOGIC RELEASE

Plasma levels of ANP and BNP are extremely low (5–10 and 0.5–1.0 fmol/mL, respectively) and rise in response to any interventions that increase venous return, and therefore atrial pressure and stretch. There remains controversy over whether the stimulus for cardiocyte release of natriuretic peptide is pressure as opposed to stretch; however, the importance of the distinction is perhaps only minor. Pressor agents can release ANP in vivo and some even act in isolated tissues in vitro, suggesting direct cellular effects inde-

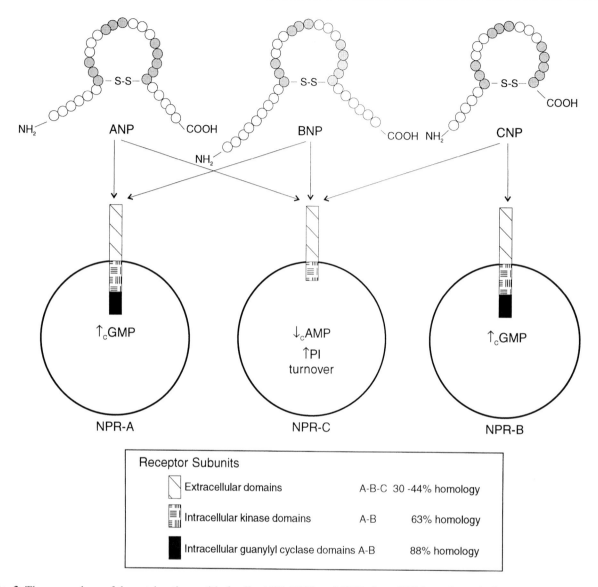

Fig. 3. Three members of the natriuretic peptide family ANP, BNP, and CNP share 65% homology (indicated by darkened circles) in the biologically active ring structure formed by the disulfide links, and vary in the amino acid composition and lengths of their N- and C-terminal extensions. All three peptides are recognized by the natriuretic peptide C (clearance) receptor (NPR-C); however, the A receptor (NPR-A) prefers ANP and BNP. The B receptor (NPR-B) recognizes with relative preference CNP. Activation of the three receptors has been reported to generate the indicated changes in intracellular levels of cGMP of cAMP and/or phosphoinositol (PI) turnover.

pendent from increased venous return. The natriuretic effects of ANP and BNP are mirrored by the ability of hyperosmolality to stimulate directly, and indirectly via volume expansion, hormone secretion. In addition to secretion from the heart, these peptides are produced in and secreted into or from a variety of other tissues where distinct biological actions have been characterized. The absolute contribution of those release sites to circulating levels of the hormones is in all likelihood minor; however, the potential importance of paracrine effects of the natriuretic peptides in those other tissues makes the study of regulation of release in those noncardiac sites extremely important. Indeed, renal, central nervous system, gonadal, and thymic production sites suggest a diversity of functions for the peptides, and the mechanisms responsible for the regulation of secretion first must be elucidated before the physiological or pathological relevance of those production sites is fully understood. Within the central nervous system, some of the same circulating factors that can stimulate ANP release from myocytes (i.e., vasopressin and endothelin) similarly stimulate neuronal production and release of the peptide.

Endothelial cell production of CNP has been clearly established and the control of peptide release partially characterized. A variety of cytokines and growth factors (including interleukin 1-α and 1-β, tumor necrosis factor [TNF]-α, and transforming growth factor [TGF]-β), as well as ANP and BNP can stimulate significant release of CNP from endothelial cells. Thus, the endothelial cell can, via CNP secretion, both transduce the antimitogenic effects of circulating ANP and BNP, and buffer the proliferative effects of circulating cytokines and growth factors.

2.2.2. States of Hypersecretion

Elevations of circulating natriuretic peptides have been reported in a variety of pathophysiologic states. CNP is remarkably elevated in septic shock, but not in congestive heart failure or hypertension. This again points to the more likely paracrine actions of CNP within the endothelial cell interface with the vascular smooth muscle cell. Congestive heart failure, myocardial ischemia, and hypertension all result in increased ANP and BNP secretion, reflecting possible compensatory mechanisms called into play during those conditions. Plasma BNP levels in the cardiac overload states exceed those of ANP. Plasma levels of ANP and BNP may become useful indicators of cardiac dysfunction and predictors of the progression of cardiac failure. Although elevated during these overload states, the bioactivity of ANP and BNP appears to be reduced owing to a possible combination of effects, including reduced renal perfusion, receptor downregulation, or simultaneous activation of the renin-angiotensin system. The increased circulating levels of ANP in critically ill trauma patients is thought to be a potential cause of suppressed ACTH levels frequently observed, since ANP can act at both the hypothalamic and pituitary levels to inhibit corticotropin secretion.

2.3. Sites of Action

Three natriuretic peptide receptor subtypes have been identified (Fig. 3). Two of these proteins contain intracellular, guanylyl cyclase domains, and

activation results in the formation of cGMP. Their extracellular domains share 44% structural homology, whereas the intracellular domains share 63% homology in the kinase domains and 88% homology in the C-terminal cyclase domains. The kinase domains are thought to play a role in the regulation of the cyclase activity via interactions with ATP. These two receptors have been designated the GC-A and GC-B receptors, and are alternatively called the NPR-A and NPR-B receptors. A third receptor subtype, called the clearance or NPR-C receptor, shares approx 30% homology with NPR-A and NPR-B, but lacks the intracellular kinase and cyclase domains. This receptor was originally thought to have no biologic activity other than to sequester or clear natriuretic peptides from the extracellular fluid; however, it is now known that the NPR-C receptor plays important biologic roles, and signals via a reduction in cAMP levels and possibly a stimulation of polyinositol phosphate turnover. A distinct hierarchy of binding affinities characterizes these receptors with all three forms of natriuretic peptides binding equally to the NPR-C receptor, whereas the NPR-A receptor prefers ANP and then BNP, and the NPR-B receptor recognizes CNP most readily (Fig. 3). Thus, the sites of action of the natriuretic peptides are determined by the relative distributions of the various receptors with the NPR-B receptor predominating in brain and muscular component of the vasculature, whereas the NPR-A receptor predominates in the kidney, endothelium, and adrenal gland. The NPR-C receptor is present throughout the body and most recently it has been determined that this receptor transduces the antimitogenic effects of the natriuretic peptides in the central nervous system. The NPR-B receptor is more abundant than the NPR-A or NPR-C forms in the hypothalamo-hypophyseal system, suggesting a primary role for CNP in neuroendocrine function.

2.4. Biologic Actions

Originally CNP was thought to act only in a paracrine fashion to regulate vascular tone and growth; however, CNP can also exert cardiovascular, renal, and adrenal actions when infused intravenously. This may simply be a reflection of the fact that CNP is produced in a variety of tissues, and therefore multiple paracrine actions may occur. CNP levels are elevated in chronic renal failure, and the peptide is produced in the kidney, where it exerts

Table 1
Peripheral Actions of the Natriuretic Peptides

Tissue system	Biologic response
Kidney	Diuresis, natriuresis, inhibition of renin secretion
Adrenal gland	Inhibition of aldosterone secretion
Heart	Decreased cardiac output, negative ionotropism
Vasculature	Vasodilation, antimitogenesis, increased permeability, release of paracrine vasoactive/antimitogenic agents (NO, CNP), inhibition of release of paracrine mitogenic factors (endothelin)
Thyroid gland	Decreased hormone secretion
Gonads	Increased testosterone and progesterone secretion
Immune system	Priming of neutrophils, enhancement of natural killer cell toxicity, activation of thymic and bone-derived macrophages

diuretic and natriuretic effects. One can recognize the sites of action of the natriuretic peptides by locating receptors, but the assignment of biologic activity is not as simple. Two reagents that have clarified the receptor subtype responsible for a variety of natriuretic peptide actions are the clearance receptor ligand C-ANF$_{4-23}$, which binds preferentially to the NPR-C receptor, and the GC receptor antagonist HS-142-1, which blocks the ability of the natriuretic peptides to signal via activation of guanylyl cyclase. Using a combination of methodologic approaches, it has been realized that although the NPR-C receptor controls the antimitogenic effects of the natriuretic peptides centrally, the NPR-B receptor performs a similar function in the vascular compartment. Within the kidney, multiple receptor subtypes are found, explaining the ability of both ANP and CNP to act as natriuretic and diuretic agents. The multiple peripheral effects of the natriuretic peptides are summarized in Table 1. Although not all these actions seem related to the regulation of fluid and electrolyte homeostasis, some may instead be related to the antiproliferative effects of these peptides.

Within the central nervous system, similar and diverging actions of ANP and CNP have been described. In most species, more CNP is produced within the brain than ANP or BNP and, for the most part, the NPR-B and NPR-C receptors predominate within the brain interstitium; however, it should be recognized that ANP may exert its biologic actions in brain indirectly by displacing CNP from the shared clearance receptor. This has been demonstrated to be the case in the neuroendocrine hypothalamus. There are other examples where interactive

effects via the shared NPR-C receptor cannot underlie the effects observed. Thus, the ability of ANP to inhibit the behavioral (water drinking) and endocrine (prolactin secretion) aspects of fluid and electrolyte homeostasis is opposed by the stimulatory effects of CNP. Certainly in these cases, activation of the NPR-A receptor must underlie the effect of ANP, whereas the NPR-B receptor must be responsible for the stimulatory effects of CNP. In the absence of antagonists that can distinguish between these two GC receptor subtypes, other methodologies had to be created to make these distinctions. One such approach is receptor-specific cytotoxin cell targeting using the plant lectin ricin. With this approach, evidence for the involvement of the NPR-A receptor in the physiologic regulation of salt appetite has been obtained, and the importance of the NPR-B receptor in the hypothalamic mechanisms controlling neuroendocrine function has been established. The central nervous system actions of the natriuretic peptides are summarized in Table 2.

How can the multiple pharmacologic effects of exogenous natriuretic peptide administrations be examined for physiologic significance? Several experimental methodologies now are available, and a combination of approaches can address this question. A selective ligand for the NPR-C receptor, C-ANF$_{4-23}$, is available and has been utilized to establish the importance of the clearance receptor in astrocytes. The above-mentioned antagonist of the guanylyl cyclase receptors, HNS-142-1, has demonstrated that endogenous natriuretic peptides play a role in the maintenance of glomerular filtration and sodium excretion under normal conditions.

**Table 2
Central Nervous System Actions
of the Natriuretic Peptides**

ANP	Action	CNP
Decrease	Water drinking	Increase
Decrease	Prolactin secretion	Increase
Decrease	Salt appetite	Unknown
Decrease	AVP secretion	Decrease
Decrease	Basal ACTH secretion (rodents and humans)	Unknown
Increase	Hemorrhage-induced ACTH secretion (sheep)	Increase
Decrease	Astrocyte proliferation	Decrease
Decrease	LH secretion	Decrease
Decrease	Neurotransmission	Decrease

Additionally, selective cytotoxin cell targeting can eliminate cells responsive to CNP or ANP, or both in the case of the clearance receptor, and together with subsequent application of exogenous peptide, clarify the physiologic roles of natriuretic peptides signaling via specific receptor subtypes in cellular function. This technique has identified the physiologic relevance of endogenous CNP in the hypothalamic control of prolactin and luteinizing hormone secretion, and the involvement of ANP in regulation of salt appetite. Passive immunoneutralization approaches have been largely uninformative, perhaps because of the inherent problem of getting sufficient immunoglobulin to the site of release in order to sequester the peptide prior to its exposure to the receptor. This approach, however, has successfully identified the physiological relevance of ANP in brain mechanisms controlling thirst. Finally, the enzyme system responsible for the degradation of endogenous natriuretic peptides has been identified. Pharmacologic inhibition of this neutral endopeptidase (NEP, EC 3.4.24.11) results in increased circulating levels of natriuretic peptide and biological effects that mirror those seen after administration of exogenous peptide. Although this approach alone does not establish the physiologic relevance of endogenous peptide, it can be used in concert with other experimental strategies to examine the pathophysiology of the natriuretic peptides and their potential therapeutic advantages.

Recently two molecular techniques have provided additional insight into the physiology of the natriuretic peptides. Transgenic mouse models of ANP and BNP overexpression have been created. In the case of the ANP transgene, homozygotes displayed significantly lower blood pressure under basal conditions than nontransgenic littermates; however, sodium excretion was not different. In response to volume expansion, the renal excretory function of transgenic mice exceeded that of normal littermates. Recent reports indicate a similar scenario in BNP transgenes. These results must be interpreted with caution, since lifelong overexpression of a natriuretic peptide may in fact result in a decreased responsiveness (i.e., resetting) to its normal biologic action. Furthermore, long-term overexpression may in fact recruit counterregulatory factors, such as endothelin, a peptide whose production and release are significantly altered by exogenous natriuretic peptide administration. The second molecular approach to the study of the physiological relevance of the natriuretic peptides is the generation of null mutations (knockouts), which result in the absence of a given peptide. Homozygous mice lacking ANP have been created, and it has been demonstrated that these animals are more susceptible to the hypertensive consequences of high salt ingestion. This important advance in the study of the natriuretic peptides reveals two important facts. First, ANP is not apparently necessary for normal embryologic and postnatal development. Second, endogenous ANP must play some role in the physiological mechanisms that protect against the development of high blood pressure.

2.5. Potential Therapeutic Uses

Although the action of the natriuretic peptides appears to be blunted in edematous states, such as congestive heart failure, cirrhosis, and the nephrotic syndrome, therapeutic usage of the peptides in these states may prove at least acutely advantageous. Certainly, if the mechanism by which the biological activity of the peptides has been reduced in these states can be elucidated, strategies might be employed that may overcome those deficits. In particular, it has already been demonstrated that in congestive heart failure, administration of pharmacologic doses of ANP and urodilatin can lower preload and increase diuresis and natriuresis, providing significant benefit in this life-threatening situation. Perhaps a similar strategy can be used to induce mineralocorticoid escape, since a role for endogenous ANP in this phenomenon has been demonstrated. Interest in the potential use of pharmacologic doses of ANP and urodilatin in the postoperative setting to pre-

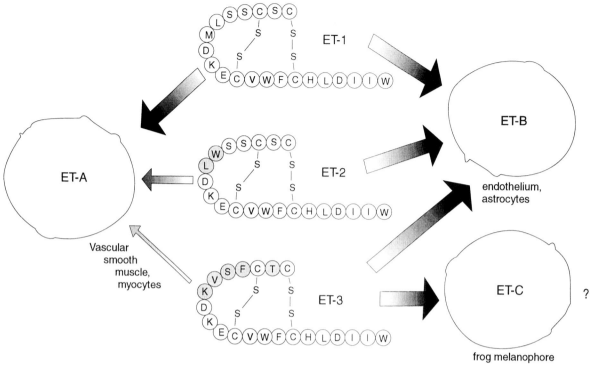

Fig. 4. Three members of the endothelin (ET) peptide family have been identified, each sharing remarkable homology in amino acid compostion. Differing amino acids are indicated in darkened circles. Three receptor subtypes have been characterized. The ET-A receptor binds ET with the relative preference indicated by the thickness of the arrows (ET-1 ≥ ET-2 > ET-3). The ET-B receptor recognizes equally all three forms of ET. The third ET receptor, ET-C, found to date only in nonmammals prefers ET-3. Sites of receptor expression are indicated.

vent acute renal failure has been stimulated by preliminary results, which demonstrated that such infusions can in some patients obviate the need for hemodialysis/hemofiltration.

Most promising in a therapeutic sense is the potential for the natriuretic peptides to be employed as antiproliferative agents. In a rabbit model of vascular lesions caused by balloon catheter injury, CNP administration significantly lowered the resultant intima-to-media ratios, providing direct evidence for a paracrine action of the peptide to suppress intimal thickening. Furthermore, local CNP antagonizes the growth-promoting effects of angiotensin II and the vascular consequences of cyclosporine A induction of endothelin release and subsequent mitogenesis, again predicting a significant avenue for the prevention of vascular lesions. With the realization that both ANP and BNP can stimulate local production of CNP, the antiproliferative agent that acts locally to suppress mitogenesis, we are perhaps closer to a manipulation that will stimulate endogenous protective mechanisms in the vasculature.

3. THE ENDOTHELINS

3.1. Gene Structure and Regulation

In addition to the production of endothelial-derived relaxing factors in the vasculature, it had been known for some time that the cells lining the blood vessels produced potent vasoconstrictive substances as well. In 1988, the sequence of a powerful, endogenous vasoconstrictor substance produced in endothelial cells was identified. This 21 amino acid peptide was named endothelin. It is now recognized that there are three forms of endothelin (ET-1, ET-2, and ET-3), all 21 amino acid peptides differing by only two to five amino acids in the 15-membered ring structure formed by two internal disulfide bonds (Fig. 4). Each are products of unique genes and are processed similarly into first a preprohormone form of 203 amino acids, in the case of ET-1, and then posttranslationally modified into the 39 amino acid prohormone intermediate, big ET. In states of hypersecretion, the prohormone form appears in plasma; however, under normal conditions the mature 21 amino acid form is the major secretory product. The final cleavage of the prohormone is thought to occur at secretion and to be catalyzed by a phosphorami-don-sensitive metalloproteinase designated endothelin-converting enzyme (EC 3.4.24.11). Knowledge of this important conversion enzyme's presence has led to potential therapeutic intervention strategies for the interruption of endothelin action in states of hypersecretion, since the prohormone big ET has limited biologic activity.

The human ET-1 gene has five exons and four introns, with the peptide coded in the second exon. The gene is transcriptionally regulated via cis-elements, including a GATA-2 protein-binding site and an AP-1 site that is activated by thrombin, angiotensin II, epidermal growth factor (EGF), basic fibroblast growth factor (bFGF), insulin-like growth factor (IGF-I), and transforming growth factor-β (TGF-β). Other transcriptional regulators include vasopressin, the interleukins, tumor necrosis factor-α (TNFα), and NO, which apparently mediates the ability of heparin to stimulate ET production. Physical factors also activate transcription, including pressure and anoxia. Translational regulation is exerted by a variety of factors that also regulate secretion, since little hormone is stored intracellularly. High-density lipoproteins stimulate production and secretion, whereas insulin not only stimulates production and secretion, but also augments ET binding and action. Negative regulation of production and secretion is exerted at the transcriptional level by NO, and at the translational event, by prostaglandins, prostacyclin, adrenomedullin, and ANP (Table 3).

3.2. Hormone Secretion

Fortunately, the majority of the endothelin produced is secreted abluminally, away from the vessel lumen, to act in an autocrine or paracrine fashion. Although levels of the hormone do rise in certain pathologic conditions, probably reflecting tissue damage in most cases, in general, this peptide should be kept out of the circulation because of its potent vasoconstrictive properties and the fact that in experimental animals, elevation in circulating ET results in respiratory failure and/or cerebral vasospasms and aneurysms. Thus, a knowledge of production sites predicts biologic actions. The major site of ET-1 production is the endothelium (Fig. 2) where upon release it causes vasoconstriction. Additional production sites include the brain, uterus, kidney mesangial cells, sertoli cells,

Table 3
Factors That Regulate Endothelin Production

Stimulatory	Stimulatory	Inhibitory
Angiotensin II	Vasopressin	NO
Thrombin	Insulin	Prostaglandin E$_2$(PGE$_2$)
HDL and LDL	Catecholamines	Prostacyclin (PGI$_2$)
Calcium	Cytokines	Atrial natriuretic peptide
Growth factors (TGF-β, IGF-1, EGF, bFGF)		Adrenomedullin

and breast epithelial cells. ET-3 production occurs mainly within the central nervous system, where a role for the peptide in neuronal and astroglial development and proliferation has been suggested. What little ET-2 is produced in the body is found in kidney, intestine (hence, the alternative name vasoactive intestinal contractor, VIC), myocardium, and uterus. The endothelins have a relatively short half-life in plasma, about 4–7 min, and are released predominantly in response to hypoxia, ischemia, and shear stress.

3.3. Sites and Mechanisms of Action

Two mammalian endothelin receptor subtypes have been cloned, and they are members of the G-protein-linked, seven-transmembrane-spanning domain superfamily of biologic receptors (Fig. 4). The ET-A receptor displays a rank order of binding affinity with ET-1 being the preferred ligand (ET-1 $\geq$ ET-2 $>>$ ET-3). This receptor predominates on vascular smooth muscle cells and cardiac myocytes. Activation of this receptor results, depending on tissue site, in the activation of a variety of signaling cascades, including in the lung the production of prostanoids via stimulation of phospholipase D and A$_2$ activities resulting in bronchoconstriction and in the scenario of hypersecretion, pulmonary hypertension (Fig. 5). In vascular smooth muscle cells, ET stimulates contraction and mitogenesis via multiple signaling pathways, including activation of phospholipase C with the resultant formation of diacylglycerol (DAG) and inositol triphosphate (IP$_3$). The DAG formed activates the kinase cascade via protein kinase C, and IP$_3$ mobilizes intracellular calcium initiating the contractile event. ET-A receptor activation also in these cells has been reported to open potassium channels and to activate

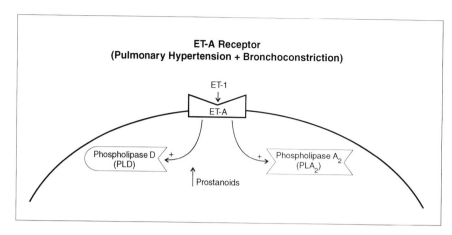

Fig. 5. Schematic representation of the role of activation of the ET-A receptor in pulmonary hypertension and bronchocon-striction. Activation of the ET-A receptor leads to stimulation of the production of prostanoids.

adenylate cyclase (Fig. 6). In the myocardium, the ET-A receptor is thought to be activated by endogenous ET released in response to ischemia following myocardial infarction. The resultant opening of potassium channels causes a decrease in electrical activity of the myocyte and closes the chloride channel, resulting in a suppression of catecholamine activation of contractile function (Fig. 7).

The ET-B receptor predominates in the endothelium itself and in the central nervous system. This receptor binds all three isoforms equally and is responsible for the ability of circulating ET to stimulate a transient vasodilatory response in the periphery, via acute release of such vasodilators as NO and CNP (Fig. 2). The signaling cascade that follows activation of the ET-B receptor is multifaceted. G-protein-coupled activation of phospholipase C results in activation of protein kinase C and mobilization of intracellular calcium. NO synthase activity is stimulated with the resultant production of the potent vasodilator NO, which can act within the endothelial cell to activate soluble guanylyl cyclase or diffuse across to the smooth muscle cells to perform the same function. Additionally, ET-B activation results in opening of the sodium-hydrogen antiporter and inhibition of adenylate cyclase (Fig. 8). The mitogenic effects of ET are thought to be transduced via PKC activation and tyrosine phosphorylation-initiated activation of the MAP-kinase system. In mesangial cells the mitogenic effect of ET is mediated via transcriptional activation of immediate early genes. Activation of *Ras* proteins and downstream induction of the kinase activity of *Raf*-1

result in transcriptional induction of the c-*fos* serum response element, perhaps providing a mechanism for the mitogenic effects of ET. One hallmark characteristic of the biologic effects of the ETs is their profound tachyphylaxis. Although some data indicate this to be the result of chronic membrane effects or overloading of the cytosolic calcium pool, evidence also exists for rapid internalization of the ligand–receptor complex and continued signaling from the internalized aggregate.

3.4. Biologic Actions

Although multiple pharmacologic effects of the endothelins have been reported, there is a need to establish which of those have biologic significance and physiologic relevance. In this case, multiple pharmacologic tools are available, such that selective antagonism of the ET-A receptor is possible and isoform-specific activation of the ET-B receptor can be accomplished. Also available are antagonists that affect both the ET-A and ET-B receptor, and a new generation of relatively specific ET-B antagonists. Much interest continues in the possible existence of a unique, ET-3-selective ET-C receptor in mammals similar to that found in frog melanophores, and it is hoped that eventual cloning of that protein will permit generation of similarly selective receptor antagonists.

Surprising results from molecular approaches have provided new insight into the biology of the endothelins. As discussed below, it was anticipated that these potent vasoconstrictive peptides would be found to play an important role in the development

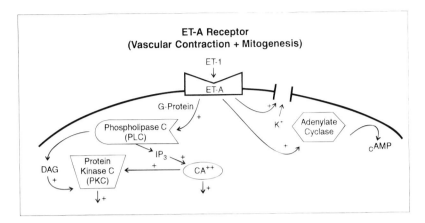

Fig. 6. Schematic representation of the effects of ET on VSMC and mitogenesis. Activation of the ET-A receptor results in multiple signaling pathways, including production of DAG and IP_3, opening of potassium channels, and activation of adenylate cyclase.

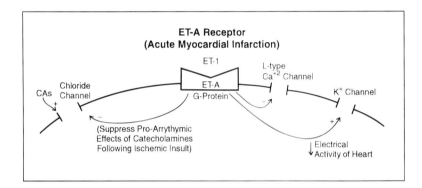

Fig. 7. Schematic representation of the role of ET in tissue damage secondary to acute myocardial infarction. Activation of the G-protein-linked ET-A receptor can block the ability of catecholamines to open chloride channels, close calcium channels, and open potassium channels leading to decreased electrical activity in the heart.

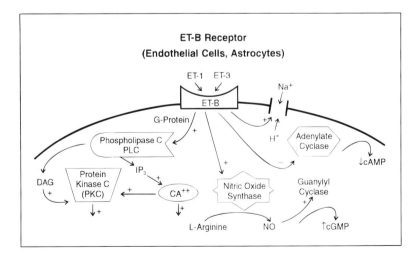

Fig. 8. ET-B receptors signal via a variety of mechanisms, including production of DAG and IP_3, production of NO, opening of the sodium/hydrogen antiporter, and activation of adenylate cyclase.

of hypertension; however, gene knockout homozygotes have, if anything, slightly elevated blood pressure, not the expected hypotension. Unexpected results accrued from these null mutation strategies. Mice lacking expression of the normal ET-1 gene are born with severe craniofacial malformations, suggesting a developmental role for the peptide in pharyngeal arch structures. Additionally these animals succumb to respiratory failure, suggesting an important embryogenic role of the peptide in the preparation of respiratory structures for postnatal life. Knockouts of the genes encoding the ET-B receptor or ET-3 itself result in a postnatal phenotype similar to that observed in Hirschsprung's disease (congenital megacolon), suggesting the importance of ET in the development of the intrinsic nervous system of the gut and the regulation of gastrointestinal smooth muscle function. Multiple central nervous system actions of the endothelins have been reported ranging from mitogenic effects on astrocytes mediated via the ET-B receptor to effects on descending sympathetic activity. The presence of ET peptide and ET receptors during fetal development indicates a potential embryogenic role in central nervous system structures, which may mirror the situation uncovered by the ET-3 and ET-B receptor knockouts in the intrinsic nervous system of the gut, and indeed loss of neurotropic effects of the endothelins may be responsible in part for the respiratory failure seen in the immediate postpartum interval. With regard to neuromodulatory effects of the endothelins, antagonist studies have revealed the physiologic relevance of the antidipsogenic effects of ET; however, the day-to-day significance of the neuroendocrine actions of the peptide (including activation of the hypothalamic mechanisms controlling anterior pituitary function and vasopressin secretion) and the effects of the peptides on sympathetic function have yet to be established. A final central nervous system consequence of ET administration is potentially disastrous. ET infusion results in some species in rupture of the basal artery, and a role for endogenous ET in vasospasm subsequent to subarachnoid hemorrhage has been established by the observation that pretreatment with an ET antagonist can prevent this event. This has led to the hypothesis that ET antagonists may prove therapeutically advantageous to prevent or lessen ischemic damage downstream from damaged, hypoxic endothelium of cerebral vessels after thrombosis or infarct.

3.5. Pathophysiology of the Endothelins

Because of the multiple pharmacologic activities of the endothelins, their involvement in numerous pathologic states has been hypothesized (Table 4). These hypotheses were based largely on elevated hormone levels or responses seen in these conditions and, under many circumstances, it remains unclear whether the associations are causal or coincidental in nature.

As mentioned above, the most predicted role for the endothelins in pathophysiology was that in hypertensive states. Indeed, plasma levels are not consistently found to correlate with blood pressure, and although they may be elevated in some animal models of hypertension, null mutant mice actually had elevated pressures. Just the same, there may instead be a hyperresponsiveness to the peptide in certain states, so the controversy continues. Similarly controversial is the potential role for ET in reperfusion injury, where one group using an isolated perfused rat heart model argued against a causative role and another utilizing isolated ventricular myocytes argued in favor. In vivo evidence favoring a role for endogenous ET in reperfusion injury comes from studies in pigs where both myocardial ischemia and infarction resulted in significantly elevated ET production and release. In rats receiving infusion of antiserum directed against ET-1 prior to coronary artery ligation, damage distal to the ligation was marked reduced. Similar results were obtained with the ET-A receptor antagonist in a canine, myocardial infarction model. These data provide the best evidence for a role for ET in reperfusion injury and ischemia.

Endothelin antagonists improve renal function in a genetic model of hypertension, the spontaneously hypertensive rat, and ET has been invoked in the pathogenesis of acute renal failure (postischemia renal failure). Cyclosporine A-induced nephrotoxicity has been identified at least in part to be owing to endothelin-induced vasoconstriction of the afferent arteriole, since the renal toxicity of immunosuppressant therapy was blocked by ET antagonist pretreatment. The mitogenic actions of ET are thought to underlie the development of graft arteriosclerosis in cardiac allografts, the establishment of atherosclerotic plaques, and the development of diabetes-related vascular lesions. Its role in vasospasm secondary to subarachnoid hemorrhage has been

Table 4
Potential Pathologic Roles for the Endothelins in Disease States

Evidenced	*Proposed*
Myocardial damage owing to vascular insult	Acute vascular insult (brain)
	Patent ductus arteriosus
Cyclosporine-induced nephrotoxicity	Pulmonary hypertension and fibrosis
Postischemic renal failure	Gastric ulceration
Vasospasm secondary to subarachnoid hemorrhage	Heart failure manifestations
	Hepatorenal syndrome (cirrhosis)
Hirschsprung's disease	Unstable angina
	Raynaud's disease
	Shock
	Glomerulonephritis
	Inflammatory bowel disease
	Dysmenorrhea
	Asthma
	Pre-eclampsia

established in animal models. Within the lung, roles for endothelin in asthma and pulmonary hypertension have been proposed on the basis of measurement levels of the hormone. Although still much more data are needed to establish a pathophysiologic role for the endothelins in a variety of clinical settings, the current literature promises therapeutic advantage following manipulation of endogenous ET systems with antagonist administration in the setting of vascular disease and ischemia. Perhaps the most promise lies in the development of therapies that will interdict the mitogenic actions of these hormones.

4. ADRENOMEDULLIN: A NOVEL VASOACTIVE PEPTIDE

4.1. Gene Structure and Regulation

Utilizing a bioassay system that monitored the accumulation of cAMP in platelets, the group from the Miyazaki Medical College and the Japanese National Cardiovascular Center Research Institute identified in 1993, a novel vasoactive peptide in extracts of a human pheochromocytoma. This peptide (52 amino acids in humans, 50 in the rat) is produced in normal chromaffin cells of the adrenal gland, as well as a variety of other tissues, including brain, kidney, endothelial cells, and vascular smooth muscle cells. Posttranslational processing of the precursor (185 amino acids in humans) results in the production and secretion of the mature form, designated adrenomedullin, and a 20 amino acid fragment from the N-terminal prohormone designated proad-

renomedullin N-20 terminal peptide (PAMP), a peptide with some similar biological activity to that of adrenomedullin. Although activation of adenylate cyclase was used as a screening bioassay during the initial phases of work on this peptide, the hallmark bioassay is the potent hypotensive action when infused intravenously (Table 5).

Adrenomedullin production in vascular smooth muscle cells and endothelial cells is regulated at the transcriptional level by a variety of cytokines, including interleukin 1-α and 1-β, TNF-α, and TNF-β. Production of adrenomedullin in these cells was also reported recently to be stimulated by thrombin, aldosterone, cortisol, retinoic acid, and thyroid hormones. To a lesser degree, stimulation of production in vascular smooth muscle cells also was seen in response to angiotensin II, epinephrine, platelet-derived growth factor (PDGF), EGF, and FGF. Inhibition of production was observed in the presence of TGF-β and cAMP. Subtle differences in the kinetics of the effects of the various factors that elevate adrenomedullin production may underlie unique transcriptional regulation. Additionally, the regulation of gene transcription in other tissues has yet to be characterized.

4.2. Hormone Secretion

Many of the same factors that stimulate adrenomedullin production also activate secretion in isolated cell systems, leading to the hypothesis that this peptide may be responsible for the hypotension of inflammation, endotoxic shock, and atherosclerosis. Circulating levels in humans have been reported to be

Table 5
Pharmacologic Actions of Adrenomedullin/PAMP

Tissue system	Effect
Blood vessels	Hypotension
	Decreased total peripheral resistance
	Increased renal blood flow
Lung	Pulmonary vasodilation
Adrenal gland	Inhibition of cholinergic stimulation of catecholamine release
	Inhibition of stimulated aldosterone secretion
Kidney	Diuresis
	Natriuresis
Pituitary gland	Inhibition of ACTH secretion
Central nervous system	Inhibition of water drinking (antidipsogenesis)

similar to those of other vasoactive hormones (about 3 fmol/mL plasma), suggesting that like other vasoactive substances, the actions of adrenomedullin may be predominantly autocrine or paracrine in nature. One group failed to observe elevations in plasma adrenomedullin during hypertensive attacks in patients with pheochromocytomas; however, cosecretion of adrenomedullin and catecholamines from cultured bovine adrenal medullary cells has been observed. In fact, the cosecretion of PAMP and catecholamines from these cells is calcium-dependent and induced by carbachol activation of nicotinic receptors. Those studies also pointed to an autocrine or paracrine action of the peptide, since PAMP acted as an anticholinergic inhibiting sodium influx and reducing the magnitude of catecholamine response to carbachol.

4.3. Sites of Actions

Some of the pharmacologic actions of adrenomedullin can be prevented by prior administration of the calcitonin gene-related peptide antagonist, $CGRP_{8-37}$. Adrenomedullin and CGRP share considerable structural homology. Both activate adenylate cyclase in a variety of tissues and can displace each other in binding assays. Mesenteric vasodilatory responses to adrenomedullin are antagonized by $CGRP_{8-37}$ in vitro, but in vivo vasodilatory responses are not. Additionally, the increase in cAMP levels

observed in response to adrenomedullin in endothelial cells in culture is not blocked by $CGRP_{8-37}$. Until a unique receptor for adrenomedullin is cloned, the controversy over whether these peptides act through similar receptors will not be silenced.* It remains possible that the CGRP affects merely reflect pharmacologic activation of endogenous adrenomedullin receptors and not vice versa. Additionally, the effects of adrenomedullin in nonvascular sites, such as renal tubules, pituitary gland, and brain, have been reported not to be via a receptor similar to that for CGRP.

4.4. Biologic Actions

Intravenous infusion of adrenomedullin in doses calculated to double circulating levels has resulted in profound, long-lasting hypotension with attendant reflexive increases in heart rate. The vasoactive effect of adrenomedullin is blocked by false substrates for NO synthase, suggesting a role for the soluble gas in transduction of the adrenomedullin signal. Indeed, in cultured bovine aortic endothelial cells, adrenomedullin stimulates, via a cholera toxin-sensitive G-protein mechanism(s), signal transduction by at least two parallel pathways, one involving to elevation of cAMP levels and the other resulting in inositol triphosphate production, mobilization of intracellular calcium and activation of NO synthase. Adrenomedullin also increases cAMP levels in rat mesangial cells and in hepatic stellate cells, perhaps reflecting circulatory effects in those tissues as well. Signaling downstream to protein kinase C activation recently has been demonstrated in rat mesangial cells where adrenomedullin decreased MAP-kinase activation by vasopressin.

The increase in renal perfusion seen in response to intravenous adrenomedullin infusion is the result of a decrease in renal vascular resistance subsequent to dilation of both the afferent and efferent arterioles. This effect is also NO-mediated. The increased perfusion of the glomerulus after adrenomedullin may not be responsible for the profound natriuretic and diuretic effects of the peptide. Adrenomedullin-like immunoreactivity is present in the canine glomerulus, cortical collecting tubules, and medullary collecting duct, suggesting direct, distal tubule actions underlying its effect on fractional sodium excretion. These effects are not blocked by NO synthesis blockade.

*See Note Added in Proof at end of chapter.

Another action of adrenomedullin that does not appear to be the result of its ability to activate NO synthase is in the pituitary gland. Although the peptide failed to stimulate NO production, it did significantly inhibit basal and CRH-stimulated corticotropin secretion in vitro. An adenylate cyclase-dependent mechanism for the selective inhibition of ACTH secretion is unlikely, since adrenomedullin failed to alter basal or CRH-stimulated cAMP accumulation. This ability of adrenomedullin to inhibit pituitary ACTH secretion may be another mechanism by which the peptide functions to regulate sodium homeostasis. Adrenal effects to inhibit stimulated aldosterone secretion have also been reported, again suggesting a role in fluid and electrolyte homeostasis.

Within the central nervous system, adrenomedullin acts to suppress water intake and salt appetite. Although no significant effects on basal water drinking in the sated state or on locomotor activity or blood pressure in the conscious rat were observed at the doses tested (22–88 pmol), drinking in response to angiotensin II or two physiologic stimuli (overnight water deprivation, hyperosmotic challenge) was inhibited in a dose-related manner by exogenous adrenomedullin. Thus, the diuretic effects in kidney appear mirrored by CNS actions on water intake. The natriuretic effects of the peptide are mirrored as well by CNS actions to inhibit salt appetite, an effect that has recently been demonstrated by passive immunoneutralization studies to have physiologic relevance. Although the CNS sites and mechanisms of action are still being characterized, it is already apparent that this novel vasoactive peptide can exert effects within the brain that complement those expressed in the periphery and, as with other vasoactive hormones, a central theme is emerging for the physiology of adrenomedullin, that of a volume regulatory factor that assists in unloading an expanded vascular tree. Indeed, many of the effects of adrenomedullin oppose those of angiotensin II and support those of the natriuretic peptides, further expanding the growing concept of multiple endocrine factors controlling fluid and electrolyte homeostasis and cardiovascular function.

4.5. Pathophysiology of Adrenomedullin

Just as the multiple pharmacologic properties of adrenomedullin are being described, already some insight into potential pathophysiologic actions are being gained. Plasma levels of the hormone are elevated in hypertension, more so in those patients with renal failure. In an experimental model of hypertension, the DOCA-salt-sensitive hypertensive rat, the ability of adrenomedullin to decrease vascular resistance is attenuated, suggesting the loss of an important local regulatory effect of the peptide subsequent to vascular damage. Plasma adrenomedullin levels correlate well with circulating ANP, epinephrine, and cAMP, suggesting that it may be part of a compensatory mechanism by which the integrity of the cardiovascular system is maintained. Certainly the ability of a host of cytokines to stimulate adrenomedullin production and secretion at the endothelial cell–vascular smooth muscle interface justifies an examination of the role it may play in the pathology of shock and inflammation. Just as the knowledge bases for the natriuretic peptides and endothelins expanded rapidly in the first years following their discovery, so too are the fields of adrenomedullin pharmacology, physiology, and pathophysiology expanding in the early exponent.

5. INTERACTIVE EFFECTS OF THE CARDIOVASCULAR HORMONES

It is apparent that individual vasoactive hormones can act in a coordinate fashion in a variety of tissues to affect cardiovascular status. Additional, noncardiovascular effects have been demonstrated, and their relation to the vascular and renal actions of the peptides is unclear. All the same, the peptides represent excellent models for an integrated regulatory system controlling important physiologic functions, and it is now clear that multiple factors interact in such a manner that a push and a pull on volume homeostasis, vascular remodeling and permeability, and endocrine regulation are being expressed. Our limitations in the realization of the physiological relevance of these interactions is merely the techniques now employed. Novel approaches are being devised with which the significance of any one of these factors can be elucidated; however, in their interactions with the other vasoactive factors, loss of the function of one peptide may be compensated by another or, alternatively, the activity of that remaining factor altered substantially. Thus, although it is imperative that the molecular mechanisms underlying the production, release, and action of the various hormones must be determined, it is in the whole-animal, integrative setting that the importance of one or more of these hormones to normal physiology and the progress of disease will ultimately be understood and capitalized on.

NOTE ADDED IN PROOF

A unique adrenomedullin receptor has been cloned and sequenced since the original composition of this manuscript (Kapas et al., 1995).

SELECTED READINGS

Baldi E, Maggi M, Cameron IT, Dunn MJ, eds. Endothelins in endocrinology: new advances. In: *Frontiers in Endocrinology*, vol 15. Rome: Ares-Serano Symposia Publications, 1995.

Brandt RR, Wright RS, Redfield MM, Burnett JC. Atrial natriuretic peptide in heart failure. *J Am Coll Cardiol* 1993; 22:86A.

Feng CJ, Kang B, Kaye AD, Kadowitz PJ, Nossman BD. L-NAME modulates responses to adrenomedullin in hindquarters vascular bed of the rat. *Life Sci* 1994; 55:433.

Haynes WG. Endothelins as regulators of vascular tone in man. *Clin Sci* 1995; 88:509.

Hirata Y, Hayakawa H, Suzuki Y, Suzuki E, Ikenouchi H, Kohmoto O, Kimura K, Kitamura K, Eto T, Kangawa K, Matsuo H, Omata M. Mechanisms of adrenomedullin-induced vasodilation in the rat kidney. *Hypertension* 1995; 25:790.

Inagami T, Naruse M, Hoover R. Endothelium as an endocrine organ. *Annu Rev Physiol* 1995; 57:171.

John SWM, Krege JH, Oliver P, Hagaman J, Hodgin JB, Pang SC, Flynn TG, Marda N, Smithies O. Genetically decreased levels of atrial natriuretic peptide and salt-sensitive hypertension. *Science* 1995; 267:679.

Kapas et al. *J Biol Chem* 1995; 270:25344.

Kitamura K, Kangawa K, Matsuo H, Eto T. Adrenomedullin. Implications for hypertension research. *Drugs* 1995; 49:485.

Koller KJ, Goeddel DV. Molecular biology of the natriuretic peptides and their receptors. *Circulation* 1992; 86:1081.

Levin ER, Frank HJ. Natriuretic peptides inhibit rat astroglial proliferation: mediation by the C-receptor. *Am J Physiol* 1991; 261:R453.

Naruse M, Naruse K, Demura H. Recent advances in endothelin research on cardiovascular and endocrine systems. *Endocr J* 1994; 41:491.

Nazario B, Hu RM, Pedram A, Prins B, Levin ER. Atrial and brain natriuretic peptides stimulate the production and secretion of C-type natriuretic peptide from bovine aortic endothelial cells. *J Clin Invest* 1995; 95:1151.

Richards AM. The natriuretic peptides and hypertension. *J Int Med* 1994; 235:543.

Samson WK, Huang FLS, Fulton RJ. C-type natriuretic peptide mediates the hypothalamic actions of the natriuretic peptides to inhibit luteinizing hormone secretion. *Endocrinology* 1993; 132:504.

Samson WK, Murphy T, Schell DA. A novel vasoactive peptide, adrenomedullin, inhibits pituitary adrenocorticotropin release. *Endocrinology* 1995; 136:2349.

24 Adrenal Medulla (Catecholamine and Peptides)

William J. Raum, MD, PhD

Contents

1. DEVELOPMENTAL ORIGIN

Some primitive autonomic ganglia transform into neurons, some into satellite and neurolemma cells associated with neurons, and others become distinct endocrine elements. The latter stain brown with chrome salts and are thus designated chromaffin cells. This reaction is the result of the presence of the hormone, epinephrine, contained within the cells. The chromaffin system consists of various aggregates of these cells throughout the body. The adrenal medulla is the most prominent member of the group.

Paraganglia, aptly named, consist of chromaffin cells that collect in close approximation to autonomic ganglia and plexuses. They begin to form at about 2 mo of gestation and attain a diameter of about 1 mm by birth.

Chromaffin bodies are chromaffin masses that arise along the course of the aorta. Chromaffin cells are intermingled with strands of connective tissue and enclosed in a connective tissue capsule. They develop first at the root of the inferior mesenteric artery at about 2 mo of gestation. At birth, they are about 1 cm in diameter. The largest complex in the abdomen, the organ of Zuckerkandl, occurs near the bifurcation of the aorta into the iliac arteries. After birth, chromaffin bodies begin to decline in size and nearly disappear by puberty.

Carotid bodies begin as a mesodermal condensation on the wall of each internal carotid in the seventh week. Chromaffin cells and nonchromaffin autonomic ganglion cells invade and branches of the glossopharengeal nerve innervate the bodies. When mature, the organ functions in the reflex regulation of blood pressure.

The adrenal gland is actually two distinct glands combined in a common capsule. The cortex is derived from mesoderm and secretes steroid hormones. The medulla is derived from ectodermal chromaffin tissue and secretes catecholamines. In lower animals, such as fish, the cortex and medulla present as separate organs. During the seventh week of gestation, chromaffin cells from the celiac plexus collect on the medial side of the already prominent primordial cortex and migrate inward. By the fourth month, the chromaffin tissue occupies a central position in the gland. The tissue becomes organized into cords and masses permeated with a profuse network of sinusoidal capillaries.

The link between the autonomic nervous system and the adrenal medulla is both embryologic and functional. The adrenal medulla functions much like

From: *Endocrinology: Basic and Clinical Principles* (P. M. Conn and S. Melmed, eds.), Humana Press Inc., Totowa, NJ.

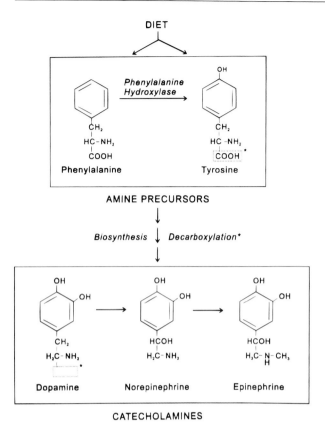

DIET

*Phenylalanine
Hydroxylase*

Phenylalanine

Tyrosine

AMINE PRECURSORS

Biosynthesis ↓ *Decarboxylation**

Dopamine   Norepinephrine   Epinephrine

CATECHOLAMINES

Fig. 1. APUD is a feature characteristic of endocrine and neuroendocrine tissues. The amino acids, phenylalanine and tyrosine, are the amine precursors that are decarboxylated and subsequently become catecholamines in sympathetic neurons and chromaffin tissue. Both amino acids are derived from the diet, but tyrosine may also be synthesized from phenylalanine in the liver.

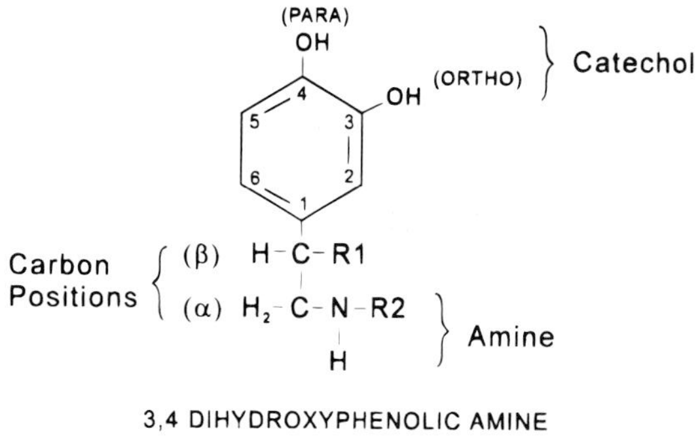

(PARA)
OH

(ORTHO) } Catechol

Carbon
Positions { (β) H–C–R1
           (α) H₂–C–N–R2 } Amine
                    H

3,4 DIHYDROXYPHENOLIC AMINE

	Substitutions	
Product	β(R1)	α(R2)
Dopamine	-H	-H
Norepinephrine	-OH	-H
Epinephrine	-OH	-CH₃

Fig. 2. Catecholamine structure. The catecholamines are 3,4-dihydroxyphenolic amines. The benzene ring structure numbering is counterclockwise with carbon-1 being bonded to the aliphatic side chain. The catechol group consists of two adjacent hydroxyl groups, one at position-4 or *para* with respect to position-1, and the second at position-3 or *ortho* with respect to the hydroxyl at position-4. The aliphatic side-chain carbon atoms are labeled β and α. As illustrated, the substitutions on these carbons define each of the three most prominent catecholamines.

the postganglionic sympathetic neuron, but the neurotransmitter (epinephrine) is released into the bloodstream rather than the synaptic junction. The receptors and effector cells are located throughout the body rather than just across the synapse. An appreciation of their similarities and differences aids in understanding how one influences the other in both normal and pathophysiologic processes.

2. CATECHOLAMINES

The principal catecholamines found in the body, norepinephrine, epinephrine, and dopamine, are formed by hydroxylation and decarboxylation of the amino acids phenylalanine and tyrosine (Fig. 1). The process of amine precursor uptake and decarboxylation (APUD) is a feature common to a variety of endocrine and neuroendocrine tissues that are emby-

rologically related and secrete polypeptide hormones, hormone precursors, and catecholamines. All three of these catecholamines act as neurotransmitters in the central nervous system. Norepinephrine also functions as a neurotransmitter in the sympathetic nervous system. Although there are dopamine receptors outside the central nervous system, the role of dopamine as a hormone or neurotransmitter peripherally is not fully described. Epinephrine is the circulating hormone secreted by the adrenal medulla and influences processes throughout the body.

2.1. Catecholamine Biosynthesis

Catecholamines are 3, 4-dihydroxyated phenolic amines (Fig. 2). The most prevalent of these are dopamine, norepinephrine, and epinephrine. The biosynthesis (Fig. 3) begins with tyrosine, which consists of a benzene ring hyroxylated in the 4-(*para*) position to the two-carbon side chain at the 1-position. The β-carbon, closest to the ring, is sat-

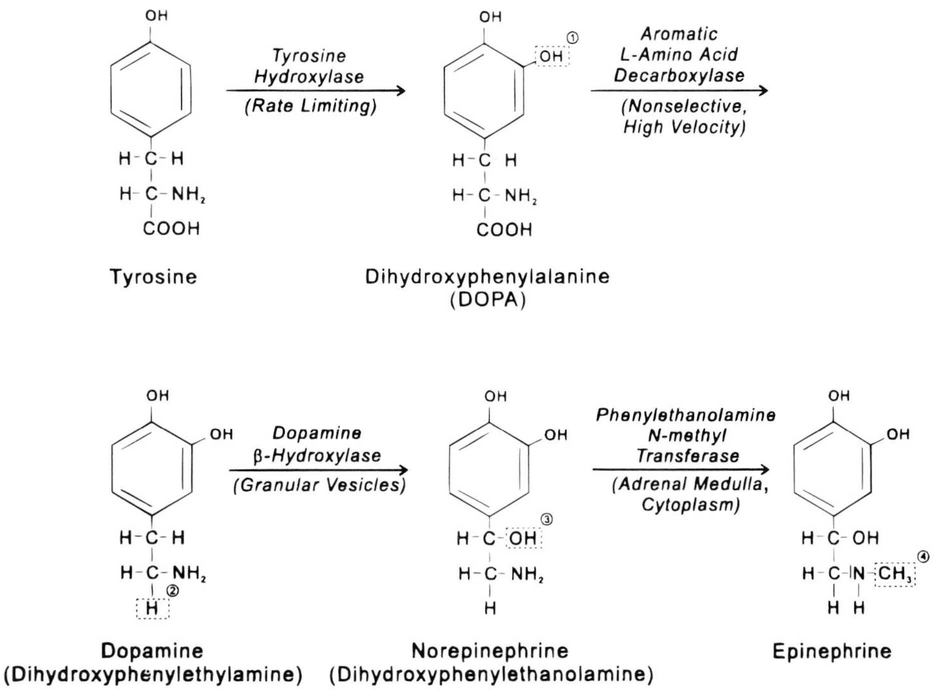

Fig. 3. Catecholamine biosynthesis. Tyrosine hydroxylase catalyzes the (1) *para*-hydroxylation of tyrosine to form DOPA and is the rate-limiting step in the biosynthesis of catecholamines. The other major steps include (2) decarboxylation of DOPA, (3) β-hydroxylation of dopamine, and (4) *N*-methylation of norepinephrine to form epinephrine.

urated with hydrogen and is single bonded to the α-carbon. The α-carbon is bonded to the amino and carboxylic acid groups that define the amino acids. The rate-limiting enzyme, tyrosine hydroxylase, 3-hydroxylates (*ortho* with respect to the 4-position hydroxyl) tyrosine to dihydroxyphenylalanine (DOPA). The α-carbon is decarboxylated by aromatic L-amino acid decarboxylase to form the first catecholamine, dopamine (L-dihydroxyphenylethylamine). Hydroxylation of the β-carbon of dopamine (by dopamine β-hydroxylase) results in the formation of norepinephrine. Norepinephrine can be converted to epinephrine by methylation of the amino group on the α-carbon by phenylethanolamine-*N*-methyl transferase.

Tyrosine hydroxylase activity is the rate-limiting step in catecholamine synthesis. Control is achieved through several mechanisms that maintain the synthesis rate of catecholamines proportional to their release. The reaction requires tyrosine (substrate), oxygen, and a reduced pteridine cofactor. Norepinephrine exerts negative feedback with a sensitivity that is inversely proportional to the level of pteridine cofactor. The usual rate of catecholamine production is, therefore, influenced by three factors. First is the intraneuronal (or intracellular) transport of tyrosine, which may be altered by certain drugs that inhibit active transport, other amino acids that compete for the transport system, or other amino acids that act as competitive inhibitors, such a α-methylparatyrosine. Second is the activity of dihydropteridine reductase and subsequent concentration of reduced pteridine cofactor. Third is the cytoplasmic concentration of norepinephrine. A high intracellular concentration of norepinephrine is attained by transport of catecholamines out of the cytoplasm, away from tyrosine hydroxylase, and into storage vesicles. In response to a stimulus, catecholamines are released from storage vesicles, not from activation of tyrosine hydroxylase and *de novo* synthesis. However, as stores are replaced and cytoplasmic norepinephrine is depleted, feedback inhibition of tyrosine hydroxylase is removed. The released norepinephrine binds to a synaptic membrane receptor linked to cyclic adenosine monophosphate (cAMP), which activates a protein kinase that phosphorlyates and activates tyrosine hydroxylase. Gene activation of tyrosine hydroxylase occurs after prolonged stimulation (hours). It has been reported that both cholinergic ganglionic stimulation of sympathetic nerves or the adrenal medulla, and intracellular depletion of catecholamines by reserpine result in an increase in tyrosine hydroxylase gene transcription rate. Four types of tyrosine hydroxylase mRNAs have been described, produced by a single gene. The multiple forms may provide an additional level of regulation of the enzyme through differential phosphorylation and activation of each subtype. Glucocorticoids and cyclic AMP also stimulate transcription, and cyclic AMP may also stabilize mRNA and prolong its activity.

Aromatic L-amino acid decarboxylase is found in many tissues and defines them as part of the APUD (decarboxylation) system as described in the beginning of this chapter. This enzyme is found in high concentrations and requires a cofactor, pyridoxal 5-phosphate. The affinity for its substrate, DOPA, is very high as is its capacity (maximum velocity). It is relatively nonselective, but even potent inhibitors (α-methyldopa) have little effect on the synthesis rate of catecholamines.

Dopamine β-hydroxylase is a copper-containing oxidase that requires ascorbic acid and oxygen to hydroxylate dopamine to norepinephrine. The enzyme in both soluble and insoluble forms is found within granular storage vesicles. The granule consists of ATP, chromogranin A (a macromolecule), dopamine β-hydroxylase, norepinephrine, or epinephrine. Dopamine must be actively transported into the vesicle to be converted to norepinephrine. The transport process requires ATP and is inhibited by reserpine. Stimulation results in fusion of the vesicular membrane with the plasma membrane and release of the entire contents. Thus, dopamine β-hydroxylase, chromogranin A, and catecholamine plasma levels increase with sympathetic stimulation. Exocytosis results from calcium ion (Ca^{2+}) entry at the plasma membrane via nicotinic or voltage-activated channels. The rise in cytosolic Ca^{2+} leads to a reorganization of the cortical actin network and triggering access of the granule to its exocytotic sites. Calpactin, the Ca^{2+} and phospholipid-dependent annexin protein, has been strongly implicated in the interaction of the granule with the plasma membrane. Calcium channel-blocking agents, such as nifedipine and verapamil, inhibit catecholamine secretion. Because the enzyme is lost when excreted with the granule, it must be synthesized and replaced in response to the release of catecholamines. There is little substrate

specificity despite its name. Many phenylethylamines (Fig. 4) can be hydroxylated, including the monohydroxylated amine, tyramine (from the decarboxylation of tyrosine) forming octopamine, α-methylparatyramine (from the decarboxylation of α-methylparatyrosine) forming α-methyloctopamine, and α-methyl dopamine (from the decarboxylation of α-methyl DOPA) forming α-methyl norepinephrine. The lack of substrate specificity by aromatic L-amino decarboxylase and dopamine β-hydroxylase can be utilized to ameliorate high catecholamine states by virtue of two effects. One effect involves competitive inhibition decreasing the rate the production of the biologically active catecholamines, and the other involves the storage and release of false neurotransmitters. This latter effect is based on the fact that the α-methyl derivatives described above can displace norepinephrine from sites within the storage vesicles and be released in place of norepinephrine. For the most part, these derivatives have significantly less biologic activity than the catecholamines that they replace.

Phenylethanolamine-N-methyl transferase (PNMT) is found in the adrenal medulla and chromaffin cells near the adrenal cortex. Although some PNMT activity can be found in a few brain cells, the marked prevalence of enzyme activity in close proximity to the adrenal cortex is the result of the effects of glucocorticoids. Although it is not clear how glucocorticoids regulate enzyme activity, the mechanism does not involve gene activation. It has been speculated that glucocorticoids may regulate a cosubstrate or act to stabilize the enzyme. Whatever the mechanism, it also does not involve the classical (Type II) glucocorticoid receptor. Although norepinephrine is the preferred substrate, the enzyme is aptly named because it is nonselective and will N-methylate any phenylethanolamine, including octopamine, α-methyloctopamine, α-methyl-norepinephrine, and structurally related compounds (*see* Fig. 4). PNMT requires S-adenosylmethionine for a methyl-group donor, oxygen, and magnesium. Noncompetitive inhibition by its product, epinephrine, is its most potent immediate regulator of activity. Cholinergic stimulation will cause PNMT gene activation in the adrenal medulla. Although angiotensin and imidazolines (clonidine, cimetidine) have been shown to increase PNMT mRNA in adrenal medullary chromaffin cells, the physiological implications of this effect are unclear at this time.

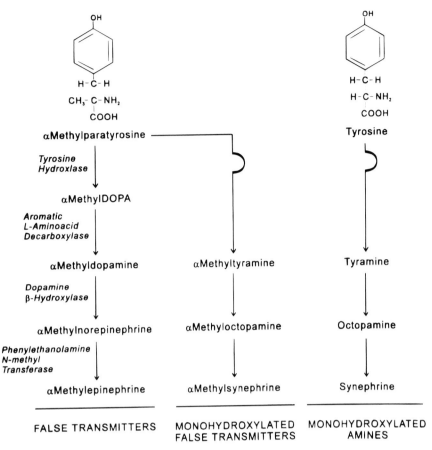

Fig. 4. The synthesis of false transmitters and monohydroxylated amines. Because of the lack of specificity, a host of other compounds can be produced by the enzymes involved in catecholamine synthesis. α-Methylparatyrosine, a competitive inhibitor of tyrosine hydroxylase, may be administered to patients with pheochromocytoma to treat excess catecholamine secretion. As a result of interaction with tyrosine hydroxylase, the less biologically active α-methyl derivatives or false transmitters are synthesized instead of the normal, active compounds. Both naturally occurring monohydroxylated amines and α-methyl derivatives are produced when the initial reaction with tyrosine hydroxylase is bypassed.

2.2. Catecholamine Catabolism

There are two primary pathways for the degradation of catecholamines (Fig. 5), one near the sites where catecholamines are synthesized and stored (chromaffin cells and sympathetic neurons) and the second deactivates primarily circulating catecholamines. Monoamine oxidase (MAO) catalyzes the first and catechol-*O*-methyltransferase (COMT) the second. MAO, a mitochondrial enzyme, cleaves off the terminal aliphatic amine and oxidizes the α-carbon to carboxylic acid. The product, 3,4-dihydroxymandelic acid is the same for epinephrine and norepinephrine, because the *N*-methyl group, which distinguishes the two, is removed. COMT using the methyl-group donor, *S*-adenosylmethionine, methylates the 3-hydroxy group producing

metanephrine and normetanephrine, respectively, from epinephrine and norepinephrine. *O*-methylation of 3,4-dihydroxymandelic acid by COMT or oxidative deamination of the metanephrines by MAO produces vanillylmandelic acid (VMA). Most of the substrates and products of these reactions may be conjugated to sulfate (primarily) or glucuronide, which reduces further metabolism and enhances excretion.

2.3. Adrenal Medullary Catecholamine Physiology

2.3.1. BIOSYNTHESIS AND RELEASE

Most of the catecholamine synthetic steps up to norepinephrine are not significantly different in the adrenal medulla compared to sympathetic nerves

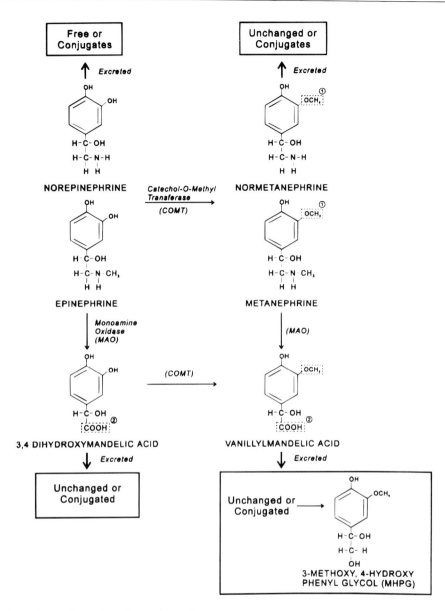

Fig. 5. The catabolism of catecholamines. Regardless of the first step (1) methylation of the 3-position hydroxyl group or (2) oxidative deamination, the end product of the sum of the reactions is VMA, which is excreted in the urine or may be further reduced to be excreted as MHPG. Epinephrine and norepinephrine may be excreted in the free form (the source of urinary total catecholamines), or be converted to metanephrine and normetanephrine (the source of urinary metanephrines), respectively by COMT. Interaction of the catecholamines or metanephrines with (2) MAO results in deamination, and therefore, eliminates any further ability to differentiate the contribution of epinephrine or norepinephrine to the product.

(Fig. 6). Biosynthesis begins with tyrosine, which can be obtained from the diet or synthesized from phenylalanine by phenylalanine hydroxylase, which is found in the liver. Tyrosine is actively transported from the bloodstream into the adrenal. Tyrosine is converted to DOPA by the rate-limiting mitochondrial enzyme, tyrosine hydroxylase. Feedback inhibition is exerted by norepinephrine.

Decarboxylation of DOPA to dopamine is catalyzed by the cytosolic enzyme, aromatic L-amino acid decarboxylase. Dopamine must then be actively transported into granulated vesicles, which contain dopamine β-hydroxylase, to be converted to norepinephrine. For most chromaffin tissue and neurons, the synthesis ends with norepinephrine binding to the granule, which is made

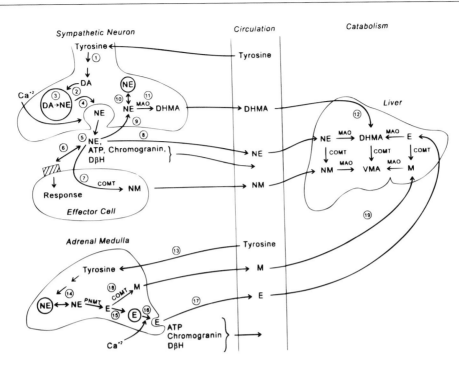

Fig. 6. A comparison of the biosynthesis, release, and catabolism of catecholamines in the sympathetic neuron and the adrenal medulla. (1) Tyrosine is converted to dopamine (DA), which is (2) actively transported into storage granules to be (3) converted to norepinephrine (NE). During depolarization, calcium (CA^{2+}) moves into the neuron, exocytosis (4) occurs, and (5) NE is released into the synapse along with ATP, chromogranin, and dopamine β-hydroxylase (DβH). NE may then (6) bind to a receptor to produce a response, be internalized (7) and metabolized COMT to normetanephrine (NM), (8) leak out of the synapse to reach the blood stream, or (9) be taken up into the neuron to be transported back into (10) a storage granule or metabolized (11) to dihydroxymandelic acid (DHMA). NE, NM and DHMA can be transported by the circulation to the liver and (12) metabolized to VMA. Tyrosine (13) is taken up by the adrenal medulla and converted to NE, which is then released back into the cytoplasm (14) to be converted to epinephrine (E) by (PNMT). E can then be taken up by storage granules (15) and released (16) by exocytosis into the bloodstream (17) along with ATP, chromogranin, and DβH. E can then be transported to distant receptors to produce a hormonal response or be transported (19) to the liver along with M to be metabolized to VMA.

up of dopamine β-hydroxylase, a macro-molecule, chromogranin A, and ATP. In the noradrenergic neuron, this granule containing norepinephrine is secreted into the synapse during depolarization. As with other chromaffin tissue, the adrenal medulla stores and releases norepinephrine in granules. However, the adrenal medulla is the body's primary source of epinephrine and the cytosolic enzyme, PNMT, which produces epinephrine from norepinephrine. Because PNMT activity is so dependent on glucocorticoids (cortisol in humans), it is also dependent on pituitary ACTH and the rest of the hypothalamic–pituitary–adrenal cortical axis. ACTH also has a trophic effect on adrenal medullary tyrosine hydroxylase activity. In order for the enzymatic reaction to occur, norepinephrine must be released from its storage granule, combine with PNMT in the cytoplasm to produce epineph-

rine, and then be transported back into another granule. The storage granules in the adrenal medulla contain epinephrine or norepinephrine, and the release can be selective. That is, epinephrine can be released independently from norepinephrine, but how this is accomplished is not known. Approximately 80% of the catecholamine output from the adrenal medulla is epinephrine under the usual physiological circumstances.

2.3.2. PHYSIOLOGIC FUNCTION

Although derived from neural tissue, which characteristically induces a discrete sympathetic response in one organ, the adrenal medulla's function is to produce a similar sympathetic response in all organs at approximately the same time. Epinephrine, secreted by the adrenal medulla, is the hormonal equivalent of the sympathetic neuron's neurotransmitter, norepinephrine. Epinephrine provides a rapid physiologic response to cold, fatigue, shock, hypoglycemia, and other emergencies.

2.4. Mechanism of Action

2.4.1 TYPE AND DISTRIBUTION OF ADRENERGIC RECEPTORS

Catecholamines exert their effects through receptors located on the target organ's cell membrane. A representative listing of the receptors and their responses is presented in Table 1. There are two main grouping of receptors, α and β. Each of these is divided into two or perhaps three subgroups labeled α_1, α_2, β_1, and so on. The classification of the receptor types is determined by examining the effect of a defined concentration (dose–response) curve of a series of pharmacologic derivatives of the catecholamines (agonists and antagonists) on certain tissue response systems, which act as the standards to which the unclassified drug or tissue response is compared against. β_2-Receptors are predominantly found in smooth muscle and glandular cells, and β_1-receptors are most prevalent in the myocardium. However, some tissues possess both types in different proportions. β_1-Receptors or α_1-receptors predominate at postsynaptic sites, and convey the primary neuronal signal to the effector cell. α_2-Receptors are located at presynaptic nerve terminal sites and mediate feedback inhibition of neuronally released norepinephrine. Although certain generalizations can be made about the effect and relative potencies of various sympathomimetic amines on certain receptor subtypes, there are usually several exceptions to each generalization. The physiologic state of the tissue, the relative ratio of one receptor type compared to another, aging, temperature, and the presence or absence of other seemingly unrelated drugs or hormones can alter adrenergic responses. Many drugs may not even act directly on an adrenergic receptor, but cause an increase or decrease in catecholamine levels, or release of endogenous catecholamines that will influence receptor responses. The number of active receptors may decrease during agonist stimulation, resulting in a progressively less maximal response to progressively higher levels of stimulation, termed downregulation or tachyphylaxis. Exhaustion of a second messenger like c-AMP or its intermediates may result in loss of a response.

Table 1
Responses Mediated by α-Adrenergic and β-Adrenergic Receptor Stimulation

Tissue or organ response	Receptor type
Cardiac	
Increase rate (chronotropy)	β
Increase contractility (inotropy)	β
Increase A-V node conduction	β
Vascular	
Constriction (arteries and veins)	α
Dilatation (only arteries)	β
Pulmonary	
Dilatation bronchial smooth muscle	β
Liver	
Gluconeogenesis, glycogenolysis	β
Pancreas	
Exocrine—decrease secretion	α
Endocrine (insulin, glucagon)	
Inhibit secretion	α
Stimulate secretion	β
Fat cells	
Increase lypolysis	
(increase free fatty acids)	β
Salivary glands	
Increase amylase secretion	β

2.4.2. RECEPTOR CHARACTERISTICS: DIFFERENTIAL EFFECTS OF EPINEPHRINE AND NOREPINEPHRINE

The physiologic response to epinephrine or norepinephrine is dependent on the relative sensitivity of the receptor to that catecholamine and the range of physiologic concentrations that can be attained at the receptor site. For example, epinephrine and norepinephrine both stimulate β_1-receptors in the heart and increase heart rate and contractility. Epinephrine can elicit these effects at 1–2 nm, which is equivalent to the normal concentration of epinephrine in the blood. In contrast, >20 nM norepinephrine are required to obtain a response from β_1-receptors, which is four- to fivefold higher than normal plasma levels. Only certain pathologic conditions generate circulating norepinephrine to a level that will stimulate cardiac β_1-receptors. On the other hand, sympathetic noradrenergic neurons innervating the myocardium will readily produce intrasynaptic concentrations exceeding the threshold needed to elicit a β_1-receptor response. Both epinephrine and norepinephrine are secreted by the adrenal medulla, but only epinephrine conveys the biologic response to stimulation. The adrenal medulla produces virtually all of the circulating epinephrine and practically none of the circulating norepinephrine. Plasma norepinephrine is primarily derived from a "leak" of norepinephrine from sympathetic neurons and their synaptic discharges.

The principal effects of epinephrine are to vasodilate arterioles in skeletal muscle and vasoconstrict arterioles in the skin, stimulate the rate and force of myocardial contractions, cause the relaxation of the smooth muscles of the gut, lungs, and urinary bladder, and contraction of the sphincters, stimulate the breakdown of glycogen and inhibit insulin to elevate blood sugar, and stimulate lipolysis to elevate fatty acids and glycerol. The latter two effects provide fuel for muscle action (fatty acids) and glucose for the central nervous system. Most of these effects are mediated by β-receptors and cAMP.

2.5. Pathophysiology

2.5.1. ADRENAL MEDULLARY INSUFFICIENCY

Adrenal medullary insufficiency is associated with no known disease. After bilateral adrenalectomy, urinary epinephrine secretion falls, but <10% of norepinephrine and its metabolites are lost, and this has no significant physiologic impact. The contribution of the adrenal medulla to circulating norepinephrine is insignificant compared to the sympathetic nervous system, because most adrenergic receptors, the mediators of secreted norepinephrine, are associated with synapses. The synaptic concentration of norepinephrine during a stimulus is several orders of magnitude above that in the circulation. Is it the leak of norepinephrine from the neurons and synapses that is the major contributor to plasma norepinephrine levels. This source of norepinephrine is the result of adrenergic stimulation and not the cause.

2.5.2. INTRA- AND EXTRAADRENAL HYPERFUNCTION

Conditions are generally pathologic where circulating levels of norepinephrine are higher than synaptic concentrations. Under these circumstances, circulating levels of norepinephrine are high enough to elicit symptoms of increased sympathetic stimulation. Tumors of chromaffin tissues can produce clinically important syndromes and lead to life-threatening clinical disease. Pheochromocytoma is

the term applied to catecholamine-secreting tumors of the adrenal medulla. Paraganglioma is the term that has been used to describe catecholamine-secreting tumors that arise in extra-adrenal chromaffin tissue, such as paraganglia, chromaffin bodies, and carotid bodies. It would be preferable to designate all catecholamine-secreting tumors as pheochromocytoma and qualify the description with the anatomical location. The is no advantage to using separate terms, because the pathophysiology and treatment of excess catecholamine secretion are changed little by whether the source of the catecholamines is intra- or extra-adrenal.

2.5.3. PHEOCHROMOCYTOMA

Catecholamine-secreting tumors of chromaffin tissue, pheochromocytomas, are a rare cause of a common disease, hypertension. Less than 0.1% of the hypertensive population have pheochromocytoma. Finding this "needle in the haystack" has several important clinical aspects. The hypertension caused by pheochromocytoma is usually curable, whereas essential hypertension can ordinarily only be controlled. Administration of the wrong antihypertensive or surgery on a patient with unrecognized pheochromocytoma can be fatal. These tumors may be associated with other potentially fatal, but curable diseases. Pheochromocytoma may mimic other diseases, such as diabetes mellitus, thyrotoxicosis, severe anxiety, coronary artery disease, or carcinoid syndrome. The high incidence of pheochromocytoma in families as a primary disease, in association with multiple endocrine neoplasia, or in association with other familial diseases indicates the need for genetic counseling in these families. Finally, there is a rational and specific approach to diagnosis and treatment.

2.5.3.1. *Pathophysiology.* Pheochromocytoma occurs 80% of the time as a benign tumor in one of the adrenal glands. Twenty percent are extra-adrenal with half (i.e., 10%) below the diaphragm in such areas as along the aorta, near the urinary bladder, and in the organ of Zuckerkandl, and the other half above the diaphragm in areas along the aorta, in the lungs or heart, or in the neck or carotid bodies. Ten percent occur in children. In nonfamilial disease, 10% of patients have bilateral adrenal tumors and 10% have multiple extra-adrenal tumors, but in familial disease, more than 80% are bilateral or multiple sites. Malignant pheochromocytoma occurs in 10% of patients. Pheochromocytoma is evenly distributed between the sexes and can occur at any age, although the incidence peaks between the fourth and sixth decades.

Catecholamines are mostly responsible for the signs and symptoms of pheochromocytoma. It is unusual that a tumor will grow large enough or be so invasive as to interfere with the function of surrounding organs, such as the liver, kidneys, or spinal cord. The manifestations of pheochromocytoma are primarily the result of the excessive secretion of norepinephrine, epinephrine, and dopamine. The most common mix is predominately norepinephrine with epinephrine. Some tumors secrete only norepinephrine, but <10% secrete only epinephrine. Dopamine and its metabolite, HVA, derived from the combined activities of MAO and COMT, have not been measured in the routine laboratory examination of pheochromocytoma. When dopamine levels have been reported, they rarely exceed the concentration of norepinephrine. Dopamine and HVA are more likely to be significantly elevated in children with pheochromocytoma or in malignancy.

The reasons for increased production and secretion of catecholamines are not clear. Abnormally high turnover rates have been noted in small tumors, but the granules and storage mechanisms appeared normal, leading to the logical, but as yet unproven conclusion that there is a defect in the systems regulating synthesis and release.

Perhaps the negative-feedback mechanism of norepinephrine on tyrosine hydroxylase is altered so that sensitivity to feedback is decreased, or metabolism or release is so rapid that feedback does not occur. One animal study has shown that increased cell contact in pheochromocytoma increases the tyrosine hydroxylase transcription rate, leading to higher concentrations of the enzyme. In some tumors, secretion occurs at a relatively constant high rate, some in bursts in between periods of normal secretion, or in others a combination of the two. Small tumors tend to secrete high levels of free catecholamines. With more intracellular metabolism occurring in large tumors, high levels of metabolites tend to be released, and free catecholamine secretion is reduced.

Some patients are more symptomatic that others. Approximately 50% of patients with pheochromocytoma have sustained hypertension, whereas 45% are normotensive with paroxysms of hypertension, and only 5% are normotensive or even hypotensive.

Part of the reason for these differences relate to the patterns of catecholamine secretion. Bursts produce hypertensive episodes. Sustained hypertension and some normotensive patients can have high or normal levels of norepinephrine. How high sustained levels of norepinephrine result in sustained hypertension is readily understood. However, if an elevated secretion rate persists, α- and β-receptors may become desensitized or downregulated. Hemo-dynamic mechanisms will no longer respond to the elevated levels of norepinephrine, and blood pressure will be normalized. In this way, two patients with the same plasma concentration of norepinephrine could result in one being normotensive and the other hypertensive. Some investigators have reported this finding as indicating that there is no correlation between blood pressure and catecholamine levels. This has been misinterpreted by some to imply that catecholamines do not affect blood pressure in patients with pheochromocytoma. This is not the case. The normotensive patient with elevated levels of norepinephrine is capable of responding to an additional burst of catecholamines with a hypertensive episode. Before catecholamines could be measured reliably, this was the observation and rationale for the stimulation tests. Catecholamine levels and blood pressure may not correlate well between patients, but within an individual, a significant change in catecholamine concentration will elicit a blood pressure response. The rare, exclusively epinephrine-secreting tumors, can present with normotension or hypotension owing to the predominantly vasodilating effects of epinephrine. Another cause of hypotension is orthostatic hypo-tension, resulting from the ganglionic blocking activity of excessive amounts of catecholamines that prevent the normal sympathetic response to upright posture.

The pathophysiology of pheochromocytoma has been described primarily in relation to the effects of the catecholamines on blood pressure, because of the ease and accuracy of blood pressure measurements, and its rapid response to changes in catecholamine levels. The excessive secretion of catecholamines have many other important pathophysiological consequences that will be examined in the subsequent sections.

2.5.3.2. Clinical Manifestations. Most symptoms of pheochromocytoma can be readily attributed to the pharmacologic effects of catecholamines. The

Table 2
The Frequency of the Symptoms of
Pheochromocytoma

Frequency >50%
  Headache
  Sweating
  Palpitations
Frequency >50% and >25%
  Pallor
  Nausea
  Tremor
  Anxiety
  Abdominal pain
  Chest pain
Frequency <25% and >10%
  Weakness
  Fatigue
  Dyspnea
  Weight loss
  Flushing

Table 3
Diseases Mimicked by Pheochromocytoma

Anxiety states, psychoneuroses, panic attacks
Carcinoid
Diabetes mellitus
Drug abuse (cocaine, amphetamines)
Essential hypertension
Hyperthyroidism
Malignant hypertension
Megacolon, chronic constipation
Migraine and other vascular headaches
Primary cardiac disease (coronary insufficiency,
  congestive cardiomyopathy)
Toxemia of pregnancy

most frequent symptoms associated with pheochromocytoma are headache, sweating, and palpitations, and these and other symptoms, listed in Table 2, are usually paroxysmal even if the hypertension is persistent. The paroxysms can be precipitated by certain drugs or physical activity, such as straining, lifting, or even micturition (provoking secretion from a tumor on or near the bladder), or be spontaneous.

Many patients present with more subtle signs and symptoms that mimic and can be confused with other diseases (*see* Table 3). Pheochromocytoma and these diseases may need to be differentiated from one another.

Pheochromocytoma could be familial or sporadic. As a familial disease, it may be associated with a variety of other familial endocrine tumors, which are mostly all autosomal-dominant. Table 4 contains a listing of these diseases. Identified families should be screened for pheochromocytoma.

2.5.3.3. Diagnosis. A careful history is essential to eliminate indiscriminate laboratory testing. Although measuring catecholamines and their metabolites is very sensitive, they are not very specific. There are many conditions (*see* Table 5) and drugs (*see* Table 6) that can significantly elevate catecholamines. Therefore, unless these conditions are controlled or resolved, and interfering drugs eliminated, false-positive tests will be obtained that will

require additional expensive and possibly more invasive tests. Catecholamines are not a specific tumor marker, nor is any level of catecholamines diagnostic of pheochromocytoma.

If the conditions listed in Table 5 have been eliminated or stabilized, the drugs listed in Table 6 have been discontinued or dosage minimized, and the history and physical examination are strongly suggestive of pheochromocytoma, then biochemical testing should be done. Other conditions where biochemical testing is appropriate include families with multiple endocrine neoplasia (MEN) or familial pheochromocytoma, or other associated diseases listed in Table 4. Finally, incidental adrenal tumors from abdominal computerized tomography (CT) or magnetic resonance (MR) scans require screening tests to eliminate the presence of a hormone-secreting tumor, including pheochromocytoma.

The specificity of the most sensitive tests for pheochromocytoma depends in a large part on the proper selection of a symptomatic, hypertensive patient where other confounding conditions and drugs have been eliminated. The most sensitive tests for pheochromocytoma are a 24-h urine collection for metanephrines (metanephrine and normetanephrine) and free epinephrine and norepinephrine by high-pressure liquid chromatography (HPLC) with electrochemical detection. Total urinary catecholamines by fluorometric methods remain an adequate substitute when HPLC methods are not readily available. If catecholamine levels are greater than threefold above the upper limit of normal in a symptomatic and hypertensive patient, then imaging is indicated. If catecholamine levels are <1.5-fold of the upper limit of

Table 4
Associated Familial Diseases

MEN Type II and Type III
Neurofibromatosis
von Hipple-Lindau
Sturge-Weber
Tuberous sclerosis

Table 5
Conditions That Increase Catecholamine Secretion

Increase greater than fivefold
    Acute myocardial infarction
    Congestive heart failure and pulmonary edema
    Diabetic ketoacidosis
    Hypoglycemia
    Pheochromocytoma
Increase greater than twofold
    Burns
    Hypoxia
    Depression
    Shock (hemorrhagic, septic)
    Mental stress
    Stroke

normal, then it is unlikely that the patient has pheochromocytoma. If the levels are marginally elevated, between 1.5-fold and threefold above the upper limit of normal, then a 12-h, nighttime collection of urine for catecholamines and metanephrines is indicated. The collection at night eliminates the effects of stress and upright posture on the production of catecholamines that occurs during the day in normal patients and will not affect the secretion of catecholamines in pheochromocytoma. If levels remain marginally elevated or higher, then proceed to imaging. If levels are normal, then discontinue testing. If patient has only brief paroxysms that occur only a few times per day or less frequently, then obtain the tests as a timed urine collection (2–4 h) during a prominent symptomatic hypertensive episode. If values exceed threefold, then proceed to imaging, and if less than threefold, depending on the level of clinical suspicion, either discontinue testing or repeat the test during another episode. This combination of urinary catecholamines and metanephrines measurement has been reported by most investigators for many years to be a sensitive (98–100%) and specific (96–98%) biochemical test for pheochromocytoma.

The purpose of making the diagnosis of pheochromocytoma is to enable the surgical excision of the source of the excessive secretion of catecholamines causing the patient's hypertension and symptoms. If significantly elevated catecholamines cannot be demonstrated during a hypertensive, symptomatic episode, then catecholamines are not causing the problem and testing should not proceed to imaging. If a high degree of suspicion remains despite the negative biochemical testing, then the patient should be treated medically and re-evaluated at a later date.

Pharmacologic tests developed to elicit or inhibit catecholamine secretion from a pheochromocytoma bear a significant risk and are generally less specific and sensitive than urinary collections.

Other biochemical testing offers little or no advantage over measurement of urinary cate-cholamines and metanephrines. Urinary VMA by colorometric methods is less specific, and by HPLC is equivalent to metanephrines, but is more costly and less readily available. Plasma catecholamines measurements produce more false positives, and are more expensive to obtain and analyze. Theoretically, plasma catecholamines would be a more sensitive method of documenting elevated catecholamine secretion during a brief hypertensive, symptomatic episode. The logistics required to obtain such a sample without prolonged hospitalization are problematic. Chromogranin A and dopamine β-hydroxylase are released with catecholamines during exocytosis. Both are frequently elevated in pheochromocytoma, but are less specific than urinary catecholamine measurement.

The diagnosis will have been made prior to imaging based on the history, physical findings, and biochemical measurements. The purpose of localization, imaging, is to find the tumor and plan the approach for surgical removal. Finding a mass with characteristics that are consistent with a pheochromocytoma helps to confirm, but does not make the diagnosis. MR imaging is the preferred method of tumor detection. The sensitivity and specificity of MR are at least equal to or greater than CT, and do not expose the patient to ionizing radiation. Pheochromocytoma on T_2-weighted imaging (MR) presents an especially bright mass in comparison to most other tumors. CT provides no similar distinguishing characteristics of pheochromocytoma compared to other masses. MR of the abdomen and pelvis is the first examination to be

Table 6
Drugs Reported to Increase Catecholamine Levels

Increase greater than twofold
    Caffeine
    Clonidine (abrupt withdrawal > 3 fold)
    Clozepine
    Cocaine
    Hydrochlorthiazide
    Insulin
    Marijuana
    Nifedipine
    Phenoxybenzamine
    Prazosin
Increase less than twofold
    Amphetamine
    Hydralazine
    Nitroglycerin
    Propranolol
    Nicotine

performed, because 90% of tumors are found below the diaphragm. If no tumor is found below the diaphragm, then the chest and neck should be imaged. If no mass is found, then CT imaging with contrast should be performed of the same areas and in the same order. If still no mass is found, then the ^{131}I-metaiodobenzylguanidine (MIBG) scan could be considered. Although this scan is highly specific (100%), it is considerably less sensitive (80%) than either the MR or CT scans (>98%). The isotope is specifically concentrated in intra- and extra-adrenal pheochromocytomas. Because it is an ^{131}I-based isotope, it has a short half-life (9 d). It is expensive and not readily available.

There is a high incidence of gallstones in pheochromocytoma, and ultrasound examination of the gallbladder and ducts is warranted prior to surgery.

2.5.3.4. Management. The definitive treatment for pheochromocytoma is surgery. The early, coordinated team effort of the endocrinologist, anesthesiologist, and surgeon helps, to ensure a successful outcome. The goals of preoperative medical therapy are to control hypertension, obtain adequate fluid balance and treat tachyarrythmias, heart failure, and glucose intolerance. The nonselective and long-acting α-adrenergic blocker, phenoxybenzamine, is the principal drug used to prevent hypertensive episodes. Optimal blockade requires 1–2 wk of therapy. Shorting-acting α_1-blockers, such as

prazosin, could be used as well. The effects of the calcium channel blocker, nifedipine, on the inhibition of calcium-mediated exocytosis of storage granules are also moderately effective in controlling hypertension. Adequate hydration and volume expansion with saline or plasma are used to reduce the incidence of postoperative hypotension. The addition of α-methyltyrosine (Demser), a competitive inhibitor of tyrosine hydroxylase and catecholamine biosynthesis, to α-adrenergic blockade provides several important advantages. Control of hypertension can be obtained with a lower dose of α-blocker, which minimizes the duration and severity of hypotensive episodes. β-Blockade should never be instituted prior to α-blockade. The inability to vasodilate (β-receptors blocked) and unopposed α-receptor-stimulated vasoconstriction could precipitate a hypertensive crisis, congestive heart failure, and acute pulmonary edema. If β-blockade is needed, propranolol or a more cardioselective β_1-antagonist, atenolol, can be used. α-Methyltyrosine may reduce the need for β-blockers and is the drug of choice to treat catecholamine-induced toxic cardiomyopathy. Hyperglycemia is best treated with a sliding scale of regular insulin in the immediate preoperative period to maintain blood glucose between 150 and 200 mg%. Glucose intolerance usually ends abruptly after the tumor's blood supply is isolated during surgery. Hypoglycemia during anesthesia is to be avoided.

The advantages of a coordinated team approach are most apparent during surgery. The selection of premedications, induction anesthesia, muscle relaxant, and general anesthetic to be used in pheochromocytoma is based on those that do not stimulate catecholamine release or sensitize the myocardium to catecholamines. These drugs include diazepam or pentobarbital, meperidine, and scopolamine for premedications. Thiopental is the preferred drug for induction and vecuronium for neuromuscular blockade. Isofluane and enflurane are excellent volatile general anesthetics, but the newest member of this family, desflurane, has the distinct advantage of being very volatile and thus very short-acting. Increasing the inhaled concentration of desflurane will rapidly reduce blood pressure (2 min) during a hypertensive episode, and hypotensive effects dissipate just as quickly by reducing the inhaled concentration. The achievement of rapid, stress-free anesthesia reduces the risk of complications during surgery. During surgery, tumor manipulation and isolation of the vessels draining the tumor can result in changes in plasma catecholamine concentrations of 1000-fold within minutes. With modest α-receptor blockade, α-methyltyrosine, and desflurane, the need for the urgent application of nitroprusside or phentolamine to control blood pressure during surgery may be eliminated. Pheochromocytomas are very vascular by nature, and significant hemorrhage is a potential hazard. Advanced preparation reduces the impact of these complications. Whole-blood, plasma expanders, nitroprusside and esmolol, a short-acting β-Blocker, should be immediately available.

When bilateral adrenalectomy is being performed, adrenal cortical insufficiency should be treated with stress doses of hydrocortisone intraoperatively and postoperatively until stable. Mineralocorticoid should be replaced postoperatively.

Hypotension is the most common complication encountered in the recovery room. The loss of the vasoconstrictive and iontropic effects of catecholamines, persistent α-receptor blockade, downregulated adrenergic receptors, and perioperative blood loss all contribute. The treatment is aggressive volume expansion. Sympathomimetic amines are rarely indicated. Hypoglycemia may result from administered insulin or be reactive. Dextrose should be given during the immediate postoperative period and blood glucose monitored regularly for several hours.

2.5.3.5. Prognosis. Most patients become normotensive within a week or two after surgery. Hypertension persists in about a third of the patients either because they have an underlying essential hypertension or they have residual tumor. Patients with essential hypertension no longer have the symptoms of pheochromocytoma, and their blood pressure is usually easily controlled with conventional therapy. If a patient has a residual tumor, an unidentified second site, or multiple metastases, then the signs and symptoms of pheochromocytoma will gradually or abruptly recur in proportion to the level of catecholamines being secreted.

There are no characteristic histologic changes on which to base the diagnosis of malignancy. The clinical course showing an aggressive, recurrent tumor, or finding chromaffin cells in nonendocrine tissue, such as lymph nodes, bone, muscle, or liver,

makes the diagnosis. Extra-adrenal tumors, large size, local tumor invasion, family history of pheochromocytoma, associated endocrine disorders, and young age are significant in predicting a malignant course.

The primary approach to the treatment of malignant pheochromocytoma is surgical debulking with medical management similar to that used for preoperative preparation. All treatment is palliative, there is no cure. Chemotherapy with a combination of cyclophosphamide, vincristine, and dacarbazine produced a 57% response with a median duration of 21 mo. High doses of ^{131}I-MIBG have been used to shrink tumors and decrease catecholamine secretion in some patients who demonstrate high-grade uptake of this compound.

3. PEPTIDES

3.1. Developmental Origin

The cells of the adrenal medulla have a pluripotential capacity to secrete a variety of other peptide hormones, which are usually biologically active. A great deal is known about the development and regulation of the catecholaminergic properties of these cells, but relatively little is known about developmental control of their peptidergic properties. Evidence suggests that glucocorticoids derived from an intact hypothalamic–pituitary–adrenal cortical axis and splanchnic innervation are essential to the developmental expression of these peptides. The list of neuropeptides discovered continues to grow and includes Met-enkephalin, Leu-enkephalin, neurotension, substance P, vasoactive intestinal peptide (VIP), and neuropeptide Y.

3.2. Potential Physiologic or Pathophysiologic Roles

Some peptide hormone secretion may be only pathophysiologic and derived from a neoplastic process, like pheochromocytoma. Alternatively, normal physiologic processes can be operative, but have yet to be discovered. VIP, ACTH, and a PTH-like hormone can be produced by pheochromocytoma, and produce symptoms of watery diarrhea, Cushing's syndrome, and hypercalcemia, respectively. Neuropeptide Y is secreted in sympathetic storage vesicles along with norepinephrine, chromogranin, dopamine β-hydroxylase, and ATP. Like chromogranin, it is not taken back up into the neuron after release, and measured levels may be used as another marker of sympathetic activity. Neuropeptide Y appears to mediate vasoconstriction through potentiating noradrenergic stimulation of α-receptor responses, and secretion is increased in severe hypertension. Endothelin-1 is another potent vasoconstrictor peptide that has been found along with its mRNA in pheochromocytomas. Both of these peptides could be involved in normal circulatory regulation, contribute to the pathophysiology of sympathetically mediated hypertension, or even be responsible for the unusual hypertensive episodes of pheochromocytoma that do not correlate well with catecholamine levels.

Another role suggested for some of the neuropeptides, Met-enkephalin (also synthesized in chromaffin tissue, stored and released in sympathetic granules), and VIP, is to increase adrenal blood flow in response to cholinergic stimulation and thus enhance the distribution of epinephrine into the bloodstream. In contrast, neuropeptide Y released by cholinergic stimulation inhibits adrenal blood flow and could, therefore, function to inhibit the distribution of epinephrine.

SELECTED READINGS

Burgoyne R D, Morgan A, Robinson I, Pender N, Cheek T R. Exocytosis in adrenal chromaffin cells. *J Anat* 1993; 183:309.

Evans D B, Lee J E, Merrell R C, Hickey R C. Adrenal medullary disease in multiple endocrine neoplasia type 2. Appropriate management. *Endocrin Metab Clin North Am* 1994; 23:167.

Graham P E, Smythe G A, Lazarus L. Laboratory diagnosis of pheochromocytoma: which analytes should we measure? *Ann Clin Biochem* 1993; 30:129.

Hinson J P, Cameron L A, Purbrick A, Kapas S. The role of neuropeptides in the regulation of adrenal vascular tone: effects of vasoactive intestinal polypeptide, substance P, neuropeptide Y, neurotensin, Met-enkephalin, and Leu-enkephalin on perfusion medium flow rate in the intact perfused rat adrenal. *Regul Pep* 1994; 51:55.

Nagatsu T. Genes for human catecholamine-synthesizing enzymes. *Neurosci Res* 1991; 12:315.

Nativ O, Grant C S, Sheps S G, O'Fallon J R, Farrow G M, van Heerden J A, Lieber M M. The clinical significance of nuclear DNA pattern in 184 patients with pheochromocytoma. *Cancer* 1992; 69:2683.

Raum WJ. Pheochromocytoma. In: Bardin C W, ed. *Current Therapy in Endocrinology and Metabolism*, 5th ed. St. Louis, MO: Mosby, 1994:172.

25 Kidney Hormones

The Kallikrein-Kinin and Renin-Angiotensin Systems

Gordon H. Williams, MD, Julie Chao, PhD, and Lee Chao, PhD

CONTENTS

1. INTRODUCTION

The tissue kallikrein gene family is a subset of closely related serine proteinases that exhibit a narrow range of substrate specificities. Members of the family are involved in processing of polypeptide precursors to generate biologically active peptide hormones and growth factors. The best-known physiological function of tissue kallikrein is the cleavage of low-mol-wt kininogen substrate to release the vasoactive kinin peptide. Kinin binds to its receptor in target tissues and exerts a broad spectrum of biological activities, including vasodilation, blood pressure reduction, smooth muscle relaxation and contraction, pain induction, and inflammation. There are two types of kinin receptors, B_1 and B_2, which differ in pharmacological properties, biological activities, and primary structures. The B_2-receptor has a greater affinity to intact kinin than to kinin's metabolites. The B_1-receptor binds weakly to intact bradykinin (a

From: *Endocrinology: Basic and Clinical Principles* (P. M. Conn and S. Melmed, eds.), Humana Press Inc., Totowa, NJ.

nonapeptide), but strongly to the metabolites desArg[9]-bradykinin and des-Arg[10]-kallidin (Lys-bradykinin), which are generated by kininase I (Fig. 1).

The renin-angiotensin (RA) system is a closely knit group of enzymes with a single initial substrate (Fig. 2). In contrast to the kallikrein gene family where the major biological action is mediated by a paracrine action, this system has both classical endocrine and paracrine actions. Similar to the kallikrein family, the major products of the RA system are biologically active small peptides, the most important of which is the octapeptide angiotensin II (Ang II). In many respects, the actions of the angiotensins on the vascular system and renal function are the opposite of the actions of kinins. Thus, these two systems serve as a "yin-yang" approach to regulate vascular tone and renal function at the local level. Additionally, the RA system plays a major role in regulating aldosterone secretion and, thereby, sodium homeostasis. Similar to kinins, there are in humans two separate Ang II receptors. One, the AT_1-receptor, mediates most of its biological effects. The other, the AT_2-receptor, appears to have a relatively

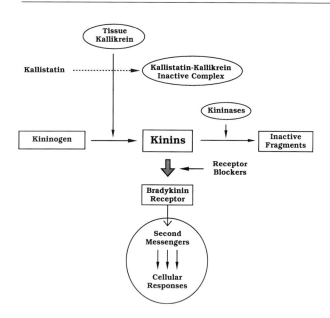

Fig. 1. The tissue kallikrein-kinin system.

limited role in adults, but is widely expressed in fetal tissue. In addition to the biologically opposite effects on renal function and vascular tone, the kallikrein-kinin and RA systems share a common component: kininase II (which inactivates kinins) is identical to the angiotensin-converting enzyme (ACE) (which converts the biologically inactive decapeptide angiotensin I [Ang I] into the biologically active Ang II).

Mechanisms involved in the regulation of kallikrein gene and RA family members operate at both transcriptional and posttranscriptional levels. The activity and metabolism of kallikreins are modulated by kallikrein binding protein (kallistatin). While a similar renin binding protein has been described, it is unclear whether this serves a substantial functional role.

2. THE COMPONENTS OF THE KALLIKREIN-KININ AND RA SYSTEMS

The vasodilatory effects of the tissue kallikrein-kinin system counterbalance the vasoconstricting effects of the RA system. Figure 3 shows interrelationships of the tissue kallikrein-kinin and RA systems. Tissue kallikrein cleaves kininogen to produce the vasodilator kinin. Renin cleaves angiotensinogen to produce Ang I, which is converted by ACE to Ang II, a potent vasoconstrictor. Both systems are closely linked by the function of the dipeptidase, ACE, which is also called kininase II. Kininase II degrades bradykinin or kallidin at the Pro-Phe bond to release a

dipeptide fragment, Phe-Arg, from the carboxyl-end of the intact kinin peptide. In addition, tissue kallikrein has been shown to convert angiotensinogen to Ang II at slightly acidic pH. Tonin, a kallikrein gene family member in rats, is capable of cleaving angiotensinogen or Ang I to produce Ang II.

2.1. The Tissue Kallikrein-Kinin System

2.1.1. Tissue Kallikrein

The tissue kallikrein gene family consists of a large number of closely related and tandemly arranged genes. The sizes of the kallikrein gene family vary among different species, with 15–20 members in the rat, 23–30 members in the mouse, and 3–5 genes in the human. The structure and organization of tissue kallikrein genes from rat, mouse, monkey, and human are similar to those of other trypsin-like serine proteinases, consisting of five exons and four introns. The tissue kallikrein gene is located on human chromosome 19q13.3–13.4, rat chromosome 1, and mouse chromosome 7. These gene family members exhibit highly homologous sequences, which strongly suggest that they share a common ancestral gene. The current gene families are likely derived from gene duplications. The expression of the kallikrein gene is regulated by cis-acting elements and trans-acting factors. Hormonal responsive elements have been identified in the 5′-flanking region of the kallikrein gene promoter, and include cAMP, estrogen, progesterone, and glucocorticoid responsive elements. Such factors as steroid hormones, thyroxin, isoproterenol, dopamine, dietary proteins, and salt intake are known to affect the expression levels of tissue kallikrein in various tissues. The kallikrein gene encodes a preproenzyme comprised of a signal peptide, a profragment and an active protein. A well-characterized member of the gene family is true tissue kallikrein (glandular kallikrein) (EC 3.4.21.35). Tissue kallikreins isolated from different species are acidic glycoprotein with an apparent molecular mass of 25–43 kDa. They contain the active site triad histidine, serine, and aspartic acid, which are encoded by separate exons, and kallikrein-like cleavage specificity at basic amino acids.

2.1.2. Kallistatin, a Kallikrein-Binding Protein

The structure and organization of kallistatin are similar to those of other serpin gene family members. The cDNA and genes encoding kallikrein-binding

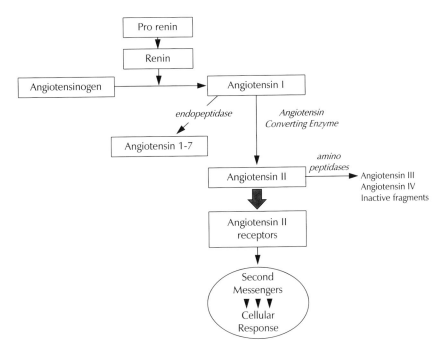

Fig. 2. The renin-angiotensin system.

proteins from humans and rodents are encoded by four introns and five exons. The first exon is noncoding, and the reactive center is encoded by the fifth exon. Two consensus promoter sequences in the human and rat kallistatin genes have been identified and one promoter is located in the 5′-flanking region, whereas the other is in the first intron. Both promoters contain consensus TATA boxes and CAAT boxes as well as hormonal response elements. Kallistatin is a newly identified serpin (serine proteinase inhibitor). It shares 44–46% sequence identity with other serpins, such as human α1-antichymotrypsin, protein C inhibitor, α1-antitrypsin, and thyroxin-binding globulin. The kallistatin gene is located on human chromosome 14q32, rat chromosome 6, and mouse chromosome 12, the same region containing other serpins. The expression of kallikrein-binding protein in rats is upregulated by estrogen, progesterone, growth hormone, and thyroxin, and downregulated during acute-phase inflammation. Kallistatin forms a covalent and SDS-stable complex with tissue kallikrein, and inhibits kallikrein's activity. Kallistatins from humans and rodents are acidic glycoproteins with p*I*s of 4.6–5.2 with an apparent molecular mass of 58–60 kDa. After forming an equimolar enzyme–inhibitor complex with kallikrein, a small carboxylterminal fragment from kallistatin is cleaved by kallikrein. The cleavage site is unique among serpins with P1-P1′-residues being Phe-Ser. Human kallistatin is a secretory protein, and is present in the circulation, bodily fluids, blood cells, and a wide variety of tissues.

2.1.3. KININ RECEPTORS

There are two types of kinin receptors, B_1 and B_2, which were classified according to the relative potency of kinin agonist on isolated smooth muscle preparations. The existence of B_1- and B_2-receptors was confirmed by cloning and characterization of the cDNAs and genes encoding these two receptors. The human B_2-receptor gene shares a high degree of identity with rat and mouse B_2 genes in both the nucleotide sequence and exon–intron arrangement. It contains three exons separated by two introns. The first and second exons are noncoding, whereas the third exon encodes a protein of 364 amino acids, including seven-transmembrane domains, a structure common to the G-protein-coupled receptor superfamily. A consensus TATA box, IL-6, and cAMP response elements have been identified in the 5′-flanking region. The human and rat B_2-receptor cDNAs have been expressed in *Xenopus* oocytes and Chinese hamster lung CCL39 fibroblasts. Furthermore, the recombinant B_2-receptor showed

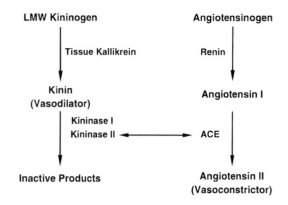

Fig. 3. Interrelationships of the kallikrein-kinin and the RA systems.

specific affinity to bradykinin, activating a transmembrane signaling pathway on binding to bradykinin. Both human B_1- and B_2-receptor genes are located on chromosome 14q32, close to that of the kallistatin gene. At the amino acid level, the human B_1- and B_2-receptors share only 36% sequence homology. It is uncertain whether these two receptors belong to a gene family or if they are linked by their functions. The B_1-receptor is generally absent in normal mammalian tissues, but appears in pathological states, such as inflammation and trauma, whereas the B_2-receptor is widely distributed in many tissues. Binding of the B_1-receptor has been shown to be induced by interleukin-1, endotoxin, and epidermal growth factor. The expression of the B_2 receptor is upregulated by *Ras* and *dbl* oncogenes and cAMP, but downregulated by salt restriction, water deprivation, dexamethasone, and bradykinin.

2.2. The RA System

2.2.1. RENIN

In contrast to the kallikrein-kinin system, the RA systems consist of relatively few genes. The principal enzyme, renin (EC 3.4.25.15), is synthesized as a preproprotein. The gene is located on the short arm of chromosome 1 (1q32–1q42). In the mouse, there are two renin genes, both located on chromosome 1, whereas in the rat, the renin gene is located on chromosome 13. In each species, the nucleotide sequence is approx 12 kb, with 10 exons and 9 introns. The transcription product from the gene is a 1.5-kb mRNA. The enzyme product of this gene is a member of the aspartyl proteinase family of enzymes. The gene product consists of 340 amino acids, of which

the first 43 are a prosegment, which is cleaved to produce the active enzyme. The N- and C-terminal halves of the enzyme are similar, and therefore, renin is a "double-domain" enzyme. Each domain contains a single aspartic acid residue, which is essential for its catalytic activity. Its three-dimensional structure has been characterized by X-ray crystallography, which has assisted in the development of inhibitors. Angiotensinogen is the only known substrate for renin. Indeed, apparently minor differences in the structure of angiotensinogens from different species render the substrate relatively inactive. Thus, rat and mouse angiotensinogens are not very efficient as substrates for human renin. Hormonal responsive elements have been identified in the 5′-flanking region of the renin gene and include consensus elements for cAMP and steroids (estrogen, progesterone, and glucocorticoids).

2.2.2. ANGIOTENSINOGEN

Angiotensinogen is the only known substrate capable of releasing angiotensin peptides. It is the exclusive substrate for renin. In humans, it belongs to the serpin superfamily of proteins. There is a single gene for angiotensinogen located on the human chromosome 1q42.3 very near the renin gene. Analyses of GT microsatellite repeats at the renin locus and at the angiotensinogen locus in pedigrees have reported linkage between these two loci (lod score Z = 4.89) with a recombination estimate Θ = 0.30. Thus, the probability of recombination between these two genes is different than what one would expect if they were randomly occurring. Yet, this close association between the angiotensinogen and renin genes does not seem to be universal, since the mouse angiotensinogen is located at the distal end of chromosome 8, whereas the rat's is located on chromosome 19, not on the same chromosomes where the renin genes are located. The angiotensinogen gene consists of five exons and four introns and is ~13 kb in length. The cDNA consists of 1455 nucleotides and codes for 485 amino acids, of which 33 appear to be a presegment. The first 10 amino acids of the mature protein correspond to Ang I. The angiotensinogen gene has several consensus sequences in the 5′-promoter region for steroids (glucocorticoids and estrogens) and cytokines. Of interest, S-1 nuclease mapping has shown several sites of polyadenylation, although the relevance of this in regulating the RA system is unclear.

Angiotensinogen's primary site of production is the liver. However, a number of other tissues also synthesize angiotensinogen.

2.2.3. ACE

ACE is a dipeptidyl carboxyl zinc metallopeptidase (EC 3.4.15.1), which is bound to cell membranes with its catalytic sites exposed to the extracellular surface. It has a mol wt of ~170 kDa and a repetitive structure with two homologous domains with consensus sequences for zinc metallopeptidases in each domain, thus suggesting there are two active sites in each molecule. It is extensively glycosylated. Since it is associated with vascular endothelial cell membranes, it is ubiquitously distributed. There are two molecular forms of ACE (somatic or endothelial and germinal). Germinal ACE is found only in the testes. It is an ~90 kDa peptide consisting of 732 amino acids, translated from a 3-kb mRNA. Somatic ACE consists of 1306 amino acids transcribed from a 4.3-kb mRNA. In contrast to somatic ACE, germinal ACE contains only one catalytic site. The germinal ACE was probably the primordial ACE with gene duplication producing the somatic form. This is supported by the finding of an ACE-like enzyme in the housefly, whose physical and chemical characteristics are similar to germinal rather than somatic ACE. In humans, the ACE gene is located on chromosome 17q23. There is a single gene in humans, rats, mice, and rabbits. In humans and mice, the gene is composed of 26 exons and 25 introns. The two forms of the enzyme are under different control mechanisms. Even though they are products of a single gene, they have separate promoter regions. The somatic promoter is located 5′ upstream from the first exon, whereas the germinal promoter is located upstream from the 13th exon. The 13th exon encodes a unique leader sequence for germinal ACE, not found in the somatic ACE.

2.2.4. ANGIOTENSIN RECEPTORS

There are at least two primary forms of angiotensin receptors, termed "AT_1 and AT_2." Preliminary data suggest that there may be a separate receptor for angiotensin IV. The receptor that serves as the mediator for most of Ang II's known biologic effects is the AT_1. In humans, there is a single gene for this located on chromosome 3. In rats, there are at least two subtypes, AT_{1a} located on chromosome 17, and AT_{1b} located on chromosome 2. Although in humans the AT_1 receptor structurally appears similar to AT_{1b} in rats, functionally, it behaves closer to the AT_{1a} receptor. The AT_1 gene consists of three or four exons in the rat, and of at least five exons in humans. The 5′-flanking region contains a functional receptor with at least three putative glucocorticoid-responsive elements—only one of which appears to be functional. The AT_1 receptor consists of 359 amino acids with a relative mol wt of 41 KDa. The number of amino acid residues is similar in bovine, rat and humans. The receptor consist of a classical seven-transmembrane regions, with a disulfide bridge linking the first and the fourth extracellular segments. Uniquely, the first cytosolic loop has a number of hydrophobic amino acids residues, suggesting that this loop may indeed be within the plasma membrane rather than in the cytosol. Genomic DNA of mouse and human AT_2-receptor consists of three exons and two introns, with the entire coding region contained within the third exon. The AT_2-receptor is also a seven-transmembrane domain structure, likely coupled to a G-protein, although it may also be coupled to a phosphotyrosine phosphatase. Both receptor subtypes bind Ang II with high affinity. However, structurally the binding domains of the AT_2- and AT_1-receptors are sufficiently different that specific antagonists and agonists for the two receptor subtypes have been developed. Some data support the concept that the common binding site is located in the fifth putative transmembrane domain, with receptor specificity being conferred by interaction with other extracellular domains. The principal signaling mechanism involved in the AT_1-receptor is through a G_Q-mediated activation of phospholipase C with consequent release of inositol 1,4,5-trisphosphate. However, the protein tyrosine kinase pathway may also be involved.

Regulation of angiotensin receptor gene expression is complicated, depending on the species, the tissue, and the receptor subtype. In general, AT_1-receptors in vascular smooth muscle are downregulated by phorbol esters and Ang II, and upregulated by glucocorticoids. In the rat adrenal, low-sodium and high-potassium diets increase the AT_1-receptor. However, the majority of the AT_1 in the rat adrenal is AT_{1b} as opposed to AT_{1a}, which predominates in the vascular smooth muscle. The relationship of these differences to functional effects and the specific role of the AT_2-receptor have yet to be defined.

2.2.5. ANGIOTENSINS

There are at least four biologically active angiotensin peptides (Table 1). Ang I, the decapeptide cleaved from angiotensinogen, is not biologically active. However, its primary decapeptide product, Ang II, does demonstrate full biologic activity in all target tissues for Ang II. Ang II can be further modified by aminopeptidase A to form the seven amino acid product, angiotensin III (Ang III). Ang III has less vasoconstrictor activity, but equivalent efficacy to Ang II on aldosterone secretion and modification of renal blood flow. An additional amino acid can be cleaved by aminopeptidase B from angiotensin III to form angiotensin 3–8 (Ang IV). This peptide appears to bind to a separate, as yet unidentified, receptor that, at least in the cerebral and renal circulations, seems to have the opposite effect of Ang II, i.e., it is a vasodilator. A fourth biologic compound produced from Ang I by the action of a propyl endopeptidase is angiotensin 1–7. The function of this peptide is unclear. It is primarily found in mammalian heart tissue.

3. EXPRESSION AND LOCALIZATION

3.1. Components of the Circulating and Tissue RA Systems

The RA system produces its effects using two approaches, one of which is an endocrine circulating system. This system primarily derives renin from the juxtaglomerular apparatus of the kidney and angiotensinogen from the liver. They interact in the circulation to form Ang I. The K_m of the RA reaction is ~1 $\mu M/L$—~the plasma concentration of angiotensinogen, at least in rats and humans. Thus, ~10 times the normal concentration of the substrate would be necessary to reach zero-order kinetics. This has led some investigators to speculate that variations in the angiotensinogen concentration may actually modify Ang I generation under physiologic conditions. Angiotensin I is rapidly converted to the biologically active Ang II by ACE located ubiquitously in the endothelial cells throughout the vasculature. Ang II's half-life in the circulation is very short (probably less than a minute). It is rapidly either degraded by enzymes in the circulation or taken up into cells through a receptor-mediated mechanism. Ang II circulates in the picomolar range. Interestingly, its affinity for its receptor is in the nanomolar range, suggesting that a number of

Table 1
Angiotensin Peptides

Ang I	Asp-Arg-Val-Tyr-Ile-His-Pro-Phe-His-Leu
Ang II	Asp-Arg-Val-Tyr-Ile-His-Pro-Phe
Ang III	Arg-Val-Tyr-Ile-His-Pro-Phe
Ang IV	Val-Tyr-Ile-His-Pro-Phe
Ang 1–7	Asp-Arg-Val-Tyr-Ile-His-Pro

Ang II's effects are likely mediated by its local generation.

The adrenal, the kidney, the heart, and the brain all can synthesize the three major components necessary to generate Ang II: renin, angiotensinogen, and ACE. In the adrenal, the glomerulosa cell can synthesize all these proteins and therefore secretes Ang II *de novo* rather than forming it in the extracellular milieu. In contrast, Ang II generated in the heart and brain may primarily be formed extracellularly, with individual components of the RA system synthesized by different cells. Other tissues may synthesize only one component of the RA system, relying on other cells and/or circulating components to complete the processing to Ang II. For example, fat cells synthesize angiotensinogen, but not renin or ACE. Presumably, the renin used comes from the circulation, whereas the ACE used is located on endothelial cells lining the blood vessels. The tissue distribution of the components of the RA system is given in Table 2. Although other mammalian species have relatively similar distributions for renin, angiotensinogen, and ACE, there is considerable species-specific variability in the distribution of the AT_1- vs AT_2-receptors.

3.2. Components of the Kallikrein-Kinin System in the Kidney, Adrenal Gland, and Vasculature

True tissue (or glandular) kallikrein was first discovered in human urine for its hypotensive effect in anesthetized dogs. Since urinary kallikrein originates in the kidney, altered urinary kallikrein levels reflect abnormalities in renal function. Renal kallikrein is produced in cells of the tubules, and released into the urine and vascular compartment. Urinary excretion of renal kallikrein has been used as an index for the activity of the renal kallikrein-kinin system, which is altered in several disease states. The expression of tissue kallikrein has been identified in the kidney as

Table 2
Tissue Distribution of Peptide Components of the RA System in Humans

Tissue	Renin	Angiotensinogen	ACE	Angiotensin receptor	
				AT_1	AT_2
Hepatocytes	−	+++++	−	+	−
Brain					
Pituitary	+	−	+	+	−
Basal ganglia	−	−	++	+	±
Hypothalamus	−	++++	++	+	+
Cerebral cortex	++	±	±	±	±
Cerebellum	−	+++	++	±	±
Spinal cord	±	+++	−	+	−
Choroid plexes	−	±	++	+	−
Kidney					
JG apparatus	+++++	±	±	−	−
Cortex	−	+++	++	++	+
Medulla	−	++	±	±	−
Adrenals					
Cortex	++	++	+	++	−
Medulla	−	±	−	±	+
Adipose tissue					
Brown	−	++	−	±	−
White	−	+	−	−	−
Vessels					
Endothelium	+	+	++++	+	−
Media	+	+	−	++	−
Adventitia	+	+	−	−	−
Heart					
Atria	+	++	+	+	+
Ventricles	+	+	±	+	+
Gonadal tissue					
Female	+	+	?	−	+
Male	+	±	+	+	−

well as in the pancreas, salivary gland, blood vessels, pituitary gland, heart, adrenal gland, colon, and many other tissues.

Since renal kallikrein occupies a "strategic" position in the kidney tubules, colocalization of kallikrein with other components of the system, such as kininogen, kallistatin, and bradykinin receptors, has provided the anatomical basis for understanding the mechanisms through which the system exerts its effects on blood flow and blood pressure regulation. Table 3 summarizes cellular localization of the site of synthesis of the kallikrein-kinin system in human kidney and adrenal gland by *in situ* hybridization histochemistry and RT-PCR Southern blot. The transcripts of these components are colocalized in both cortex and medulla of human kidney with minor differences in their distri-bution. High expression levels of the tissue kallikrein, kallistatin, kininogen, and B_2-receptor were found in the distal tubules of the cortex and the collecting ducts of the medulla. Expression of these genes was also found in other regions of the kidney and in endothelial cells of blood vessels. In the adrenal cortex, the human B_2-receptor mRNA was localized in zona glomerulosa, zona fasciculata, and zona reticularis, whereas the B_1-receptor transcript was identified in zona fasciculata, but not in zona glomerulosa and zona reticularis. The B_1-receptor mRNA was present at a high level, whereas the B_2-receptor had a low level of expression in the adrenal medulla. Kallikrein, kallistatin, and kininogen transcripts were all found in the adrenal medulla, but they are differentially distrib-uted in the adrenal cortex.

Table 3
**Cellular Localization of the Kallikrein-Kinin System in Human Kidney
and Adrenal Gland by *In Situ* Hybridization and RT-PCR Southern Blot**

Tissues	Kallikrein	Kallistatin	Kininogen	B_2-receptor	B_1-receptor
Kidney					
Cortex					
Juxtaglomerular cells	+	+	+	+	–
Endothelial cells	+	+	+	+	–
Mesangial cells	–	–	+	+	–
Bowman's capsule (Parietal)	+	+	+	+	+
Bowman's capsule (Visceral)	–	–	+	–	–
Proximal tubules	+	+	+	+	–
Distal tubules	+	+	+	+	–
Medulla					
Henle's loop—thin segments	+	+	+	+	+
Henle's loop—thick segments	+	+	+	+	–
Collecting ducts	+	+	+	+	–
Adrenal gland					
Cortex					
Zona glomerulosa	–	–	+	+	–
Zona fasciculata	+	+	+	+	+
Zona reticularis	+	–	+	+	–
Medulla	+	+	+	+	+

"The sections were hybridized with digoxigenin-labeled antisense riboprobes and the signals were detected with antidigoxigenin Fab fragments. The sense riboprobes were used as controls under the same experimental conditions. + = presence; ND = not detectable.

4. PHYSIOLOGIC EFFECTS OF KININ AND ANG II

4.1. Primary Effects

Ang II has five primary functions related to maintaining normal extracellular volume and blood pressure homeostasis:

1. Increasing aldosterone secretion;
2. Constricting vascular smooth muscle, thereby increasing blood pressure and reducing renal blood flow;
3. Enhancing the activity of the sympathetic nervous system by increasing central sympathetic outflow, thereby increasing norepinephrine discharge from sympathetic nerve terminals;
4. Releasing norepinephrine and epinephrine from the adrenal medulla; and
5. Promoting the release of vasopressin.

Other potential functions include:

1. A role in modifying ACTH release from the pituitary;
2. Other as yet poorly defined central nervous system functions;
3. Involvement in cellular growth in its target tissues; and
4. Potential involvement in regulating ovarian and placental function by, for example, modifying follicular maturation and atresia.

Kinins have prominent effects in the cardiovascular, pulmonary, gastrointestinal, and reproductive systems. Kinins are involved in the regulation of blood pressure and local blood flow, smooth muscle contraction and relaxation, electrolyte and glucose transport, pain, ovulation, sperm mobility, and cell proliferation. These peptide hormones produce biological effects via binding to kinin receptors with subsequent release of various mediators, such as nitric oxide, prostaglandins, platelet-activating factor, leukotrines, catecholamines, cytokines, and substance P. Kinins induce contraction of smooth muscles in the vein, ileum, uterus, bladder, and bronchiolus, whereas they cause relaxation in the artery and duodenum. After acute myocardial infarction, kinins can improve cardiac function and metabolism, and may produce beneficial effects by reducing or limiting the size of the myocardial infarct. Kinins' beneficial effects may be secondary to improved perfusion, oxygenation, and transport of glucose to the affected tissues. They also play a major role in inflammation by enhancing vascular permeability, thereby causing protein and fluid leakage from the microvascular system, and causing local vasodilation and edema.

4.2. Transgenic Analysis of the Kallikrein-Kinin and RA Systems

Transgenic technology has been instrumental in providing new insights into the mechanisms of development, gene regulation, and the physiological function of many genes. Transgenic mice expressing exogenous genes, such as tissue kallikrein, kallistatin, renin, or angiotensinogen, have become valuable animal models for studying human hypertensive diseases. Transgenic mice lines overexpressing either rat renin or rat angiotensinogen have been developed. In neither line is there any pathophysiologic effects of the transgene. However, when the lines were mated, significant hypertension developed. Similar results have been reported for human renin and angiotensinogen. However, when mouse renin alone is overexpressed in rats, severe hypertension develops within 10 wk. These animals' hypertension is responsive to ACE inhibitors and/or sodium restriction, and there is substantial overexpression of the transgene in the adrenal with derangements in both corticosterone and aldosterone secretion. Finally, inserting an antisense angiotensinogen fusion gene in mice causes a significant reduction in blood pressure. Taken together, these studies provide strong support for the critical role of the RA system in regulating blood pressure.

Hypotensive transgenic mice were created when the human tissue kallikrein gene under the control of the metallothionein metal-responsive element (MRE) or albumin promoter were introduced into the germ line of the mice. These transgenic mice have high kallikrein levels in the circulation, and the hypotensive effect of these mice can be reversed by injection of aprotinin, a potent tissue kallikrein inhibitor, or Hoe 140, a bradykinin receptor blocker. These results

are consistent with earlier clinical studies showing that oral administration of pig pancreatic kallikrein can temporarily reduce the blood pressure of hypertensive patients, suggesting that a continuous supply of human tissue kallikrein can have a prolonged effect on blood pressure reduction. These findings establish a direct link between tissue kallikrein and blood pressure regulation, and implicate tissue kallikrein as a powerful vasodepressor that may counterbalance the vasoconstrictive RA system.

5. REGULATION OF SECRETION OF THE CIRCULATING RA SYSTEM

Renal renin release is controlled by four independent factors:

1. Juxtaglomerular cells act as miniature pressure transducers sensing renal perfusion pressure and corresponding changes in efferent arteriolar perfusion pressure. Reduction in pressure results in the release of renin.
2. The macular densa cells of the distal convoluted tubule are in direct apposition to the juxtaglomerular cells. They function as chemoreceptors, monitoring the sodium and/or chloride load present in the distal tubule.
3. The sympathetic nervous system regulates the release of renin in response to assuming the upright posture.
4. A number of circulating factors also influence renin.

Increasing dietary potassium directly decreases renin release; Ang II administration suppresses renin release independent of alterations in renal blood flow pressure or aldosterone secretion. Atrial natriuretic peptides also inhibit renin release. The tissue RA systems sometimes do not follow a similar pattern of regulation. For example, high potassium intake increases adrenal renin secretion where it reduces renal renin secretion. Plasma angiotensinogen levels are increased by steroids (estrogens and glucocorticoids), thyroid hormone, and Ang II itself. As might be anticipated, angiotensinogen mRNA levels in the liver are increased by sodium depletion and decreased by sodium loading. Angiotensinogen is secreted constituitively. In contrast, renin secretion at least from the juxtaglomerular apparatus is primarily secreted via a regulated pathway.

6. PATHOPHYSIOLOGY

6.1 Renal Kallikrein and Hypertension

The observation that urinary excretion of kallikrein is significantly reduced in hypertensive patients was recorded as early as 1934, and this finding was confirmed more than three decades later. Extensive studies have shown that an association of reduced urinary kallikrein excretion exists in hypertensive human and animal models. Epidemiologic studies showed that urinary kallikrein levels are inversely correlated with blood pressure in infants, children, and parents. A study involving a large Utah family pedigree concluded that a dominant allele, expressed as high urinary kallikrein excretion, may be associated with a decreased risk of essential hypertension. Reduced urinary kallikrein excretion has also been described in a number of genetically hypertensive rats. Rat tissue kallikrein has been linked with blood pressure regulation by restriction fragment-length polymorphisms and cosegregation studies in genetically hypertensive rats. Collectively, these findings are consistent with the notion that genetic factors causing a decrease in renal kallikrein activity might contribute to the pathogenesis of hypertension.

6.2 RA System and Hypertension

Ang II infused chronically in experimental animals increases blood pressure. Likewise, unilateral renal artery stenosis, a condition that increases endogenous Ang II production, is accompanied by hypertension. The hypertension is reversed by administration of a converting enzyme inhibitor that blocks the formation of Ang II. The rare renin-secreting tumor also causes hypertension. Finally, there have been described two functional derangements in target tissue responses to Ang II. (1) In nonmodulators, a condition afflicting 20–25% of the essential hypertension population, there is decreased adrenal and renal vascular response to infused Ang II. (2) Some patients with low renin hypertension have an enhanced adrenal response to Ang II on a high-sodium intake. In both circumstances, these functional derangements may explain why the individual has an increase in blood pressure.

7. GENETIC FACTORS

7.1. Genetic Differences in the RA System and Cardiovascular Disease

Linkage and association studies have been performed using polymorphic markers of ACE, angio-
tensinogen, and renin. In humans, there is no indication of any linkage or association of ACE or renin with hypertension. However, there is for angiotensinogen. Using severely affected sib pairs, there was a highly significant linkage between hypertension and the polymorphic marker. Additionally, a variant in the angiotensinogen gene at codon 235 (a change from methionine to threonine) was associated with hypertension. The 235T subjects also have higher angiotensinogen levels. In contrast to the studies in humans, in rats, polymorphism of the renin gene has been linked to hypertension in at least in two genetic strains. However, there has been no linkage of the angiotensinogen gene to hypertension in rats.

An ACE gene polymorphism, the presence or absence of a DNA fragment located in the 16th intron, has a substantial effect on circulating ACE levels. The deletion allele is associated with increases in circulating ACE levels and an increased conversion of infused Ang I to Ang II. However, there is no evidence that this polymorphism is associated with hypertension. On the other hand, this polymorphism may be associated with a predisposition to develop both nephropathy and myocardial infarction.

7.2. Potential of Kallikrein Gene Therapy in Human Hypertensive Diseases

Intravenous infusion of purified tissue kallikrein or kinin into animals causes a transient reduction of blood pressure. The blood pressure lowering effect cannot be sustained because of the presence of tissue kallikrein inhibitors in the circulation. The half-life of kinins in the blood is <30 s, since circulating kinins are inactivated mainly during their passage through the lung by a number of kininases. Clinical studies have shown that blood pressures of hypertensive patients can be temporarily lowered by oral administration of porcine pancreatic kallikrein. However, to achieve this hypotensive effect, repeated administration of purified tissue kallikrein is required, since tissue kallikrein is absorbed by the gut in small amounts. Epidemiological studies suggest that a genetically determined decrease in renal kallikrein activity, relative to the sodium intake, may contribute to the pathogenesis of hypertension. The hypothesis that hypertension can develop in patients with impaired sodium excretion because of abnormalities in the kallikrein-kinin system forms the basis for treating hypertension with exogenous kallikrein. Oral kallikrein administration reduces blood pressure levels only in salt-sensitive hypertensives, but not in salt-resistant hypertensives. In both the salt-sensitive and salt-resistant groups, a marked increase in the urinary excretion of sodium was observed after kallikrein treatment. Therefore, the enhanced antihypertensive effect of oral kallikrein therapy observed in the sodium-sensitive patients is not only owing to its natriuretic action, but also to other kallikrein-related effects.

Hypertension associated with cardiovascular diseases causes one-quarter of the deaths in the US. The management of hypertension by conventional drug therapy has been generally successful, but has limitations. By altering the RA system, the control of hypertension is possible. For instance, ACE inhibitors are effective in reducing blood pressure in more than 50% of patients with essential hypertension. Efforts to develop other approaches involving renin inhibitors and angiotensin receptor antagonists are currently under intense investigation. Treating hypertension by gene therapy is very appealing, because a single dose could have a lasting effect without the side effects of conventional pharmaceuticals. Antisense inhibition of Ang II Type 1 receptor and angiotensinogen genes in the brain with synthetic antisense oligonucleotides has been shown to lower blood pressures in spontaneously hypertensive rats (SHR). An alternative approach to treating hypertension is to stimulate or increase the activities of the tissue kallikrein-kinin system by direct gene delivery. Additional benefits of kallikrein gene therapy include the potential cardioprotective and renal effects of kinin. Somatic gene delivery of human tissue kallikrein by intravenous, intramuscular, and intraperitoneal injections caused significant reduction of blood pressures for several weeks in SHR. Animals injected with human tissue kallikrein DNA constructs did not develop antibodies to human tissue kallikrein or kallikrein DNA, and showed normal growth and development. The findings that somatic kallikrein gene therapy in hypertensive rats and transgenic mice overexpressing human tissue kallikrein induces a sustained reduction of blood pressure suggest the potential of kallikrein gene therapy for treating human hypertensive diseases. Investigating the feasibility of kallikrein gene therapy could open a new avenue of pharmacological intervention in treating human hypertension.

SELECTED READING

Kallikrein-Kinin System

Berry TD, Hasstedt SJ, Hunt SC, Wu LL, Smith JB, Ash KO, Kuida H, Williams RR. A gene for high urinary kallikrein may protect against hypertension in Utah kindreds. *Hypertension* 1989; 13:3.

Bhoola KD, Figueroa CD, Worthy K. Bioregulation of kinins: kallikreins, kininogens, and kininases. *Pharmacol Rev* 1992; 44:1.

Chai KX, Chen LM, Chao J, Chao L. Kallistatin: a novel human serine proteinase inhibitor. Molecular cloning, tissue distribution, and expression in *Escherichia coli. J Biol Chem* 1993; 268:24, 498.

Clements JA. The glandular kallikrein family of enzymes: tissue-specific expression and hormonal regulation. *Endocr Rev* 1989; 10:393.

Farmer SG. Biochemical and molecular pharmacology of kinin receptors. *Annu Rev Pharmacol Toxicol* 1992; 32:511.

MacDonald RJ, Margolius HS, Erdos EG. Molecular biology of tissue kallikrein. *Biochem J* 1988; 253:313.

Margolius HS. Tissue kallikreins and kinins: regulation and roles in hypertensive and diabetic diseases. *Ann Rev Pharmacol Toxicol* 1989; 29:343.

Murray SR, Chao J, Lin FK, Chao L. Kallikrein multigene families and the regulation of their expression. *J Cardiovasc Pharmacol* 1990; 15:S7.

Overlack A, Stumpe KO, Kolloch R, Ressel C, Krueck F. Antihypertensive effect of orally administered glandular kallikrein in essential hypertension. Results of double blind study. *Hypertension* 1981; 3:118.

Pravenec M, Kren V, Kunes J, Scicli AG, Carretero OA, Simonet L, Kurtz TW. Cosegregation of blood pressure with a kallikrein gene family polymorphism. *Hypertension* 1991; 17:242.

Regoli D, Barabe J. Pharmacology of bradykinin and related kinins. *Pharmacol Rev* 1980; 32:1.

Scicli AG, Carretero OA. Renal kallikrein-kinin system. *Kidney Int* 1986; 29:120.

Wang C, Chao L, Chao J. Direct gene delivery of human tissue kallikrein reduces blood pressure in spontaneously hypertensive rats. *J Clin Invest* 1995; 95:1710.

Wang J, Xiong W, Yang Z, Davis T, Dewey MJ, Chao J, Chao L. Human tissue kallikrein induces hypotension in transgenic mice. *Hypertension* 1994; 23:236.

Woodley-Miller C, Chao J, Chao L. Restriction fragment length polymorphisms mapped in spontaneously hypertensive rats using kallikrein probes. *J Hypertens* 1989; 7:865.

Zhou GX, Chao L, Chao J. Kallistatin: a novel human tissue kallikrein inhibitor. Purification, characterization and reactive center sequence. *J Biol Chem* 1992; 267:25, 873.

RA System

Baxter JD, Dunkin K. Chu W, et al. Molecular biology of human renin gene. *Recent Prog Horm Res* 1991; 47:211.

Chen M, Harris MP, Rose D, Smart A, et al. Renin and renin mRNA in proximal tubules of the rat kidney. *J Clin Invest* 1994; 94:237.

Corvol P, Jeunemaitre X, Charru A, et al. Role of the renin-angiotensin system in blood pressure regulation and in human hypertension: New insights in molecular genetics. *Recent Prog Horm Res* 1995; 50:287.

Gilbert MT, Sun J, Yan Y, Oddoux C, Lazarus A, Tansey WP, et al. Renin gene promoter activity in GC cells is regulated by cAMP and thyroid hormone through pit-1-dependent mechanisms. *J Biol Chem* 1994; 269:28, 049.

Hate T, Takimoto E, Murakami K, Fukamizua A. Comparative studies on species-specific reactivity between renin and angiotensinogen. *Mol Cell Biochem* 1994; 131:43.

Inagami T. Recent progress in molecular and cell biological studies of angiotensin receptors. *Curr Opinion Nephrol Hypertens* 1995; 4:47.

Jeunemaitre X, Soubrier F, Kotelevtsev YV, Lifton RP, Williams CS, Charru A, Hunt SC, Hopkins PN, William RR, Lalouel J-M. Molecular basis of human hypertension: Role of angiotensinogen. *Cell* 1992; 71:169.

Morris BJ. Molecular biology of renin. I: Gene and protein structure. Synthesis and processing. *J Hypertens* 1992; 10:209.

Paul M, Wagner J, Dzau VJ. Gene expression of the renin-angiotensin system in human tissues. Quantitative analysis by the polymerized chain reaction. *J Clin Invest* 1993; 91:2582.

Raizada MK, Phillips MI, Sumners C, eds. *Cellular and Molecular Biology of the Renin-Angiotensin System*. Boca Raton: CRC, 1993.

Ueda S, Elliot HL, Morton JJ, Connell JM. Enhanced pressor response to angiotensin I in normotensive men with the deletion genotype (DD) for angiotensin converting enzyme. *Hypertension* 1995; 25:1266.

Williams GH, Dluhy RG, Lifton RP, Moore TJ, Gleason R, Williams R, Hunt SC, Hopkins PN, Hollenberg NK. Nonmodulation as an intermediate phenotype in essential hypertension. *Hypertension* 1992; 20:788.

26 Reproduction and Fertility

Alan C. Dalkin, MD, and John C. Marshall, MD, PhD

CONTENTS

1. INTRODUCTION

The control of reproduction includes a series of hormonal interactions between the central nervous system (hypothalamus and pituitary) and gonads. Gonadotropin-releasing hormone (GnRH) is a decapeptide produced by a few hundred hypothalamic neurons. These cells extend termini to the median eminence to secrete GnRH in a pulsatile fashion into the hypophyseal-portal venous system. GnRH is then carried to the anterior pituitary where the gonadotropes (which comprise 5–7% of the total cell population) respond to GnRH via high-affinity cell-surface GnRH receptors by effecting the synthesis and secretion of the gonadotropins, luteinizing hormone (LH), and follicle-stimulating hormone (FSH). LH and FSH are dimeric peptides, comprised of a common α subunit and distinct β subunits, the latter conferring biological activity. Both LH and FSH are released in pulses into the systemic circulation, and act on the gonads in concert, with FSH predominantly regulating gamete development, but also being required to induce hormonal responses to LH. Thus, the combined actions of LH and FSH control both hormonogenesis (estradiol and progesterone from the ovary, testosterone from the testes, and inhibin, activin, and follistatin in both sexes) and gametogenesis. These steroid and peptide hormones have both local effects to promote gamete formation, and exert feedback regulation at the hypothalamus and pituitary.

In recent years, there have been a series of important advances in our understanding of the reproductive axis, adding to its complexity. In particular, the peptide hormones inhibin, activin, and follistatin (an activin-binding protein) have been identified initially in gonadal extracts and later in extra gonadal tissues. The recombinant production and study of these hormones suggest that they serve two broad types of regulatory functions. First, inhibins, activins, and follistatins are released from the gonads into the circulation to effect feedback actions predominantly on FSH at the pituitary gland. Additionally, these peptides may form important autocrine/paracrine feedback loops in the gonads, as well as in the pituitary, to alter local cellular functions. It is the purpose of this chapter to review the established actions of GnRH and gonadal steroids, and then to describe the emerging physiologic roles of inhibin, activin, and follistatin in the regulation of reproduction.

From: *Endocrinology: Basic and Clinical Principles* (P. M. Conn and S. Melmed, eds.), Humana Press Inc., Totowa, NJ.

2. HORMONAL PATTERNS IN REPRODUCTION

2.1. GnRH/GnRH-Receptor Signaling

The pulsatile nature of GnRH secretion is crucial for maintenance of gonadotrope secretory function. This was initially shown in hypothalamic lesioned monkeys (deficient in endogenous GnRH), where a continuous GnRH stimulus elicited LH release for a few hours, but a pulsatile (1 pulse/h) GnRH stimulus was required to maintain gonadotropin secretion over days to weeks. The pulsatile release of GnRH appears to be an inherent function of the hypothalamic neurons, as isolated neurons (in vitro) secrete bursts of GnRH at consistent intervals. This in turn suggests that variations in the GnRH secretory pattern in vivo result from suprahypothalamic regulation. Catecholamines promote GnRH release, whereas opioid peptides exert an inhibitory tone to slow the frequency of pulsatile secretion. Progesterone (in the presence of estradiol) and testosterone act to slow GnRH pulse secretion by mechanisms that involve increased hypothalamic opioid tone, and it is likely that additional central nervous system pathways also impact on GnRH-secreting neurons, resulting in dynamic GnRH pulse patterns during reproductive cycles.

GnRH acts at the gonadotrope cell via a high-affinity cell-surface GnRH receptor (GnRH-R). GnRH-R expression appears to be intimately tied to the responses of the gonadotrope. GnRH-R mRNA increase in response to GnRH pulses, and the number of GnRH-binding sites vary during the reproductive cycle. Moreover, GnRH-R numbers correlate well with LH secretory responses. GnRH/GnRH-R binding results in the activation of protein kinase C, calcium/calmodulin kinase, and perhaps protein kinase A, though increases in cAMP occur much later than activation of the other second messenger pathways. Although the exact functional role of each of the signaling pathways is uncertain, GnRH both induces hormone secretion and stimulates expression of the genes encoding the LH and FSH subunits and the GnRH-R (*see* Section 2.2.3. and Figs. 3 and 4).

2.2. Gonadotropin Synthesis and Secretion

2.2.1. Estrous Cycle

During the rat estrous cycle, both coordinate and differential regulation of gonadotropin secretion and gonadotropin subunit mRNAs is observed (Fig. 1).

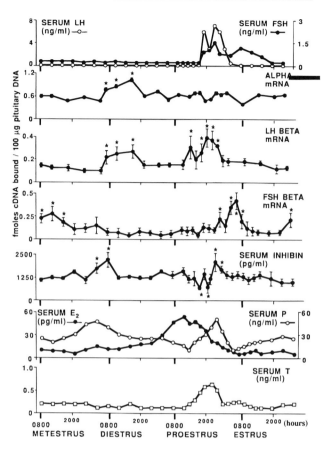

Fig. 1. Serum gonadotropins, gonadotropin subunit mRNA concentrations, serum inhibin and serum gonadal steroids (estradiol [E$_2$], progesterone [P] and testosterone [T]) during the 4-d estrous cycle in rats. *p < 0.05 vs basal values. (Reproduced with permission from Marshall et al., 1991.)

Early on the day of proestrus, the circulating concentration of estradiol (E$_2$) rises to a level that enhances gonadotrope responses to GnRH, the positive feedback action of E$_2$. In the late afternoon, GnRH secretion increases to a nearly continuous secretory pattern, which in concert with the enhanced gonadotrope response, induces the gonadotropin surge. A transient increase in the ovarian release of androgens (testosterone, T) and progesterone (P) is also seen on the afternoon of proestrus, which is followed approx 1 d later by a second rise in P secretion from the ovarian corpora lutea. The increase in P continues through metestrus when, failing conception, levels decline to basal values.

Changes in gonadotropin β subunit gene expression generally parallel those of gonadotropin secretion, though times of independent regulation are also present. During the proestrus gonadotropin surge,

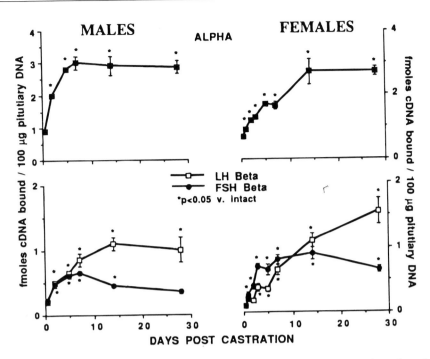

Fig. 2. Pituitary gonadotropin subunit mRNA concentrations following gonadectomy in male and female rats.

increases in LH β are coincident with maximal LH release, and the rise in FSH β is seen a few hours later during the secondary FSH secretory surge. Although these increases in secretion and β mRNA expression are likely related (at least in part) to GnRH, the α subunit mRNA (which increases in response to a wide range of GnRH pulse profiles— *see* Section 2.2.3. and Fig. 3) is not changed during proestrus. On estrus/metestrus, only the expression of FSH β mRNA is increased, without measurable changes in FSH secretion. The factor(s) responsible for this selective FSH response remains uncertain, but may reflect slow-frequency GnRH secretion in the presence of low concentrations of serum inhibin. On the following day, diestrus, both α and LH β mRNAs rise in the absence of significant changes in LH release, also supporting the notion that gene expression and hormone secretion can be independently regulated.

2.2.2. GONADECTOMY

Data obtained following gonadectomy in both male and female rats have revealed differential regulation of gonadotropin subunit gene expression (Fig. 2). Since rats lack a sex-steroid-binding globulin, the decline in plasma T, E_2, and P is rapid (minutes-hours). GnRH pulse frequency increases over hours

in males and days in females, from an interpulse interval of 2–4 h, to approx 30 min intervals. In males, the three gonadotropin subunit mRNAs increase within 24 h. α and LH β continue to increase for several days. However the rise in FSH β is not maintained in long-term castrated animals. Administration of a GnRH antagonist or T replacement at the time of castration prevents the increases in gonadotropin subunit gene expression, though T effects on FSH β mRNA are complex. Specifically, androgens reduce FSH β via hypothalamic feedback on GnRH, but also increase FSH β mRNA half-life via an action directly at the pituitary gland. It has been postulated that these dual mechanisms serve as a means for T (the production of which is predominantly under the control of LH) to feed back and reduce further LH drive without simultaneously reducing circulating FSH to levels that could impair gamete production. Although the mechanism(s) by which T changes FSH β mRNA stability is unknown, it is possible that despite increased GnRH secretion, the later postcastration decline in FSH β mRNA is related to the loss of T and reduced FSH β mRNA half-life.

In females, FSH β mRNA increases within 30–60 minute (and serum FSH within 2–4 h), whereas α and LH β mRNAs and serum LH rise more slowly (over 1–2 d). Administration of a GnRH antagonist or replacement with E_2 and P prevents the increase in α and LH β, but only partially prevents the increase in FSH β. This likely reflects the loss of inhibitory nonsteroidal gonadal factors, and the early increase in FSH β and FSH secretion has been attributed to a fall in circulating inhibin, as passive immunoneutralization can reproduce the initial post-ovariectomy changes. This effect is GnRH-independent and not prevented by GnRH blockade. Of interest, circulating inhibin levels in adult male rats are low and may account, in part, for the slower FSH responses in males.

2.2.3. EXOGENOUS GnRH PULSES

It is clear that alterations in gonadotropin subunit gene expression during the estrous cycle and following castration reflect changes in the GnRH signal pattern. Using GnRH-deficient rat models, we have characterized the effects of GnRH pulse amplitude and frequency in male and female rats. GnRH pulses given every 30 min (to mimic the postcastration GnRH pulse interval) to GnRH-deficient male rats increase GnRH-R, α, LH β, and FSH β mRNAs over a wide range of pulse amplitudes, 5–250 ng/pulse (shown in Fig. 3). In contrast, in GnRH deficient female rats, α mRNA was increased over this range of GnRH pulse doses, with GnRH-R and FSH β mRNA selectively responding to lower doses of GnRH. Of interest, LH β mRNA concentrations were not altered by exogenous GnRH, suggesting that other factors are needed in addition to GnRH to increase LH β gene expression. Recently, we have shown that T (which is transiently increased during the proestrus increase in β subunit mRNAs) is required to facilitate acute GnRH-induced increases in LH β mRNA.

For the study of pulse frequency (Fig. 4), a 25-ng GnRH dose/pulse was used since it produces serum levels of GnRH (250 pg/mL) that are similar to hypophyseal-portal levels. In males, faster pulse frequencies favored α and LH β, slower frequencies favored FSH β, whereas expression of GnRH-R mRNA was increased by all pulse intervals studied. In females, we observed a pattern similar to that observed in males with the exception that increases in LH β mRNA were not seen as the study was performed in the absence of T.

Thus, variations in GnRH pulse frequency and amplitude may provide a mechanism for differential

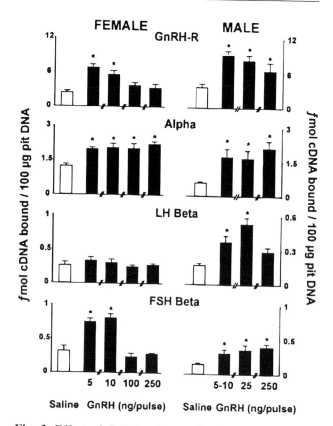

Fig. 3. Effect of GnRH pulse amplitude on gonadotrope responses.

regulation of gonadotropin production. As in the estrous cycle, infrequent GnRH pulses are associated with predominantly FSH synthesis and secretion. Conversely, at least in the male animal model, fast frequency GnRH (at intervals seen after castration and on proestrus) increases gonadotropin subunit gene expression. Elucidation of the role of GnRH pulse patterns on LH β mRNA expression in female rats awaits studies in the presence of T to reproduce the hormonal milieu of proestrus.

The mechanisms by which GnRH increases gonadotropin subunit gene expression appear to involve both mRNA synthesis (transcription) and mRNA degradation (stability). In GnRH-deficient male rats, GnRH pulses increase the transcriptional rates for the three gonadotropin subunit genes within 1 h. Moreover, the activation of transcription is frequency-dependent with an 8-min pulse interval increasing α, 30-min pulses stimulating α, LH β, and FSH β, whereas slower frequencies selectively increase FSH β mRNA synthesis. Interestingly, despite the continued rise in gonadotropin subunit

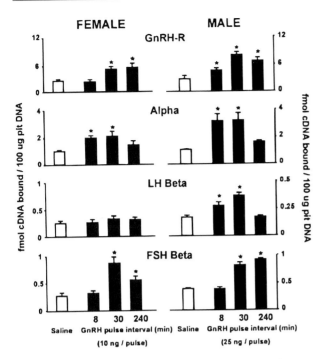

Fig. 4. Effect of GnRH pulse frequency on gonadotrope responses.

mRNA concentrations while pulsatile GnRH is maintained, LH β and FSH β subunit transcription did not remain elevated and returned to basal levels by 24 h. This suggests that GnRH may also regulate gonadotropin subunit gene expression via nontranscriptional mechanisms. In support, studies have reported that GnRH increases gonadotropin subunit mRNA polyadenylation, suggesting that GnRH, either directly or via unknown intermediate proteins, also may alter mRNA stability.

2.2.4. GONADAL STEROIDS

E_2 has actions at both the hypothalamus and pituitary. E_2 replacement at the time of ovariectomy acts via GnRH to prevent the increase in serum LH and LH β mRNA, and partially prevents the rise in α and FSH β mRNAs and serum FSH. This partial efficacy may reflect residual endogenous GnRH secretion, since diurnal changes in α mRNA and serum LH are observed in ovariectomized rats replaced with physiologic levels of E_2. When given to longer-term ovariectomized animals, E_2 reduces gonadotropin subunit gene transcription, an action presumably via GnRH, since E_2 does not alter transcriptional rates in vitro. Conversely, E_2 also can stimulate GnRH secretion. Maximal GnRH secretion during the proestrus

gonadotropin surge is preceded by an increase in serum E_2. Similarly, the frequency of pulsatile LH increases during the late follicular phase in humans as E_2 concentrations rise. Thus, the actions of E_2 are biphasic, and likely depend on time and dose relations.

The actions of P depend on the preceding steroid milieu with some differences between species also apparent. In the anestrus sheep, progesterone inhibits GnRH (and hence LH) secretion. In contrast, in the female rat P treatment alone has little effect on either GnRH secretion or gonadotropin subunit gene expression. However, the addition of P to E_2 is more effective than E_2 alone in preventing the postcastration increases in gonadotropin subunit mRNAs. In vitro, P transiently augments LH and FSH secretion in response to GnRH in E_2 pretreated rat pituitaries. P may also act directly at the pituitary to increase FSH β mRNA levels, further supporting the notion that like E_2, P has numerous sites of action.

T administration at the time of castration prevents the increase in gonadotropin secretion and subunit mRNA concentrations via inhibition of GnRH. However, when T is given to pituitary cells in vitro, or in vivo either to GnRH-deficient animals or in pharmacologic doses to long-term castrated animals, FSH β mRNA concentrations are selectively increased via a nontranscriptional mechanism. This action can be reproduced by dihydrotestosterone (DHT), but not E_2. Whether androgens directly interact with the FSH β mRNA to prevent degradation is unknown.

2.2.5. SUMMARY

Overall, the regulation of the reproductive system is complex and involves a number of hormonal interactions reflecting both dynamic signal patterns (e.g., variations in GnRH pulse amplitude and/or frequency) and dynamic cellular response systems (e.g., changes in GnRH receptor numbers). GnRH increases gonadotropin subunit gene expression at the transcriptional level and potentially via alterations in mRNA half-life. Subsequent gonadal responses include a series of steroid feedback systems to modulate GnRH and gonadotrope responses. At the gonadotrope cell, there appear to be mechanisms that preserve FSH synthesis and secretion independently of LH. Specifically, both ovarian and testicular steroids can selectively increase FSH β mRNA half-life. Furthermore, the gonadal peptides inhibin, activin, and follistatin (*see* Section 3.) act predominantly on FSH β mRNA half-life. With the identification of these "gonadal" peptides in extragonadal tissues, including the pituitary, it appears that pituitary-derived activin and follistatin regulate FSH directly, and may also may serve as moderators of GnRH and steroid hormone signals. Thus, we will next review the gonadal aspects of inhibin, activin, and follistatin and then describe their extragonadal production.

3. GONADAL PEPTIDES: ENDOCRINE REGULATION

3.1. Inhibins

The existence of gonadal nonsteroidal factors that inhibit FSH has long been postulated, after reports that testicular irradiation increased FSH secretion without reducing plasma T. Once isolated, the inhibins were found to be members of the transforming growth factor (TGF)-β superfamily of polypeptides. There are at least 18 proteins in this superfamily sharing a dimeric structure with disulfide bonds, Asn-linked glycosylation sites, and protein homologies of 25–90%, with a wide array of biological actions involving cell growth, differentiation, and cell–cell signaling. Included are the TGF-βs, Mullerian inhibiting substance, decapentaplegic product gene complex (*Drosophila*), Vg1 (*Xenopus laevis*), bone morphogenetic proteins, and the inhibins/activins. These compounds are synthesized as a precursor polypeptide that is cleaved to form active hormones.

The activity of the mature products also appears to be regulated in a common manner. Specifically, noncovalent binding to another protein to induce latency or block activity (e.g., a portion of the TGF-β prohormone interacts with mature TGF-β protein; the follistatins, a family of unrelated proteins, bind to activin) has been reported. The isolation of the inhibin α (Iα), β-A, β-B, and follistatin cDNAs and genomic elements, and the production of these proteins by recombinant DNA technology have allowed for detailed study of the regulation and action of these peptides. A schematic representation of these peptides is shown in Fig. 5.

The dimeric combination of an Iα and either β-A or β-B subunit results in the formation of inhibin A or inhibin B, respectively. If two β subunits are combined (β-A β-A; β-A β-B; β-B β-B), the activins A, AB, and B are produced. Inhibin A and B and activin A and AB have been isolated in testic-

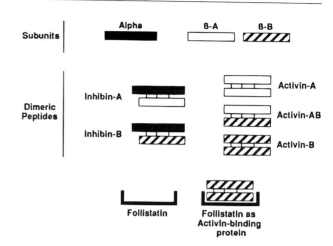

Fig. 5. Structural representation of the inhibins, activins, and follistatins.

ular and/or ovarian extracts. Activin B has been produced in vitro through recombinant DNA technology. The human, porcine, bovine, and rat ovarian cDNAs as well as the human and rat testicular cDNAs have been isolated. Each inhibin subunit is encoded by a separate gene, and analysis of their regulatory elements and mRNA concentrations suggests independent control. In general, the bioactivities of the inhibins (as well as activins and follistatins) are similar, and hence, in the subsequent text, we will refer to each peptide in the singular (e.g., inhibin).

3.1.1. GENE REGULATION

3.1.1.1. Iα Subunit. The Iα gene is >3 kb in length with a single intron of approx 1.5 kb, and codes for a peptide of 44–50 kDa, which is cleaved to form a mature protein of 18 kDa (132 amino acids). There is approximately an 80% homology between rat and human Iα protein. The Iα mRNA is the most abundant of the three inhibin subunit mRNAs in the gonads, and levels of Iα (as well as β-A and β-B) vary during embryogenesis, sexual maturation, and the estrous cycle (*see* Section 3.1.2.1.).

Iα subunit mRNA expression, found predominantly in ovarian granulosa cells and to a lesser extent in thecal cells, is regulated by both pituitary and gonadal hormones. In granulosa cell cultures, FSH, pregnant mare serum gonadotropin (PMSG) and E_2 increase Iα mRNA concentrations. In Sertoli cell cultures, Iα mRNA levels are also stimulated by FSH, but not by T. Regulation of Iα subunit gene expression is likely of physiologic significance, since cotransfection studies have shown that high levels of Iα favor Iα-β dimerization, whereas low levels favor β-β dimers. Further, changes in gonadal inhibin secretion generally parallel changes in Iα mRNA concentration.

Granulosa cell secretion of inhibin is stimulated by FSH, forskolin, PMSG, E_2 and somatomedin-C. E_2 can also augment the inhibin response to FSH. Rat granulosa cells express GnRH receptors (the physiologic significance of which is unknown), and pharmacologic levels of GnRH in static culture may block the inhibin response to FSH. In males, testicular inhibin secretion is stimulated by FSH, cholera toxin, forskolin, and dibutyryl cAMP, but not by T or DHT. However, T may partially prevent the Sertoli cell response to low levels of FSH. In contrast to females, E_2 has no effect on inhibin secretion in males. Though the significance is unclear, β-endorphin has been shown to attenuate FSH-induced inhibin secretion. Thus, in both the ovary and testis, Iα subunit mRNA levels and inhibin secretion respond in a similar fashion, suggesting that the availability of this subunit may be rate-limiting in the formation of inhibin.

3.1.1.2. Inhibin β-B Subunit.
The gene for the inhibin β-B subunit is approx 6 kb in size with a single 3-kb intron. The propeptide is 40 kDa, which is cleaved to the mature protein of 14 kDa (114 amino acids). In species studied to date, the homology for β-B protein is ≥97%. β-B mRNA is present in both testes and ovary in two predominant species of 4.3–4.4 and 3.1–3.3 kb, perhaps related to alternate splicing or differences in polyadenylation. In granulosa cells, FSH and E_2 increased β-B mRNAs, suggesting coordinate regulation of the Iα and β-B subunits. In the rat testes, β-B mRNA concentrations peak prepubertally and decline to lower levels in adults. This pattern is similar to that seen for Iα and in keeping with data showing that circulating inhibin levels are low in adult male rats. Of interest, hypophysectomy in adult male rats increased β-B mRNA levels, and replacement of either FSH or T had no effect.

3.1.1.3. Inhibin β-A Subunit.
A single mRNA species (≈6 kb) has been observed in the ovary, and is either present in very low amounts or absent in the testis. The β-A propeptide is 40 kDa, with a mature subunit of 15 kDa (115 amino acids). The β-A subunit is highly conserved between species, with a

homology of nearly 100%. Like ovarian Iα and β-B, FSH increase β-A mRNA levels in granulosa cell culture, whereas E_2 has no effect. Taken together, these findings suggest that ovarian β-A and β-B mRNAs may be independently regulated by E_2, and that different inhibin/activin species may be present in males and females.

3.1.2. Actions of Inhibin

3.1.2.1. Studies in Females.
During sexual maturation in female rats, inhibin levels rise steadily in an inverse relationship to serum FSH, which is followed by cyclic variation during the estrous cycle (Fig. 1). Serum inhibin levels rise throughout the day of proestrus, reaching maximal levels late on that evening. This secretory pattern is paralleled by changes in ovarian Iα mRNA, which, although present at all stages of follicular maturation, increase to maximal levels in preovulatory follicles late on proestrus. A decline in Iα mRNA is seen thereafter, coincident with the subsequent decline in circulating inhibin and the secondary FSH surge. Regulation of the β subunits appears distinct from that noted for the Iα gene. Throughout the day of estrus, the mRNAs for the β-A and β-B subunits in the granulosa cells of secondary and tertiary follicles remain at high levels despite diminished Iα. Whether these changes in ovarian inhibin subunit expression on the day of estrus reflect a change from inhibin to activin production remains unknown, but is suggested by the fact that FSH β mRNA levels increase during estrus-metestrus.

These data are consistent with the hypothesis that FSH is the primary stimulus for granulosa cell inhibin subunit gene expression/secretion, which then exerts feedback inhibition on FSH, independent of GnRH. In response to exogenous inhibin, FSH β mRNA levels rapidly declined in a GnRH-deficient ewe model. Similar results are seen using dispersed pituitary cells where inhibin has suppressive effects on FSH synthesis and content, as well as in reducing basal and GnRH-stimulated release. Inhibin may reduce GnRH receptor numbers, but does not appear to alter hypothalamic GnRH secretion in rats. Of interest, inhibin-induced alterations in FSH β mRNA concentrations precede FSH secretory changes. Passive immunoneutralization of circulating inhibin in female rats increases FSH β mRNA within 2 h and serum FSH within 12 h. This rise in FSH secretory activity is physiologically important. Since a subsequent increase in ovulatory rate has been documented following passive immunoneutralization. It is unclear if alterations in FSH β mRNA directly result in reduced levels of FSH β peptide production and then FSH secretion. Regardless, in the female rat, circulating inhibin acts in an endocrine feedback fashion to regulate physiologic FSH secretion.

The effects of inhibin on LH biosynthesis and secretion are less clear, with some studies reporting a decline in basal LH release, others an effect only on GnRH stimulated release, and still others showing no effect of inhibin on LH secretion. Inhibin does not appear to alter LH β mRNA concentrations, suggesting its primary action is on FSH biosynthesis and secretion.

3.1.2.2. Studies in Males. Interestingly, although both adult male and adult female rats respond similarly to exogenous inhibin, the physiologic importance of gonadal-derived inhibin may differ between the sexes. In vivo studies administering recombinant human (rh) inhibin to gonadectomized male rats have shown a dose-related decrease in FSH secretion, lasting for 8–12 h. Despite this response to exogenous inhibin, levels of circulating inhibins in adult male rats are less than in adult females. In immature male rats, circulating inhibin levels are elevated, but fall to low or immeasurable values at maturity. Furthermore, passive immunoneutralization of inhibin in immature male rats increased serum FSH, an effect that was lost in adult animals. This relationship may differ in primates, since the male rhesus monkey appears to have biologically active circulating inhibin. Less information is available in humans, though immunoreactive inhibin peptide appears to be present in adult men. Thus, species-specific differences in testicular inhibin production are apparent and, in the rat testicular inhibin, may not serve the endocrine functions observed in the female.

3.1.2.3. Mechanism of Inhibin Action. It is generally believed that inhibin regulates FSH β mRNA expression at the level of mRNA stability (degradation) rather than mRNA synthesis (transcription). Studies documenting increased FSH β gene expression following ovariectomy or inhibin immunoneutralization, in the absence of altered FSH β transcriptional rates, support such an action for inhibin. The mechanism by which inhibin acts is unknown, but administering the protein synthesis inhibitor cyclohexamide can mimic the effects of

inhibin, suggesting a role for intermediate intracellular polypeptides in inhibin responses. Whether actual inhibin receptors exist remains speculative. Specific binding sites appear to be present on the gonadotrope and in the gonads, but to date, attempts to isolate a functional inhibin receptor have been unsuccessful.

3.2. Activins

3.2.1. Actions of Activin

The activins are known to have diverse actions in multiple tissues. These include paracrine effects on granulosa cell function, regulation of follicular development, modulation of testicular androgen production, stimulation of erythropoesis, and modulation of corticotropin-releasing hormone (CRH), adrenocorticotropic hormone (ACTH), and growth hormone (GH) secretion. Unfortunately, our understanding of endogenous activin action is very incomplete, since a reliable assay for the activins has not yet been developed. Whereas both inhibin dimers possess the Iα subunit and thus both inhibin A and B are detected with a single Iα-directed antibody, measurement of the three dimeric combinations for activins requires double-antibody systems directed to the β-chains to ensure that the inhibin α-β dimer is not crossreacting in the assay. Moreover, because abundance of the β subunits may differ in normal physiology, measurement of changes in activin levels would necessitate assay systems for all three activin species (A, AB, and B). Hence, the role of activin in the physiologic regulation of gonadotrope function has generally been inferred from studies of the actions of exogenous activin.

Activin increases FSH β mRNA within 2–4 h and FSH secretion increases thereafter. Changes in LH secretion, α or LH β mRNAs are not consistently observed. Like inhibin, activin acts independently of GnRH, and can induce FSH secretion in GnRH-desensitized pituitary cells and augment GnRH-induced FSH secretion. Activin has also been shown to alter the gonadotrope cell population by selectively increasing the number of measurable FSH secreting cells. The half-life of FSH β mRNA has been shown to increase following the addition of activin to dispersed pituitary cells treated with actinomycin D (a transcriptional inhibitor). Thus, activin has been postulated to regulate FSH β mRNA and subsequently FSH synthesis, and secretion by a nontranscriptional mechanism. In vivo, activin increased FSH β mRNA and FSH secretion within 4 h in immature female and OVX/E$_2$-treated adult female rats, whereas little or no effect was observed in immature or adult male rats. These data suggest that activin regulates FSH β mRNA concentrations and subsequently FSH synthesis, an effect that appears to be more important in females.

3.2.2. Activin Receptors

Activin acts via specific membrane receptors with serine kinase activity. At least three members of the activin receptor (ActR) family have been identified to date. As with the TGF-β receptors, there are Type I and Type II receptors, with two Type II subunits (A and B) for the activins (shown in Fig. 6). Dimeric combination of the subunits is needed for formation of a functional receptor, and likely involves the interaction of the Type I receptor peptide with either of the Type II peptide chains. The physiologic significance of two Type II receptors is unknown, but data showing selective expression in a variety of tissues and at different stages of fetal development suggest that the different ActRIIs may support diverse actions of activin.

3.2.2.1. ActRIIA.
Mathews and Vale initially isolated a mouse ActR similar to the TGF-β Type II receptor. This activin receptor (ActRIIA), when expressed in COS cells, binds activin with a K_d of ≅ 200 pM. The ActRIIA also binds inhibin, though the affinity is 10–50-fold less compared to activin, suggesting that a separate inhibin receptor must also exist. Subsequently, cDNAs for the rat, human, and *Xenopus laevis* ActRIIA have been published with nucleotide homologies in rats, mice, and humans of ≥97%.

The ActRIIA receptor gene is expressed in the later stages of fetal development and/or in adult tissues, in contrast to ActRIIB, which is more prevalent in fetal development. ActRIIA gene expression occurs in a variety of adult tissues, including brain, pituitary, prostate, placenta, and gonads. During testicular development in the rat, ActRIIA mRNA levels increase, but then decline in the adult testes. Alterations in ActRIIA mRNA are also seen during fetal development in the chick, and ActRIIA mRNA has been detected in murine embryos. Limited physiologic studies of pituitary ActRIIA mRNA expression have been reported. Following ovariectomy, ActRIIA mRNAs increase within 8 h, a response that is not altered by steroid replacement or GnRH blockade. These findings suggest that a yet to be deter-

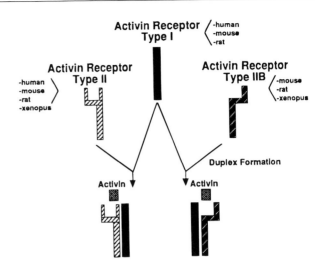

Fig. 6. Schematic representation of activin receptor subunit dimerization. The species in which the subunits have been characterized are listed.

mined gonadal factor(s) inhibits ActRIIA gene expression in the adult rat.

3.2.2.2. ActRIIB.
A second, highly homologous Type II ActR was identified in the mouse by Attisano and colleagues, which appears to be expressed as four separate isotypes and has been termed ActRIIB1–4. Regional amino acid homologies between ActRIIA and ActRIIB are 51% in the ligand-binding region, 42% in the transmembrane region, and 75% in the intracellular region. Affinities (K_d) of the ActRIIB receptors (when in complex with a Type I receptor) for activin range from 100–300 pM and, as with ActRIIA, displacement of activin by inhibin is observed only when inhibin is present in 50–100-fold excess. ActRIIB cDNAs have been reported in the rat and in *Xenopus laevis* with >95% nucleotide homology between rat and mouse. The ActRIIB 5-regulatory element(s) have yet to be identified.

The presence of ActRIIB mRNA in rodent fetal development has been reported. ActRIIB mRNA has a wide tissue distribution in the embryo and can be detected within the first 9–10 d in some tissues. In studies that have examined both ActRIIA and IIB mRNAs in adult tissues, levels of IIB gene expression appear to be less abundant. Overall, there are both fetal and adult tissues that possess both Type II receptors (such as pituitary), whereas other adult tissues (such as the prostate gland and ovary) predominantly express the ActRIIA.

3.2.2.3. ActRI. Most recently, a Type I Activin Receptor (ActRI) has been isolated in the mouse, human (also termed ALK-2), and the rat. The ActRI shows approximately a 40% sequence homology with the Type II receptors, which is greatest in the intracellular regions, since the ActRI also encodes a serine-threonine kinase domain. In contrast, the extracellular domains of the Type I and Type II receptors show minimal overlap. ActRI mRNA is expressed in brain, pituitary, lung, and to a lesser extent in kidney, testes, and liver. A second potential Type I ActR has been reported called ActRIB (ALK-4 in humans), though its expression in physiology has not been studied.

Of interest, ActRI does not appear to bind activin ligand, but rather associates with either Type II receptor in forming an active receptor complex and allowing postreceptor signal transduction. Conversely, the ActRIIA peptide alone is capable of binding activin ligand, but is unable to generate the postreceptor events associated with a fully functional receptor. The means by which the receptor peptide chains dimerize and the factor(s) regulating receptor activation are unknown at this time. Although some postreceptor events, such as receptor autophosphorylation have been reported, the intracellular events that produce activin-induced increases in FSH β mRNA half-life have not been identified.

3.3. Follistatin

3.3.1. Regulation of Follistatin Expression

Follistatins (FS) are a family of glycosylated monomeric proteins with FSH-suppressing activity. The rat, human, and porcine cDNAs and rat genomic sequence for the FS have been reported, and the protein sequences are highly (98%) conserved between species. As a result of alternative mRNA splicing, three different FS proteins are encoded (315, 300, and 288 amino acids) with the 288 amino acid protein having slightly greater bioactivity than either the 300 amino acid species (the predominant form in follicular fluid) or the 315 amino acid species. Little is known regarding how differential regulation of the three isoforms occurs.

Gonadal FS is likely regulated by gonadotropins, since PMSG can increase ovarian FS production. Studies of the rat FS promoter also support the importance of gonadotropin regulation. The FS promoter contains three distinct TATA-like sequences,

each associated with a separate transcriptional start site. There are also a number of potential cis-regulatory sites, including two potential AP-2 sites, which are of particular interest for gonadotropin action, since AP-2-mediated transcription is thought to be involved in both the cAMP and TPA pathways.

3.3.2. Actions of Follistatin

FS exerts its physiologic action by binding to activin, thereby preventing activin binding to its receptor. This may explain why FS is more effective than inhibin in blocking the effect of activin on FSH β mRNA and FSH secretion. FS binds activin via its β subunit, and hence, FS can theoretically also bind inhibin. However, FS/inhibin binding does not neutralize the biological effects of inhibin. The binding of FS to activin is rapid and irreversible with a Kd of approx 50 pM, similar to the affinity of activin for activin receptors, suggesting that FS competes for activin binding with the cell-surface activin receptors.

Recent data from Weiss and colleagues (Crowley et al., 1991) have expanded our thoughts regarding the physiologic actions of FS. As expected, concomitant treatment of pituitary cells (in perifusion) with FS and activin blocked the ability of activin to increase FSH β mRNA. Of interest, limiting the FS treatment to the period preceding activin administration augmented the activin-induced increases in FSH β gene expression. The authors hypothesized that, since FS is known to associate with heparin sulfate chains of proteogylcans, FS could bind to these cell-surface sites and serve to position/assist activin binding to its receptors (as opposed to the action of "free" FS, which would compete for available activin and prevent its binding to activin receptors). Thus, the actions of FS are complex with the "net" effect perhaps being determined by prevailing levels at the gonadotrope cell surface.

3.3.3. Follistatin Secretion

The development of a reliable assays to measure circulating FS has only recently been reported. FS does not appear to be the only circulating activin-binding protein, Since α-2 macroglobulin also binds activin, although at a reduced affinity when compared to FS. Results are conflicting regarding the relative contributions of α-2 macroglobulin and FS in the circulation. Significantly, some FS does appear to circulate unbound to activin, and hence, changes in FS could modify the effects of activin at a variety of target tissues where locally derived activin may be produced.

4. GONADAL PEPTIDES: AUTOCRINE/PARACRINE REGULATION

4.1. Gonadotrope

In addition to the gonads, inhibin subunit mRNAs are present in brain, placenta, bone marrow, kidney, adrenal gland, and pituitary. In particular, Iα and β-B (but not β-A) mRNAs were identified in the rat pituitary gland (gonadotrope), with the Iα mRNA being more abundant than the β-B subunit mRNA in females. Moreover, the expression of these two mRNAs appears to be inhibited by gonadal factors that are yet to be determined. Pituitary inhibin subunit gene expression increases after ovariectomy with changes in β-B mRNA seen within 2 d and Iα within 3 wk, with only the latter being prevented by E_2 replacement.

Despite the technical limitations preventing the direct measurement of activin in the pituitary, there is sufficient evidence to conclude that the pituitary translates these mRNAs into bioactive peptides. Although it is unknown if gonadotropes synthesize inhibin, pituitary production of activin does occur. Following treatment of dispersed adult male pituitaries with a monoclonal antibody (MAb) to the β-B subunit, FSH secretion and FSH β mRNA decline, whereas LH release and α or LH β mRNAs are unchanged. This suggests that pituitary-derived activin exerts an autocrine/paracrine stimulatory effect on FSH secretion and synthesis. Furthermore, pituitary production of activin is necessary to maintain basal FSHβ mRNA levels in vitro. Immunohistochemistry has confirmed pituitary production of activin B (β-A protein was not detected), and activation of either protein kinase A or protein kinase C stimulated β-B protein production. Potentially, regulation of activin production at both the gonads and/or the pituitary could result in a dynamic regulation of FSH. Moreover, the levels of activin receptors could impact on activin responses, and serve to alter FSH mRNA and secretory responses.

As with activin, follistatin is produced in a number of sites outside the gonads, and both follistatin mRNA and protein have been identified in the pituitary. Pituitary FS mRNA levels rise following gonadectomy in rats, an effect that is inhibited by T replacement (males), whereas E_2 replacement in females may actually induce further increases.

Also, pituitary FS mRNA concentrations rise on the afternoon of proestrus, suggesting that pituitary-derived FS may regulate FSH secretion during the gonadotropin surge.

Factors that regulate pituitary FS and potentially mediate the physiologic changes in FS production noted above have only recently been recognized. Activin increases pituitary FS mRNA and protein, an effect that would serve as a short-loop feedback to limit activin action. GnRH also increases pituitary FS gene expression with the pattern of pulsatile GnRH providing differential regulation. Specifically, pituitary FS mRNA increased when GnRH was given at the fast-physiologic pulse intervals (8 and 30 min), but was not elevated after slower pulse frequencies. In contrast, FSH β mRNA levels are only increased at pulse intervals between 30 and 480 min (see Fig. 2). Assuming that the increase in pituitary FS mRNA results in similar changes in FS protein, these results proved a novel mechanism whereby GnRH can differentially regulate gonadotropin subunit gene expression. More specifically, since GnRH pulse frequency increases after castration, pituitary production of FS may increase and bind to locally produced activin, thereby limiting FSH β mRNA responses to GnRH. Increased FS after gonadectomy may account for the early plateau in FSH β mRNA in females and/or the later decline in FSH β in males. In summary, pituitary production of FS is dynamic, and predictions regarding activin's actions must account for the presence of FS. The potential roles of GnRH, activin, and FS on the gonadotropes are shown in Fig. 7.

4.1.1. HORMONOGENESIS

Inhibin, activin, and FS are important autocrine and paracrine regulators of gonadal function, modulating both hormone biosynthesis and gamete maturation (Fig. 8). In vitro studies with isolated granulosa cells have shown that activin directly stimulates Iα and β-B mRNAs, inhibin secretion, and FSH receptor expression. Furthermore, activin augments FSH-induced increases in cAMP, inhibin subunit gene expression secretion, E_2 production, and LH receptor numbers, all physiologic characteristics of developing follicles. Activin also inhibits P production, further demonstrating its antiluteinization effects. In contrast, activin directly attenuates LH-stimulated thecal cell androgen synthesis. Since androstenedione and dehydro-epiandrosterone are E_2

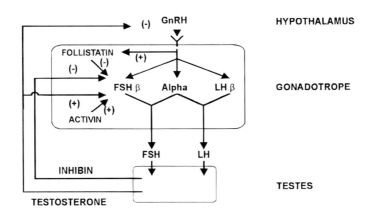

Fig. 7. Schematic representation of gonadotropin subunit mRNA regulation.

precursors, activin can induce opposing effects on E_2 production with an overall action perhaps determined by which cell type receives the greater activin stimulus. As would be predicted, the effects of FS on granulosa cells contrast that of activin. FS prevents activin/FSH-induced increases in aromatase activity, E_2 biosynthesis, and inhibin secretion, while favoring P production and luteinization. To date, studies detailing clear actions of inhibin on ovarian hormone release are currently lacking. In summary, activin appears to play a role in the hormonal secretory patterns associated with developing follicles, actions that may be attenuated by FS.

4.1.2. Gametogenesis

Both in vitro and in vivo studies have investigated the effects of gonadal peptides on gamete formation. In oocyte cultures, inhibin reduced meiotic maturation, whereas activin was either stimulatory or ineffective. This local action of inhibin could combine with its feedback inhibition of FSH release and prevent follicular recruitment. Conversely, as inhibin levels decline before the LH/FSH surge, a new round of follicular maturation would begin after ovulation. Unexpectedly, FS appears to have the opposite effect of inhibin and can induce oocyte maturation in vitro. In vivo studies have been performed by injecting microgram amounts of inhibin or activin directly into the ovarian bursa, likely resulting in supraphysiologic concentrations. In contrast to results from in vitro studies, these data reveal that inhibin stimulates and activin inhibits follicular development. Therefore, further studies are needed to provide a clearer delineation of gonadal peptide actions on gamete maturation.

5. GONADAL PEPTIDES IN DISEASE STATES

5.1 Neoplasia

5.1.1. Inhibin-α Gene Deletions

Activins and inhibins, as members of the TGF-β family, in certain cell systems can act as regulators of growth and differentiation. For example, activin induces differentiation of erythroid cell precursors and was originally termed erythroid differentiation factor (EDF) when isolated from the bone marrow. Potentially, reproductive tissues may respond to activin, inhibin, and FS with altered cell growth. To address this question, studies utilized embryonic stem cell technology to create a mouse with the inhibin α gene deleted, which has provided intriguing data on the role of activin (and by inference inhibin) on cell proliferation. Animals homozygous for the mutation are characterized by marked reduction in fertility, increased serum FSH, no measurable circulating inhibin, a 200-fold increase in testicular β-A subunit mRNA, and the early development of gonadal sex cord-stromal tumors. Thus, it is hypothesized that inhibin is a tumor repressor and that unopposed activin is tumorogenic. Moreover, in a clonal testes tumor cell line derived from these animals, exogenous activin stimulated tumor growth and thymidine incorporation into DNA, which was attenuated by FS or an activin antibody. If the animals are gonadectomized prior to tumor formation, adrenal tumors develop later, suggesting that nonreproductive tissues may respond to activin and inhibin in a similar fashion.

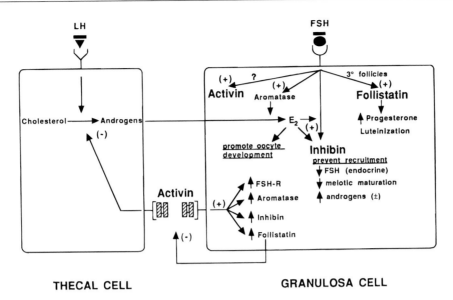

Fig. 8. Endocrine and autocrine/paracrine regulation of ovarian steroid and female gamete production.

5.1.2. PITUITARY TUMORS

Several investigators have examined pituitary tumor tissue for the expression of the inhibin subunits and FS. In general, most pituitary tumors appear to express the β-B subunit mRNA and to a lesser extent the α subunit. Data are conflicting on the β-A subunit, which, if present, is in low abundance. Interestingly, inhibin subunit mRNAs can be detected in nonfunctioning (presumably gonadotrope-derived), somatotroph-, corticotroph-, and lactotroph-derived neoplasms. Since the majority of functional gonadotrope-derived adenomas secrete FSH, it is possible that activins may have effects on pituitary tumors both in terms of secretory function and cell proliferation.

5.2. Polycystic Ovarian Syndrome

A few reports have addressed whether inhibin subunit gene expression is altered in women with polycystic ovarian syndrome (PCOS). In brief, women with PCOS have ovarian hyperandrogenism with end-organ effects, such as acne and hirsutism, an increased LH:FSH ratio (in a approx 75% of individuals), obesity, and menstrual disturbances. Although a full discussion of PCOS is beyond the scope of this chapter, these women would be candidates for altered ovarian inhibin and activin production. Results from the limited number of studies to date are conflicting. Some reports have suggested that there is no change in the patterns of ovarian

inhibin subunit mRNAs, whereas others have shown that the small antral follicles in women with PCOS have reduced levels of inhibin α and FS mRNAs, which could indicate a relative increase in the production/response to activin.

REFERENCE

Crowley WF Jr, Whitcomb RW, Jameson JL, Weiss J, Finkelstein JS, O'Dea LSL. Neuroendocrine control of human reproduction in the male. *Rec Prog Horm Res* 1991; 47:27.

Marshall JC, Dalkin AC, Haisenleder DJ, Paul SJ, Ortolano GA, Kelch RP. Gonadotropin releasing hormone pulses: regulators of gonadotropin synthesis and ovulatory cycles. *Rec Prog Horm Res.* 1991; 47:155.

SELECTED READINGS

DePaolo LV, Bicsak TA, Erickson GF, Shimasaki S, Ling N. Follistatin and activin: a potential intrinsic regulatory system within diverse tissues. *Soc Exp Biol Med* 1991; 198:500.

Findlay JK. An update on the roles of inhibin, activin, and follistatin as local regulators of folliculogenesis. *Biol Reprod* 1993; 48:15.

Gharib SD, Wierman ME, Shupnik MA, Chin WW. Molecular biology of the pituitary gonadotropins. *Endo Rev* 1990; 11:177.

Haisenleder DJ, Dalkin AC, Marshall JC. Regulation of gonadotropin gene expression. In: Knobil E, Neill JD eds. *The Physiology of Reproduction*, 2nd ed. New York: Raven, 1994:1793.

Ling N, DePaolo LV, Bicsak TA, Shimasaki S. Novel ovarian regulatory peptides: inhibin, activin, and follistatin. *Clin Obstet Gynecol* 1990; 33:690.

Marshall JC. Hormonal regulation of the menstrual cycle and mechanisms of anovulation. In: DeGroot LJ, Besser M,

Burger H, Jameson JL, Loriaux DL, Marshall JC, Odell WD, Potts JT Jr., Rubenstein AH eds. *Endocrinology.* Philadelphia: W.B. Saunders, 1995:2046.

Marshall JC. Regulation of gonadotropin secretion. In: DeGroot LJ, Besser M, Burger H, Jameson JL, Loriaux DL, Marshall JC, Odell WD, Potts JT Jr, Rubenstein AH eds. *Endocrinology.* Philadelphia: W.B. Saunders, 1995:1993.

Mathews LS, Activin receptors and cellular signalling by the receptor serine kinase family. *Endo Rev* 1994; 15:310.

Savoy-Moore RT, Schwartz NB, Duncan JA, Marshall JC. Pituitary gonadotropin-releasing hormone receptors during the rat estrous cycle. *Science* 1980; 209:942.

Ying SY. Inhibins, activins, and follistatins: gonadal proteins modulating the secretion of follicle-stimulating hormone. *Endo, Rev* 1988; 9:267.

27 Regulation of Pregnancy, Parturition, and Lactation

John R. G. Challis, PhD, DSc, FRSC

CONTENTS

1. INTRODUCTION

It is during our intrauterine development that many of the traits and characteristics that will affect our postnatal performance are established. At the time of fertilization, our genotype is established, but during fetal life, our further growth and development are influenced by many factors, including fetal genotype, placental function, local growth factors, circulating hormones, and the maternal environment. In North America, growth retardation leading to babies that are small for gestational age occurs in about 6% of all pregnancies. Preterm delivery occurs in 8–10% of all deliveries. Birth too soon of an infant that is very immature may be associated with conditions, such as cerebral palsy, and with respiratory distress syndrome in the newborn. In the US, the cost of preterm delivery—reflected in the cost of caring for these babies in Neonatal Intensive Care Units (NICUs)—has been estimated at $5–6 billion annually. The emotional cost for parents and families is substantial. Babies born too small may have additional longer-term problems. Recently, David Barker and colleagues have demonstrated that weight at birth is a powerful indicator of predisposition to disease in adult life (*see* Barker, 1994). The infant who is born inappropriately small has a much higher risk of developing high blood pressure, Type II diabetes, and of dying from cardiovascular disease in adult life. This relationship is particularly strong if the fetal growth reduction is asymmetrical and the placenta is disproportionately large. These relationships—small birthweight and subsequent hypertension—can be reproduced in the offspring of rats fed low-protein diets or treated with glucocorticoids during pregnancy. Thus, understanding factors regulating pregnancy and pregnancy outcome as well as fetal growth and development are crucial for understanding, and potentially treating and preventing, diseases that may continue to affect us lifelong.

From: *Endocrinology: Basic and Clinical Principles* (P. M. Conn and S. Melmed, eds.), Humana Press Inc., Totowa, NJ.

In this chapter, we begin by reviewing the formation of the placenta, since it forms both the communication channel and barrier between mother and fetus. Next, we examine factors regulating production of steroid and peptide hormones by the placenta, and the variations in these that may reflect or dictate fetal growth and development *in utero*. Our understanding of the process of birth has been increased considerably through animal studies, particularly with species, such as sheep. In these animals, it is clear that the fetus provides the signals leading to birth, and expression of that signal may be altered in a hostile or compromised uterine environment. Collectively, these aspects allow us to understand the mechanisms of myometrial quiescence, activation, and contractility at birth.

2. ESTABLISHMENT OF PLACENTATION

2.1. Types of Placenta

Placental classification may be based on shape, the type of feto-maternal interdigitation, and the nature of the placental membrane or barrier. The latter describes the nature and number of cell layers that separate maternal and fetal vascular systems, and may also be referred to as the interhemal membrane. Placentation is called epitheliochorial, where invasion of the maternal endometrium by trophoblast has not occurred. Maternal and fetal blood are separated by six layers of cells. Three, fetal endothelium, chorionic connective tissue, and trophoblast epithelium, are of fetal origin, and three, maternal endometrial epithelium, endometrial connective tissue, and maternal capillary endothelium, are of maternal origin. This maximum barrier is progressively eroded by the invasiveness of the blastocyst. In syndesmochorial placentation, the endometrial epithelium is lost, but the remaining tissue layers are intact. Placentation of this type may occur in regions of the sheep and goat placenta, although most authors have characterized the placenta of these species as epitheliochorial. Direct contact between trophoblast epithelium with maternal capillary endothelium (i.e., four tissue layers to the interhemal membrane) is called endotheliochorial placentation, and is found in carnivores. When invasiveness progresses further so that maternal blood vessels are eroded, the trophoblast epithelium becomes bathed in maternal blood. This hemochorial placentation is found in rodents and higher primates, including humans.

2.2. Hemochorial Placentation

In women, the early blastocyst is divided into an inner cell mass or embryoblast and outer cell mass or trophoblast. Implantation is interstitial, and the trophoblast invades the uterine epithelium and underlying stroma. As it does so, the uninucleate cytotrophoblast cells form an inner cellular layer. These cells express adhesion molecules and growth factors, and are mitotically active. By fusion, cytotrophoblast gives rise to an outer layer that lacks cell boundaries and is called syncytiotrophoblast. The mass of syncytiotrophoblast increases at the implantation pole, and it expands further over the surface of the implanting blastocyst. Primary villi of blind ending syncytium are invaded by cytotrophoblast. With further proliferation, these give rise to villous trees, with anchoring villi maintaining contact to the outer tropho- blastic shell.

Thus, in the human placenta, the syncytiotrophoblast normally forms a relatively uninterrupted layer that extends over the surface of the villous tree and lines the intervillous space. The syncytiotrophoblast expresses key enzymes for steroid, peptide, and glycoprotein synthesis; the intervillous space becomes filled with maternal blood from basal spiral arterioles. Villous cytotrophoblast (Langhan's cells) are the generally undifferentiated stem cells that in early pregnancy form a layer beneath the syncytium. The numbers of Langhan's cells become depleted in the term placenta. Cytotrophoblast gives rise to syncytiotrophoblast by syncytial fusion, a process initiated by formation of gap junctions that bridge the intercellular gap between syncytium and cytotrophoblast cells. Cytotrophoblast proliferation and syncytial fusion are influenced by a number of factors, including oxygen tension and paracrine growth factors. The villous stroma is made up of a network of connective tissue, reticular cells, fibroblasts and macrophages (Hofbauer cells), and fetal capillaries. Polyhedral, mononuclear, or binuclear intermediate trophoblasts, identified by positive cytokeratin immunostaining, are abundant extravillous components of the placenta. Extravillous cytotrophoblast cells invade the decidua to reach the uterine vessels where they displace the maternal endothelium and vascular smooth muscle. Failure of this latter process appears to be associated with such conditions as pre-eclampsia.

The amniotic cavity and umbilical cord are lined with amnion. Over the surface of the placenta, amnion covers the underlying chorionic plate, through which traverse branches of the umbilical vessels before they dip down into the major divisions of the placenta, the cotyledons. In the membranes, amniotic epithelium sits on a layer of connective tissue (mesoderm) that is separated from chorionic mesoderm by an intermediate (spongy) layer. Recent studies have suggested a close paracrine relationship between mesenchymal cells in the amniotic mesoderm and amniotic epithelium. Chorionic mesoderm contains variable numbers of fibroblasts. It is separated by a basal lamina from the trophoblast layer of chorion. This layer, of variable thickness and containing multiple polygonal cells, has many of the differentiated properties of syncytiotrophoblast and of extravillous intermediate trophoblast cells. It produces steroids, peptides, and eicosanoids, and expresses enzymes for the synthesis and metabolism of these compounds. Atrophic villi are present throughout the chorionic trophoblast layer. This layer forms an irregular border with the underlying decidua.

2.3. Epitheliochorial Placentation

In such species as sheep, implantation is central. The trophoblast expands rapidly before implantation so as to come into contact with a large area of uterine lumenal epithelium. The ovine placenta is made up of about 100–130 separate placentomes. Each of these is made up of interdigitating maternal tissue (caruncle) and fetal tissue (cotyledon). Caruncles are recognized in the nonpregnant uterus as raised areas of endometrium, and their presence as prospective maternal attachment sites at implantation can be exploited experimentally by their removal prior to pregnancy (carunclectomy) to produce fetal growth restriction.

In the placentomes, the trophoblastic villous epithelium is in contact with the syncytial epithelium of the interdigitating maternal tissue. Cytotrophoblast cells may be mononuclear or binuclear. Several authors have reported that the maternal syncytium of the sheep is formed by fusion with trophoblast binucleate cells (placental lactogen-positive cells). Between the placentones, in the intercotyledonary areas, the chorion adheres to the endometrium apparently through the trophoblast brush border, but there are no chorionic villi formed.

3. STEROID HORMONES IN PREGNANCY

3.1. Progesterone

The effects of progesterone in maintaining uterine quiescence during pregnancy are well established in most species, except humans. In some animals, such as rabbit, rat, and goat, the primary source of progesterone during pregnancy is the corpus luteum; in others, it is the placenta. Maintenance of the corpus luteum for a critical period, even in animals with later placental progesterone synthesis, is essential for early pregnancy establishment and maintenance. This process, termed the maternal recognition of pregnancy by Roger Short in the 1960s, depends on the production of a luteotrophic substance, such as chorionic gonadotrophin in primates, or the antiluteolytic effect of the embryo in such species as sheep. Here, the trophoblast produces a Type I interferon (IFN), which depresses expression of endometrial oxytocin receptors, and increases expression of endometrial β2-microglobulin, MHC class I antigens, and other proteins. In nonpregnant sheep, luteal regression is associated with increased production of uterine prostaglandin $F_{2\alpha}$, in response to stimulation by luteal oxytocin. Downregulation of the uterine oxytocin receptor by IFN in early pregnancy prevents this, resulting in rescue of the corpus luteum.

3.1.1. HUMAN

In human pregnancy, the corpus luteum continues to produce small amounts of progesterone for the duration of pregnancy, but this capacity decreases after the sixth to seventh week. By this time, placental progesterone production is adequate to maintain gestation, the so-called luteo-placental shift. Thus, ovariectomy or regression of the corpus luteum in women leads to abortion only during the first 2 mo of pregnancy; there is no effect on pregnancy outcome of these procedures performed after the ninth week. The importance of progesterone in the establishment of human pregnancy is apparent from the abortifacient action of the progesterone receptor antagonist RU-486 administered during early pregnancy.

In human pregnancy, plasma progesterone concentrations rise progressively, reflecting increasing output from the placenta. Placental progesterone production depends mainly on the availability of LDL-associated cholesterol from the maternal circulation and adequate uteroplacental blood flow. Trophoblast tissues contain

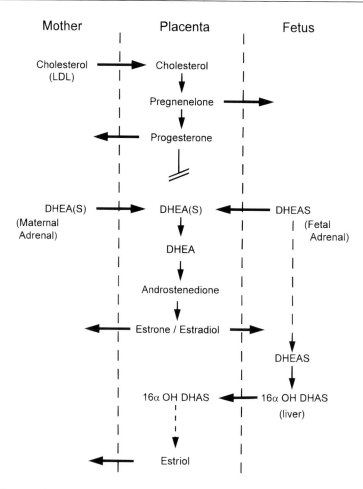

Fig. 1. Pathways of steroid production in mother, placenta, and fetus during human pregnancy.

LDL receptors. Uptake of LDL by syncytiotro-phoblast, numbers of LDL receptors, and levels of LDL receptor mRNA are all increased by estrogen. Pepe and Albrecht (1995) have shown in the baboon that trophoblast LDL receptor mRNA levels were approximately four fold higher in late than in midgestation. Placental LDL uptake was suppressed in animals treated with the antiestrogen MER-25, and in animals in which maternal estrogen concentrations were reduced after fetectomy. Conversely, in animals treated with androstenedione, the estrogen precursor, specific LDL uptake was restored.

After LDL is bound, it is internalized by active endocytosis. LDL becomes incorporated within lysosomes, and then broken down to amino acids and cholesterol esters. After hydrolysis, the cholesterol ester gives rise to cholesterol. In mitochondria, cholesterol is the substrate for the P_{450} side-chain cleavage ($P_{450\ SCC}$) enzyme to yield pregnenolone. In turn,

pregnenolone is substrate for the placental Type I 3β-hydroxysteroid dehydrogenase: Δ5-4 isomerase enzyme (3βHSD) to yield progesterone (Fig. 1).

Activity of $P_{450\ SCC}$ is also influenced by estrogen. Levels of mRNA for the primary transcript of $P_{450\ SCC}$ increase in syncytiotrophoblast from the baboon placenta in late gestation, and $P_{450\ SCC}$ activity is inhibited after treatment of baboons with antiestrogen. Type I 3βHSD immunoreactivity localizes by immunohistochemical staining to syncytiotrophoblast, extravillous cytotrophoblast in the placenta, and to chorionic trophoblast in human fetal membranes. Levels of mRNA for Type I 3βHSD are greater in placenta than in chorion-decidua, and levels in this tissue are greater than in amnion. However, there are no differences in 3βHSD mRNA levels in placental villous tissue or fetal membranes in association with labor at term or preterm in the absence of infection. Thus, alterations in the expression of this enzyme or levels of its activity do not occur in the placenta or membranes prior to the onset of labor in women.

In tissue culture, levels of type I 3βHSD increase with time as cytotrophoblast cells form a syncytium over 48–72 h. Output of progesterone by the cells, and levels of 3βHSD mRNA are increased by treatment with cyclic AMP agonists, insulin-like growth factor-1 (IGF-1), and with β-agonists. These effects appear to be at the level of transcription. 8-Bromo cAMP also increases mRNAs for $P_{450 \; SCC}$ and adrenodoxin in cultured trophoblast cells in vitro.

These data are consistent with progesterone output exerting an effect on myometrial activity, but whether this is via a systemic or paracrine action remains unclear. There is no good evidence for withdrawal of progesterone action on the human myometrium in late pregnancy. However, the recent possibility that progesterone actions may be inhibited by locally generated transforming growth factor-β (TGF-β) in intra-uterine tissues, or by competition for receptor-binding sites by reduced progestagen metabolites seems worthy of further exploration. Activity of 3βHSD is also inhibited by steroids, such as progesterone and 20α-dihydroprogesterone (20αdiHP). In addition, progesterone is interconverted to the inactive 20αdiHP by the enzyme 20αHSD, which is particularly active in amnion and chorion. At labor, conversion of progesterone to 20αdiHP in amnion increases, perhaps providing an additional mechanism for progesterone withdrawal.

The importance of progesterone in maintaining myometrial activity in pregnancy is well established in many species. Its effects are mediated through suppression of the spontaneous generation and propagation of action potentials. The myometrium under progesterone dominance is refractory to stimulation by oxytocin, prostaglandins, and an extrinsic electrical field. Myometrial excitability is increased after progesterone withdrawal, which in species other than higher primates appears to be a characteristic of the endocrine events surrounding parturition.

3.1.2. Sheep

Progesterone production during ovine pregnancy is primarily of placental origin after day 50 of gestation (term ~145 d). Maternal peripheral plasma progesterone concentrations increase progressively during late pregnancy, and then fall within 1–5 d of parturition at term. This fall in systemic progesterone can be provoked by the administration of ACTH or glucocorticoids to the fetus *in utero* (*see* Section 5.1.2.). In the ovine placenta, the 3βHSD enzyme is present in trophoblast mononuclear or binuclear cells. Detailed studies on the regulation of the activities of purified populations of these cells are still lacking.

The fall in placental progesterone output at term occurs in response to the rise in fetal cortisol that occurs prepartum (*see* Section 5.1.2.). In vitro incubation studies with sheep placental tissue have shown that glucocorticoids induce expression of $P_{450 \; c17}$ mRNA and activity. Thus, at term, C21 steroids are metabolized in the placenta to form C19 steroids, predominantly through the Δ5 pathway. In this way, they are diverted away from progesterone production. The metabolite 17α, 20αdiHP rises in systemic plasma concomitant with the fall in progesterone. Upregulation of $P_{450 \; C17}$ expression also generates more substrate for estrogen biosynthesis, leading to the concurrent rise in maternal plasma estradiol concentrations. The importance of progesterone withdrawal in mechanisms leading to labor in sheep is well established. Exogenous progesterone given in high amounts will block myometrial activity in late pregnant animals. More convincingly, the administration of the progesterone receptor antagonist RU486 or a 3βHSD inhibitor, such as trilostane or epostane, results in rapid evolution of uterine contractility and premature delivery.

3.1.3. Lower Primates

Ovariectomy can be performed in the rhesus monkey early in pregnancy without inducing abortion. Plasma concentrations of progesterone remain at about mid-luteal levels during the second half of gestation and then rise immediately prepartum. This latter effect is attributable to an increase in ovarian progesterone production at term. "Rejuvenation" of the corpus luteum at this time is owing to an increase in 3βHSD activity in the corpora lutea, rather than through alterations in $P_{450 \; SCC}$. The finding of similar maternal plasma progesterone levels in intact and ovariectomized monkeys in late pregnancy suggests the presence of some compensatory mechanism to placental progesterone production after ovariectomy. The role of systemic progesterone in the control of myometrium activity in the monkey is unclear, and as in the human, the evidence linking progesterone to myometrial quiescence through pregnancy is less than convincing.

3.2. Estrogens

3.2.1. HUMAN

Estrogen production in human pregnancy is dependent on the biochemical interdependence of anatomically distinct compartments, the fetus, the placenta, and maternal adrenal gland (Fig. 1). More specifically, the human placenta lacks $P_{450\ C17}$ activity, and is therefore unable to convert C21 steroids (such as progesterone) to C19 steroids (androgens). However, the placenta expresses abundant aromatase activity and is able to utilize C19 precursor steroids in the manufacture of estrogen. The fetal zone of the fetal adrenal gland, which occupies 85% of the fetal adrenal cortex, has a relative deficiency of Type II 3βHSD. Therefore, it secretes predominantly Δ5 rather than Δ4 steroids. Because of the high sulfotransferase activity in the fetal adrenal, these compounds, predominantly dehydroepiandrosterone (DHA) are secreted as sulfoconjugates (DHAS). Some of the fetal adrenal DHAS passes directly to the placenta, where it is ultimately converted to estrogen. Much of the fetal adrenal DHAS, however, passes to the fetal liver, where it is converted by a 16α hydroxylase enzyme to form 16α hydroxy-DHAS. This compound then passess to the placenta, where it is aromatized to form the 16-hydroxylated estrogen, estriol (Fig. 1). Maternal estrogen concentrations rise progressively through the course of pregnancy. Approximately 50% of maternal plasma estrone and estradiol is derived from fetal adrenal C19 precursor steroids, with the remaining component being derived from maternal adrenal C19 steroids. On the other hand, approx 90% of maternal estriol is derived from precursors originating through 16α hydroxylation in the fetal liver. It is important to note that the maternal adrenal production of DHA(S) increases during pregnancy, but this does not result in an increase in maternal plasma concentrations of these steroids. This is pertinent because the placenta utilizes progressively increasing amounts of DHAS from the maternal side in the synthesis of estrogen.

The human fetal adrenal gland is divided into an outer adult cortex that produces predominantly cortisol and an inner fetal zone that produces predominantly Δ5 steroids. In culture, these cells utilize LDL to derive cholesterol, and uptake of LDL by fetal adrenal cortical cells is promoted by ACTH treatment. Recent studies have shown that in vitro culture of fetal zone cells with ACTH results in increased ACTH receptor mRNA accumulation, as well as increases in mRNA for steroidogenic enzymes along the pathway to cortisol production. Thus regulation of adrenal function in the human fetus appears to be associated with mechanisms similar to those described in the ovine fetus (*see* Section 5.1.2.).

In the placenta, conversion of sulfoconjugated C19 steroids to estrogen requires activities of sulfatase, 3βHSD, aromatase, and 17βHSD enzymes. Using immunohistochemistry, these enzymes have been shown to be associated with the syncytiotrophoblast layer of the placental villi. Absence of sulfatase leads to inability of the placenta to utilize sulfoconjugated precursors from the fetus, and results in lowered estrogen concentrations in the mother. Although patients with placental sulfatase deficiency may progress to term, the development of uterine activity at labor is impaired.

Placental Type I 3βHSD, which catalyzes conversion of Δ5 to Δ4 steroids, is associated with both mitochondrial and microsomal fractions. Regulation of this enzyme by cyclic AMP (cAMP) and IGF was discussed above. Since trophoblast cells express abundant IGF-1 and IGF-2, their effects on 3βHSD expression may be through similar mechanisms. Recent studies have characterized the $P_{450\ arom}$, and shown that this belongs to a functionally related multigene family. $P_{450\ arom}$ is upregulated by cAMP and by activators of the protein kinase C pathway.

Thus, output of estrogens by the placenta depends on availability of precursors from the maternal and fetal compartments, and from activities of placental enzymes, including placental sulfatase. In conditions of anencephaly and fetal adrenal hypoplasia, there are reduced concentrations of estrogen in maternal plasma. Similarly, administration of synthetic glucocorticoids into the maternal compartment leads to suppression of fetal hypothalamic-pituitary-adrenal (HPA) function, after transplacental passage. Since the supply of fetal adrenal precursors falls, maternal estrogen concentrations are reduced. This is particularly marked for estriol. Endogenous glucocorticoids appear also to influence the activity of fetal HPA function. During the third trimester of pregnancy, maternal estriol concentrations are highest between 2200 and 0400 h, at the time when the endogenous rhythm of maternal cortisol concentration is at its nadir. As maternal cortisol concentrations increase during the morning hours, so maternal estriol concentrations decrease. Interpretation of these results suggested that at physiologic concentrations, maternal cortisol can cross the human placenta during the latter third of gestation into the fetus and exert some negative-feedback action at the level of the fetal hypothalamus and pituitary. This results in decreased fetal pituitary secretion of ACTH, diminished drive to the fetal adrenal, and a reduction in the secretion from the fetal adrenal of C19 precursor steroids for 16 hydroxylation in the fetal liver, and subsequent aromatization in the placenta.

Estrogens are also produced within the fetal membranes, although here aromatase activity is limited, and the major precursor is estrone sulfate. Estrone sulfatase activity is present in amnion, chorion, and decidua, and is greatest in choriodecidual tissue. In intact cells and in subcellular fractions, the conversion of estrone sulfate to estrone was greater in tissue collected from patients after spontaneous labor than in tissue from patients at elective cesarean section at term. The rise in maximum velocity (V_{max}) of the enzyme was associated with a decrease in its K_d for estrone sulfate substrate. In contrast, there was no change in V_{max} or K_d for DHAS conversion to DHA with labor. Estrone sulfate was also converted to E_2, thereby demonstrating the presence of 17βHSD activity in chorio-decidua. These studies raise the intriguing possibility that local production of estrogen from sulfoconjugated precursors may increase in patients at the time of labor. Preliminary studies suggested that a similar change occurred in patients in preterm labor in the absence of infection. Immunohistochemistry has been used to localize the estrone sulfatase enzyme to the trophoblast cells of the chorion, and studies are now required on the regulation of this enzyme in extravillous trophoblasts.

3.2.2. SHEEP

In sheep, the concentration of unconjugated estrogens in maternal plasma is low during most of the pregnancy and rises significantly only during the final 24 h before spontaneous parturition. This increase follows a rise in the concentration of estrone sulfate (E_1S) in maternal plasma and of estrogen sulfates in fetal plasma. Unconjugated E_1 and E_2 also rise in amniotic fluid during the last 3–6 d of pregnancy. Because similar increases in maternal and fetal estrogen levels occur in sheep induced to deliver prematurely by the administration of dexamethasone to the fetus, even after fetal adrenalectomy, it has been argued that the fetal adrenals do not provide the

precursors for placental aromatization. Although it is clear that the prepartum rise in maternal estrogen concentrations can occur in the absence of, or during suppression of, fetal adrenal function, these findings do not preclude a role for an activated fetal adrenal at term pregnancy in providing C19 estrogen precursor steroids. It has been established that incubation of sheep fetal adrenal tissue with placental tissue produces more estrogen than from placental tissue alone. Concentrations of androstenedione and testosterone rise in fetal sheep plasma before parturition, and androstenedione infused into the circulation of the chronically catheterized fetal sheep is converted into estrogen, measurable in the fetal and maternal circulation. Indeed, it has been estimated that up to 30% of maternal estrogens at term might be formed in the placenta from fetal adrenal precursors.

At present, however, it is believed that the main source of estrogen production at term, and the site of action for the prepartum rise of fetal cortisol, is the placenta. Several studies have shown that fetal cortisol increases placental $P_{450\,C17}$ gene expression and activity. Thus, as discussed earlier, at term, the sheep placenta, under the influence of fetal cortisol, has the potential to convert C27 steroid (cholesterol) through to estrogen. This step provides a key link allowing maternal expression of endocrine events that have been initiated in the fetus. Fetal membranes of the sheep also produce estrogens from conjugated precursors. It is possible that this steroid may have local bioactivity, but this suggestion has not been explored experimentally at the present time.

3.2.3. RHESUS MONKEY

In the rhesus monkey, the maternal plasma concentrations of estrogen are much lower than in higher primates, but increase progressively during the last month of gestation to reach highest values at the time of parturition. This rise corresponds to a progressive increase in concentrations of DHAS in the fetal circulation, which presumably reflects increased activation of fetal adrenal function. Maternal estradiol concentrations fall after fetal death, fetectomy, or administration of dexamethasone to the mother or fetus. All these observations therefore suggest that estrogens in the maternal plasma of the monkey are of fetal placental origin as in human gestation. Peter Nathanielsz and colleagues have shown that infusion of androstenedione to monkeys during late gestation results in increases of maternal plasma estrogen concentrations, labor-like uterine contractions, and premature delivery (Guissani et al., 1996). Previously, this group had shown that birth in the monkey was heralded by 24-h patterns of uterine contractility, with maximum activity overnight. In monkeys treated with constant androstenedione infusion, the magnitude of the overnight increase in myometrial contractility was greater at an earlier time in pregnancy than in saline control animals.

These studies provide compelling information linking fetal-placental estrogen production to the onset of parturition in primates. As discussed below, the mechanism of estrogen action is likely brought about through increased expression of a cassette of responsive genes within myometrial tissue and in decidua. During pregnancy, estrogen is also responsible for the increases in uterine blood flow that provide the substrate and metabolic demands of the growing uterus and fetus. In primates, estrogen stimulates production of the high-affinity binding protein for cortisol, corticosteroid-binding globulin (CBG), from the maternal liver, and this may be important in regulating the delivery of glucocorticoids to uterine target tissues, as well as affecting glucocorticoid negative feedback. Other effects of fetoplacental steroid hormones in primate gestation are discussed at length in the elegant review by Pepe and Albrecht (1995).

3.3. Corticosteroids

3.3.1. HUMAN

Mean concentrations of cortisol in maternal peripheral plasma rise progressively through human pregnancy. The normal diurnal pattern of cortisol concentration change is maintained, and the rise in concentration appears attributable to a progressive increase in levels of CBG. As discussed above, maternal corticosteroids may have important effects on the level of activity of the hypothalamic–pituitary–adrenal (HPA) axis in the fetus. However, recent studies have shown that the action of maternal cortisol on fetal HPA function is modified through the activity of the enzyme 11βHSD in the placenta. In late gestation, the human placenta contains predominantly Type 2 11βHSD activity. This converts cortisol to its biologically inactive metabolite cortisone. By Northern blotting, levels of Type 2 11βHSD mRNA in placenta far exceed those of other intrauterine tissues, and reach amounts found only in kidney.

In this issue, activity of 11βHSD-2 is thought to protect mineralocorticoid receptors from high circulating cortisol concentrations, by converting cortisol to the inactive cortisone. In placenta, 11βHSD-2 localizes predominantly to syncytiotrophoblast. The bidirectional 11βHSD-1 enzyme, which operates at a much lower $(\mu M)K_m$ for cortisol-to-cortisone conversion is absent from syncytiotrophoblast. It is however present in fetal membranes, including amnion and chorionic trophoblast, and in endothelial cells of fetal blood vessels in the placenta.

Recent studies have suggested a direct correlation between levels of placental Type 2 11βHSD and fetal weight. The thesis has been advanced that placental 11βHSD-2 protects the fetus from adverse effects of high maternal cortisol concentrations. In pregnancies where the enzyme activity is diminished, excessive maternal cortisol crosses to the fetus and contributes to growth restriction, perhaps through suppression of IGF-2 expression in susceptible fetal tissues. This paradigm has been reproduced experimentally in rats.

The regulation of placental 11βHSD-2 has been studied in vivo by Pepe and Albrecht (1995) in the baboon. In this species, at midgestation, placental 11βHSD activity favors formation of cortisol. It is likely that maternal cortisol crossing the placenta exerts relative negative-feedback action on the fetal HPA axis, and prevents precocious stimulation of fetal adrenal function. In late gestation, under the influence of estrogen, 11βHSD-2 activity in the baboon placenta is increased. Maternal cortisol is now metabolized to biologically inactive cortisone. In this way, the maternal inhibition on fetal HPA function is removed, and the fetal pituitary begins to secrete increasing amounts of ACTH. In turn, ACTH increases secretion from the fetal adrenal of C19 estrogen precursor steroids, resulting in a further increase in estrogen output from the placenta.

During human pregnancy, there is also an increase in concentrations of deoxycorticosterone (DOC) in maternal plasma. DOC is potent mineralocorticoid. Its increased levels result from the conversion of plasma progesterone to DOC in the kidney through increased activity of renal 21-hydroxylase. This enzyme also appears to be stimulated by rising concentrations of estrogen. Previously it had been postulated that elevated concentrations of maternal DOC might play a role in pre-eclampsia. However, plasma DOC levels are not further elevated in such patients.

4. PROTEIN HORMONES

4.1. Placental Interactions

The human placenta produces a wide variety of peptide and glycoprotein hormones. In addition to human chorionic gonadotrophin (hCG) and placental lactogen (hPL), the placenta synthesizes a wide variety of cytokines, neuromodulators, and growth factors. These may act in an autocrine, paracrine, or endocrine fashion. Interestingly, placental peptide and glycoproteins appear in part to replicate production of analogous hormones from the hypothalamus and pituitary. Thus, it has been suggested that local feedback control mechanisms, analogous to those between the hypothalamus and pituitary, may exist between cell types within the placenta. For example, gonadotrophin-releasing hormone (GnRH) produced from cytotrophoblast may stimulate output of chorionic gonadotrophin (analogous to LH) from syncytiotrophoblast. Similarly, the placenta synthesizes increasing amounts of corticotropin-releasing hormone (CRH) during late gestation. This affects expression of proopiomelanocortin (POMC) and output of POMC-derived peptides (*see* Section 5.1.2.). It is beyond the scope of this chapter to cover all of these peptides in detail. In this section, we discuss briefly the role of chorionic gonadotrophin and of CRH. Placental neurohormones and cytokines are discussed later in relation to the onset of parturition.

4.2. hCG

hCG is a glycoprotein consisting of a 92 amino acid α subunit noncovalently bonded to a 145 amino acid β subunit. There is a single gene for the α subunit. The gene for βhCG is contained within a cluster of 7 hCG-β-like genes on chromosome 19. hCG is produced by syncytiotrophoblast and secreted into the intervillous space. Concentrations rise rapidly immediately following implantation to reach peak values by about the ninth week of gestation. Values then decline toward the end of pregnancy.

Trophoblast secretes not only intact hCG, but also uncombined α and β subunits. Other forms of hCG, including a low-mol-wt form of the β subunit called β-core fragment are also present during pregnancy. The hCGβ core fragment is unable to combine with α subunit and is therefore devoid of biological activity.

In tissue culture, hCG output is stimulated by cyclic AMP, which increases mRNA levels for both α and β subunits. Production of hCG is also stimulated by pla-cental GnRH in a dose-dependent fashion, and GnRH receptors have been isolated on syncytiotrophoblast membranes. In addition, peptides, such as inhibin, appear to suppress hCG output, whereas others, such as activin, augment GnRH-induced hCG output.

As discussed earlier, the production of hCG in early human pregnancy is critical for rescue of the corpus luteum of pregnancy. hCG also stimulates testosterone production from the fetal testes and steroid output from the fetal adrenal gland. The biochemistry of hCG synthesis and control of its secretion are discussed in detail in the excellent chapter by Ogren and Talamantes (1994).

4.3. CRH

The concentrations of CRH in maternal peripheral blood rise during the third trimester of normal pregnancy. This increase correlates with an increase in the content of CRH and prepro-CRH mRNA in the placenta. From the umbilical vein–umbilical artery concentration differences, it is clear that the placenta is a major source of CRH output in human pregnancy. In the placenta, CRH has been localized to the syncytiotrophoblast. In the membranes, it is present in the amniotic epithelium, extravillous trophoblast, and decidual stromal tissue. The rise in maternal plasma CRH concentrations in normal pregnancy may be associated with an increase in the concentration of a circulating CRH-binding protein (CRH-BP). This is thought to antagonize the biological effects of CRH at the level of the maternal pituitary gland (Petraglia et al., 1996). Maternal CRH concentrations are elevated in preterm labor in the absence of an infective process. Longitudinal studies have shown that the concentrations of CRH-BP in maternal plasma decrease at this time, so that concentrations of unbound CRH are presumably markedly elevated. CRH output and CRH mRNA levels in placental tissue are increased by glucocorticoids and decreased by progesterone. Hypoxemia does not affect placental CRH output directly in vitro. However, in vivo, hypoxemia that is known to activate fetal HPA function may well stimulate placental CRH output indirectly. This happens because hypoxia provokes ACTH release from the fetal pituitary, which in turn drives fetal adrenal cortisol output. We have suggested elsewhere that in response to stresses, such as hypoxemia, the human infant, particularly when at risk of growth restriction, activates HPA function in a manner that might lead to increased CRH output from the placenta. In the placenta, CRH is a vasodilator. Its effects may be modulated by nitric oxide. If the hypoxic stimulus to CRH production is sustained, then a second level of interactions may ensue, leading to premature delivery. CRH stimulates output from placental and decidual tissue of prostaglandins. CRH acts in synergy with prostaglandins and oxytocin to promote myometrial contractility. In turn, these substances, and others including catecholamines, vasopressin, and neuropeptide Y, induce further CRH synthesis and release. Thus, increased production and action of CRH may have an important role to play in the etiology of preterm labor in the absence of infection.

A recent study has shown that maternal peripheral plasma CRH concentrations are elevated early in pregnancy in those patients destined to deliver prematurely. Interestingly, maternal peripheral plasma CRH concentrations were lower in patients that went on to deliver post dates. Because these changes were detectable during the second trimester of gestation, the study, if substantiated, suggests that mechanisms leading to premature delivery may be activated much earlier than had been previously assumed.

5. PARTURITION

5.1. Role of the Fetus

5.1.1. Human

In 1933, Malpas concluded from a study of the relationship between gestation length and fetal anomalies, such as anencephaly, that the fetus "especially the fetal pituitary and adrenal glands was responsible for the trigger to the neuromuscular expulsive mechanisms that led to the onset of labor." Although later studies, especially in such species as sheep have provided strong support for the proposal of Malpas, definitive evidence for a role of the human fetus in controlling gestational length remains elusive. Later workers reported in a larger series of patients that the mean length of pregnancy in anencephaly was not significantly different from pregnancies with normal fetuses, although the variability around that mean gestational length was much greater. This distribution is similar to that reported subsequently after experimental anencephaly in the monkey. Studies such as these led to the conclusion that the human fetus plays a role in the fine-tuning of gestational length, rather than providing the trigger mechanism, as in the sheep. (*see* Challis and Lye, 1994).

Later studies clearly showed that there was activation of the HPA axis in the human fetus in late gestation, and these observations have been supported by more recent measurements in subhuman primates. CRH and arginine vasopressin (AVP)-like immunoreactivities are present in human fetal hypothalamic tissue by the first week of gestation. The immunoreactivity present as CRH separated into CRH 1–41 and a large-mol-wt compound on gel chromatography. This material stimulated ACTH release by dispersed anterior pituitary cells. In the baboon, Albrecht and Pepe (1995) have shown clearly that POMC mRNA is expressed in the fetal pituitary, at least by mid gestation, and that the levels of POMC mRNA increase near term, as in the ovine species.

ACTH appears to be the predominant steroidogenic stimulus to the human fetal adrenal gland. Effects of ACTH are mediated through increased uptake of LDL and increased expression of a cassette of responsive genes. TGF-β also influences human fetal adrenal steroidogenesis by inhibiting the binding and use of LDL, and it seems that steroidogenic expression by the gland is dependent on a balance between these different endocrine/paracrine influences. There is substantial evidence for increased glucocorticoid output by the primate fetal adrenal during late gestation. However, as mentioned previously, the likely role of the human and subhuman primate fetal adrenal in the initiation of parturition is through provision of C19 estrogen precursors, such as DHA or DHAS.

5.1.2. Sheep

Our understanding of the role of the fetus in the initiation of parturition stems from pioneering studies of Mont Liggins in the middle 1960s. In this species, fetal hypophysectomy or adrenalectomy results in prolongation of gestation, whereas infusion of ACTH or glucocorticoids into the fetus provokes early delivery. Evidence that the sheep fetus initiated the onset of parturition through activation of HPA function was provided by the seminal observation of Bassett and Thorburn in 1969 of a progressive increase in the concentration of cortisol in the plasma of the fetal lamb during the last 15–20 d of pregnancy. Subsequently, many groups have examined in detail the cellular and molecular mechanisms responsible for activation of fetal HPA function in the sheep (Fig. 2).

In this species, it is now clear that there are increased levels of mRNAs for CRH and AVP in the

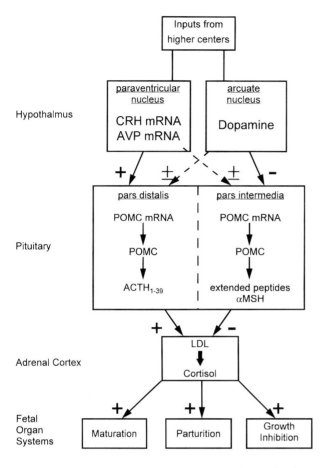

Fetal
Organ
Systems

Fig. 2. Summary of factors leading to maturation and activation of hypothalamic–pituitary–adrenal (HPA) function in the sheep fetus during late gestation. CRH, corticotrophin-releasing hormone; AVP, arginine vasopressin, POMC, proopiomelanocortin.

form of the enzyme. In vitro studies suggest greater conversion of cortisol to cortisone in pituitary tissue from term animals, thereby providing a mechanism by which bioactive cortisol may be inactivated in the pituitary and negative-feedback inhibition averted. Second, CBG rises in the plasma of the late gestation fetus. By RT-PCR, CBG expression has also been identified in fetal pituitary tissue. We have provided evidence that CBG binds cortisol and prevents it from exerting negative feedback on basal and CRH-stimulated ACTH release by pituitary cells in vitro. It is now clear that there are changes in posttranslational processing of POMC in fetal pituitary cells in late pregnancy. Currently, there is no information available on expression or activity of the prohormone convertase enzymes. However, histologically, the distribution of corticotrophs in the fetal pituitary changes during late gestation and after glucocorticoid treatment to a cell type that appears to secrete more bioactive ACTH 1–39. The pars intermedia of the fetal pituitary expresses much greater amounts of POMC mRNA than the pars distalis, but appears to process this to α-MSH and to large-mol-wt ACTH-related peptides. These may be present as circulating antagonists of ACTH action (Fig. 2). A change in the ratio of these compounds to bioactive ACTH 1–39 immediately before parturition has been suggested as a mechanism for increasing the drive to fetal adrenal maturation.

The rise in plasma cortisol of the late gestation ovine fetus is associated not only with an increase in trophic drive to the gland, but also with an increase in responsiveness of the gland to ACTH stimulation. As in the human fetal adrenal, responsiveness can be provoked by administration of ACTH to the fetus or addition of ACTH to ovine adrenocortical cells. The mechanism appears to involve upregulation of ACTH receptor mRNA and ACTH receptor number. In turn, there is increased expression of most of the enzymes on the biosynthetic pathway to cortisol production. In particular, $P_{450\,C17}$ mRNA, protein levels, and activity are increased, thereby ensuring metabolism of C21 steroids through the 17-hydroxy pathway leading to cortisol. The increase in $P_{450\,C17}$ expression is somewhat greater than for enzymes, such as Type 2 3βHSD, which appears to be distributed throughout the cortex of the fetal adrenal for much of pregnancy. Several investigators have shown that cortisol itself may participate in the change in adrenal responsiveness through local feed-

hypothalamus during late gestation. There are increases in POMC mRNA in the fetal pituitary over the same time period. The finding that CRH stimulates increased levels of POMC mRNA in late gestation fetal pituitary cells maintained in culture, and also stimulated ACTH output, indicated clearly the importance of CRH in the activation of this axis. During late pregnancy in the fetal lamb, rises in plasma cortisol occur in parallel with an increase in fetal plasma ACTH concentrations. This apparent override of the negative-feedback effects of glucocorticoids may be attributable to a number of factors. First, 11βHSD mRNA and activity in the fetal pituitary increase in late gestation and appear to be accounted for primarily by the Type I bidirectional back on fetal adrenal cortical cells and modulation of ACTH-induced activation of fetal adrenal function. This action does not appear to be at the level of expression or activity of steroidogenic enzymes, but rather is an influence on ACTH receptor coupling through G_s and adenylate cyclase activity.

ACTH also stimulates fetal adrenal blood flow, and this is an additional important factor, particularly as an adaptive response to stress in utero. Hypoxemia is known to increase HPA function, and leads to elevated fetal plasma ACTH and cortisol concentrations. During hypoxemia, fetal adrenal blood flow rises. The increase in blood flow to the fetal adrenal cortex, but not to the medulla was suppressed by concurrent glucocorticoid administration. This suggested that ACTH, release of which was inhibited by the concurrent glucocorticoid, promoted adrenal cortical blood flow, but that medullary blood flow responses were independent of ACTH action. Short-term hypoxemia also increased levels of CRH mRNA in the paraventricular nucleus of the hypothalamus, and POMC mRNA in the fetal pituitary. We have suggested (*see* Section 5.1.1.) that this response may contribute to the fetal escape from a compromised intrauterine environment.

5.2. Prostaglandins

In sheep, the rise in fetal cortisol leads to a decrease in progesterone output from the placenta, and a concurrent increase in estrogen secretion. The steroid changes are associated temporally with an increase in uteroplacental production of prostaglandin F2α ($PGF_2\alpha$). Recent studies using *in situ* hybridization showed that elevated prostaglandin output occurs in response to upregulation of cyclooxygenase Type 2 (the inducible form of cyclooxygenase) in the trophoblast component of the placentome at term. The cellular mediators of this response are not known, but likely involve the action of products of early response genes such as c-*fos*, or cytokines, such as interleukin-1β (*see* Section 5.3.).

The role of increased production of prostaglandins as stimulators of myometrial activity at the time of parturition is widely accepted. Prostaglandin concentrations in amniotic fluid and maternal plasma, and prostaglandin metabolite levels in maternal urine increase in association with labor. Administration of prostaglandin synthase (cyclooxygenase) inhibitors suppresses myometrial activity in women and in animal models. Further, the stimulatory effects of

prostaglandins on the myometrium, particularly in primates, is well established.

Although the placenta appears to be the major site of prostaglandin production in the sheep before parturition, the situation in the human is quite different. Here, prostaglandin synthesis and metabolism are discretely compartmentalized within the pregnant uterus. Amnion is a major site of prostaglandin synthesis, particularly of PGE2, and this activity increases at the time of term labor. Production of PGE2 by amnion presumably accounts, to a large extent, for the increase in PGE2 concentrations of human amniotic fluid that correlates with progressive dilatation of the cervix during labor. Chorion contains prostaglandin synthase and 15-hydroxy prostaglandin dehydrogenase (PGDH) activity (Fig. 3). Through much of pregnancy, PGDH activity predominates in chorion. Thus, in women, chorion may be regarded as a barrier preventing the passage of prostaglandin synthesized in the membranes from reaching decidua and myometrium. As discussed later, a deficiency in this PGDH activity may be causal to preterm labor in a substantial subset of patients, even in the absence of infection. Decidual tissue contains predominately prostaglandin synthase activity, and forms both PGE2 and PGF2α. It is currently believed that decidual activation, through mechanisms discussed below, leads to increased production of PGE2 and PGF2α at term, and this provides the major paracrine stimulus to myometrial contractility. For much of pregnancy, the myometrium produces predominantly PGI2, an inhibitory eicosanoid. At the time of parturition, the effects of PGI2 may be opposed, and overcome, by increased amounts of stimulatory uterotonins, including PGE2 and PGF2α.

Regulation of prostaglandin production may occur at different points along the biosynthetic and metabolic pathways. Arachidonic acid, the obligate precursor for prostaglandins, is formed from membrane glycerophospholipids. It is liberated through the activities of phospholipases C and A_2. This step has often been regarded as rate-limiting to prostaglandin formation. Phospholipase C exists as a number of isozymes, distributed throughout amnion, chorionic trophoblasts, and decidual stromal cells. The major form of phospholipase A_2 (PLA_2) most likely involved in prostaglandin production at parturition is the 85–110 kDa cytoplasmic isozyme. $cPLA_2$ activity increases gradually in intrauterine tissue throughout human pregnancy. mRNA for Type 2

PG metabolism at term and pre-term

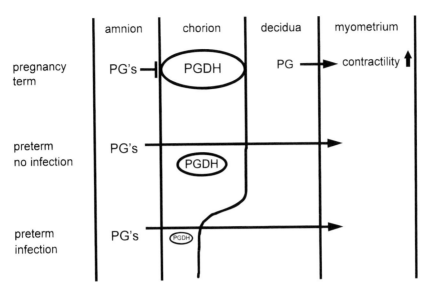

Fig. 3. Diagram to show how changes in the activity of PGDH in human chorion at term pregnancy, and preterm delivery in the absence or presence of infection affect the passage of prostaglandins derived from amnion (or chorion) to the decidua and myometrium. Note that in term pregnancy, the presence of the PGDH barrier in chorion implies the necessity of prostaglandin production through decidual or myometrial activation, whereas in preterm delivery, prostaglandins reaching myometrium could also originate from amnion and/or chorion.

PLA_2 (14 kDa, secretory PLA_2, $sPLA_2$) increases in placental tissue at the time of labor, although there are no changes in the mRNA levels of this enzyme in choriodecidual tissue. Recent studies with cultured amnion cells have shown that $sPLA_2$ activity and mRNA are increased in a dose- and time-dependent fashion by cytokines, at the same time as increases in prostaglandin synthase (PGHS)-2 mRNA.

Primary prostaglandins are formed from arachidonic acid through the activity of PGHS enzyme, which has both cyclooxygenase and peroxidase activities. There are constitutive (Type 1) and inducible (Type 2) forms of PGHS. These are different gene products. PHGS-2 increases in response to stimulation by cytokines, growth factors, and phorbol esters; it is inhibited by glucocorticoids. Both PGHS-1 mRNA and PGHS-2 mRNA have been measured in amnion, chorion, and decidual tissue using RT-PCR. Although initially no major differences were described in these mRNA levels between tissues obtained before or after labor, later studies have demonstrated increased levels of expression, protein, and activity of PGHS-2 in amnion and choriodecidual tissue obtained from patients after labor.

Arachidonic acid may also be metabolized through the lipoxygenase pathway to form leukotrienes and hydroxyeicosatetranoeic acids (HETEs). These compounds are weak uterotonins in in vitro assays. However, in amnion cells, the ratio of cyclooxygenase products formed from arachidonic acid compared to lipoxygenase products increases at the time of labor, suggesting differential regulation of arachidonic metabolism toward more potent eicosanoids.

Prostaglandin output from amnion or decidual tissue maintained in vitro is influenced through activators of protein kinase A, protein kinase C, or through tyrosine kinase-linked receptors. Prostaglandin output in vitro increases in response to platelet-activating factor (PAF), epidermal growth factor (EGF), and cytokines, such as interleukin-1 (IL-1), IL-6, and TNF. The bacterial endotoxin lipopolysaccharide (LPS) also stimulates prostaglandin output by cultured amnion and decidual cells, but this action may be mediated through cytokines. Early studies showed that prostaglandin production was inhibited by various agents, including members of the annexin family. Removal of these inhibitory influences, and decreased levels of annexin-1 mRNA in amnion at parturition may allow increased phospholipase activity and an increased supply of substrate for prostaglandin biosynthesis.

5.3. Preterm Labor

Preterm labor (birth before 37 wk of completed gestation) in women occurs in association with an underlying infective process in about 30% of cases. Ascending infection may lead directly to release of phospholipases from the bacterial organisms or to stimulation by LPS of cytokines from cell types, such as macrophages in decidua and in amnion mesoderm. In turn, these cytokines stimulate release of prostaglandins from decidual stromal cells and from amniotic epithelial cells. Recent studies have suggested that chorion is a more potent source of IL-6 and IL-8 than either amnion or decidua. Output of these cytokines is stimulated by IL-1β and TNF. The effect is at a transcriptional level, and is associated with concentration-dependent increases in levels of IL-6 and IL-8 mRNA.

We referred earlier to the possibility of increased placental production of CRH as a mediator leading to preterm delivery. We proposed that the fetus responds to a hypoxic intrauterine environment with HPA activation, and that fetal adrenal cortisol upregulates CRH expression in the placenta. CRH stimulates prostaglandin output and synergizes with prostaglandins to stimulate myometrial activity.

Other recent studies have shown that a significant portion of patients in preterm labor have a relative deficiency of the prostaglandin-metabolising enzyme PGDH (Fig. 3) in chorionic trophoblasts. This enzyme normally serves as a metabolic barrier, preventing passage of primary prostaglandins from amnion and chorion to decidua and myometrium. In its absence, prostaglandin synthesized from these sources, in response to any stimulus, can access the decidual and myometrial tissue, and promote contractility. Mean levels of PGDH mRNA were lower in patients in preterm delivery without infection. PGDH mRNA and activity were lower still in patients in preterm labor with an underlying infective process. Subsequently, it was found that during infection, leukocyte infiltration of the chorion is associated with loss of trophoblast cells, and hence loss of PGDH activity. Thus, with infection, prostaglandin synthesis is increased, and prostaglandin metabolism is reduced, resulting in a rapid increase of biologically active prostaglandin.

Recently, Claudia van Meir and colleagues (1996) have examined the regional distribution of PGDH within the fetal membranes of the pregnant uterus. They found that the activity of this enzyme was lower in chorion overlying the internal os of the cervix than in other areas of the uterus, in patients at cesarean section in labor. It was speculated that the differential loss of activity from this region could allow PGE-2 generated in amnion to act on the cervix and promote cervical dilatation. There is good evidence that PGDH activity is normally maintained by progesterone. This suggests a possible strategy by which administration of a progesterone receptor antagonist placed in the cervix could be used to enhance cervical ripening in the patient with a low Bishop's score alone or more likely as a supplement to intracervical PGE2 gel.

6. PATTERNS OF UTERINE ACTIVITY THROUGHOUT PREGNANCY

Uterine activity is relatively quiescent through much of pregnancy. Inhibition is maintained through the actions of progesterone, prostacyclin, the polypeptide hormone, relaxin, nitric oxide, and parathyroid hormone related peptide (PTHrP) (Fig. 4).

The human genome contains two relaxin genes, H1 and H2, which code for polypeptides significantly different in amino acid sequence. The full spectrum of biologic activities of these peptides has not been examined, but transcription appears to be limited to the H2 relaxin gene in the human corpus luteum, the classic site of relaxin synthesis. However, it is now apparent that relaxin is synthesized in a number of other sites, including the decidua, fetal membranes, and trophoblast, in human gestation. During human pregnancy, the highest plasma concentrations of relaxin are found during the first trimester, but the peptide is detectable in the circulation throughout pregnancy. The highest tissue levels of relaxin mRNA, relaxin C-peptide (a component of preprorelaxin) and mature relaxin peptide are found within decidua at term. Levels decrease rapidly after birth. The levels of relaxin mRNA are lower in decidual tissue collected after labor, compared with elective cesarean section at term, suggesting that there may be withdrawal of relaxin synthesis in association with the labor process. Processing of relaxin is effected through the prohormone convertase-1, an endopeptidase that cleaves the relaxin pro-

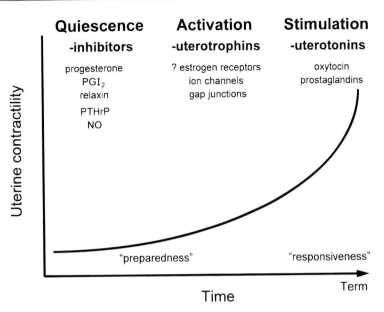

Fig. 4. Diagram to show how changes in uterine contractility through pregnancy may be influenced by factors promoting uterine quiescence, activation, or stimulation.

hormone at specific pairs of basic amino acids, to produce the mature two-chain disulfide-linked active species. Little is known about regulation of PC-1 expression and patterns of relaxin processing in human decidua.

Nitric oxide relaxes vascular smooth muscle as well as uterine smooth muscle. Decreased nitric oxide synthesis within the uterus has been found near labor in rats and rabbits. This may represent an additional component of withdrawal of a block placed on myometrial activity through gestation. However, inhibition of nitric oxide synthesis in the rat was without effect on the timing of labor.

An additional inhibitor of uterine contractions is PTHrP, an oncofetal protein. PTHrP mRNA abundance is greater in amnion than in other intrauterine tissues, and expression decreases with rupture of the membranes at term. PTHrP concentrations in amniotic fluid have been reported as significantly lower in patients at preterm labor, and this interesting possibility requires substantiation.

In preparation for parturition, the myometrium comes under the influence of a group of compounds collectively called uterotrophins. Among these estrogen is likely a major component. Steve Lye, at the University of Toronto (*see* Challis and Lye, 1994), has suggested that in the prelabor period, uterotrophins activate a cassette of regulatory genes. These include

oxytocin, oxytocin receptor, prostaglandin receptors, and connexin-43. Studies in the rat have shown clearly that connexin-43 mRNA increases in myometrium within the last 24–36 h of pregnancy. The expression of this gene is increased by treatment of animals with estrogen or after administration of a progesterone antagonist. Connexin-43 expression is inhibited in animals treated with progesterone. The expression of connexins is crucial to the optimum functioning of the myometrium during labor and its ability to develop well coordinated synchronous contractions. The cell-to-cell coupling required for these contractions is brought about through formation of gap junctions from structural entities linking adjacent cells and made up of connexins. The mechanisms that regulate the opening and closing of gap junctions in the myometrium are not well understood. Calcium ionophores and cAMP reduce cell coupling, whereas they have opposing effects on uterine contractile activity. In addition to these changes, the myometrium expresses a variety of ion-specific channels within the cell membrane, which act to regulate the excitability of the smooth muscle. These include voltage-gated sodium channels and calcium channels, which may be voltage-dependent or receptor-operated.

The final phase of uterine activity is stimulation, in which uterotonins, including prostaglandins and oxytocin, cause contraction of the activated uterus in which responsiveness has been ensured. The factors regulating prostaglandin production have been discussed above. Recent studies have suggested that at term, and perhaps preterm labor, oxytocin may be secreted not only from the posterior pituitary, but also from decidual tissue itself. In monkeys, oxytocin concentrations have a circadian rhythm in maternal plasma that correlates with changes in myometrial contractility. In the rat and human, oxytocin mRNA is present in decidua and endometrium, and there is increased oxytocin mRNA expression in decidual tissue taken from women in spontaneous labor compared to term elective cesarean section in the absence of labor. Estrogen increases oxytocin expression in decidual explants maintained in culture. Thus, the action of estrogen as a uterotrophin may be to increase further the production of potential uterotonins for myometrial contractility.

The endocrine/paracrine events of parturition affect not only myometrium, but also cervix. The cervix is made up of smooth muscle, collagen, and elastin. At term, degradation of collagen occurs through collagenase activity. Elastase, located in the granules of polymorphonuclear leukocytes, may be more associated with collagen degradation in granulocyte-dependent inflammatory reactions. Collagenase activity is dependent on the rate of its synthesis and secretion, and there is evidence that this activity may be increased by estrogen, prostaglandins, and cytokines, such as IL-8.

7. LACTATION

Development of the mammary glands in humans occurs during fetal life, at the time of puberty, and during the menstrual cycle. During pregnancy, there is additional growth and development of glandular epithelial cell proliferation during the first trimester and functional differentiation during the second half of pregnancy. In vitro and in vivo studies have demonstrated the necessity of prolactin and insulin for mitogenic activity of mammary epithelial cells. Addition of estrogen and progesterone is necessary to obtain full lobuloalveolar development. Others have suggested that estrogen alone is adequate to promote proliferation of human breast epithelial cells. The role of progesterone remains unclear, and different studies have produced conflicting results.

It is possible that the effects of steroids are direct or mediated indirectly through stimulation of peptide growth factors. Epidermal growth factor, TGF-α,

and IGFs have all been implicated as growth-promoting agents for mammary tissue. Growth factors are expressed within mammary tissue. Differences in the timing and localization of their expression suggest a high degree of specificity in their action. IGF-1 mRNA has been localized in the stromal, but not epithelial cells of the human mammary gland, and IGFs are mitogenic in breast carcinoma tissue. Clearly further studies on the expression of IGFs and IGF-BPs are required to elucidate the role of these compounds in mammary development.

8. CONCLUDING COMMENTS

It is now clear that undernutrition and other adverse influences during fetal life may have a permanent effect on the structure and physiology of the newborn. Babies who are small for dates have raised systolic and diastolic pressure as children and as adults. It is apparent that in both men and women, small size at birth correlates with increased death rates from cardiovascular disease in later life. Therefore, conditions that impair normal implantation or lead to growth restriction in intrauterine life have long-term consequences for later health. Further understanding of the factors that bring about normal growth and maturation during pregnancy, and that cause birth at term or preterm are important in enabling us to understand these different conditions.

ACKNOWLEDGMENTS

Work in the author's laboratory is supported by the Canadian Medical Research Council Group Grant in Fetal and Neonatal Health and Development. I am indebted to Jenny Katsoulakos for her help in the preparation of this manuscript.

REFERENCES

Ogren L, Talamantes F. The placenta as an endocrine organ: polypeptides. In: (Knobil E and Neill JD, eds.) *The Physiology of Reproduction*, vol. 2, 2nd ed. New York: Raven 1994:875.

Pepe GJ, Albrecht ED. Actions of placental and fetal adrenal steroid hormones in primate pregnancy. *Endoc Rev* 1995;16:608.

SELECTED READINGS

Barker DJP. *Mothers, Babies, and Disease in Later Life*. London: BMJ Publishing Group, 1994.

Bassett JM, Thorburn GD. Foetal plasma corticosteroids and the initiation of parturition in the sheep. *J Endocrinol* 1969; 44:285.

Benirschke K, Kaufmann P. *Pathology of the Human Placenta*, 2nd ed. New York: Springer-Verlag, 1990.

Challis JRG, Lye SJ. Parturition. In: (Knobil E and Neill JD, eds.) *The Physiology of Reproduction*, vol. 2, 2nd ed. New York: Raven, 1994:985.

Challis JRG, Matthews SG, van Meir C, Ramirez MM. Current topic: The placental corticotrophin-releasing hormone-adrenocorticotrophin axis. *Placenta* 1995;16:481.

Guissani DA, Jenkins SL, Winter JA, Mecenas CA, Wu WX, Umscheid CA, Farber DM, Nathanielsz PW. Differences in androstenedione (AT) and estradiol treatment (ET) in pregnant monkeys: effects on myometrial activity patterns (MyoAP), time to delivery and maternal estradiol (E$_2$) oxytocin (OT) and progesterone (P) plasma levels. *J Soc Gynecol Invest* 1996; 3(2) suppl: 86 abstract.

Liggins GC, Fairclough RJ, Grieves SA, Forster CS, Knox BS. Parturition in the sheep. In: *A Ciba Foundation Symposium. The Fetus and Birth*. The Netherlands: Mouton, 1977:5.

Matthews SG, Lü F, Yang K, Challis JRG. Hypothalamic pituitary adrenal function in the sheep fetus. *Reprod Fertil Dev* 1995;7:509.

Petraglia F, Florio P, Nappi C, Genazzani AR. Peptide signaling in human placenta and membranes: Autocrine, paracrine, and endocrine mechanisms. *Endocrine Reviews* 1996; 17:156–186.

Ramsey EM. *The Placenta, Human and Animal.* New York: Praeger, 1982.

Sangha RK, Walton JC, Ensor CM, Tai H-H, Challis JRG. Immunohistochemical localization, messenger ribonucleic acid abundance, and activity of 15-hydroxyprostaglandin dehydrogenase in placenta and fetal membranes during term and preterm labor. *J Clin Endocrinol Metab.* 1993; 78:982.

Short RV. Implantation and the maternal recognition of pregnancy. In: *Foetal Autonomy*, London: Churchill, 1969:2.

Stewart HJ, Guesdon FMJ, Payne JH, Charleston B, Vallet JL, Flint APF. Trophoblast interferons in early pregnancy of domestic ruminants. In: Brooks N, Challis J, McNeilly A, Doboroka C, eds. *Frontiers in Reproductive Biology*. Journals of Reproduction and Fertility Ltd., Cambridge: 1992:59.

van Meir CA, Matthews SG, Ramirez MM, Calder AA, Keirse JNC, Challis JRG. Chorionic prostaglandin catabolism is decreased in the lower uterine segment with term labor. *Placenta* (in press), 1996.

Yen SSC. *Endocrinology of Pregnancy.* In: Creasy R, Resnik, R. *Maternal Fetal Medicine, Principles and Practice*, 3rd ed., Philadelphia: W.B. Saunders Co., 1994:382.

INDEX

ABOUT THE EDITORS

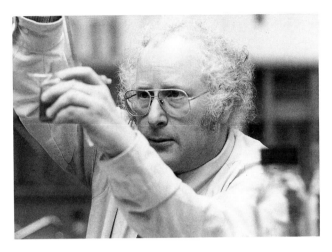

Dr. P. Michael Conn is the Associate Director and Senior Scientist of the Oregon Regional Primate Research Center, and Special Assistant to the President and Professor of Physiology and Pharmacology at Oregon Health Sciences University. Dr. Conn is presently the Editor-in-Chief of *Endocrine, Methods in Neurosciences, NeuroProtocols, Contemporary Endocrinology, Contemporary Drug Therapy*, and *Recent Progress in Hormone Research*. He is the editor of texts in pharmacology *(Essentials of Pharmacology)*, neuroscience *(Medical Neuroscience)*, and endocrinology *(Endocrinology)* as well as more than 60 volumes in endocrinology and neuroscience. The work of his laboratory has been recognized with the J.J. Abel Award of the American Society for Pharmacology and Experimental Therapeutics, the Weitzman and Oppenheimer Awards of the Endocrine Society, the Canadian Stevenson Award, and the National Science of Mexico Award (Miguel Aleman Award). Dr. Conn is currently President of the Endocrine Society.

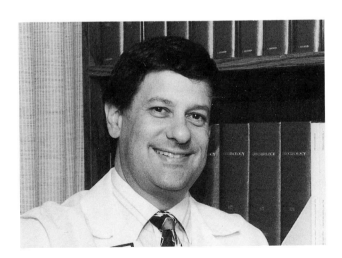

Dr. Shlomo Melmed is currently Professor of Medicine at the University of California Los Angeles, School of Medicine, where he is Director of the Division of Endocrinology and Metabolism, and Director of the Research Institute at Cedars-Sinai Medical Center, Los Angeles. Board certified in endocrinology and metabolism by the American Board of Internal Medicine, a Fellow of the American College of Physicians, an elected member of the Association of American Physicians and the American Society of Clinical Investigation, as well as a recipient of the Endocrinology Medal of the Royal Society of Medicine, he is author of more than 150 peer-reviewed manuscripts, the editor of several textbooks, including *The Pituitary,* and Editor-in-Chief of *Endocrinology* and *Endocrine Updates*.